Arthroscopic Management of Ulnar Pain

Francisco del Piñal (Editor in Chief)
Christophe Mathoulin and Toshiyasu Nakamura (Co-editors)

Arthroscopic Management of Ulnar Pain

Springer

Editors
Francisco del Piñal
Private Practice and Hospital
Mutua Montañesa
Santander
Spain

Christophe Mathoulin
Institut de la main
Clinique Jouvenet
Paris
France

Toshiyasu Nakamura
Department of Orthopaedic Surgery
School of Medicine
Keio University
Tokyo
Japan

Illustrator
Massimiliano Crespi
Milano
Italy

ISBN 978-3-662-52065-9 ISBN 978-3-642-30544-3 (eBook)
DOI 10.1007/978-3-642-30544-3
Springer Heidelberg New York Dordrecht London

Printed on acid-free paper

Springer is part of Springer Science+Business Media (www.springer.com)

To my kids Lucía, Guiller, Miguel, and Juan
To Estíbaliz
To the surgeons who are pushing the boundaries of wrist arthroscopy to the unimaginable

Paco Piñal

"This book is dedicated to all surgeons interested in wrist surgery, and especially to all EWAS members with whom we have made so much progress over the last seven years. Thanks to their contribution, we have been able to change our understanding and treatment of intrinsic ligamentous injuries of the wrist"

Christophe Mathoulin

Many thanks to my wife Yuzuka and lovely daughter Erie.
I sincerely hope this challenging book may be useful for all wrist arthroscopists. May the force be with you!

Toshi Nakamura

Preface

Ulnar pain has been considered the black hole of the wrist. As a matter of fact, one of the main aims when the scope was introduced in the wrist more than 20 years ago was to unravel ulnar pain. Yet, we still have not come up with all the answers!

The purpose of this book is to provide an update by renowned specialists in order to improve our understanding of ulnar pain. Some of the conditions can now be treated arthroscopically, and these have been profusely illustrated. Others are still not well understood. Hopefully, this book will assist us in untangling them. Each condition is covered in a fully comprehensive chapter. However, as stressed several times throughout the pages of this book, mixed conditions are frequently seen. I believe that many of our poor results in the early days were due to what is known as "satisfaction of search" (i.e., once an obvious problem is found, no others are sought). A systematic search of pathology is paramount, since combined pathology is the norm in the ulnar side. It is too simplistic to think that a traumatic event may cause *just* a 1A tear. Think about it! How is it that the injuring agent might penetrate the middle of the disc, causing a tear only here, and then leave the joint totally unscathed elsewhere? Does not this seem too simple?

I must admit that some of the conditions (if not all) can be treated equally well with open methods and at times faster. Nevertheless, there are several groups pushing hard to develop arthroscopic techniques and to make it simple for us all.... Do not stay out of the groove ladies and gentlemen! Things are changing very fast in wrist arthroscopy, and very much for the good. Think about what happened several years ago in knee meniscectomy, which was carried out open. But who is doing so now? Arthroscopy allows complex operations to be performed not only with perfect illumination and magnification but also with minimal damage to the rest of the patient's body. Who can give more for less? The corollary is that those who are still undecided as to the benefit of the scope should not rest on their laurels. What seemed to be a distant future is now a living present. It is just unthinkable what some people can achieve nowadays. If you have not yet done so, jump on the bandwagon because the number is up for open wrist surgery.

I hope this book contributes to shedding light into the black hole and helps our community to better understand and treat ulnar pain.

Secretary General. The European Wrist Arthroscopy Society Paco Piñal
Editor. *The Journal of Hand Surgery European Volumen.*
Chairperson of the IFSSH Scientific Committee on Arthroscopy.

Contents

Anatomy of the Ulnocarpal Compartment

1

Hisao Moritomo and Toshiyuki Kataoka

Developmental Anatomy

The form of the ulnar side of the human wrist represents progressive evolutionary development. In prosimians, the ulna continued to articulate with the pisiform and triquetrum, aiding in weight transmission across the wrist [1]. The monkey wrist showed the first step to change from the weight-bearing wrist to the mobile wrist (Fig. 1.1). In the gibbon, the ulna has migrated proximally and does not articulate directly with the pisiform and triquetrum. Instead, a thick meniscus was interposed between these three bones [1]. Chimpanzees developed a wrist that was similar to humans. There is a formal distal radioulnar joint that is bounded distally by the triangular fibrocartilage (TFC). In addition, a blind recess or prestyloid recess develops [1]. Humans have wrists characterized by further withdrawal of the ulnar styloid with loss of the articular cartilage from the ulnar styloid [2]. In addition, the distal ulna has evolved to allow greater pronosupination. The embryologic and clinical material suggests there is a tremendous variation in the development of the ulnar side of the wrist. The data also support the concept that evolution continues and that we are all different in terms of our ulnocarpal and distal radioulnar joints. Different configurations may require careful consideration before applying singular solutions to such a complex area [3].

H. Moritomo, M.D., Ph.D. (✉)
Department of Physical Therapy, Osaka Yukioka college of Health Science, Sojiji 1-1-41, Ibaragi-shi, Osaka, 567-0801, Japan
e-mail: hisao-moritomo@yukioka-u.ac.jp

T. Kataoka, M.D.
Department of Orthopaedics, Graduate School of Medicine, Osaka University, Suita-shi, Osaka, Japan

Anatomy

Ulnocarpal Ligaments

The ulnocarpal ligament is divided into the ulnocapitate, ulnotriquetral, and ulnolunate ligaments though, macroscopically, these three ligaments are often confluent and indistinguishable from each other [4–6] (Fig. 1.2).

Ulnocapitate Ligament

The ulnocapitate ligament is the most superficial of the three ulnocarpal ligaments [5]. It attaches not directly to the TFC but to the palmar portion of the fovea region of the ulnar head, which is a slight depression at the base of the ulnar styloid process. At the fovea, the ulnocapitate ligament merges with the deep fibers of the palmar radioulnar ligament. From the fovea, the ulnocapitate ligament passes distally, just anterior to the junction between the other ulnocarpal ligaments, and inserts on the ulnopalmar aspect of the capitate.

F. del Piñal et al. (eds.), *Arthroscopic Management of Ulnar Pain*,
DOI 10.1007/978-3-642-30544-3_1, © Springer-Verlag Berlin Heidelberg 2012

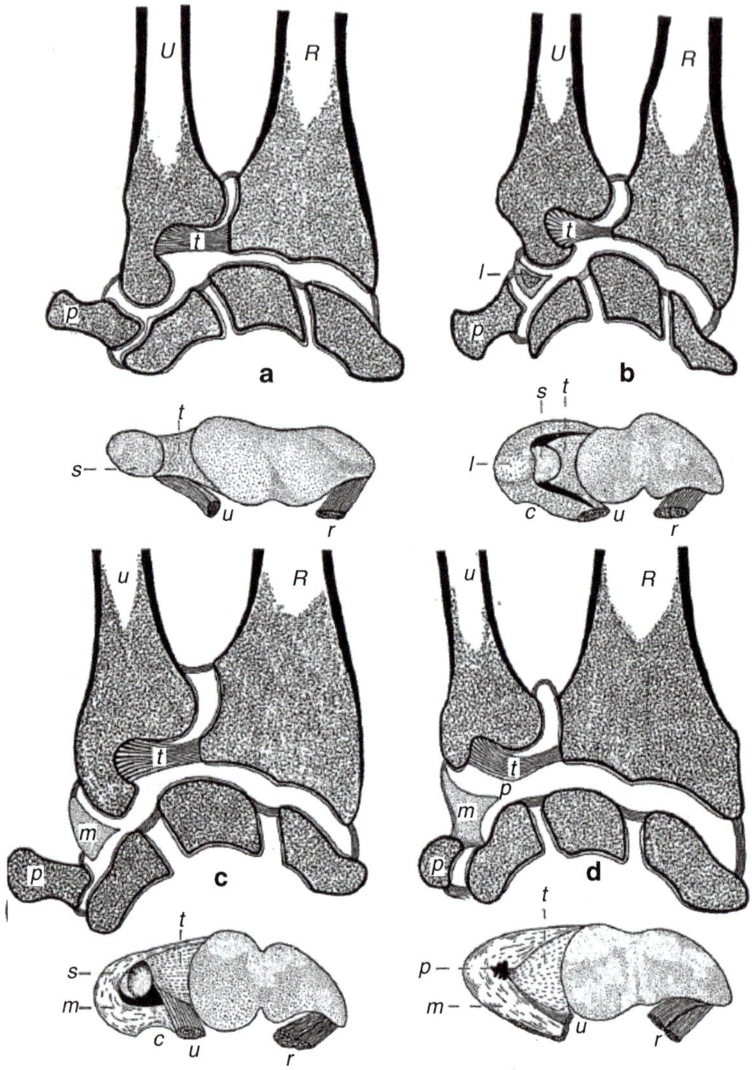

Fig. 1.1 The right wrist joint of a monkey (**a**), a gibbon (**b**), a chimpanzee (**c**), and man (**d**). In each case, the upper diagram represents a coronal section of the articulation. The lower diagram is a view of the proximal articular surface of the same articulation. *P* pisiform, *R* radius, *U* ulna, *t* triangular disk, *m* meniscus, *l* intrameniscal lunula, *u* palmar ulnocarpal ligament, *r* palmar radiocarpal ligament, *p* opening into prestyloid recess, *c* site of communication between pisotriquetral and wrist joint cavities, *s* ulnar styloid process [1]

Ulnotriquetral Ligament

The ulnotriquetral ligament originates mainly from the palmar radioulnar ligament, and some fibers originate from the palmar radial aspect of ulnar styloid process [7] (Fig. 1.2, 1.3, and 1.4). It inserts at the proximal and ulnar surfaces of the triquetrum. The ulnotriquetral ligament has a more oblique orientation than the ulnolunate ligament and is located ulnar to the ulnolunate ligament.

Ulnolunate Ligament

There is no clear demarcation between the ulnolunate and ulnotriquetral ligaments. The distinction between the two ligaments can only be made by their distal attachments. The ulnolunate ligament originates proximally from the palmar radioulnar ligament, thus attaching indirectly to the ulna. The ulnolunate ligament is continuous with the short radiolunate ligament and attaches to the palmar cortex of the lunate just as the short radiolunate ligament does. It is worth noting that unlike the monkey, in which the ulnotriquetral and ulnolunate ligaments emerge from the anterior aspect of the ulna [8], the deep ulnocarpal ligaments in the human wrist arise directly from the periphery of the TFC [9] (Fig. 1.5). Such a phylogenic modification was necessary in order to increase the range of pronosupination without impairing the ulnocarpal joint stability.

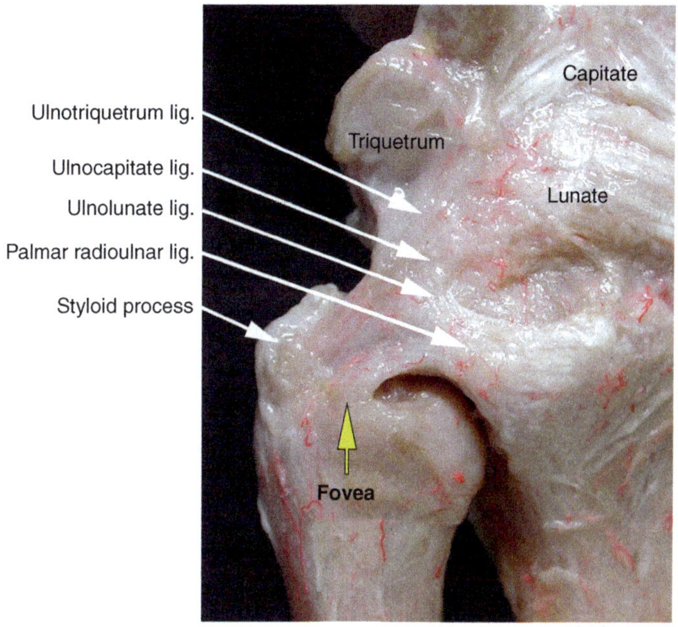

Fig. 1.2 Dissection of a human right wrist demonstrating the ulnocarpal ligament complex viewed from the palmar side. The ulnotriquetral, ulnocapitate, and ulnolunate ligaments originate together at the fovea of the ulnar head and the base of the ulnar styloid. These ligaments, along with the palmar radioulnar ligament, extend distally like a fan in the coronal plane and insert at the palmar aspects of the triquetrum, capitate, and lunate. In this case, the pisiform, ulnocarpal capsule, and flexor tendons have been excised (Courtesy of Dr. Marc Garcia-Elias)

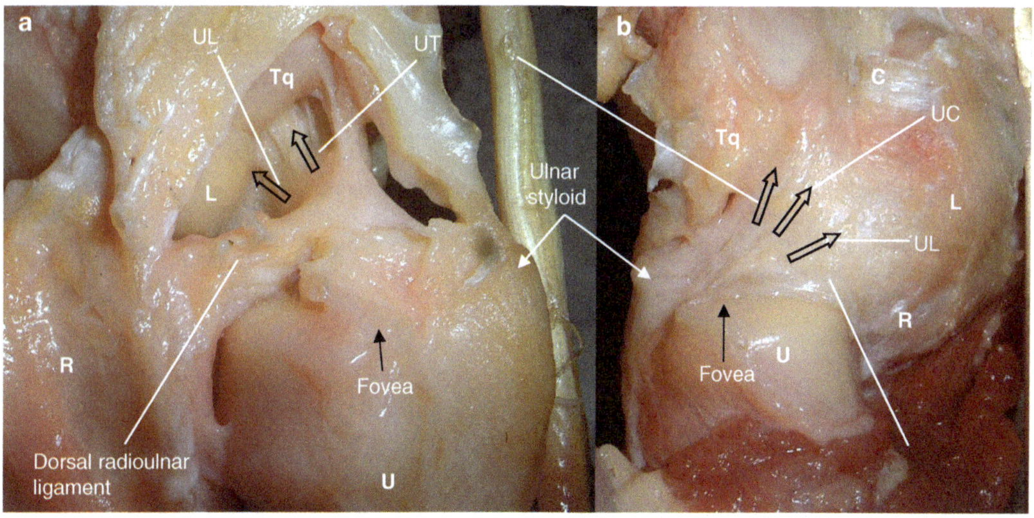

Fig. 1.3 Anatomy of the ulnocarpal ligaments in a right cadaver wrist. The ulnotriquetral ligament originates mainly from the palmar radioulnar ligament, and some fibers originate from the ulnar styloid process. Dorsal view (**a**) and palmar views (**b**). The joint capsule and the ECU sheath floor are removed. The ulnocapitate ligament is not visible from the dorsal view. *R* radius, *U* ulna, *L* lunate, *C* capitate, *Tq* triquetrum, *UT* ulnotriquetrum ligament, *UL* ulnolunate ligament, *UC* ulnocapitate ligament

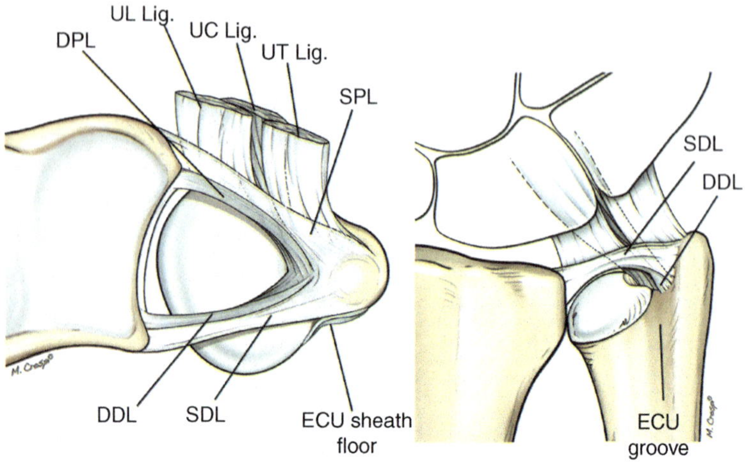

Fig. 1.4 Schematic representation of the ulnocarpal and radioulnar ligaments. The articular disk is not drawn. *DPL* deep palmar limb, *SPL* superficial palmar limb, *DDL* deep dorsal limb, *SDL* superficial dorsal limb, *UT* ulnotriquetrum, *UC* ulnocapitate, *UL* ulnolunate, extensor carpi ulnaris

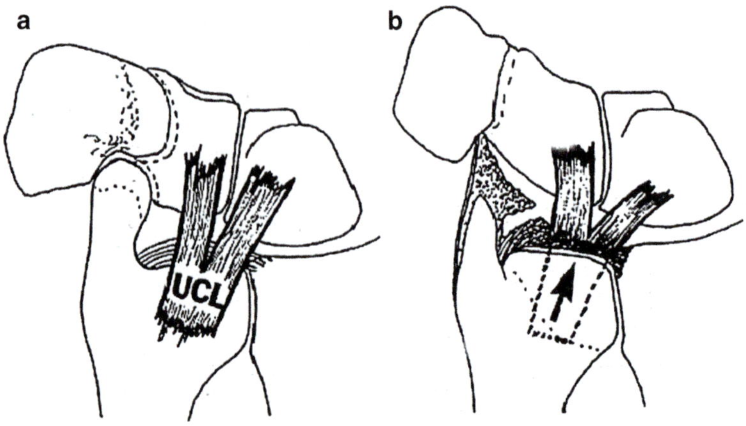

Fig. 1.5 Phylogenetic differences between the wrist of earlier apes (**a**) and that of hominoids (**b**). In hominoids, the ulnar styloid process has receded, and a meniscus-like soft tissue structure (meniscus homologue) has appeared between the styloid and the carpus. In order to achieve maximal pronosupination, the origin of the ulnocarpal ligaments (*UCL*) has migrated from the anterior aspect of the ulna to the periphery of the articular disk (*arrow*) [8]

Meniscus Homologue

The meniscus homologue is the soft tissue that is interposed between the superficial portion of the distal radioulnar joint ligaments, the triquetrum, and the ulnar capsule. When observed from distal to proximal, the meniscus homologue has a C-shaped configuration covering the peripheral fibers of the articular disk and, in most cases, englobing the tip of the ulnar styloid process [10].

The meniscus homologue is an anatomic structure that has been extensively discussed but is difficult to define its function. Bowers [11] and Taleisnik [12] both describe this as a separate structure from the TFC, but other authors have included the meniscus homologue as a part [13] or a distal extension [14] of the TFC because of its close relationship with the articular disk. From a histologic point of view, however, the meniscus homologue cannot be understood as an

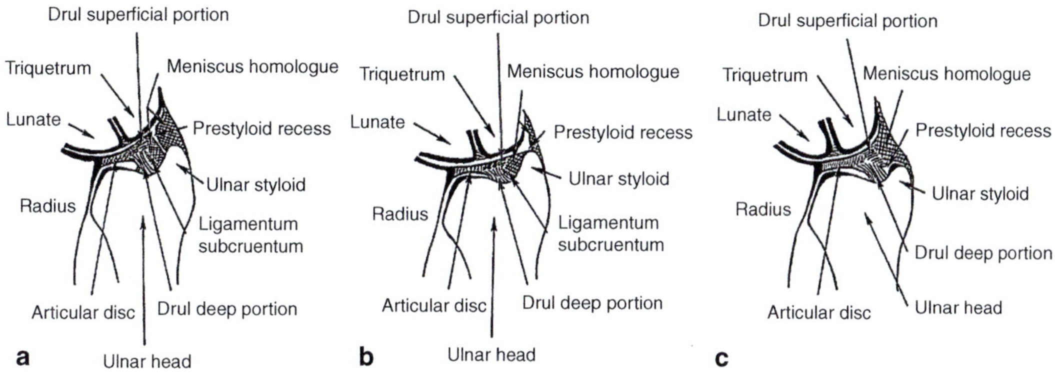

Fig. 1.6 Cross section of the TFCC illustrating the narrow opening (**a**), wide opening (**b**), and no opening types (**c**). In the narrow opening type, the prestyloid recess communicates with the ulnocarpal space by the way of a long narrow tunnel. In the wide opening type, a short, wide opening exists between the prestyloid recess and the ulnocarpal space. In the no opening type, there was no communication between the prestyloid recess and the ulnocarpal space. *DRUL* distal radioulnar ligament [7]

extension of the TFC because the meniscus homologue is not an avascular fibrocartilaginous structure, but instead, it is formed by well-vascularized, loose connective tissue [15, 16], and the inner surface of which is lined by synovial cells [6]. The meniscus homologue does not contain dense collagen fibers arranged in a parallel fashion from the ulnar styloid to the triquetrum, and the elasticity of this structure is higher than that of a true ligament [1, 6, 9].

Prestyloid Recess

Anterior to the ulnar styloid process, there is often an area where the meniscus homologue does not cover the ulnar styloid process, thereby creating a pouch, variable in size and shape, called the prestyloid recess [9, 17]. Ishii et al. revealed that the configuration of the meniscus homologue and the prestyloid recess varied in one of three ways [7] (Fig. 1.6). In 74 % of specimens, the meniscus homologue is attached to the ulnar styloid proximally to its radial, dorsal, and palmar aspects and distally to the ulnar styloid tip circumferential surface. In this type, the prestyloid recess communicates with the ulnocarpal space by way of a long narrow tunnel coming from the palmar aspect of the ulnar styloid (narrow opening type). In 11 % of specimens, the meniscus homologue is attached as in the narrow opening type but without attachment to the tip of the ulnar styloid. A short, wide opening existed between the prestyloid recess and the ulnocarpal space, coming from the tip of the ulnar styloid (wide opening type). In 15 % of specimens, the meniscus homologue was attached only to the dorsal, palmar, and ulnar aspect of the ulnar styloid. There was no communication between the prestyloid recess and the ulnocarpal space (no opening type). Instead, the prestyloid recess communicated with the distal radioulnar joint, coming from the radial aspect of the ulnar styloid.

The Extensor Carpi Ulnaris (ECU) Sheath Floor

The extensor carpi ulnaris (ECU) sheath floor is a part of the infratendinous extensor retinaculum [6], which originates from the dorsal aspect of the triquetrum and inserted on the dorsal and ulnar aspects of the ulnar styloid (Fig. 1.7a). The ECU sheath floor firmly blended with the superficial dorsal limb (SDL) of the radioulnar ligament on the dorsal ulnar aspect of the ulnar fovea (Fig.1.7b). At full pronation, the ECU sheath floor is on stretch, giving viscoelastic

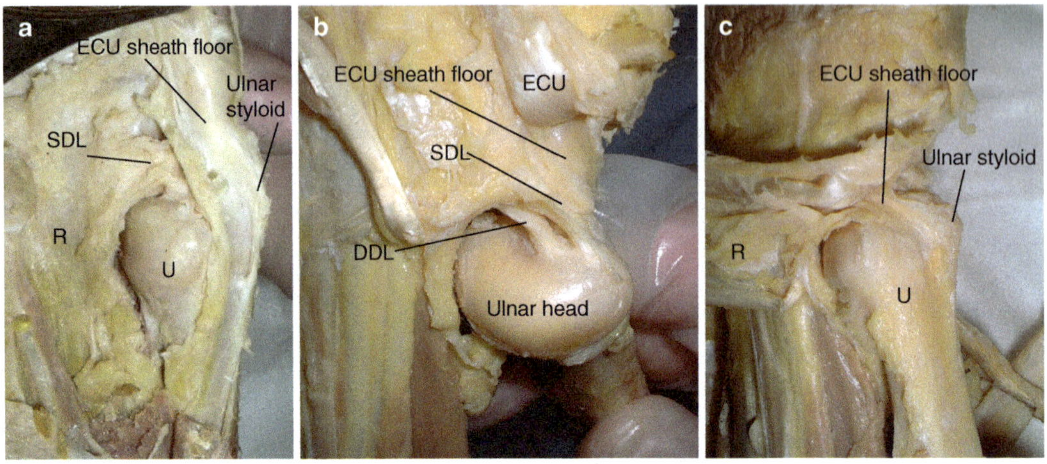

Fig. 1.7 Anatomy of the ECU sheath floor in a right cadaver wrist. Dorsal view (**a**) and distomedial view after inverting radius (**b**). The ECU sheath floor inserts on the dorsal aspect of the ulnar styloid with the superficial dorsal limb (*SDL*) of the radioulnar ligament. (**c**) At full pronation, the ECU sheath floor is on stretch. *DPL* deep palmar limb, *ECU* extensor carpi ulnaris

resistance to the tendency of the ulna toward dorsal dislocation (Fig. 1.7c) [6, 18]. In full supination, it warps, and its tension becomes loose as the ulnar styloid process approaches to the dorsal margin of the sigmoid notch of the radius. In wrist extension with supination, the ECU sheath floor is impinged between the triquetrum and the ulnar styloid process, which sometimes causes inflammation resulting in so-called *ulnar styloid impaction syndrome*.

Joint Capsule of the Distal Radioulnar and Ulnocarpal Joint

At the level of the radioulnar joint, both palmar and dorsal capsules are thin and lax and do not contain dense collagen fibers [6]. The dorsal capsule resembles the volar capsule but has major distinct features: it is much more homogeneous in thickness and is less redundant [19]. Distal to the TFC, the two capsular sheaths become thicker as they incorporate the ulnocarpal ligament and the palmar radioulnar ligament palmarly and the obliquely oriented fibers of the dorsal radiotriquetral ligament dorsally. The capsule covering the medial aspect of the joint is strongly attached to the ulnar styloid process and the external base of the meniscus homologue [9]. There is a "soft spot" between the ulnotriquetral ligament and the ECU sheath floor on the medial aspect of the ulnar capsule where the capsule is thin and used as 6U portal in arthroscopy.

Dorsal Branch of the Ulnar Nerve

The dorsal cutaneous branch of the ulnar nerve is a terminal ramus of the ulnar nerve. It separates at the distal third of the forearm and then enters the dorsal ulnar aspect. At the level of the carpus, the branch normally divides into radial and ulnar branches, which provide sensation to the dorsal aspect of the hand and to the small and ring fingers [20]. Tindall et al. reported the dorsal branch of the ulnar nerve crosses a line between the ulnar styloid and the fourth web space at an average of 2.4 cm from the ulnar styloid [21]. The authors suggest that inadvertent damage to the dorsal branch of the ulnar nerve can be avoided if care is taken to place the 6R portal in the "safe zone" found within the proximal fifth (19 %) of a line drawn from the ulnar styloid to the fourth dorsal web space. However, many variations of the ulnar nerve have been described previously [22–28]. There are differences in the

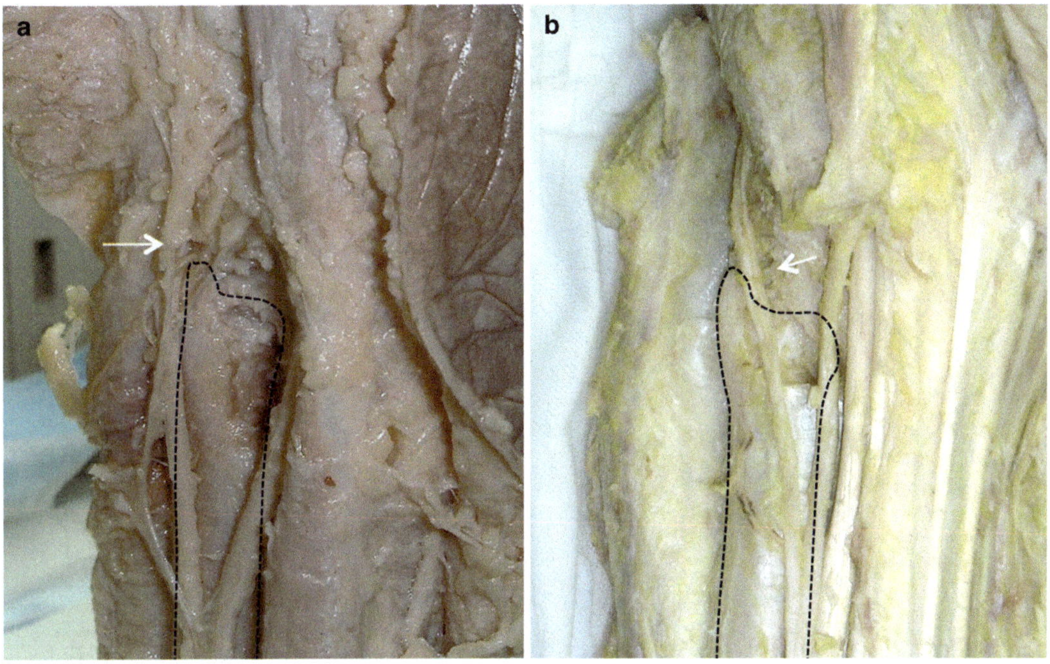

Fig. 1.8 Courses of the dorsal branch of the ulnar nerve in a right wrist viewed from the palmar side. Two division patterns of the dorsal cutaneous branch: (**a**) proximal type and (**b**) distal type. In the proximal type (70 %), the dorsal cutaneous branch goes around the ulna proximal to the ulnar styloid process (*arrow*) and directed toward the ulnodorsal aspect. In the distal type (30 %), the branch goes around the ulna and directed the ulnodorsal aspect distal to the ulnar styloid process. Note that in the distal type, the nerve passes just palmar side of the ulnar fovea (*arrow*) [28]

course of the dorsal cutaneous branch that could be separated into two types: proximal (70 %) and distal (30 %) [28] (Fig. 1.8). The proximal type goes around the ulna average 1.1 cm proximal to the ulnar styloid process and directs toward the ulnodorsal aspect. Therefore, the above mentioned safe zone can be not safe in the proximal type. The distal type goes around to the ulnodorsal aspect, average 1.7 cm distal to the styloid process. In the palmar surgical approach to the ulnar fovea in the DRUJ on either arthroscopic or open surgery, the distal type ulnar nerve can be damaged if the skin incision is put on the palmar aspect of the ulnar styloid. In order to avoid the damage, surgeon should put the incision on the ulnar margin of the flexor carpi ulnaris tendon [29]. "Kaplan's accessory branches" are also common anatomic variations in the dorsal cutaneous nerve [24–27] (Fig. 1.9). Kaplan described an aberrant branch of the dorsal cutaneous nerve that crossed the ulnar head from the dorsal to the volar side, coursing to the ulnar aspect of the pisiform to join the proximal volar sensory branch of the ulnar nerve [26]. Considering these variations, it is safe to consider the "safe zone" never exists.

Kinematics

The distal ulna and the TFCC attached to it are essential in the coordination of the distal radioulnar joint and the ulnocarpal joint. Hagert investigated ligamentous junction of the ulnotriquetral and radioulnar joints and advocated the *fixed-point concept*, where one compound ligament formed by the radioulnar and the ulnotriquetrum ligaments from a limited area in the fovea of the ulnar head extends in two perpendicular planes to insert at the palmar aspect of the triquetrum in the coronal plane and at the ulnar margin of the radius in the transverse plane [30] (Fig. 1.10). The author considers that the ulnar fovea constitutes the fixed point of the universal joint that is the

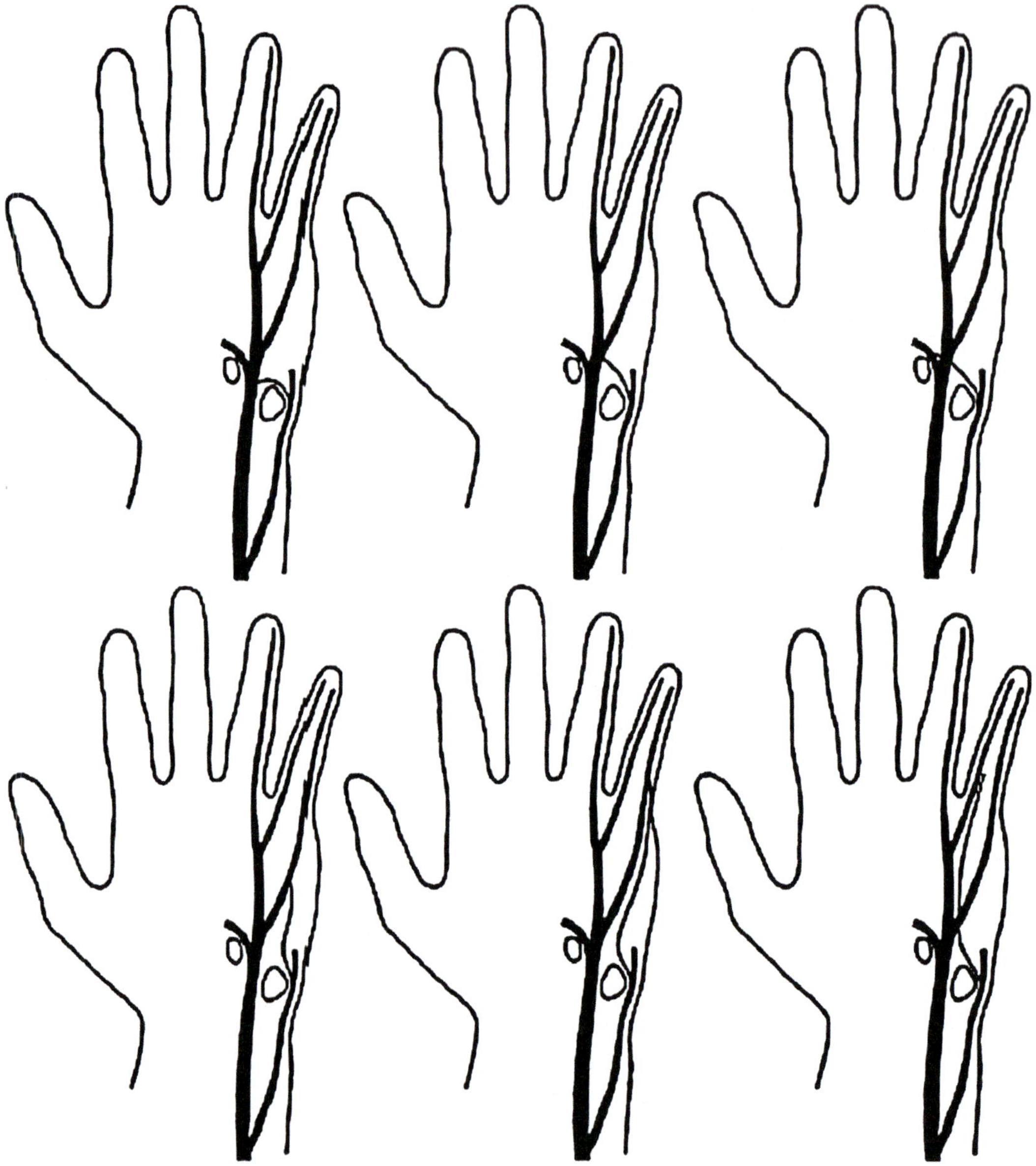

Fig. 1.9 Kaplan's accessory branches of the ulnar nerve. Type 1, branch courses to the common trunk of the ulnar nerve proximal to its bifurcation into the sensory and motor branches; type 2, branch courses to the proximal sensory branch; type 3, branch courses to the proximal motor branch; type 4, branch courses to the ulnar digital nerve to the small finger at the midportion of the hypothenar eminence; type 5, branch courses to the ulnar digital nerve of the small finger at the level of the proximal interphalangeal joint; and type 6, branch courses to the radial aspect of the volar surface of the small finger [26]

wrist joint. With the ulnar fixed, the radius can move in the transverse plane (pronation-supination), and the carpus in the sagittal plane (extension-flexion).

The ulnocarpal ligaments have an important role in stabilizing the ulnocarpal joint. Weaver et al. investigated the in situ tensions of the ulnolunate ligament in cadaver specimens and found that the tension of the ulnolunate ligament increased in ulnar deviation, supination, and extension [31]. Ritt et al. investigated the contribution of individual capsuloligamentous

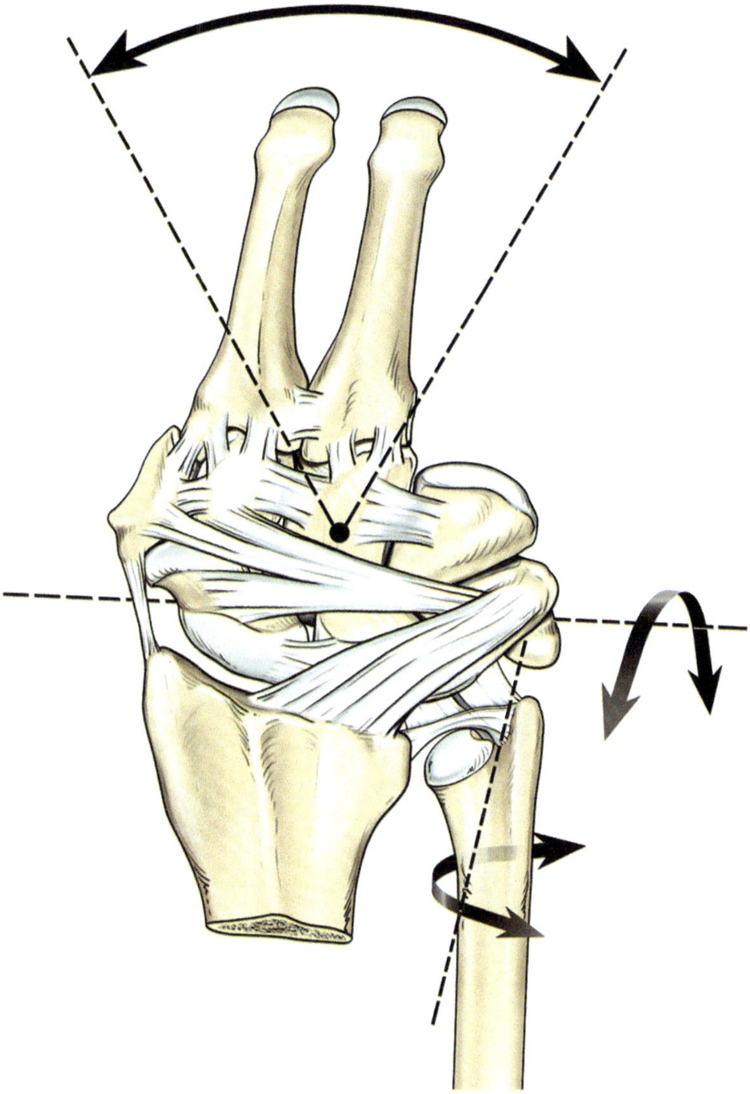

Fig. 1.10 The fixed-point concept. With the ulna flexed, the radius can move in the transverse plane (pronation-supination) and the carpus in the sagittal plane (extension-flexion) and the coronal plane (radial and ulnar deviation). The ulnar head constitutes the fixed point of the universal joint that the wrist joint is. Ultimately, stabilization of the mobile parts, in relation to the ulnar head, relies on the ulnoradial triquetral ligament [30]

structures to the rotational stability of the radiocarpal joint using fresh cadavers and reported the ulnolunate ligament is the secondary radiocarpal supination constraint [32]. From wrist ulnar deviation to radial deviation, the length of the ulnotriquetrum ligament increases, but the length of the ulnolunate ligament decreases [29] (Fig. 1.11). That is, during radioulnar deviation, the ulnotriquetrum ligament and the ulnolunate ligament show reciprocal behavior with respect to each other. These two ligaments have an opposite function in terms of carpal instability during radioulnar deviation. It is possible that these two ligaments work together to provide a continuous and stable ulnar-radial-carpal motion throughout wrist radioulnar deviation. It has also been reported that the ulnocarpal ligaments can prevent abnormal radioulnar translations of the carpus. Wiesner et al. applied progressive posteroanterior forces in the palmar direction to the carpus and found that the largest displacement was observed after the ulnar insertion of the ulnocarpal ligaments was sectioned [33].

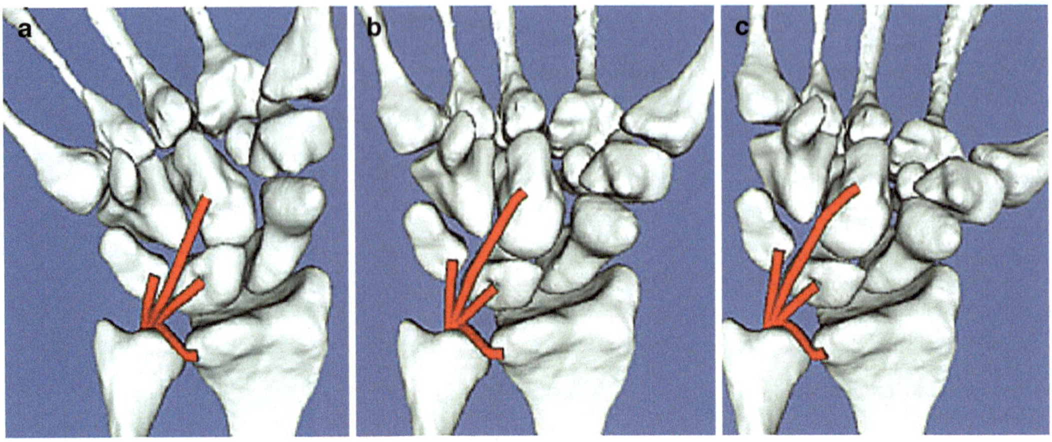

Fig. 1.11 Three-dimensional ligament paths in (**a**) ulnar deviation, (**b**) neutral position, and (**c**) radial deviation during radioulnar deviation, viewed from the palmar side in a representative case. Note that the ulnotriquetrum and ulnocapitate ligaments and the ulnolunate ligament show reciprocal behavior with respect to each other [34]

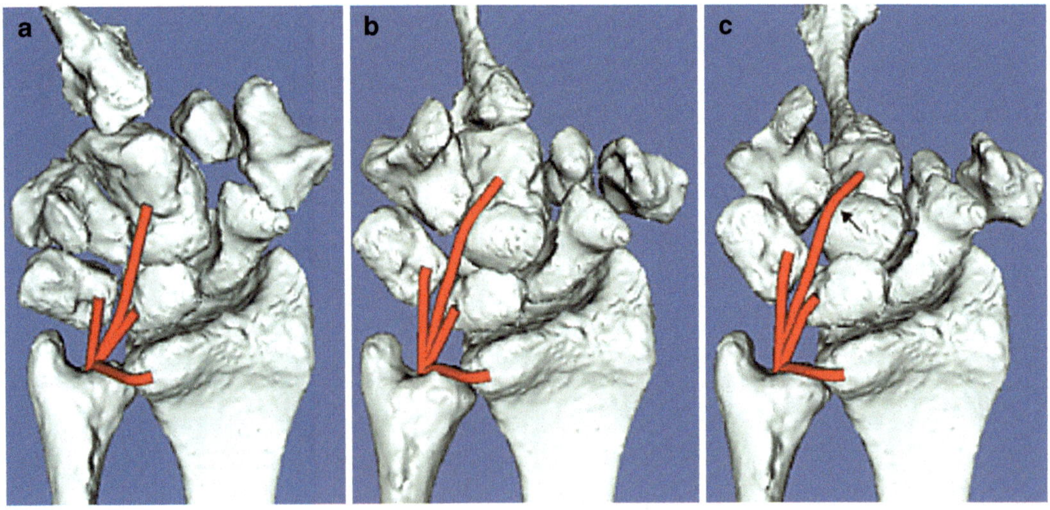

Fig. 1.12 Three-dimensional ligament paths in (**a**) ulnar flexion, (**b**) neutral position, and (**c**) radial extension during dart-throwing motion, viewed from the palmar side in a representative case. The third metacarpals are shown to indicate the global wrist position. Note that the capitate insertion of the ulnocapitate ligament shifts to the radiodorsal direction, and palmar protrusion of the capitates head made the ulnocapitate ligament detour toward the palmar side (*arrow*) [34]

In-vivo three-dimensional studies on the ulnocarpal ligaments have shown that the length of the ulnotriquetrum and ulnocapitate ligaments is maximum during wrist radial extension, which is a combination of maximal wrist extension and radial deviation, and that the ulnolunate ligament length is maximum during pure wrist extension [34]. In wrist radial extension, the capitate insertion of the ulnocapitate ligament shifts distally, and the ulnocapitate ligament gradually stretches to pass around the palmar protrusion of the capitate head (Fig. 1.12). The triquetrum also shifts distally without significant rotation, while the lunate seldom moves. These carpal movements

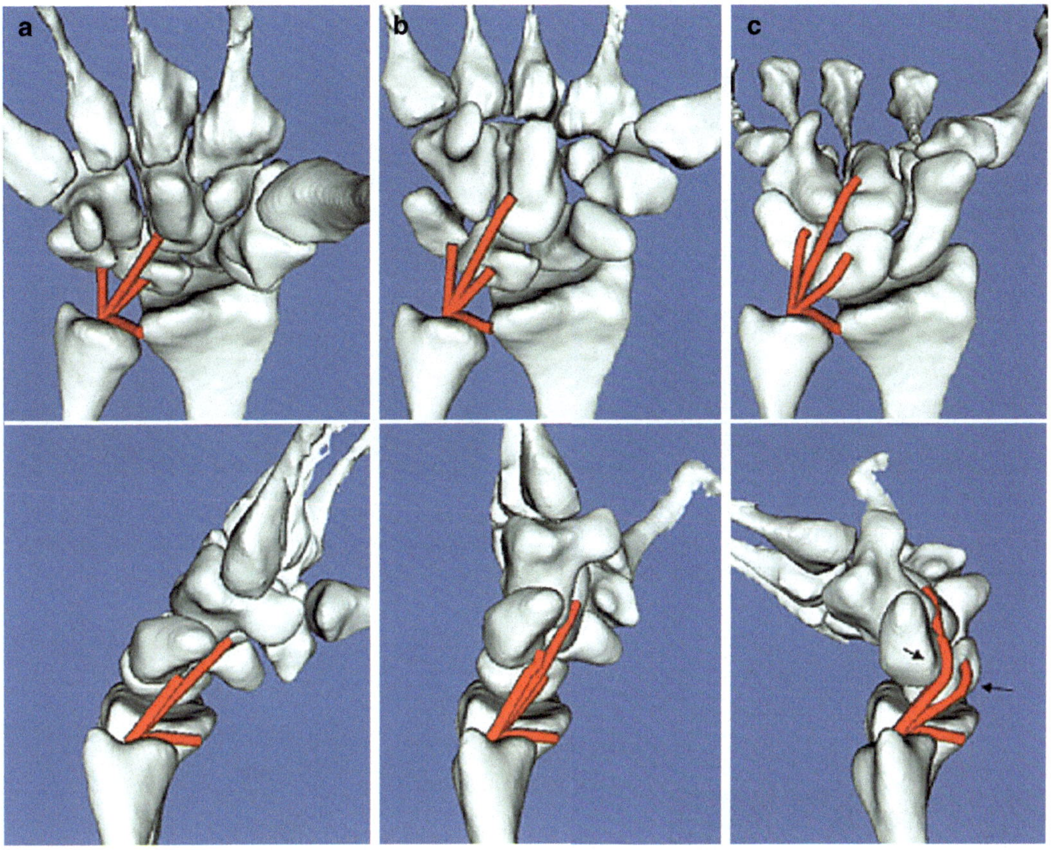

Fig. 1.13 Three-dimensional ligament paths in wrist flexion (**a**), neutral position (**b**), and extension (**c**) during flexion-extension motion viewed from the palmar side and the ulnar side in a representative case. Note that, in wrist extension, the ligament paths detour toward the palmar side because of the palmar protrusion of the triquetrum and lunate (*arrow*) [34]

that occur during wrist hyper-radial extension motion result in substantial strain to the ulnocapitate and ulnotriquetrum ligaments and on the foveal and palmar styloid insertions of the TFCC. In wrist extension, the ulnolunate ligament becomes taut and stretches the foveal insertion of the TFCC as well. In the wrist extension, the length of the ulnolunate ligament increased more than the length of the ulnotriquetrum ligament because the palmar protrusion of the proximal portion of the lunate is greater than that of the triquetrum (Fig. 1.13). Considering that the ulnotriquetral ligament has another origin on the palmar aspect of the ulnar styloid, which is eccentric from the center of forearm rotation (fovea), it is easily seen that the change in length of this fascicle would be increased by forearm supination. Strain of this fascicle during forearm supination may thus affect the tension of the foveal insertion. Based on these findings, one major injury mechanism of a TFCC foveal avulsion can be excessive traction of the ulnocarpal ligament, especially the ulnocapitate ligament, caused by wrist hyper-radial extension or hyperextension with the forearm supination (Figs. 1.14). This theory agree with the fact that more than half of the patients with traumatic TFCC foveal avulsion were caused by a fall on the outstretched hand (Fig. 1.15) and had a positive fovea sign, which is a localized tenderness on palmar aspect of the fovea and ulnar styloid (Fig. 1.16) [29].

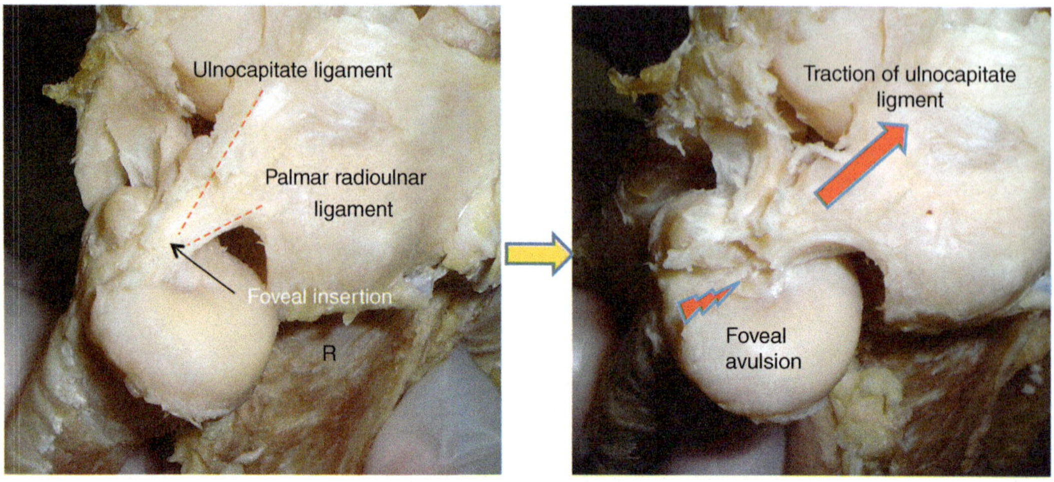

Fig. 1.14 A normal foveal insertion (**a**) and a simulated TFCC foveal avulsion (**b**) by excessive traction of the ulnocarpal ligament, especially the ulnocapitate ligament, caused by wrist hyper-radial extension. A right cadaver wrist is viewed from a distal and palmar side

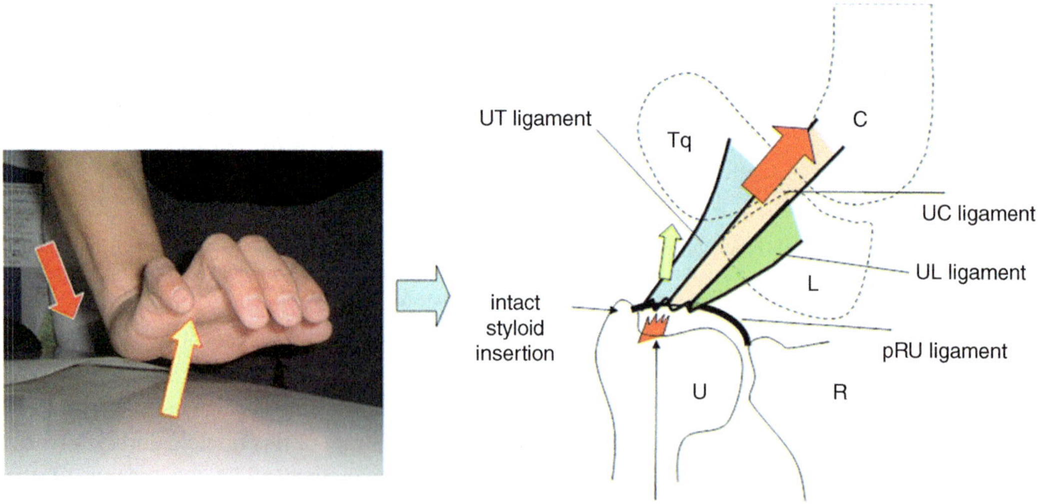

Fig.1.15 A hypothesized mechanism of a common foveal avulsion. Excessive traction of the ulnocarpal ligament caused by a fall on the outstretched hand disrupts the ulnar insertion from its palmar side leaving the DSL intact. A palmar approach allows repairing the foveal tear without damaging the DSL [34]

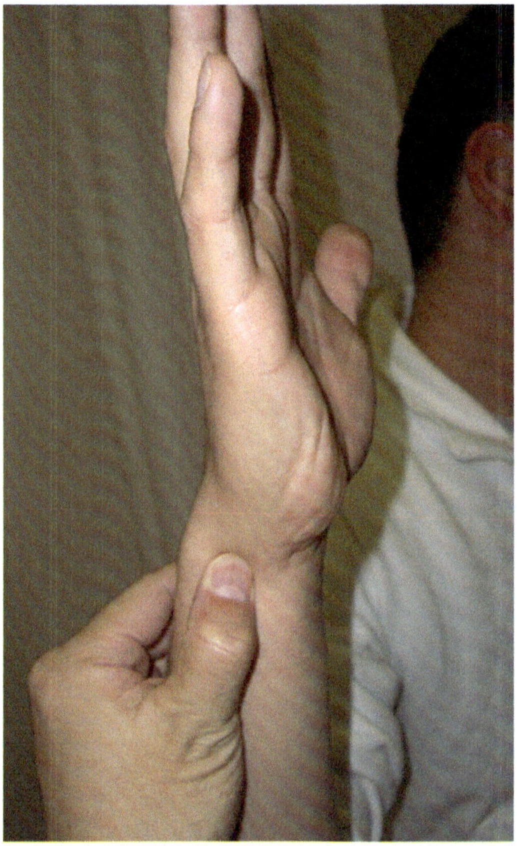

Fig. 1.16 Ulnar fovea sign test

References

1. Lewis OJ, Hamshere RJ, Bucknill TM (1970) The anatomy of the wrist joint. J Anat 106(Pt 3):539–552
2. Lewis OJ (1974) The wrist articulations of the anthropoidea. Academic, New York, pp 143–169
3. Louis DS, Jebson PJ (1998) The evolution of the distal radio-ulnar joint. Hand Clin 14(2):155–159
4. Short WH (2004) Triangular fibrocartilage complex injuries and ulnar impaction syndrome. In: Berger RA, Weiss APC (eds) Hand surgery, vol 1. Lippincott Williams & Wilkins, Philadelphia, pp 355–380
5. Berger RA (1997) The ligaments of the wrist. A current overview of anatomy with considerations of their potential functions. Hand Clin 13(1):63–82
6. Garcia-Elias M (1998) Soft-tissue anatomy and relationships about the distal ulna. Hand Clin 14(2):165–176
7. Ishii S et al (1998) An anatomic study of the ligamentous structure of the triangular fibrocartilage complex. J Hand Surg 23(6):977–985
8. Lewis OJ (1972) Osteological features characterizing the wrists of monkeys and apes, with a reconsideration of this region in Dryopithecus (Proconsul) africanus. Am J Phys Anthropol 36(1):45–58
9. Garcia-Elias M, Domenech-Mateu JM (1987) The articular disc of the wrist. Limits and relations. Acta Anat (Basel) 128(1):51–54
10. Mikic ZD (1989) Detailed anatomy of the articular disc of the distal radioulnar joint. Clin Orthop Relat Res 245:123–132
11. Bowers WH (1993) The distal radioulnar joint. In: Green DP (ed) Operative hand surgery, vol 1, 3rd edn. Churchill Livingstone, New York, pp 973–1019
12. Taleisnik J (1985) The ligaments of the wrist. The wrist. Churchill Livingstone, New York, pp 13–38
13. Palmer AK, Werner FW (1981) The triangular fibrocartilage complex of the wrist – anatomy and function. J Hand Surg Am 6(2):153–162
14. Kauer JM (1975) The articular disc of the hand. Acta Anat (Basel) 93(4):590–605
15. Bednar MS, Arnoczky SP, Weiland AJ (1991) The microvasculature of the triangular fibrocartilage complex: its clinical significance. J Hand Surg Am 16(6): 1101–1105
16. Chidgey LK (1991) Histologic anatomy of the triangular fibrocartilage. Hand Clin 7(2):249–262
17. Mikic ZD (1984) Arthrography of the wrist joint. An experimental study. J Bone Joint Surg Am 66(3):371–378
18. Nakamura T, Yabe Y, Horiuchi Y (1996) Functional anatomy of the triangular fibrocartilage complex. J Hand Surg Br 21(5):581–586
19. Kleinman WB, Graham TJ (1998) The distal radioulnar joint capsule: clinical anatomy and role in posttraumatic limitation of forearm rotation. J Hand Surg Am 23(4):588–599
20. Polatsch DB et al (2007) Ulnar nerve anatomy. Hand Clin 23(3):283–289
21. Tindall A et al (2006) The anatomy of the dorsal cutaneous branch of the ulnar nerve – a safe zone for positioning of the 6R portal in wrist arthroscopy. J Hand Surg Br 31(2):203–205
22. Botte MJ et al (1990) The dorsal branch of the ulnar nerve: an anatomic study. J Hand Surg Am 15(4): 603–607
23. Lourie GM, King J, Kleinman WB (1994) The transverse radioulnar branch from the dorsal sensory ulnar nerve: its clinical and anatomical significance further defined. J Hand Surg Am 19(2):241–245
24. Hankins CL, Flemming S (2005) A variant of Kaplan's accessory branch of the dorsal cutaneous branch of the ulnar nerve: a case report and review of the literature. J Hand Surg Am 30(6):1231–1235
25. Hoogbergen MM, Kauer JM (1992) An unusual ulnar nerve-median nerve communicating branch. J Anat 181(Pt 3):513–516
26. Kaplan EB (1963) Variation of the ulnar nerve at the wrist. Bull Hosp Joint Dis 24:85–88
27. McCarthy RE, Nalebuff EA (1980) Anomalous volar branch of the dorsal cutaneous ulnar nerve: a case report. J Hand Surg Am 5(1):19–20
28. Goto A et al (2010) The dorsal cutaneous branch of the ulnar nerve: an anatomical study. Hand Surg 15(3):165–168

29. Moritomo H, Masatomi T, Murase T, Tanaka H, Miyake J, Yoshikawa H (2010) Open repair of foveal avulsion of the triangular fibrocartilage complex and comparison by types of injury mechanism. J Hand Surg 35A:1955–1963
30. Hagert CG (1996) Current concepts of the functional anatomy of the distal radioulnar joint, including the ulnocarpal junction. Wrist instability. Martin Dunitz, London, pp 15–21
31. Weaver L, Tencer AF, Trumble TE (1994) Tensions in the palmar ligaments of the wrist. I. The normal wrist. J Hand Surg Am 19(3):464–474
32. Ritt MJ et al (1995) Rotational stability of the carpus relative to the forearm. J Hand Surg Am 20(2): 305–311
33. Wiesner L et al (1996) Experimentally induced ulno-carpal instability. A study on 13 cadaver wrists. J Hand Surg Br 21(1):24–29
34. Moritomo H et al (2008) Change in the length of the ulnocarpal ligaments during radiocarpal motion: possible impact on triangular fibrocartilage complex foveal tears. J Hand Surg Am 33(8):1278–1286

2 Anatomy and Biomechanics of the Distal Radioulnar Joint (DRUJ)

Toshiyasu Nakamura

Anatomy of the Distal Radioulnar Joint (DRUJ)

The distal radioulnar joint (DRUJ) is a cylindrical joint consisting of the sigmoid notch of the radius, the head of the ulna, the triangular fibrocartilage complex (TFCC), and the dorsal and palmar joint capsules [3, 4] (Fig. 2.1). The radioulnar ligament (RUL), which is the proximal ligamentous component of the TFCC, is considered the most important stabilizer of the DRUJ ([3, 4, 10, 13, 18]). Joint surface of the sigmoid notch of the radius with respect to the ulnar head has a concave shape on the axial plane which includes the ulnar head. The shape of the sigmoid notch of the radius on axial plane was subclassified to flat face, ski-slope, C-type, and S-type sigmoid [19]. On the coronal view, the angle of the sigmoid notch forms neutral (vertical), negative (sigmoid notch tilts ulnarly), and positive (sigmoid notch tilts radially) [17]. The positive ulnar variance wrists tend to indicate negative sigmoid notch angle, while the negative variance wrists may indicate positive sigmoid notch angles. The distal end of the ulna consists of the neck, hub, seat, fovea, and styloid process (Fig. 2.1). In the DRUJ, the radial sigmoid notch faces to the hub of the ulna, and the proximal surface of the TFCC (corresponding to the RUL) faces to the seat of the head of the ulna. The fovea and base of the ulnar styloid process is the very important portion where the RUL originates.

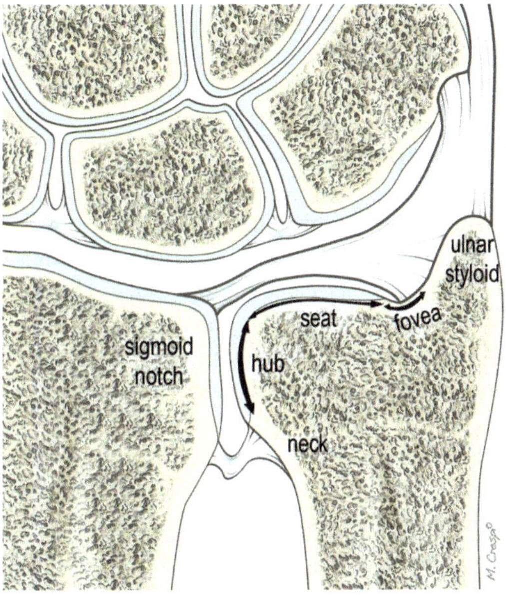

Fig. 2.1 Illustration of the DRUJ

Since the diameter of the sigmoid notch of the radius is larger than that of the ulnar seat, the DRUJ has incongruity, which indicates slight dorsopalmar translation between two bones during pronation-supination motion (Fig. 2.2) [3, 4]. This incongruity is more obvious in the neutral

T. Nakamura, M.D., Ph.D.
Department of Orthopaedic Surgery,
School of Medicine, Keio University,
35 Shinanomachi, Shinjuku-ku, Tokyo 160-8582, Japan
e-mail: tosiyasu@sc.itc.keio.ac.jp

F. del Piñal et al. (eds.), *Arthroscopic Management of Ulnar Pain*,
DOI 10.1007/978-3-642-30544-3_2, © Springer-Verlag Berlin Heidelberg 2012

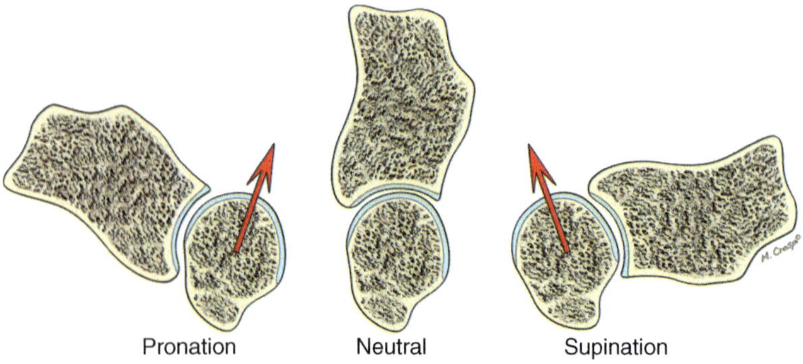

Fig. 2.2 Illustration of the normal position of the radius and ulna during pronation-supination. The ulna tends to translate dorsally in pronation and palmary in supination (*arrows*). This translation is due to incongruity between the sigmoid notch of the radius and ulnar head

and pronated position, while in supinated position, the DRUJ becomes tighter due to increased tension in extensor carpi ulnaris and pronator quadratus muscles.

DRUJ Capsule

There are dorsal and palmar joint capsules in the DRUJ. The DRUJ capsule is a thin and amorphous layer, which can be easily folded. The dorsal joint capsule is extended in the pronated position and is folded in supination like accordion pleats, while the palmar joint capsule is extended in supination and folded in pronation (Fig. 2.3). Function of the DRUJ capsule is providing limitation of the maximum pronation and supination. There were studies indicating stabilizing effect of the DRUJ joint capsule on the DRUJ stiffness in the maximum pronation and supinated position on cadaver specimen [20]. However, as it is quite difficult to achieve these maximum pronation-supination positions in a live situation, there is still a question as to the stabilizing effect of the DRUJ joint capsule.

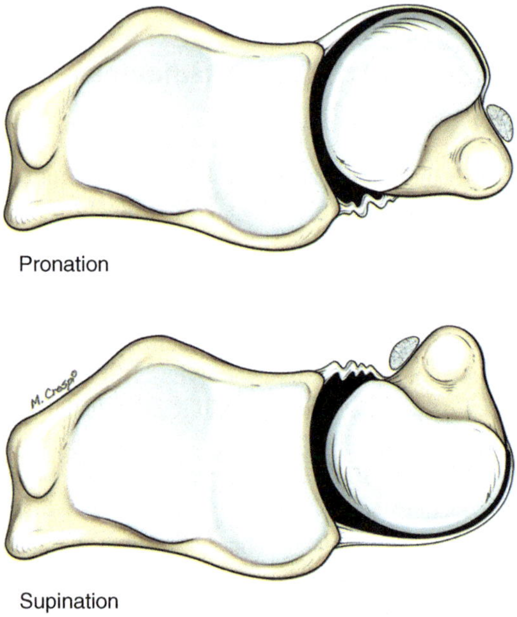

Fig. 2.3 Illustration of the dorsal and palmar joint capsule of the DRUJ. Dorsal capsule is extended in pronation, while palmar capsule is extended in supination

Triangular Fibrocartilage Complex (TFCC)

The triangular fibrocartilage complex (TFCC) consists of the triangular fibrocartilage (TFC; also termed the articular disc or disc proper) [13, 16], meniscus homologue, radioulnar ligament (RUL) [10, 13], ulnolunate ligament, ulnotriquetral ligament, sheath floor of the extensor carpi ulnaris (ECU), and ulnar joint capsule. This complex allows smooth motion of the wrist and forearm, distributes load between the ulna and ulnar carpus, and stabilizes the ulnocarpal joint as well as the DRUJ. The TFCC is divided into three components three-dimensionally: the distal hammock-like structure includes the centrally located fibrocartilage disc, meniscus homologue, ulnolunate ligament, and ulnotriquetral ligament, which supports and surrounds the ulnar carpus; the RUL, which is the proximal component of the TFCC that stabilizes the radius to the ulna directly [10]; and the functional ulnar collateral ligament which con-

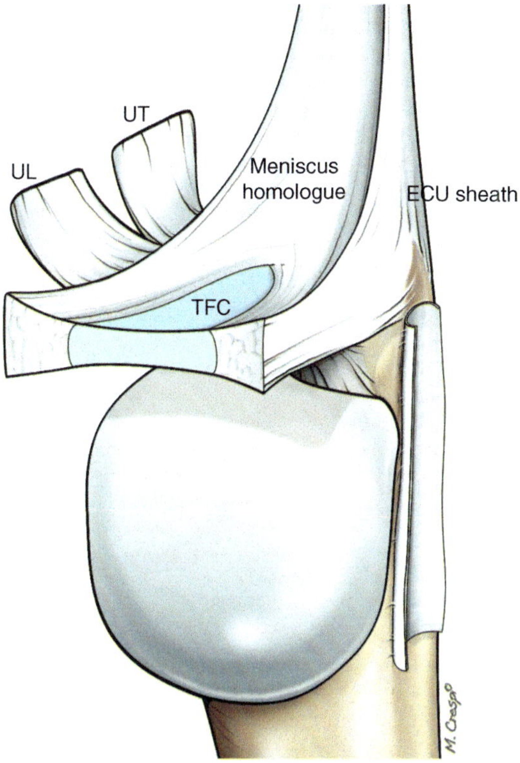

Fig. 2.4 Illustration of the three-dimensional structure of the TFCC

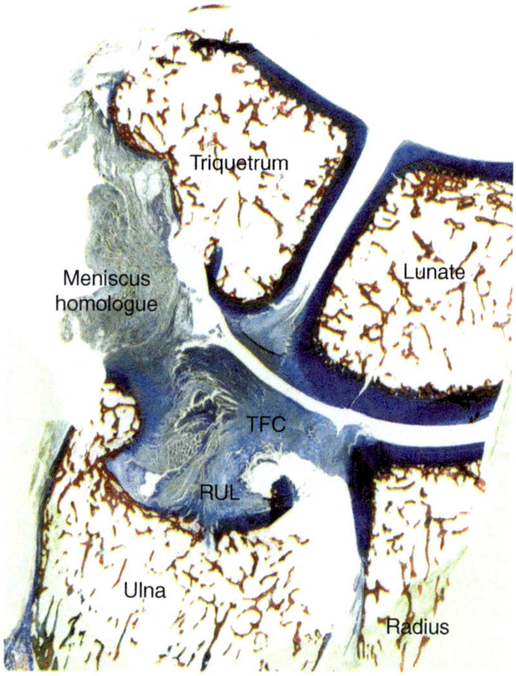

Fig. 2.5 Histological findings of the TFCC. The TFCC originates from wide area of the fovea to the base of the ulnar styloid, where the Sharpey's fibers exist. The TFC mainly faces to the ulnar carpus to support

sists of the sheath floor of the ECU and the thickened ulnar capsule (Fig. 2.4).

The histology of the TFCC shows that the RUL originates from the wide area of the fovea and base of the ulnar styloid nearly vertically (Fig. 2.5), then curls radially and separates into palmar and dorsal portions which pass through the proximal portion of the TFCC [13], and finally attaches to the radial edge of the sigmoid notch [12, 14]. The TFC mainly faces to the lunate and triquetrum. The so-called meniscus homologue, which is the inner wall of the ulnar capsule recognized as the 6U portal in wrist arthroscopy, consists of synovial tissue and elastic fibers mainly. Between the TFC and meniscus homologue, there exists a pit corresponding to the prestyloid recess. Fat-rich and loose area between the RUL and TFC and the prestyloid recess may absorb deformities of the TFCC during forearm rotation. Higher magnification histology indicated there are tight ligamentous (transition between fibers to the bone through the fibrocartilage, i.e., Sharpey's fibers) connection between the TFCC to the ulnar fovea and base of the styloid (Fig. 2.6); however, connection between the TFCC and middle to tip area of the ulnar styloid indicates transition from fibrocartilage to the hyaline-like cartilage, which shows rather weaker connection than foveal area [12, 14] (Fig. 2.7). The very dorsal and palmar attachment of the TFCC to the radial sigmoid notch also indicates ligamentous connection (Sharpey's fibers), while in most of the radial connection between the TFCC and radius, transition from fibrocartilage (TFC) to hyaline cartilage (radius), which is rather weaker connection, is noted [14] (Fig. 2.8).

Biomechanics of the TFCC

There are several paradoxes on biomechanical behavior of the TFCC during forearm rotation. The first is behavior of the RUL during forearm

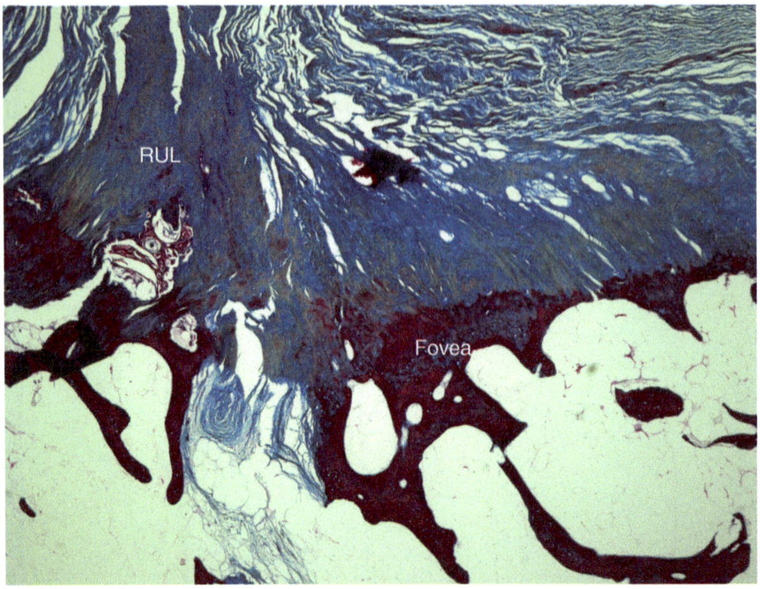

Fig. 2.6 Higher magnification indicates the strong ligamentous connection between the fovea of the ulnar and the RUL with the Sharpey's fibers

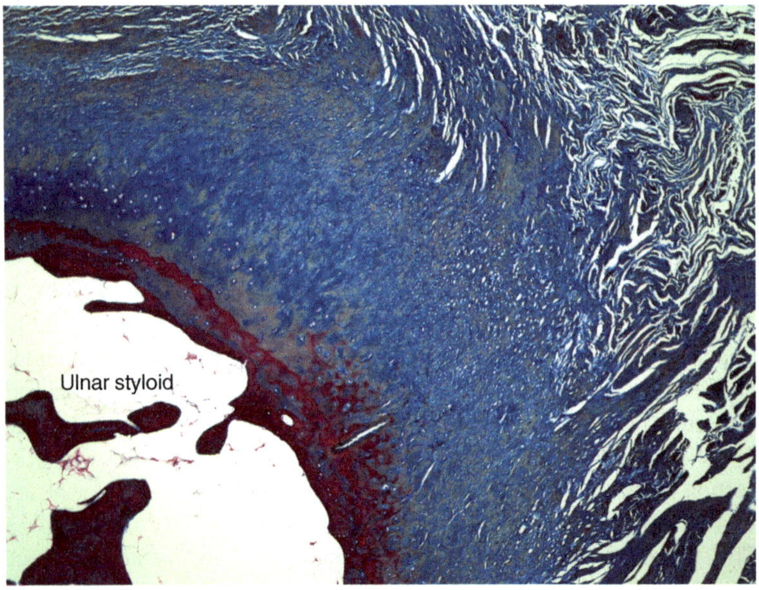

Fig. 2.7 Connection between the tip of the ulnar styloid and the TFCC is transition from the hyaline-like cartilage at the tip of the styloid to the fibrocartilage. There are no Sharpey's fibers in this connecting area

rotation. Af Ekenstam and Hagert [3] described the dorsal RUL was stretched in supination because the ulnar head tended to subluxate palmarly, and palmar RUL was stretched in pronation because the ulnar head tended to subluxate dorsally. Schuind et al. [18] described that dorsal RUL indicated longer in pronation, while palmar RUL demonstrated longer than dorsal in supination. These contradictory descriptions lied in the early 1990s as *the Schuind-Ekenstam paradox.*

Nakamura et al. [13] described from functional anatomical study that during pronation-supination, the RUL is only twisted at its origin at the fovea. Nakamura and Makita [10] described that

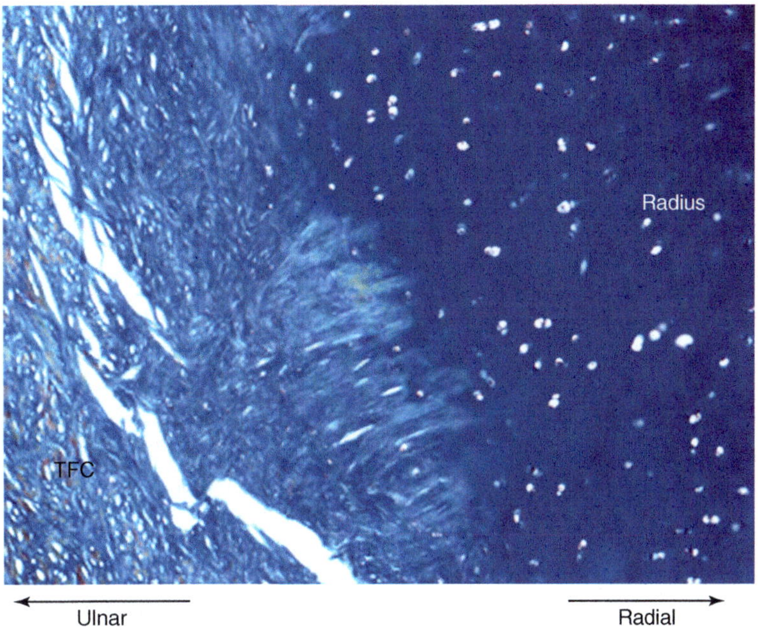

Fig. 2.8 The radial connection between the TFCC and radius indicates that transition from fibrocartilage (*TFC*) to hyaline cartilage (radius), which is rather weaker connection

centrally originating fibers from the fovea in both the dorsal and palmar portions of the RUL demonstrate a nearly isometric length pattern; however, the fibers originating from the eccentric area in the fovea and base of the ulnar styloid reveal changes in the length, where the eccentric dorsal fibers are longer in pronation and shorter in supination, while the eccentric palmar fibers are longer in supination and shorter in pronation (Fig. 2.9), as the description of Schuind et al. [18]. In repair of avulsed TFCC or reconstruction of the TFCC, theoretically avulsed fibers or reconstructing tendon(s) must be introduced to the center of the fovea.

Shape of the TFC is another issue. Kapandji [5] described that ulnar side of the TFC flexed palmary in pronation and dorsally in supination. Adams and Holley [2] indicated that the radial side of the TFC demonstrated changes in shape during pronation-supination, while the ulnar side of the TFC indicates little changes in shape. Makita et al. [6] examined this biomechanically and described that the whole structure of the TFC is stable during forearm rotation, when there is no tear in the TFC (Fig. 2.10). When the capsule or extrinsic wrist ligaments remained intact, the distal surface of the TFC always attaches to the lunate and triquetrum during pronation-supination without any distortion. Friction between the proximal surface of the TFCC and ulnar head must occur during forearm rotation.

Forearm Rotation

Forearm rotation is considered the relative circular motion between the radius and ulna [15] and its complex movement is regulated by several factors: the distal and proximal radioulnar joint surface; the ligaments connecting the radius to the ulna, i.e., the TFCC, interosseous membrane, and annular ligament; the forearm rotator muscles, i.e., the pronator quadratus (PQ), pronator teres (PT), finger flexor, supinator, and biceps brachii; and the direction of the motion, pronating or supinating. The former two factors are considered static factors and the latter two, dynamic factors [9]. Since the surfaces of the DRUJ have incongruity, it in theory allows small translation of the radius to the ulna in addition to rotation [3, 4]. Indeed, in vivo staticodynamic MR study confirmed

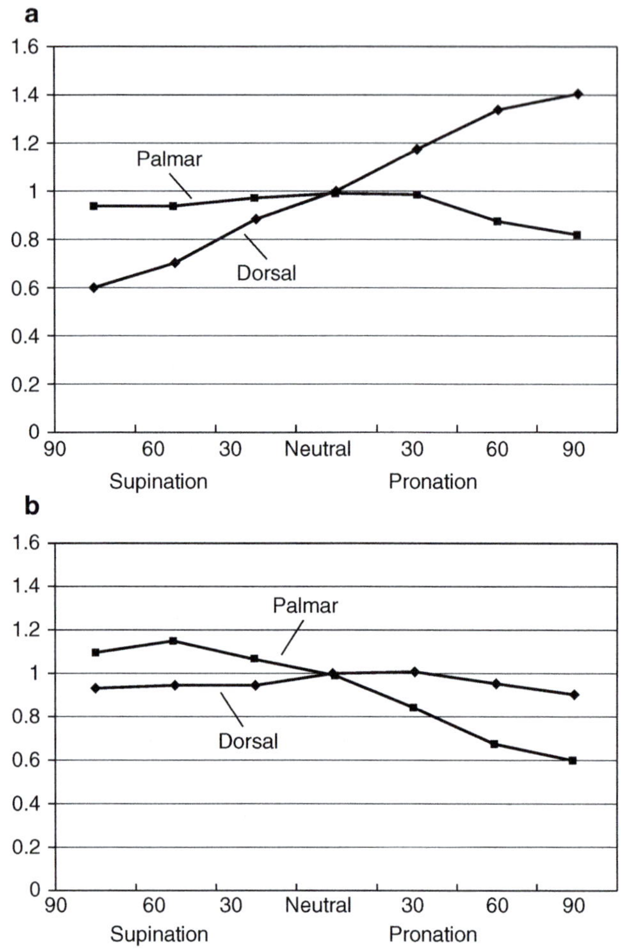

Fig. 2.9 (**a**) Length pattern of the eccentric fibers of the dorsal portion of the RUL attaching to a distance from the fovea and nearly isometric fibers of the palmar portion attaching to the center of the fovea. (**b**) Length pattern of nearly isometric fibers of the dorsal portion of the RUL attaching to the center of the fovea and eccentric fibers of the palmar portion attaching to a distance from the fovea

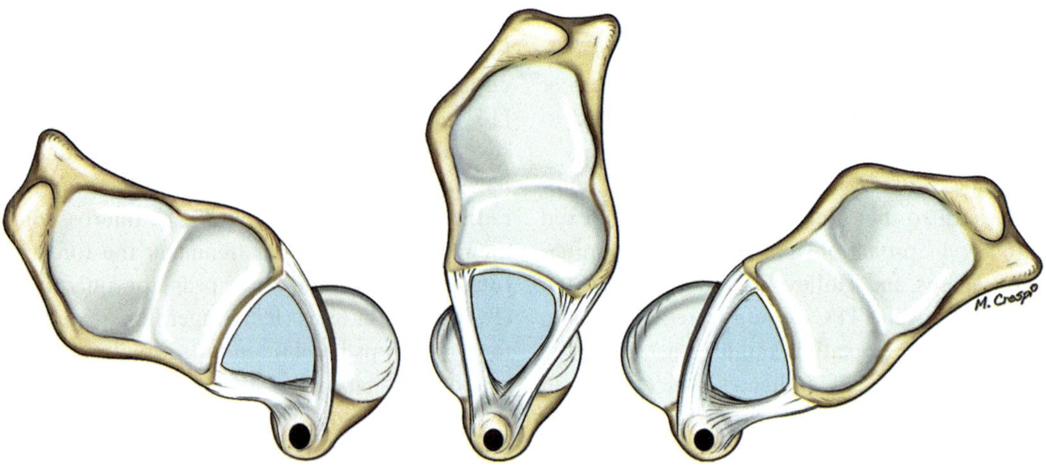

Fig. 2.10 Changes in shape of the TFC during rotation indicate stability, while ulnar side of the TFCC demonstrates changes in shape due to positional changes of the ulnar styloid (*dot*) with respect to the radius

that the forearm rotation is not a simple rotatory motion of the radius relative to the ulna, but a complex motion with axial rotation and translation [9]. During active rotational motion of the forearm or resistive motion such as twisting heavy doorknob, the dynamic factors may produce further complex combination of translation and rotation.

DRUJ Instability

Some investigators defined DRUJ instability as a static dislocation or subluxation of the joint only detected by CT [7], even though patients with the DRUJ dislocation are rarely reported. Clinically, patients with DRUJ instability do not clearly demonstrate dislocation of the DRUJ. They may usually claim "click" or "slack" during the forearm rotational motion [9]. Positive piano-key sign at maximum pronation, which indicates unstable ulnar head relative to the ulna, is usually useful, but they are not completely consistent with clinical situation. Ballottement test, which tests dorsopalmar instability in the neutral, pronated, or supinated position, is the most reliable physical test of the DRUJ instability. "Clicking" or "slacking" is probably due to small abnormal translation of the radius to the ulna during dynamic motion [9] and dislocation should represent the static situation [7]. Even though rupture of total or distal structure of the interosseous membrane (IOM) of the forearm and TFCC would be needed to produce static dislocation of the DRUJ, small abnormal movement between the radius and ulna within the DRUJ might happen at the specific position during dynamic forearm rotation in case of "dynamic" DRUJ instability [9] (Fig. 2.11).

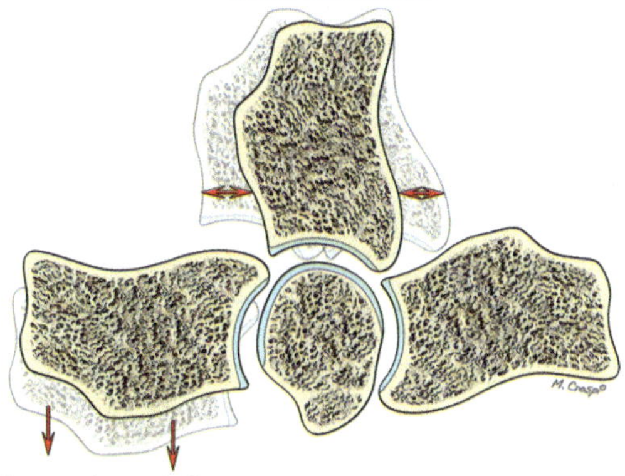

Fig. 2.11 Illustration of the abnormal motion of the radius with respect to the ulna. When the TFCC is ruptured at the fovea, abnormal clunk-like motion of the radius appears mostly in the neutral position and further abnormal translation in pronation during dynamic pronosupination motion. Arrows indicate clunk-like motion and abnormal translation

Precise mechanism of DRUJ instability has not been revealed yet. There may be bony congruity, which changes rotation axis, soft tissue problems including the TFCC and IOM, and dynamic factors deficiency including muscles, i.e., PQ and ECU [9]. Avulsion of the ulnar insertion (origin) of the RUL may be necessary for DRUJ instability ([3, 4, 10, 13, 18]. Radial avulsion of the TFCC including either the dorsal or palmar rim (where the RUL passes) also shows DRUJ instability [8]. The distal portion of the TFCC shapes a hammock-like structure which includes, surrounds, and supports the ulnar carpus, with two tight anchors to the fovea (Fig. 2.12a). Once the anchors are disrupted, the hammock is unsteady (Fig. 2.12b). DRUJ stability can be achieved by re-anchoring the RUL, such as arthroscopic or open repair [11], or reconstruction using palmaris longus ([1] and Chap. 11).

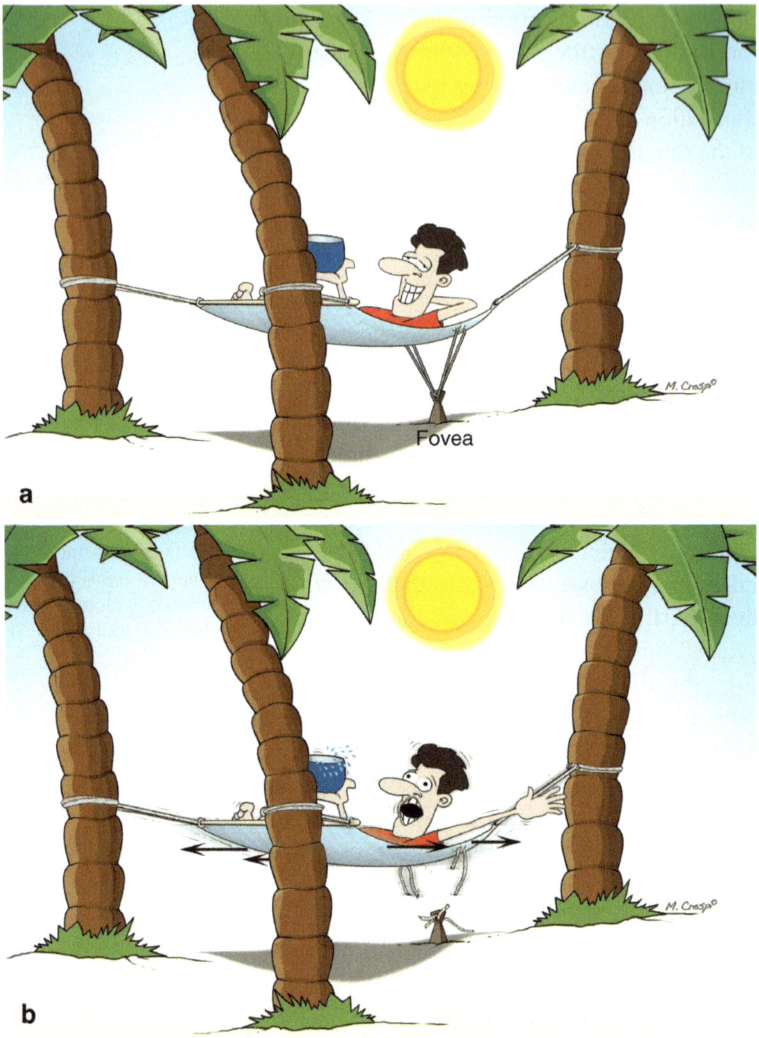

Fig. 2.12 A stable hammock (TFC) anchored to the fovea by the RUL (**a**) becomes unstable when they ruptured (**b**)

References

1. Adams BD (2000) Anatomic reconstruction of the distal radioulnar ligaments for DRUJ instability. Tech Hand Up Extrem Surg 4:154–160
2. Adams BD, Holley KA (1993) Strains in the articular disk of the triangular fibrocartilage complex: a biomechanical study. J Hand Surg 18A:919–925
3. af Ekenstam F, Hagert CG (1985) Anatomical studies on the geometry and stability of the distal radio ulnar joint. Scand J Plast Reconstr Surg 19:17–25
4. af Ekenstam F, Hagert CG (1985) The distal radio ulnar joint: the influence of geometry and ligament on simulated Colles' fracture. An experimental study. Scand J Plast Reconstr Surg 19:27–31
5. Kapandji IA (1982) The physiology of the joints: annotated diagrams of the mechanics of the human joints, vol 1, Upper limb. Churchill Livingstone, New York, pp 108–129
6. Makita A, Nakamura T, Takayama S, Toyama Y (2003) The shape of the triangular fibrocartilage during forearm rotation. J Hand Surg Br 28:537–545
7. Mino DE, Palmer AK, Levinsohn EM (1983) The role of radiography and computerised tomography in the diagnosis of subluxation and dislocation of the distal radioulnar joint. J Hand Surg 8A:23–31
8. Nakamura T (2010) Radial sided tear of the triangular fibrocartilage complex. In: Del Piñal F, Mathoulin C, Luchetti L (eds) Arthroscopic repair of fracture of the distal radius. Springer, Berlin, pp 89–98
9. Nakamura T, Berger RA, Fujita M, An K-N (2002) Distal radioulnar joint instability during forearm rotation: effect of muscle loading. J Jpn Soc Surg Hand 18:306–311

10. Nakamura T, Makita A (2000) The proximal ligamentous component of the triangular fibrocartilage complex: functional anatomy and three-dimensional changes in length of the radioulnar ligament during pronation and supination. J Hand Surg 25B:479–486
11. Nakamura T, Sato K, Okazaki M, Toyama Y, Ikegami H (2011) Repair of the foveal detachment of the triangular fibrocartilage complex: open and arthroscopic transosseous techniques. Hand Clin 27:281–290
12. Nakamura T, Yabe Y (2000) Histological anatomy of the triangular fibrocartilage complex of the human wrist. Ann Anat 182:567–572
13. Nakamura T, Yabe Y, Horiuchi Y (1996) Functional anatomy of the triangular fibrocartilage complex. J Hand Surg 21B:581–586
14. Nakamura T, Yabe Y, Horiuchi Y (2001) Origins and insertions of the triangular fibrocartilage complex – a histological study. J Hand Surg 26B:446–454
15. Nakamura T, Yabe Y, Horiuchi Y, Yamazaki N (1999) In vivo motion analysis of forearm rotation utilizing magnetic resonance imaging. Clin Biomech (Bristol, Avon) 14:315–320
16. Palmer AK, Werner FW (1981) The triangular fibrocartilage complex of the wrist -anatomy and function. J Hand Surg 6A:153–162
17. Sagerman SD, Zogby RG, Palmer AK, Werner FE, Fortino MD (1995) Relative articular inclination of the distal radioulnar joint: a radiographic study. J Hand Surg Am 20A:597–601
18. Schuind F, An KN, Berglund L, Rey R, Cooney WP, Linscheid RL, Chao EYS (1991) The distal radioulnar ligaments: a biomechanical study. J Hand Surg 16A: 1106–1114
19. Tolat AR, Stanley JK, Trail IA (1996) A cadaveric study of the anatomy and stability of the distal radioulnar joint in the coronal and transverse planes. J Hand Surg 21B:587–594
20. Watanabe H, Berger RA, An KN, Berglund LJ, Zobits ME (2004) Stability of the distal radioulnar joint contributed by the joint capsule. J Hand Surg 29A: 1114–1120

Clinical Examination of the Ulnar-Sided Painful Wrist

3

Marc Garcia-Elias

Introduction

While radial-sided wrist pain frequently results from bone or joint injury, most ulnar-sided painful dysfunctions derive from soft tissue damage, difficult to be assessed by conventional radiology. Since the introduction of arthroscopy, a good proportion of such challenging problems have had an adequate solution, but not all of them. In fact, about one fourth of all wrists with ulnar-sided wrist pain do not derive from an intracapsular derangement that could be treated arthroscopically, but from an extracapsular cause (Table 3.1) [37]. In such challenging cases, no treatment is expected to succeed unless the true origin of the problem is targeted, but to target an injury, one must first suspect and later confirm where the injury is. All this process is greatly facilitated by a methodical clinical examination.

The goals of a clinical examination are: (1) to ascertain what is the real source of the patient's pain, (2) to obtain information that facilitates deciding the most efficient treatment for each individual case, and (3) to control the cost of our clinical practice. Of course, saving costs should not be considered a goal by itself, but certainly it is a gratifying consequence of a good clinical examination. Indeed, the better the clinical examination, the less expensive the diagnostic process will be. If a patient has been thoroughly explored, the list of imaging techniques that will be required to confirm potential diagnoses will be narrower

Table 3.1 Clinical conditions which may cause ulnar-sided wrist pain

Carpometacarpal joint instability*
Enthesopathy of the extensor carpi ulnaris (ECU)*
Hook of the hamate fracture or nonunion*
Chondromalacia of the proximal pole of the hamate
Ununited dorsal chip fracture of the triquetrum
Palmar midcarpal instability
Dorsomedial midcarpal instability [45]
Capitolunate instability (CLIP syndrome)
Lunotriquetral (LTq) instability
Fracture of a partial LTq coalition (synchondrosis)
Ulnocarpal ligaments rupture or avulsion
Pisotriquetral dysfunction*
Enthesopathy of the flexor carpi ulnaris*
Ulnar styloid triquetrum impaction syndrome
TILT syndrome [42]
Synovitis in the prestyloid recess in early rheumatoid arthritis
Triangular fibrocartilage complex (TFCC) injury
Ulnocarpal impaction syndrome
Kienbock's disease
Injury to the dorsal sensory branch of the ulnar nerve*
Guyon's canal nerve entrapment*
Hypothenar hammer syndrome*
ECU tenosynovitis*
Instability secondary to injury of the ECU subsheath*
Distal radioulnar joint (DRUJ) osteoarthritis

*Extracapsular pathology

M. Garcia-Elias, M.D., Ph.D.
Hand and Upper Extremity Surgery,
Institut Kaplan, Paseo de la Bonanova, 9, 2º 2ª,
08022 Barcelona, Spain
e-mail: garciaelias@institut-kaplan.com

F. del Piñal et al. (eds.), *Arthroscopic Management of Ulnar Pain*,
DOI 10.1007/978-3-642-30544-3_3, © Springer-Verlag Berlin Heidelberg 2012

than if patient got a careless, incomplete, and disorganized clinical examination [31, 37, 44]. This chapter will review strategies to assess the most common osteoarticular problems that may cause ulnar-sided wrist pain. The ulnar-sided non-osteoarticular wrist pain will not be discussed.

History

Before being examined, the patient should provide detailed information about his/her chief complaints. The clinical history must include: age, handedness, occupation, avocational activities, previous injuries, preceding surgery, and (very important!) worker's compensation status [41]. It is important to question about the mechanism of injury and if there has been exposure to repetitive stress or vibrating tools. The patient should describe the characteristics of that pain, its location, duration, and if there is any position or movement that exacerbates or relieves the symptoms. If joint instability is suspected, it is useful asking if the wrist "gives way when loaded," or if it is "as if a screw has come loose." The first would indicate a kinetic instability, while the second would most often point to a kinematic problem [8].

Inspection

The degree of disability may be suspected by observing the way the patient uses and holds the upper limb [44]. It is important to annotate if there are abnormal movements, tremor, edema, muscle wasting, scars, skin discoloration, or tattoos. Inspection of the wrist with an acute injury may reveal the presence of skin abrasions, contusions, or ecchymosed areas indicating the presence of an internal derangement. Sometimes, chronic painful wrists exhibit bone deformities that are so characteristic of one particular condition that the diagnosis can be made almost immediately. For instance, a stiff wrist with a dorsoradial tumefaction is probably an advanced stage of a SLAC wrist. A very prominent distal ulna, associated with a forklike distal radial deformity, signifies a malunited distal radius with rupture of the radioulnar ligaments. But the most clear example of the utility of inspection in the diagnosis of wrist problems is the patient who, when asked to press down the surface of the examination table with the flat hand, shows an unusually prominent ulnar head that displaces palmarly forming a dimple on the dorsal surface of wrist [1]. It is the so-called dimple sign, a very characteristic finding in most multidirectional DRUJ instabilities.

Clinical Examination

To maximize the efficacy of a clinical examination, it is recommended that the examiner sits in front of the patient across a narrow examination table with a padded surface. The patient needs to feel comfortable with both elbows resting on the table and both forearms vertical, ready to be explored. This type of setting facilitates control of rotation of both forearms, while allowing easy comparison of findings with those of the contralateral side, and observation of the patient's face reaction to the different tests. Signs of apprehension, when performing specifics test, are important data to document.

A complete physical examination consists of: palpation, measurement of range of motion and grip strength, passive joint mobilization, and provocative tests.

Palpation

Palpation is one of the most helpful tools in the diagnosis of any wrist pathology. All palpable anatomical landmarks are to be pressed with the tip of the index finger, with the thumb, or with the tip of a ball pen, searching for areas of maximal tenderness. In the acute injury, this may not provide much information as the entire wrist is tender and swollen; nonetheless, even in such cases, palpation is useful. In all instances, and particularly in the chronic painful wrist, it is recommended to systematically follow a predetermined order of palpation and compare all findings with those from the contralateral normal side. If there

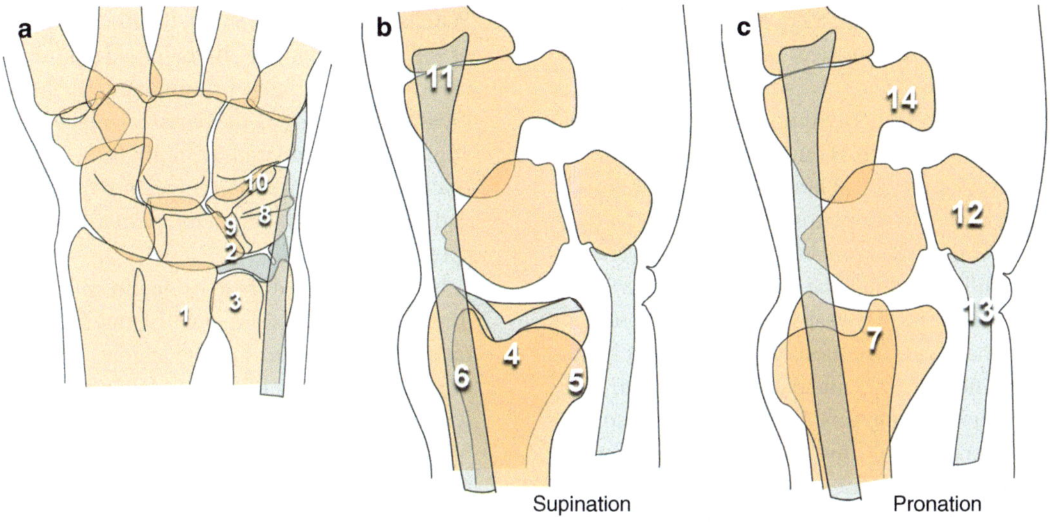

Fig. 3.1 (**a–c**) Schematic representation of the anatomical landmarks which palpation is recommended to identify the source of ulnar pain. Numbers follow the order suggested in the text. (**a**) Dorsal aspect of the wrist: *1* extensor tendons of the fourth compartment, *2* proximal ulnar corner of the lunate, *3* dorsal articular surface of the ulnar head, *8* dorsal ridge of the triquetrum, *9* dorsal aspect of the lunotriquetral joint, *10* triquetrum-hamate joint. (**b**) Ulnar aspect of the wrist with the forearm in supination: *4* foveal insertion of the triangular fibrocartilage complex, *5* anterior aspect of the articular surface of the ulnar head, *6* extensor carpi ulnaris (ECU) tendon, *11* distal insertion of the ECU into the medial aspect of the base of the fifth metacarpal. (**c**) Ulnar aspect of the wrist with the forearm in pronation: *7* ulnar styloid process, *12* pisiform bone, *13* flexor carpi ulnaris tendon, *14* hook of the hamate bone

is an area that is particularly painful, the order of palpation may have to be changed and progress from the least tender spot to the most symptomatic [3]. Complete examination of the ulnar carpus includes palpation of the following anatomical landmarks (Fig. 3.1a–c):

1. With the forearm in pronation, the dorsum of the radial metaphysis, between Lister's tubercle and the ulnar head prominence, is palpated. Swelling in this area may indicate tenosynovitis of the *finger extensors*.
2. With the wrist slightly flexed, the exploring finger is displaced distally between the fourth and fifth extensor compartments. A soft spot may be identified. Deep in that area, the *proximal ulnar corner of the lunate* can be found. If painful, a localized chondral defect, an ulnocarpal impaction syndrome, or a Kienböck's disease may be suspected.
3. Next step consists of assessing the *dorsal surface of the ulnar head*. In pronation, about two thirds of the articular surface is accessible to palpation. Tenderness while palpating that joint surface may indicate localized chondromalacia or global degenerative joint disease.
4. The forearm is then rotated into full supination. In the medial aspect of the wrist, there is a soft depression, just palmar to the extensor carpi ulnaris (ECU) tendon, between the ulnar head and the triquetrum, and slightly proximal to the location where arthroscopists would set the 6U arthroscopy portal. It is the so-called *ulnar snuffbox* [3] or *foveal area* [38]. Under the skin, the anatomical structures that fill that space, from superficial to deep, are: (1) subcutaneous fat tissue containing the dorsal branch of the ulnar nerve; (2) the prestyloid recess, a synovial fold located palmar to the styloid process; (3) the foveal attachment of the triangular fibrocartilage (TFC); and (4) the ulnocarpal meniscus homologue, distal to the foveal attachment of the TFC [7]. According to Tay et al. [38], deep compression of this area elicits exquisite tenderness in cases of foveal disruption of the TFC (positive "ulnar fovea sign"). It is important to note, however, that aside from a

foveal detachment, there are many other possible causes of a positive "ulnar fovea sign": early rheumatoid synovitis (which often starts at the prestyloid recess), chronic injury to the ulnocarpal meniscus homologue, or entrapment injury of the dorsal branch of the ulnar nerve.

5. Next step is palpation of the *volar articular surface of the ulnar head*. With the wrist still in full supination, the volar articular surface of the ulnar head is easily palpable just proximal to the foveal insertion of the TFC, just behind the flexor carpi ulnaris (FCU) tendon. Deep compression in this area, however, is not recommended, as this may result in excessive pressure onto the dorsal branch of the ulnar nerve against the unyielding ulnar head.
6. Next structure to be assessed is the *ECU tendon*. This is regularly done by maintaining the forearm in supination. In that position, the tendon is very prominent onto the top of the ulnar head. Swelling along its course indicates ECU tenosynovitis.
7. As said above, in supination, the "ulnar snuffbox" does not contain any bony structure. If we press onto that area while the wrist is brought back into pronation, a bony prominence will emerge from behind the ECU tendon and travel palmarly as the ulnar head becomes more prominent dorsally. That bony prominence is the *ulnar styloid process*. Tenderness when compressing the space between the distal tip of the ulnar styloid and the medial aspect of the triquetrum may indicate either the "ulnar styloid impaction (USI) syndrome" [40], the so-called triquetral impingement ligament tear (TILT) syndrome [42], or more likely, a carpal detachment injury, as described by Nishikawa et al. [30]. The TILT syndrome is produced by a torn portion of extensor retinaculum that has evolved into an intra-articular nucleus of scarred tissue impinging the medial border of the triquetrum and inducing painful synovitis and eburnation of the bone. A similar impingement may be produced by the tip of the ulnar styloid impacting the triquetrum, as in the USI syndrome [40]. The "ulnocarpal detachment injury" is very similar to the TILT syndrome, except that in this case, there is no extensor retinaculum split tear as found in the latter [30].
8. With the forearm pronated, the *dorsal ridge of the triquetrum* can be palpated just distal to the ulnar head prominence. To help localize that ridge, the wrist is placed in slight flexion and radial inclination. Chip fractures of the dorsal ridge are frequent and may be suspected by palpating that spot.
9. Adjacent to the dorsal ridge, in a lateral direction, the dorsal aspect of the *lunotriquetral (LTq) joint* can be palpated. This area may be particularly tender in patients with ulnocarpal impaction syndrome. Slightly proximal to this anatomical landmark is where arthroscopists place the 6R portal.
10. Immediately distal to the dorsal ridge of the triquetrum, there is another narrow transverse depression. It is the dorsal opening of the *triquetrum-hamate joint*. It is used to create the ulnar midcarpal arthroscopy portal. Isolated swelling and tenderness in that area may indicate chondromalacia of the proximal pole of the hamate [39] or a localized medial triquetral-hamate instability [45].
11. Next is the *distal insertion of the ECU tendon* at the dorsal and medial corner of the base of fifth metacarpal. Exquisite pain in that area denotes the presence of some sort of ECU tendonitis or enthesopathy.
12. The hand is now rotated into full supination, and the oval prominence of the *pisiform bone* is assessed distal to the most proximal palmar crease (Fig. 3.2).
13. Along the proximal border of the pisiform, the flexor carpi ulnaris (FCU) tendon may be palpated, searching for signs of FCU enthesopathy or tendonitis.
14. Finally, we palpate the *hook of the hamate*. It can be found at about one fingerbreadth distal and radial from the pisiform (Fig. 3.2). It is important to note that the end of this bony structure lies under a thick layer of adipose tissue plus fibers of the palmar fascia. Identifying the hook when that tissue is affected by chronic edema or fibrosis may be difficult.

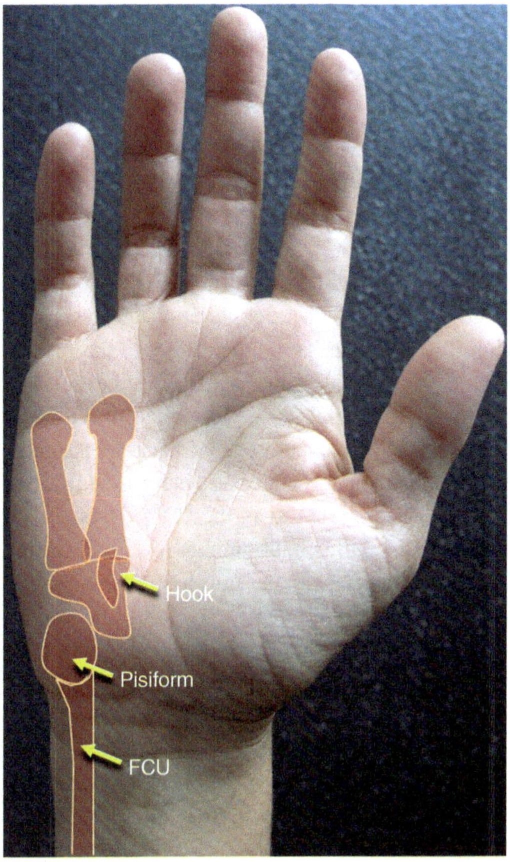

Fig. 3.2 Anatomical landmarks in the palm: flexor carpi ulnaris (*FCU*) tendon, the pisiform bone, and the hook of the hamate

Range of Motion and Grip Strength Determination

Passive and active ranges of motion, including pronosupination, are measured, usually with a standard flexible goniometer. While often limited by pain in the acutely injured wrist, motion may be normal in chronic ulnar dysfunctions. According to Watson and Weinzweig [41], if the forearm allows full-forced pronosupination without pain, it indicates that there is no injury to the TFC or the DRUJ. By contrast, loss of passive flexion consistently represents a sign of underlying carpal pathology.

As the wrist moves, actively or passively, it is important to annotate the presence of grinds, snaps, or clunks and whether such noises appear concurrently with the onset of pain. Grinding is usually caused by two rough bone surfaces rubbing against each other without good cartilage in between. An example of grinding can be found in cases with a fractured LTq partial coalition resulting in painful friction of the two bones during wrist motion [14]. A snap is a sharper sound, most often connected to a subluxing ECU coming out of its groove on the ulna during active ulnar deviation with the forearm in supination [6]. Clunking, by contrast, is a low-pitched sound produced by sudden displacement of a carpal bone in and out of its normal position.

There are different types of carpal clunking; the most frequent are the anterior midcarpal (MC) and the posterior MC clunking [12]. The anterior MC clunking is found among patients with a chronic attenuation or rupture of both the palmar MC and dorsal radiocarpal ligaments, often associated to global wrist laxity. In these cases, the proximal row remains flexed throughout the entire range of radioulnar deviation except near the end of ulnar deviation where it suddenly rotates into extension, sometimes with a palpable thud. It is the so-called catch-up clunk. The posterior MC clunking is usually present in young patients with hypermobile wrists with insufficiency or congenital absence of the dorsal intercarpal ligament. In such instances, the proximal row alignment is normal except in ulnar deviation where the capitate subluxes over the edge of the scapholunate socket inducing hyperextension of the proximal row. Included in this group are the so-called CLIP wrists reported by Louis et al. [26] and by Johnson and Carrera [17].

Grip and pinch strength also need to be investigated. Both dynamometer readings may decrease by actual loss of strength or by muscle inhibition caused by pain. In the latter case, a local anesthetic injection may rule out muscle weakness [4]. If despite local anesthesia, muscles remain weak and dysfunctional, careful evaluation of the neurovascular status is essential.

The so-called gripping rotatory impaction test (GRIT test) described by LaStayo and Weiss [20] is a quantifiable measurement which helps in suspecting an ulnocarpal impaction syndrome. It is known that the amount of load transmitted across the ulna-lunate joint is higher in pronation than in supination [36]. If there is an ulnocarpal impaction problem or a central tear of the TFC, the patient will not squeeze the dynamometer as hard in pronation as in supination because in pronation, the increased load would cause more pain than in supination. In fact, the ratio "grip strength in supination *vs*. grip strength in pronation" was found to be 1 in normal wrists, and above 1.3 in cases with ulnocarpal impaction [20].

Passive Joint Mobilization (Ballottement or Gliding Tests) (Table 3.2)

Except for tightly bound synarthroses, most articulations can be passively mobilized. By applying force in opposite directions, a joint may exhibit abnormally increased displacement. This is an important finding to note, particularly if that displacement elicits pain or crepitus reproducing the patient's chief complaint. In the ulnar column of the wrist, seven joints can be passively mobilized.

Table 3.2 Ballottement and gliding tests for ulnar-sided pain

Piano-key sign test
Distal ulna ballottement test
Distal ulna ballottement test in radial deviation
Pisiform boost test (ulnocarpal)
Reagan's ballottement test (LTq)
Pisotriquetral grinding test
Triquetrohamate shear test
Midcarpal drawer's test (anterior and posterior)
Fifth carpometacarpal stress test

Distal Radioulnar Joint

Aside from the "dimple sign" mentioned above, the so-called piano-key test is a useful tool in the diagnosis of DRUJ instability. While the patient's hand is resting flat on the exploration table in pronation, the explorer exerts pressure onto the prominent ulnar head, aiming at reducing the dorsally subluxed ulna (Fig. 3.3). Most often, the joint is passively reduced, but springs back to the start position as soon as the pressure is released [3].

Another similar test is the "DRUJ instability test" or "distal ulna ballottement test." The examiner uses both hands, one stabilizing the ulna and another mobilizing back and forth the radius [27, 31] (Fig. 3.4a, b). The test must be performed in various positions of forearm rotation. In neutral forearm rotation, up to 5 mm of translation may be normal. By contrast, in the extreme positions of supination and pronation, no translation should be noted, because the TFCC becomes taut and constrains the joint. Furthermore, if the wrist is tested in radial deviation, passive ballottement should also be reduced owing to the tightness of the ulnocarpal ligaments and the ECU tendon [34]. If there is increased displaceability of the joint at the extremes of forearm rotation and/or wrist radial deviation, DRUJ instability is present.

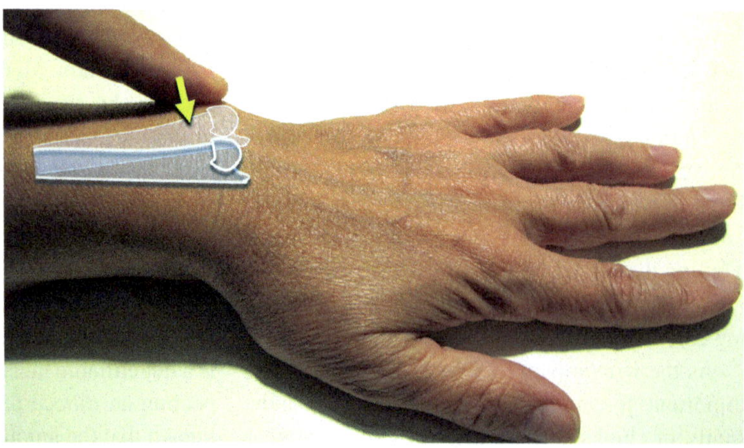

Fig. 3.3 "Piano-key test." Even though the dorsally subluxed distal ulna can be reduced (*yellow arrow*), it springs back to the start position when the reduction force is released

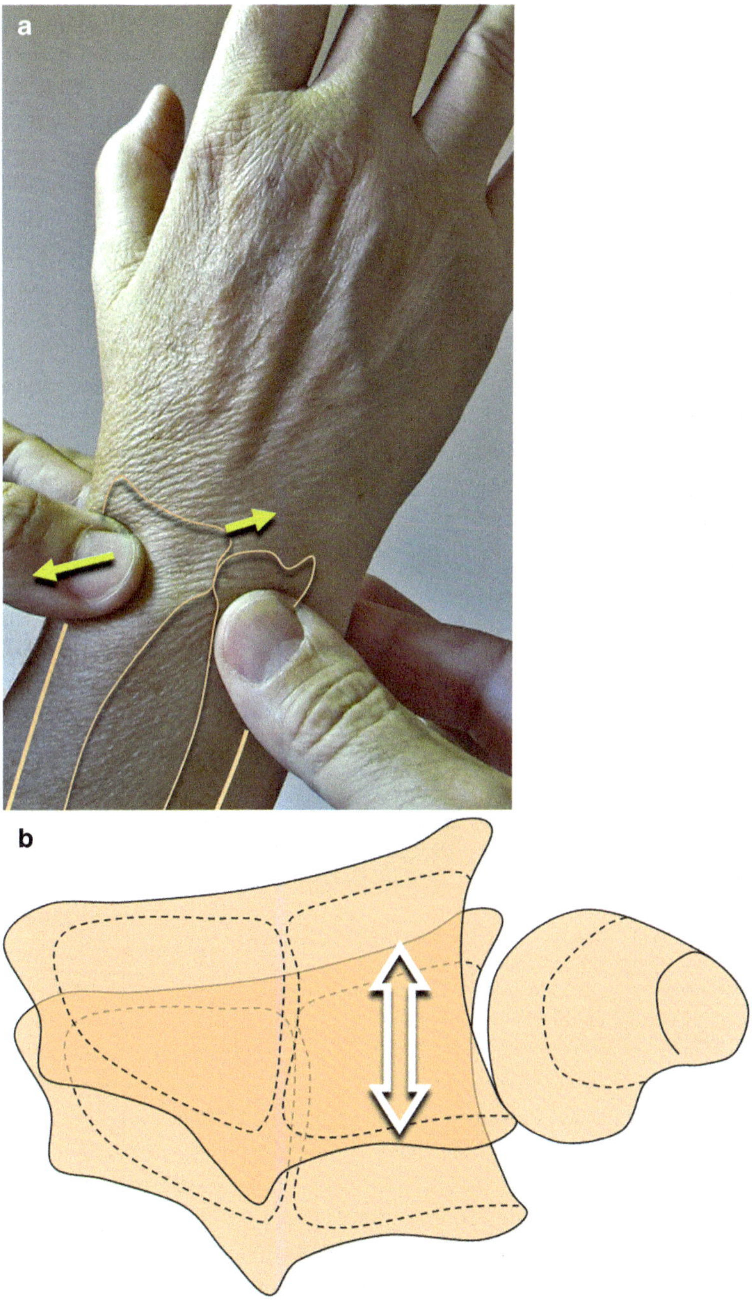

Fig. 3.4 (**a**, **b**) "DRUJ instability test," also known as "distal ulna ballottement test." (**a**) Two hands are used to mobilize back and forth the radius relative to the ulna (*yellow arrows*). (**b**) Schematic representation of the test in the transverse plane. The ulna is to be considered a fixed axis about which the radius is mobilized (*white double arrow*)

Ulnocarpal Joint

Passive mobilization of the ulnocarpal joint has also been known as "TFC shear test," "pisiform boost test," "articular disk shear test," or "ulnomeniscotriquetral dorsal glide test" [5]. Apparently similar to the "piano-key test," the goal of this maneuver is to assess the ability of the TFC and ulnocarpal meniscus homologue to resist anteroposterior shear stress. The test consists of placing the thumb over the palmar surface of the pisiform, while the ulnar head is controlled by the index and middle fingers of the same hand [16]. The examiner squeezes the thumb against the index and middle fingers to

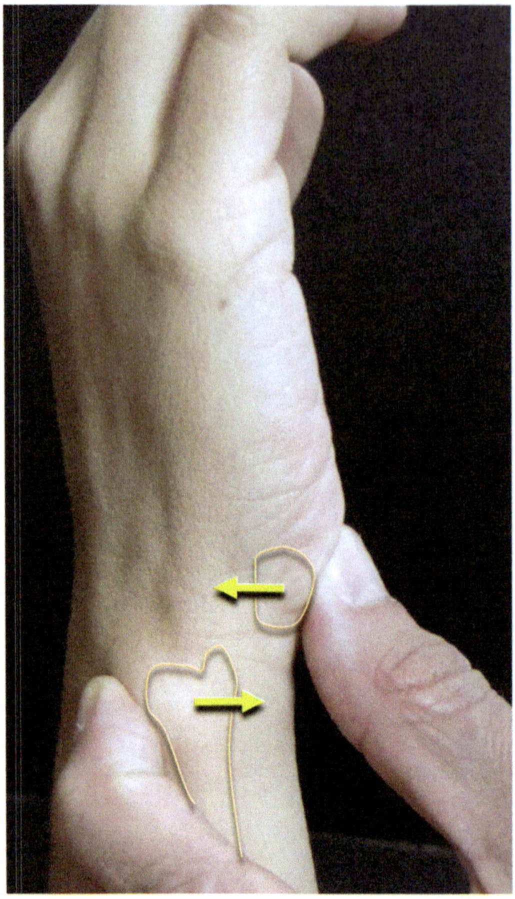

Fig. 3.5 "TFC shear test," also known as "pisiform boost test" or "ulno-menisco-triquetral dorsal glide test." The pisiform and the ulna are pushed in opposite directions, creating an anteroposterior shear stress (*yellow arrows*) to the TFC and ulnocarpal meniscus homologue

induce a dorsal translation of the pisotriquetral complex on the distal ulnar head (Fig. 3.5). With this, a shear stress to both the TFC and the ulnocarpal meniscus homologue is generated. A positive response elicits pain and crepitus, replicating the patient's symptoms. In case of DRUJ instability, increased displaceability of the ulnocarpal joint may be found. The validity of this maneuver has been reported by LaStayo and Howell [21] : two thirds of all the TFC injuries investigated gave a positive response to this test. In absence of TFC injury, this maneuver may still provoke pain and crepitus if there is a degenerative joint disease or joint incongruity in the sigmoid notch cavity.

Lunotriquetral Joint

The so-called ballottement test of the LTq joint, described by Reagan and associates [32], is said to be positive when the joint can be passively mobilized beyond normal limits, that is, more than the contralateral side (Fig. 3.6a, b). A positive test is a sign of LTq instability. The lunate is solidly stabilized with one hand, while the triquetrum and pisiform are displaced dorsally and palmarly with the other hand.

Kleinman [19] suggested an easier way to perform the "ballottement test" and called it "LTq shear test" or "shuck test" (Fig. 3.7). By stabilizing the dorsal aspect of the lunate with one finger, the pisiform is loaded in a dorsal direction with the thumb, creating the LTq shear force necessary to test for stability.

A variation of the LTq shear test is the so-called Derby test reported by Christodoulou and Bainbridge [8]. With the wrist in extension and radial inclination, the examiner uses one thumb to push dorsally the pisiform while the distal row is brought back to neutral alignment (Fig. 3.8). As long as the pisiform is kept dorsally displaced, the patient's discomfort disappears, the wrist feels more stable, and the grip strength increases. Unlike the two first tests (ballottement and shear) which are pathognomonic of LTq dissociation, the Derby test is not specific for LTq instability. Indeed, patients with a non-dissociative "volar intercalated segment instability" (VISI) pattern of carpal alignment are also likely to feel their wrists more stable and stronger with this maneuver.

Pisotriquetral Joint

The pisotriquetral joint is both highly mobile and easily movable. To assess both its stability and status of its cartilage, one may use the so-called pisotriquetral grind test [15]. To facilitate holding the pisiform, it is helpful to slightly flex and incline ulnarly the wrist (Fig. 3.9). Once the pisiform is solidly held between the thumb and the index finger, the wrist is placed back to neutral and the joint is mobilized medially and laterally. Pain and crepitus may indicate pisotriquetral degenerative joint disease. Unusual passive mobility with medial subluxation of the pisiform

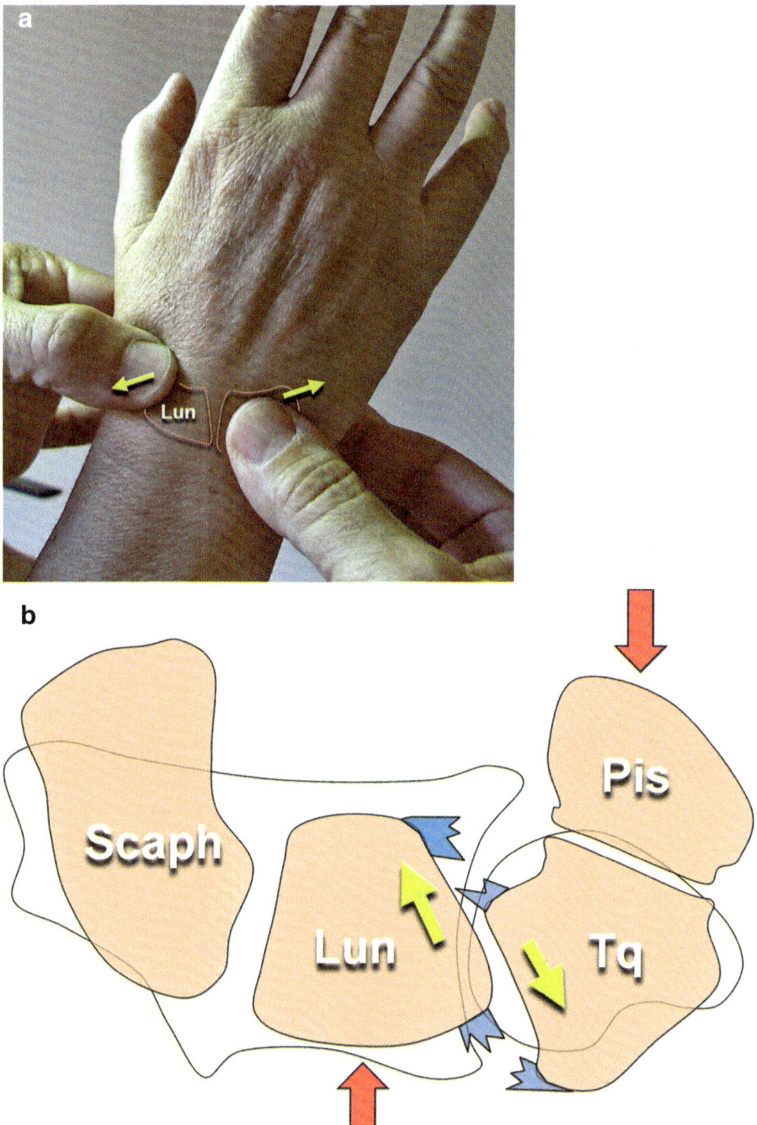

Fig. 3.6 (**a**, **b**) The "ballottement test" of the LTq joint described by Reagan and associates [32]. (**a**) With two hands, the explorer creates shear stress to the LTq joint (*yellow arrows*). (**b**) The pisotriquetral unit is pressed posteriorly, while the lunate is constrained palmarly (*red arrows*). The test is positive when the joint exhibits excessive mobility (*yellow arrows*), which may indicate LTq interosseous ligament disruption

is a rare condition which can only be diagnosed with this test.

Triquetrohamate Joint

Chondromalacia of the proximal pole of the hamate is a frequent cause of ulnar-sided pain, particularly when the wrist has a lunate type II [25]. The cartilage erosion that characterizes this problem becomes particularly painful during ulnar inclination, when this portion of bone impinges the ulnar articular facet of the lunate. To diagnose this problem, it is useful to perform the "triquetrohamate grinding (or shear) test" [5] (Fig. 3.10). With the wrist in ulnar deviation, the distal carpal row is mobilized palmarly and dorsally with one hand, while the pisotriquetral unit is solidly stabilized with the other. This creates shear stress between the lunate and the proximal pole of the hamate. Painful crepitation is what identifies this condition. Excessive mobility of the joint may point towards localized medial triquetral-hamate instability, an unusual condition

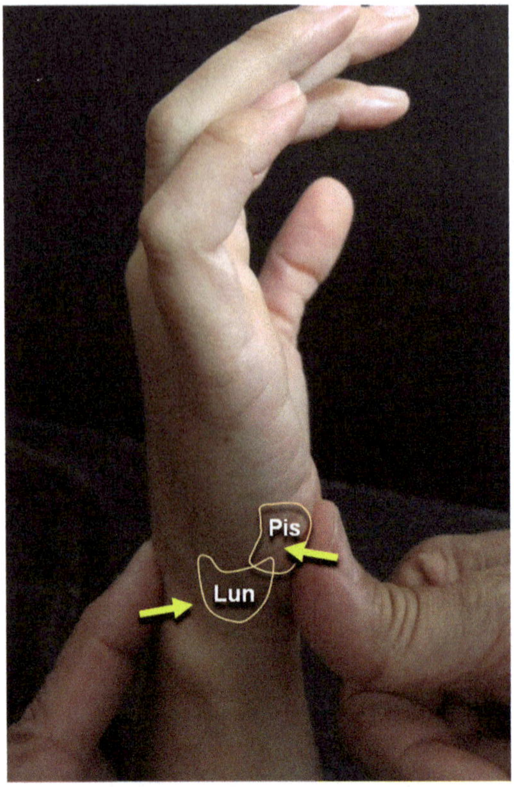

Fig. 3.7 Similar to the "LTq ballottement test," there is the "LTq shear test" or "shuck test." In this case, the two opposite forces (*yellow arrows*) onto the dorsum of the lunate (*Lun*) and the palmar convexity of the pisiform (*Pis*) are exerted by only two fingers

described by Zancolli [45] resulting from rupture of the capsular reinforcement that forms the floor of the ECU tendon sheath.

Lunocapitate Joint

Dorsal lunocapitate instability is often the result of absence or insufficiency of the more proximal thick bundle of the dorsal intercarpal ligament. Among other functions, this ligament acts as a labrum, making deeper and more stable the scapholunate-capitate ball-and-socket articulation. Should this ligament be torn or absent, the capitate may sublux dorsally, with a clunk, when the distal row is stressed dorsally with the wrist in ulnar deviation [26]. The essential difference between this type of clunking and the "catch-up clunk" described below is that, in this case, the capsular defect is dorsal midcarpal, while in the "catch-up clunk," the defect is both dorsal radiocarpal and palmar midcarpal [12, 24]. To test for the two types of midcarpal instability, the so-called drawer's tests is useful. The distal row and base of the II–V metacarpals are held and displaced dorsoradially or palmarly with one hand, while the radius is controlled by the other hand [26]. With the posterior drawer's test, the proximal row is extended, and the capitate finds an opening through which to dislocate. If the instability is palmar, the proximal row rotates into extreme flexion and the capitate subluxes anteriorly (Fig. 3.11).

Fifth Carpometacarpal Joint

Localized tenderness and swelling at the base of the fifth metacarpal is not unusual, often the result of post-traumatic instability. Mobilizing the fifth carpometacarpal joint is facilitated by holding the metacarpophalangeal joint in flexion. The metacarpal is stressed into maximal flexion-extension, internal-external rotation, and antero-posterior translation to search for articular cartilage crepitation or for abnormal displaceability. The first would indicate arthrosis; the second, instability [35].

Provocative Tests for Ulnar-Sided Pathology (Table 3.3)

To further assess the origin of the patient's pathology, a number of so-called "provocative" maneuvers have been described [5, 9, 22]. The goal of these maneuvers is to reproduce the circumstances where pain appears and based on this, to learn about the pathomechanics of that condition. Induction of the patient's symptoms not only facilitates the diagnosis and unveils the location of the offending injury but also allows the patient to confirm that the provoked symptoms are the ones that bother him/her. The following is a list of the most commonly used provocative maneuvers to investigate ulnar-sided wrist pain.

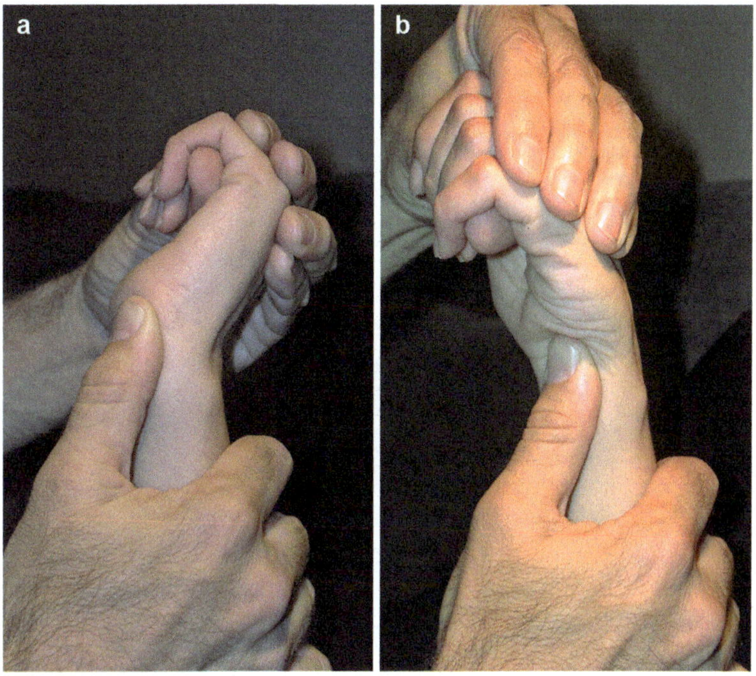

Fig. 3.8 The "Derby test" consists of reducing the VISI pattern of carpal malalignment, present both in LTq instabilities as in palmar midcarpal instabilities, by pushing dorsally the triquetrum. This generates an extension moment to the triquetrum that mitigates the patient's discomfort both in radial inclination (**a**) as in ulnar deviation (**b**)

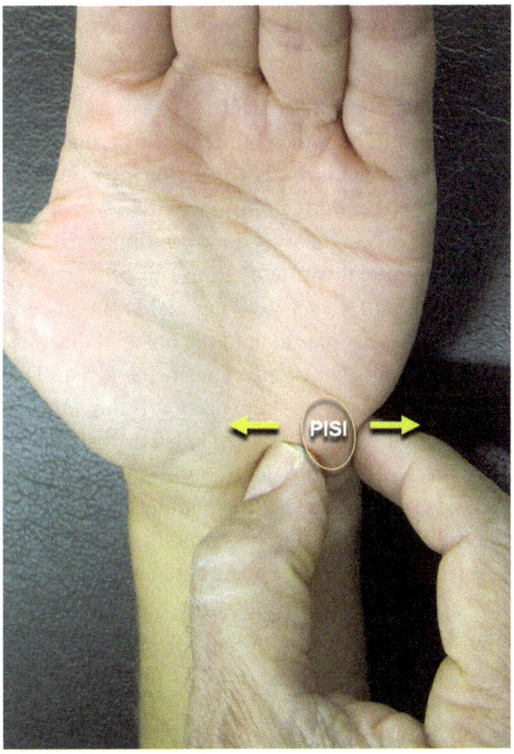

Fig. 3.9 The "pisotriquetral grind test" consists on mobilizing the pisiform laterally and medially (*yellow arrows*) searching for crepitus (osteoarthritis) or increased mobility (instability)

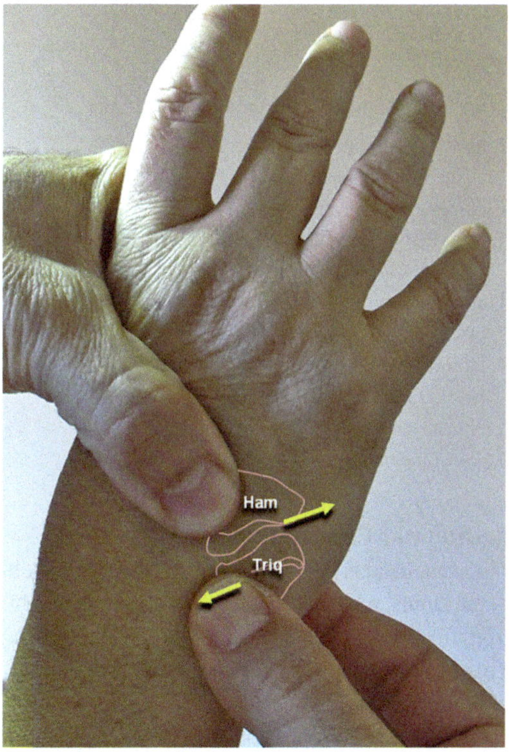

Fig. 3.10 The "triquetrohamate grinding (or shear) test" consists on mobilizing the hamate against the triquetrum (*yellow arrows*) searching for pain and crepitus, a finding that indicates the presence of chondromalacia of the proximal pole of the hamate

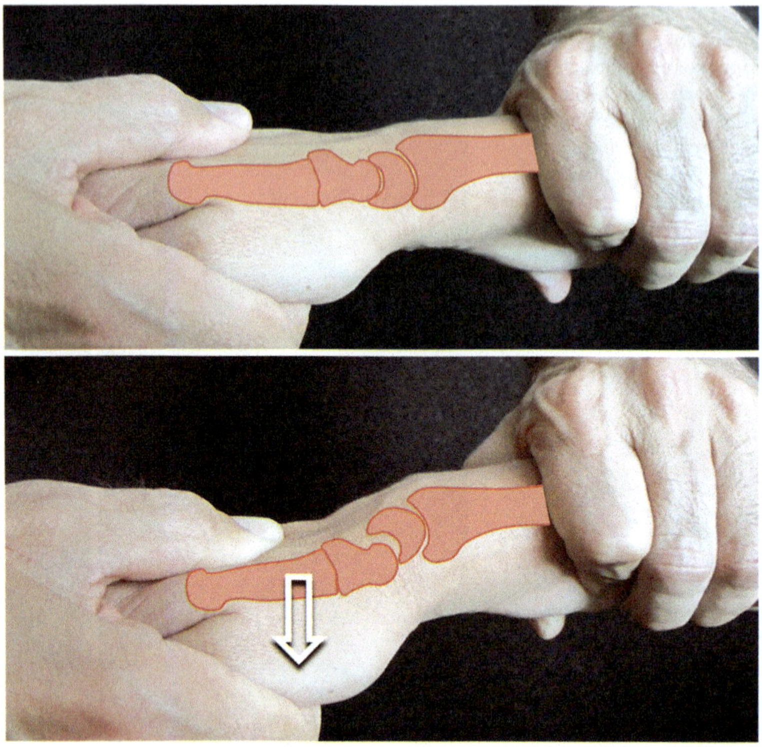

Fig. 3.11 "Anterior drawer's test." A palmar directed force (*white arrow*) to the distal row may be used to investigate the existence of a palmar midcarpal instability

Table 3.3 Provocative test for ulnar-sided pain

Radioulnar compression test
Loaded pronosupination test
ECU tendon subluxation test
ECU synergy test (Ruland and Hogan test)
TFC grind test (Nakamura's ulnocarpal stress test)
Ulnar styloid impaction test (Ruby's test)
Ulnocarpal meniscoid test (waiter's test)
Lunotriquetral compression or "ulnar snuffbox test"
Triquetral shift maneuver of Sennwald
Lichtman's midcarpal shift test
Hook of the hamate pull test

Radioulnar Compression Test

The ulnar head is pressed against the sigmoid notch of the radius, while the forearm is passively brought from full pronation to full supination [9] (Fig. 3.12). This maneuver helps assessing the status of the cartilage at both sides of the joint. If this maneuver provokes painful crepitation, the presence of localized or global degenerative osteoarthritis is likely.

Loaded Pronosupination Test

Similar to the radioulnar compression test, the "loaded pronosupination test" investigates the capacity of the ulnar head to resist transverse loading throughout the entire range of pronosupination. The test is based on using a handlebar attached to a semicircular frame with a wheel that allows a free hanging weight to continuously load the hand while this rotates from full pronation to supination and vice versa (Fig. 3.13). Loads are progressively increased until the onset of discomfort or a giving-way sensation in the wrist. The average load-bearing capability of the normal unsupported forearm is 5 kg [13]. The test allows evaluation of pathological conditions involving weakness of the pronation-supination muscles with or without joint incongruity. If a patient suffers from ulnar head chondromalacia, not only the capacity to resist transverse loading will be diminished, but also pain will appear with minimal loading.

ECU Tendon Subluxation Test

To investigate the presence of ECU tendon instability, the forearm is held in maximal supination with one hand while the other palpates the tendon [6]. The patient is then asked to deviate ulnarly the wrist against resistance. Should the ECU

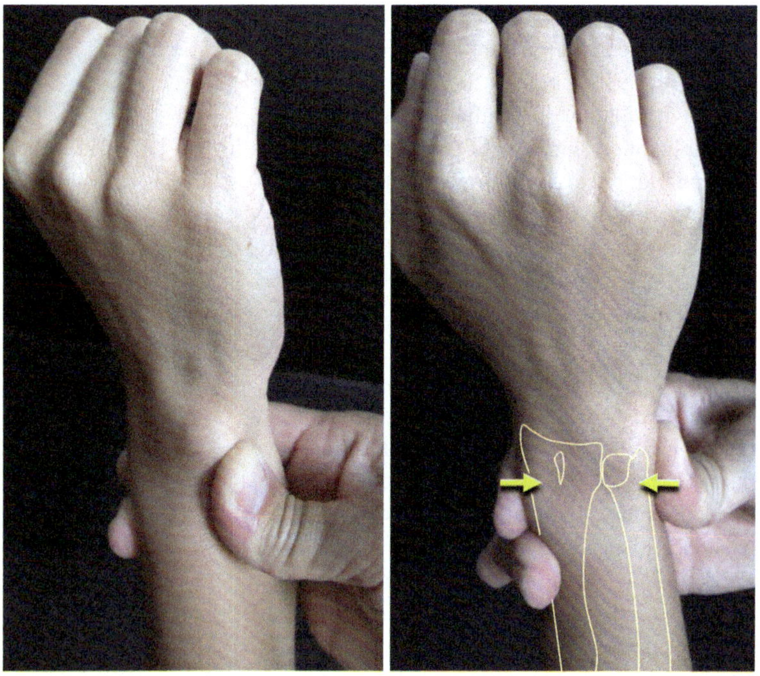

Fig. 3.12 "Radioulnar compression test." The ulna is pressed against the radius while the forearm is passively rotated. Pain and crepitus indicates degenerative osteoarthritis of the radioulnar joint

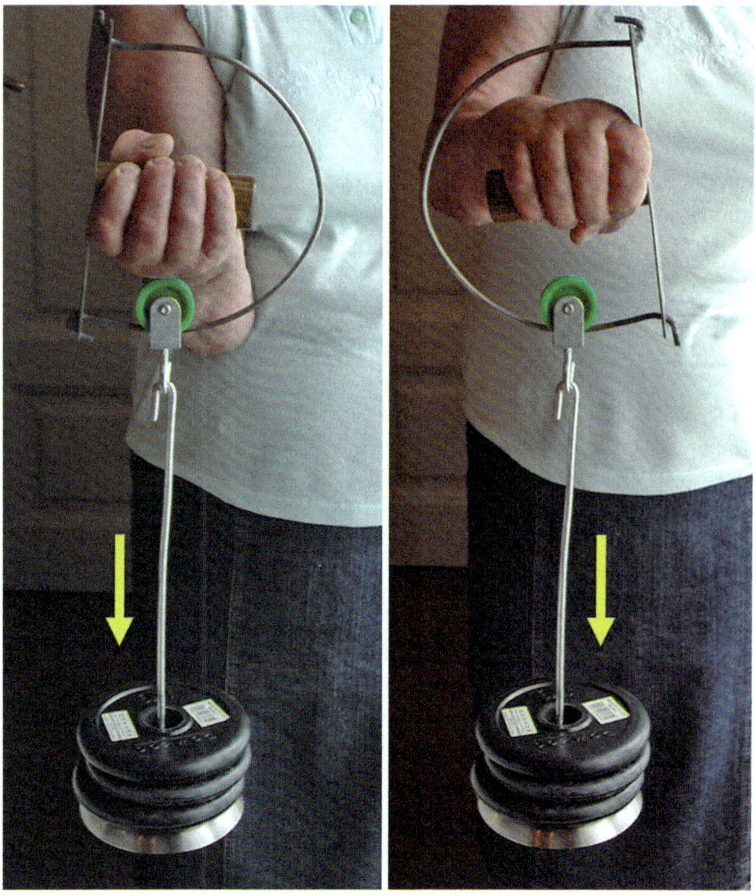

Fig. 3.13 "Loaded pronosupination test." A hanging weight (*yellow arrows*) creates a constant transverse loading to the distal radioulnar joint throughout the entire range of pronosupination. On average, the maximal load that can be tolerated without experiencing pain is 5 kg [13]. The more damaged the radioulnar joint, the less load the patient can tolerate

tendon subsheath be ruptured or elongated, the tendon would sublux palmarly out of the vertical groove that exists behind the ulnar styloid process on the dorsum of the ulnar head. Sometimes, the subluxation is not only palpable but visible and audible, provoking a typical snapping sound. It is important to note that, among hyperlax individuals, slight subluxation of the ECU may be normal and painless. As emphasized above, comparison with the contralateral side is important.

ECU Synergy Test

This test was recently described by Ruland and Hogan [33] to differentiate between ulnar-sided pain secondary to ECU tendonitis and pain secondary to intracarpal pathology. It is based on the existence of synergy between contraction of the ECU muscle and contraction of some intrinsic muscles. Certainly, isometric contraction of the abductor pollicis brevis entails a synergistic contraction of the ECU muscle in order to maintain the balance between radial and ulnar wrist forces. The test consists of placing the wrist in supination, and while the explorer is blocking the position of the thumb relative to the index finger, the patient is asked to separate the first web space (isometric contraction of the first palmar interosseous muscle and the abductor pollicis longus and brevis muscles) (Fig. 3.14). If there is ECU tendonitis, that maneuver will provoke increasing pain in the ulnar aspect of the wrist. If that painful reaction does not appear, the ulnar pain probably is not related to the ECU muscle.

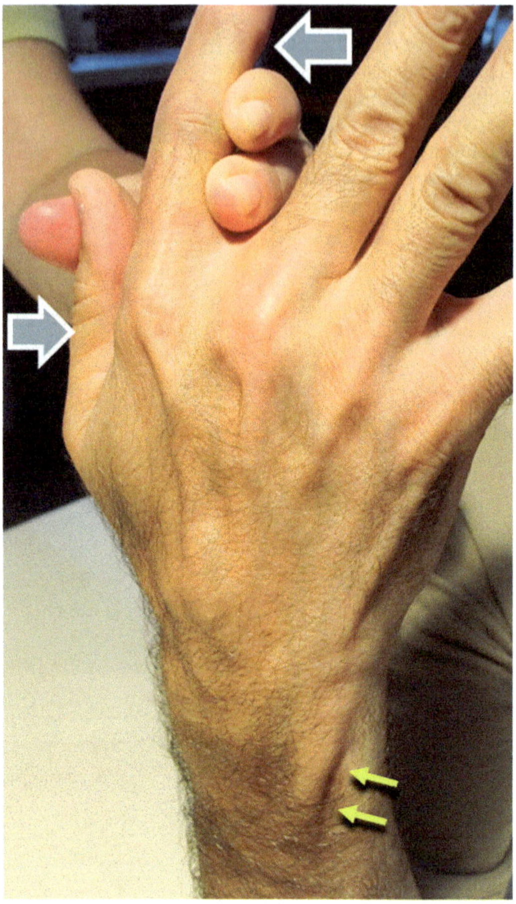

Fig. 3.14 "ECU synergy test." Described by Ruland and Hogan [33], this test is useful to differentiate between ECU tendonitis and intracarpal pathology. Isometric contraction of the abductor pollicis longus and brevis (*gray arrows*) induces synergistic contraction of the ECU tendon (*yellow arrows*). Should the latter tendon be inflamed, pain in the ulnar corner of the wrist is likely when this test is done

TFC Grind Test

Apparently similar to the abovementioned "TFC shear test," the "grind test," also known as "ulnocarpal stress test," was introduced to assess the ability of the TFC to sustain rotational shear stress [28]. The patient's hand is held by the metacarpals, while the distal forearm is stabilized in a vertical position by the other explorer's hand. The hand is then placed in ulnar deviation, and the explorer applies an axial load to the hand. In such loaded condition, the forearm is rotated from full supination to pronation (Fig. 3.15). A positive test will generate a grinding sensation to the patient with pain and crepitus, sometimes a click, indicating TFC tear or ulnocarpal impaction syndrome.

A similar provocative test was reported by Lester et al. [23]. It is the so-called press test and consists on requiring the seated patient to push his/her body weight up off a chair using the affected wrist, creating an axial ulnar load. A positive test provokes exquisite ulnar wrist pain replicating the one that led the patient to seek medical attention.

And still another similar test is the so-called screwdriver maneuver. With the hand grasping a screwdriver, the patient is asked to resist

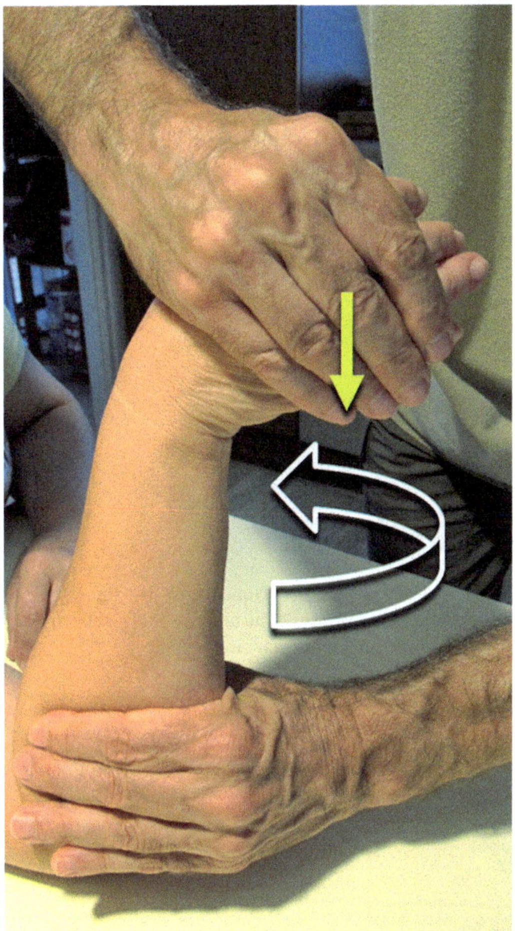

Fig. 3.15 "TFC grind test," also known as "ulnocarpal stress test." The hand is placed in ulnar deviation; the explorer applies an axial load to the hand (*yellow arrow*), and the forearm is rotated from full pronation to supination (*curved arrow*). If this causes a painful grinding sensation, either a TFC lesion or an ulnocarpal impaction syndrome is likely

pronosupination torques produced by the examiner onto the metallic end of the tool [5]. Pain and crepitus in the ulnar wrist would point to a TFC tear or ulnocarpal impaction syndrome.

Ulnar Styloid Triquetral Impaction Test

Several conditions may result in the development of the so-called ulnar styloid triquetrum impaction (USTI or USI) syndrome [40]. For the ulnar styloid process to be able to impact against the dorso-ulnar aspect of the triquetrum, aside from a size above average, the wrist needs to be maximally extended, ulnarly deviated, and the forearm needs to be in full supination. The USTI or Ruby test attempts to reproduce those circumstances and provoke the patient's pain by applying an axial load in the palm (Fig. 3.16). If the pain appears only in supination, but not in pronation, the chances of an USTI syndrome are high.

Ulnocarpal Meniscoid Test (Waiter's Test)

The ulnocarpal meniscus homologue, also known as "ulnomeniscal homologue," is a highly vascularized and innervated synovial fold extending from the inner surface of the ulnocarpal capsule into the joint space, filling the triangular space that is left between the distal surface of the TFC and the convex surface of the triquetrum [7, 11]. In frontal scans, it has a triangular configuration which reminds that of a meniscus. This structure may be injured when a sudden axial load in ulnar deviation provokes its entrapment between the triquetrum and the ulnar styloid. The injured meniscoid may become fibrotic and behave as a foreign body causing pain, comparable to that found in the above discussed USI [40], TILT [42], or ulnocarpal detachment injury [30]. The ulnocarpal meniscoid test consists of applying an axial load to the ulnar carpus, while the wrist is passively brought from extension to ulnar deviation and from there to flexion (Fig. 3.17). The goal is to create localized stress in the periphery of the ulnocarpal space, where the meniscoid is located. The test, also known as "waiter's test," is to be performed in pronation, neutral, and supination. Usually, if the meniscoid is pathologic, the test is more positive (more painful) in supination than in pronation.

Lunotriquetral Compression Test

Compression across the LTq joint with degenerative joint disease, or any other form of synovitis (instability, partial synchondrosis, etc.), is likely to induce pain proportional to the amount of load being applied. To perform the LTq compression test, also known as "ulnar snuffbox test" or "Linscheid's LTq shear test" [5], the examiner places the tip of the thumb between the FCU and ECU, slightly distal to the "ulnar snuffbox." By applying a lateral pressure over the medial border of the triquetrum, while the wrist is radially deviated,

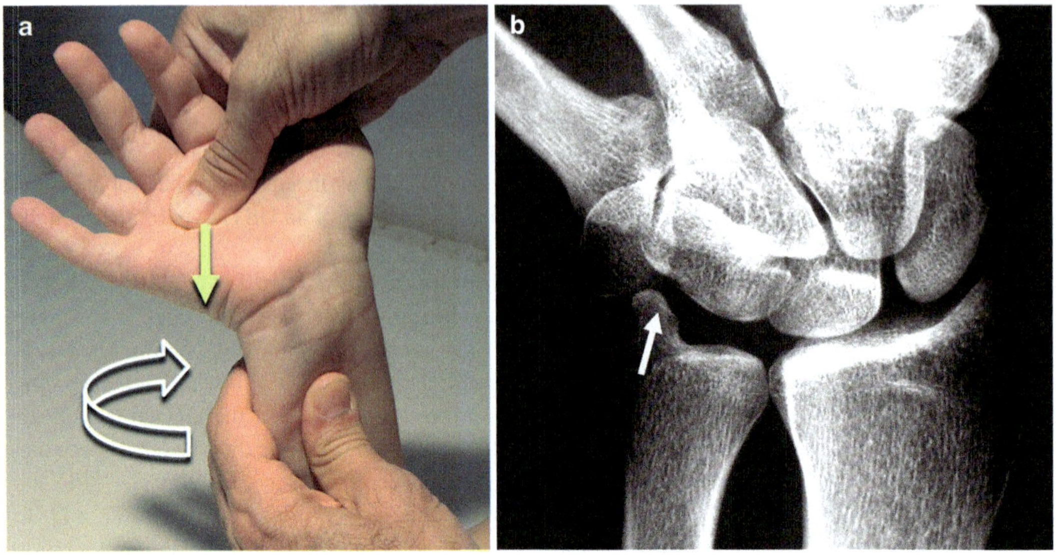

Fig. 3.16 "Ulnar styloid triquetrum impaction test." (**a**) When the wrist is in ulnar deviation and full supination (*white arrow*), if an axial compressive force (*yellow arrow*) is exerted in the palm, the ulnar styloid may contact the dorsal ridge of the triquetrum. (**b**) Radiological demonstration of how close the ulnar styloid (*white arrow*) gets to the triquetrum in such circumstances

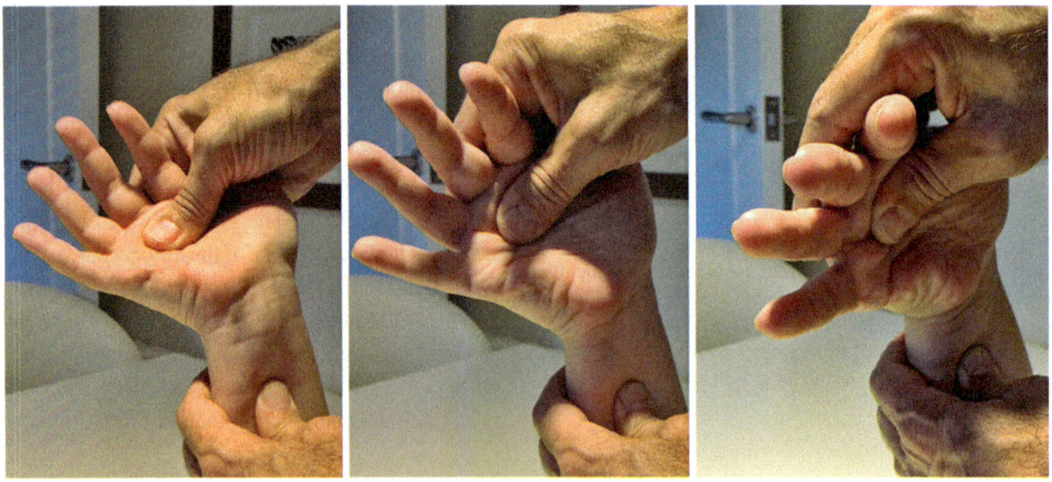

Fig. 3.17 "Ulnocarpal meniscoid test," also known as "waiter's test." An axial load is applied to the hand in extension and ulnar deviation. Without releasing pressure to the hand, this is passively brought into full ulnar deviation, and from there, into full flexion. The test is to be repeated with the forearm in pronation, neutral, and supination positions. This test investigates the integrity of the three zones of the ulnocarpal meniscus homologue: palmar, medial, and dorsal

the patient's symptoms may be reproduced [2] (Fig. 3.18). A positive test may indicate LTq injury or the TILT syndrome. When the LTq compression test is positive, the possibility of a TFCC problem is less likely.

Triquetral Shift Maneuver

It is known that the proximal row from flexion in radial deviation becomes extended in ulnar deviation. There is a smooth and progressive extension rotation of the proximal row as the wrist

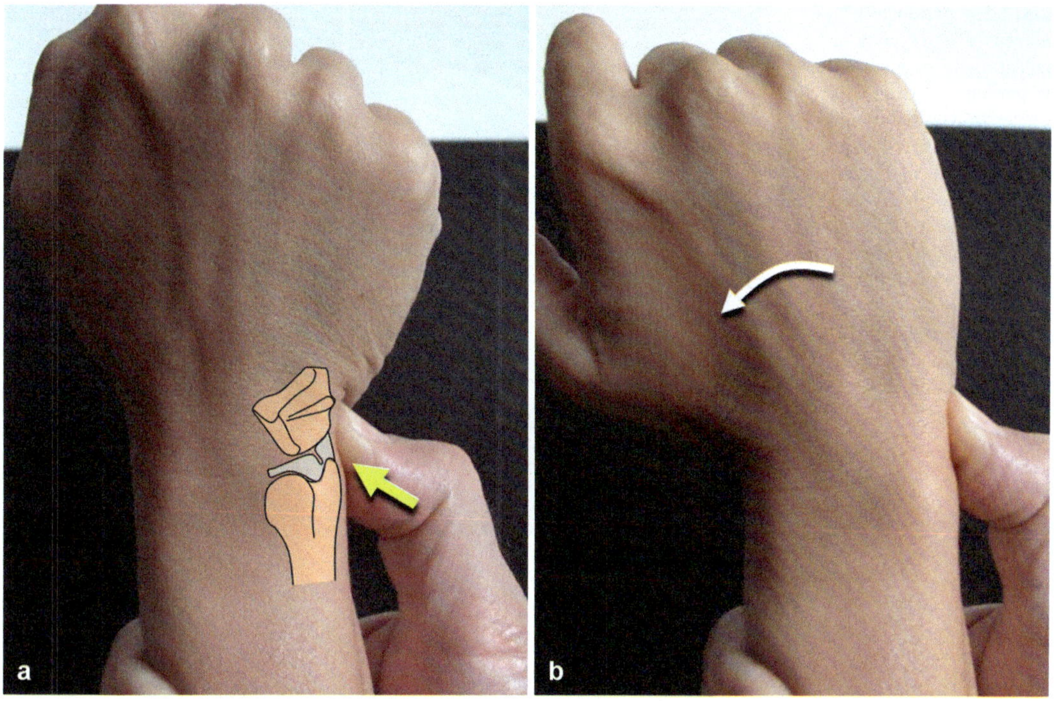

Fig. 3.18 "LTq compression test." (**a**) The wrist is in neutral position and the explorer exerts thumb pressure onto the "ulnar snuffbox" (*yellow arrow*). (**b**) If that pressure is not discontinued, the triquetrum will be forced against the lunate when the wrist is forced into radial deviation (*white arrow*). Should the LTq joint be pathological, this maneuver would provoke exquisite local pain

deviates ulnarly. The more the triquetrum extends, however, the less prominent it becomes in the dorsum of the wrist. Indeed, as the triquetrum extends, there is also slight palmar translation of the bone. This is why the bone disappears under the explorer's finger when the wrist is brought from radial to ulnar deviation. This is the basis of the "triquetral shift maneuver," first suggested by Sennwald [29] (Fig. 3.19a, b). One hand is used to support the distal radius and ulna while pressing the triquetrum palmarly with the thumb. The test starts with the wrist in ulnar deviation. In that position, the proximal row is in its maximum extended position, and the triquetrum is deep in the wrist and hardly palpable. The wrist is then brought passively towards radial deviation. The triquetrum would rotate into flexion and be more prominent dorsally, but it will not because the explorer's thumb will keep pushing it palmarly. In such circumstances, if the LTq ligaments are intact, the wrist will not be able to radially deviate. By contrast, if the LTq ligaments are ruptured or abnormally lax, the maneuver will cause shear stress in the LTq joint, with the lunate translating dorsally, this inducing pain, reproducing the patient's complaints. This maneuver is analogous to the "scaphoid shift test" described by Watson and Weinzweig [41].

Midcarpal Shift Test

The "midcarpal shift test" was described by Lichtman et al. [24] to determine the amount of midcarpal joint laxity. It consists of subluxing palmarly the midcarpal joint, while ulnarly deviating the wrist in pronation. The test is similar to the anterior "drawer's test" (Fig. 3.11) except that, in this case, the wrist is pronated and ulnarly deviated. Depending upon how much force is necessary to maintain the palmar sag in ulnar deviation, wrists are classified into five grades [10]. Grade 1 is when the distal row cannot be displaced palmarly due to the presence of strong

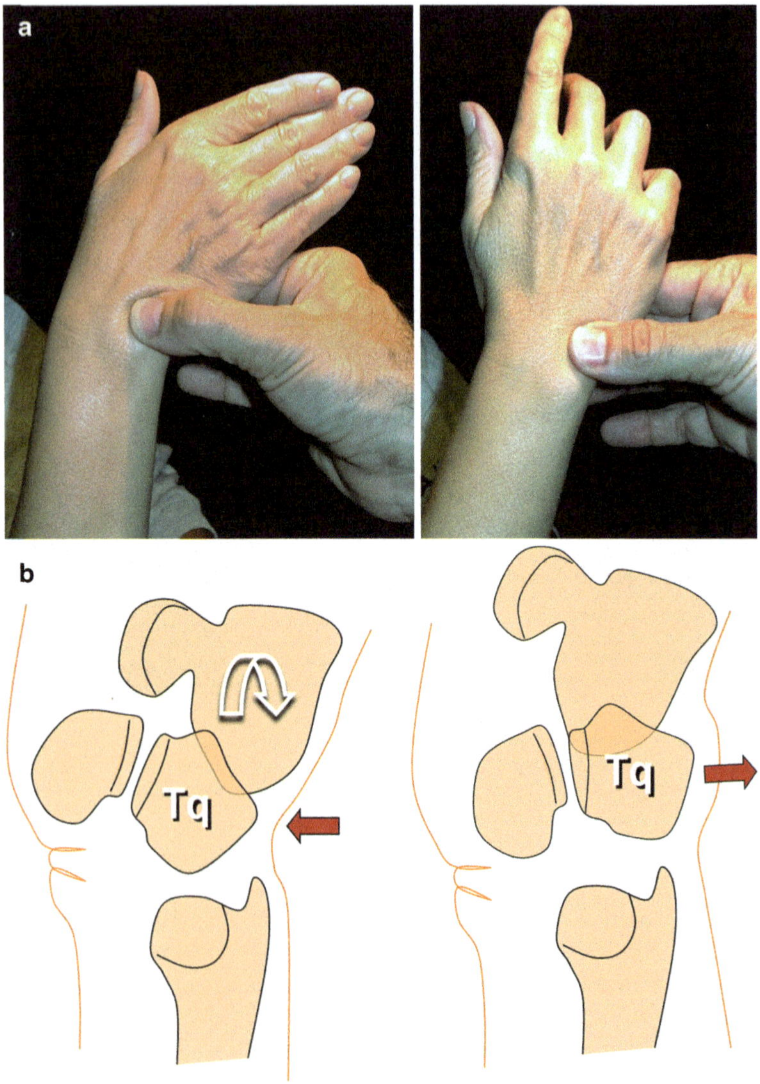

Fig. 3.19 "Triquetral shift maneuver." (**a**) It consists of palpating the dorsum of the triquetrum while the wrist rotates from radial to ulnar deviation and vice versa. (**b**) In normal conditions, the triquetral prominence disappears in ulnar deviation (*white arrow*) to become more pronounced in radial deviation (*red arrows*). If there is LTq pathology, this test induces pain and crepitus in radial deviation

and taut palmar midcarpal ligaments. Grades 2 and 3 are still found among normal individuals and represent increasing levels of midcarpal laxity. In those, the palmar sag can be obtained, but itself reduces when the force is released. Grade 4 is an abnormal level of laxity where the midcarpal joint remains subluxed when the external force is released. Grade 5 instability is when the patient is able to actively sublux the joint without assistance. This test evaluates the level of elasticity of the palmar midcarpal ligaments. High grades of instability, however, need not be interpreted as pathologic unless there is a painful unilateral dysfunction.

Hook of the Hamate Pull Test

The hook of the hamate not only should be regarded as the ulnar wall of the carpal tunnel but also as a pulley that increases the mechanical advantage of the flexor tendons of the little finger. Because the two flexor tendons change their direction at the level of the hook, any contraction of these muscles is likely to generate a laterally directed force against the hook. The "hook of the hamate pull test" is based on using these two tendons to stress the hook of the hamate [43]. The patient's wrist is placed in slight flexion and ulnar deviation. With this, the angulation of the tendons around the hook is maximal. The patient is

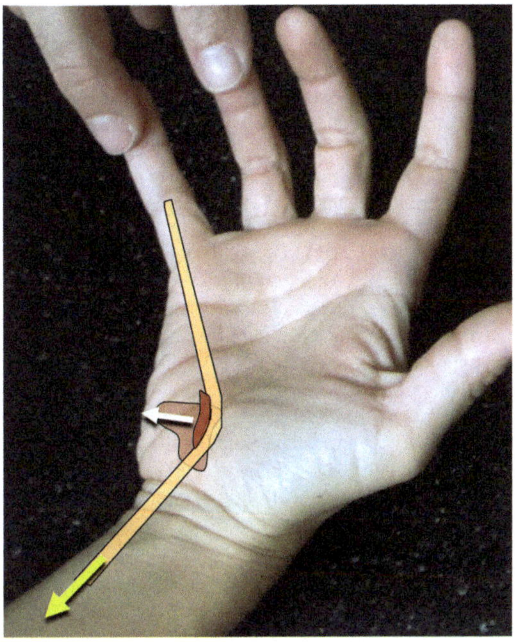

Fig. 3.20 "Hook of the hamate pull test." If there is a non-united fracture of the hook of the hamate, isometric contraction (*yellow arrow*) of the two flexor tendons of the little finger will provoke pain, as a result of the lateral directed vector generated by this tendon compressing the fracture site (*white arrow*)

then asked to contract the little finger against resistance (Fig. 3.20). By doing so, tendon tension increases, producing an ulnar-directed vector against the hook, in an attempt to widen the carpal concavity. Should the hook be fractured or nonunited, localized pain is likely to appear.

The list of provocative maneuvers described above could have been longer. There are numerous ways of provoking pain when there is pathology in the ulnar-sided carpus, but only the more widely utilized have been reviewed. All these provocative maneuvers are useful; most of them are sensitive tests but, unfortunately, poorly specific [21].

Some chronic conditions may cause pain all over the ulnar side of the wrist and may be exacerbated no matter what test is used. In such cases, it is useful to perform the so-called differential lidocaine test [18, 29]. It consists on injecting local anesthesia at the location (joint or tendon sheath) that is suspected to be the problem. If the patient claims significant reduction of pain, the targeted joint most likely is responsible for the patient's discomfort. With the anesthetic injection, not only the wrist is to become less painful but also stronger with better dynamometer readings [4]. Of course, patients who do not find significant relief with this test should have further evaluation of their problem.

References

1. Adams BD, Berger RA (2002) An anatomic reconstruction of the radioulnar ligaments for posttraumatic distal radioulnar joint instability. J Hand Surg Am 27:243–251
2. Ambrose L, Posner M (1992) Lunate-triquetral and midcarpal joint instability. Hand Clin 8:653–668
3. Beckenbaugh RD (1984) Accurate evaluation and management of the painful wrist following injury. Orthop Clin North Am 15:289–306
4. Bell SJ, Hofmeister EP, Moran SL, Shin AY (2007) The diagnostic utility of midcarpal anesthetic injection in the evaluation of chronic wrist pain. Hand 2: 39–45
5. Berger RA, Dobyns JH (1996) Physical examination and provocative maneuvers of the wrist. In: Gilula LA, Yin Y (eds) Imaging of the wrist and hand. WB Saunders, Philadelphia
6. Burkhart SS, Wood MB, Linscheid RL (1982) Posttraumatic recurrent subluxation of the extensor carpi ulnaris tendon. J Hand Surg Am 7:1–3
7. Buck FM, Gheno R, Nico MA et al (2009) Ulnomeniscal homologue of the wrist: correlation of anatomic and MR imaging findings. Radiology 253: 771–779
8. Christodoulou L, Bainbridge LC (1999) Clinical diagnosis of triquetrolunate ligament injuries. J Hand Surg Br 24:598–600
9. Cooney WP, Bishop AT, Linscheid RL (1997) Physical examination of the wrist. In: Cooney WP, Dobyns JH, Linscheid RL (eds) The wrist: diagnosis and operative treatment. Mosby, St. Louis
10. Feinstein WK, Lichtman DM, Nobel PC et al (1999) Quantitative assessment of the midcarpal shift test. J Hand Surg Am 24:977–983
11. Garcia-Elias M (1998) Soft-tissue anatomy and relationships about the distal ulna. Hand Clin 14:165–176
12. Garcia-Elias M (2008) The non-dissociative clunking wrist: a personal view. J Hand Surg Eur 33:698–711
13. Garcia-Elias M, Lluch AL, Ferreres A et al (2008) Transverse loaded prono-supination test. J Hand Surg Eur 33:765–767
14. Gross SC, Watson HK, Strickland JW et al (1989) Triquetral-lunate arthritis secondary to synostosis. J Hand Surg Am 14:95–102
15. Helal B (1978) Racquet player's pisiform. Hand 10:87–90

16. Hertling D, Kessler RM (1990) Management of common musculoskeletal disorders: physical therapy principles and methods. JB Lippincott, Philadelphia
17. Johnson RP, Carrera GF (1986) Chronic capitolunate instability. J Bone Joint Surg Am 68:1164–1175
18. Kalainov DM, Hartigan BJ, Cohen MS (2004) Lunotriquetral instability: clinical findings. Atlas Hand Clin 9:17–24
19. Kleinman WB (2007) Stability of the distal radioulnar joint: biomechanics, pathophysiology, physical diagnosis, and restoration of function; what we have learned in 25 years. J Hand Surg Am 32:1086–1106
20. LaStayo P, Weiss S (2001) The GRIT: a quantitative measure of ulnar impaction syndrome. J Hand Ther 14:173–179
21. LaStayo PC, Howell J (1995) Clinical provocative tests used in evaluating wrist pain: a descriptive study. J Hand Ther 8:10–17
22. Lee M, LaStayo PC (2011) Ulnar wrist pain and impairment: a therapist's algorithmic approach to the triangular fibrocartilage complex. In: Skirven TM, Osterman AL, Fedorczyk J et al (eds) Rehabilitation of the hand and upper extremity, 6th edn. Elsevier, Philadelphia
23. Lester B, Halbrecht J, Levy IM et al (1995) "Press test" for office diagnosis of triangular fibrocartilage complex tears of the wrist. Ann Plast Surg 35:41–45
24. Lichtman DM, Schneider JR, Swafford AR, Mack GR (1981) Ulnar midcarpal instability-clinical and laboratory analysis. J Hand Surg 6:515–523
25. Linscheid RL, Dobyns JH (1985) Athletic injuries of the wrist. Clin Orthop Relat Res 188:141–151
26. Louis DS, Hankin FM, Greene TL et al (1984) Central carpal instability – capitate lunate instability pattern. Diagnosis by dynamic displacement. Orthopedics 7:1693–1696
27. Morrissy RT, Nalebuff EA (1979) Dislocation of the distal radioulnar joint: anatomy and clues to prompt diagnosis. Clin Orthop Relat Res 144:154–158
28. Nakamura R, Horii E, Imaeda T et al (1997) The ulnocarpal stress test in the diagnosis of ulnar-sided wrist pain. J Hand Surg Br 22:719–723
29. Nelson DL (1997) Additional thoughts on the physical examination of the wrist. Hand Clin 13:35–37
30. Nishikawa S, Toh S, Miura H, Arai K (2002) The carpal detachment injury of the triangular fibrocartilage complex. J Hand Surg Br 27:86–89
31. Raskin KB, Beldner S (1998) Clinical examination of the distal ulna and surrounding structures. Hand Clin 14:177–190
32. Reagan DS, Linscheid RL, Dobyns JH (1984) Lunotriquetral sprains. J Hand Surg Am 9:502–514
33. Ruland RT, Hogan CJ (2008) The ECU synergy test: an aid to diagnose ECU tendonitis. J Hand Surg Am 33: 1777–1782
34. Sanz L, Dias R, Heras-Palou C (2009) A modification of the ballottement test in the assessment of the distal radioulnar joint instability. J Bone Joint Surg Br 91(Suppl I):80
35. Schernberg F (1990) Roentgenographic examination of the wrist: a systematic study of the normal, lax and injured wrist. J Hand Surg Br 15:210–228
36. Shaaban H, Giakas G, Bolton M et al (2004) The distal radioulnar joint as a load-bearing mechanism- a biomechanical study. J Hand Surg Am 29:85–95
37. Shin AY, Deitch MA, Sachar K et al (2005) Ulnar-sided wrist pain: diagnosis and treatment. Instr Course Lect 54:115–128
38. Tay SC, Tomita K, Berger RA (2007) The "ulnar fovea sign" for defining ulnar wrist pain: an analysis of sensitivity and specificity. J Hand Surg Am 32:438–444
39. Thurston AJ, Stanley JK (2000) Hamato-lunate impingement: an uncommon cause of ulnar-sided wrist pain. Arthroscopy 16:540–544
40. Topper SM, Wood MB, Ruby LK (1997) Ulnar styloid impaction syndrome. J Hand Surg Am 22:699–704
41. Watson HK, Weinzweig J (1997) Physical examination of the wrist. Hand Clin 13:17–34
42. Weinzweig J, Watson HK (1999) Triquetral impaction ligament tear (TILT). J Hand Surg Br 24:321–324
43. Wright TW, Moser MW, Sahajpal DT (2010) Hook of the hamate pull test. J Hand Surg Am 35:1887–1889
44. Young D, Papp S, Giachino A (2007) Physical examination of the wrist. Orthop Clin North Am 38:149–165
45. Zancolli ER 3rd (2001) Localized medial triquetral-hamate instability: anatomy and operative reconstruction-augmentation. Hand Clin 17:83–96

4 Setup, Surface Anatomy, and Portals

David J. Slutsky

Introduction

Ulnar-sided wrist pain has been the proverbial black box of the wrist. The role of wrist arthroscopy has steadily grown from a mostly diagnostic tool to a valuable adjunctive procedure in the treatment of an expanding list of ulnar-sided wrist disorders. A thorough wrist examination is integral to any arthroscopic assessment; however, although wrist arthroscopy can identify an anatomic abnormality, it cannot be used to differentiate between an asymptomatic degenerative condition vs. a pathologic lesion which is the pain generator.

Indications

The indications for the use of the standard dorsal portals are intertwined with the indications for wrist arthroscopy and are largely dependent upon the indication for surgery since this will vary considerably between arthroscopic fracture reductions as compared to performing a diagnostic procedure for chronic wrist pain. These include variable combinations of the 3–4 portal, the 4–5 portal, the 6 radial (6R), and 6 ulnar (6U) portals. Typically, the 3–4 and 4–5 portals are used interchangeably for visualizing the radiocarpal joint and for instrumentation. The 4–5 portal and the 6R portal are used to access the ulnocarpal joint. The 6U portal is typically used for outflow but can be used for instrumentation. With careful attention to surface landmarks, any portal can be used for viewing or instrumentation, however.

Midcarpal arthroscopy is essential in making the diagnosis of scapholunate and lunotriquetral instability. The grading scale reported by Geissler et al. [10] provides a means for staging the degree of instability in order to provide an algorithm for treatment. Midcarpal arthroscopy is also useful for the assessment and treatment of chondral lesions of the proximal hamate. The triquetrohamate joint can also be accessed through another special use midcarpal portal.

Volar portals for wrist arthroscopy have certain advantages over the standard dorsal portals for visualizing dorsal capsular structures as well as the palmar aspects of the carpal ligaments [14]. The volar radial (VR) portal is relatively easy to use and is an ideal portal for evaluation of the dorsal radiocarpal ligament (DRCL) and the palmar subregion of the scapholunate interosseous ligament (SLIL). It facilitates the identification of and repair of dorsal radiocarpal ligament (DRCL) tears. The VR portal also facilitates arthroscopic reduction of intra-articular fractures of the distal radius fractures by providing a clear view of the dorsal rim fragments.

D.J. Slutsky, M.D.
The Hand and Wrist Institute,
2808 Columbia Street, Torrance, CA 90503, USA

Harbor-UCLA Medical Center,
Torrance, CA, USA
e-mail: d-slutsky@msn.com

F. del Piñal et al. (eds.), *Arthroscopic Management of Ulnar Pain*,
DOI 10.1007/978-3-642-30544-3_4, © Springer-Verlag Berlin Heidelberg 2012

The volar radial midcarpal (VRM) portal may be considered as an occasional accessory portal for visualizing the palmar aspects of the capitate and hamate in cases of avascular necrosis or osteochondral fractures. This portal facilitates visualization of the palmar aspect of the capito-hamate interosseous ligament (CHIL), which is important in minimizing translational motion and has an essential role in providing stability to the transverse carpal arch.

The volar ulnar (VU) portal [15] provides unparalleled views of the dorsal radioulnar ligament and the dorsal ulnar wrist capsule, which contains the extensor carpi ulnaris subsheath (ECUS). Establishing the VU portal is more technically demanding but it has potential use in the arthroscopic diagnosis and treatment of patients with ulnar-sided wrist pain and suspected injuries to the ulnar sling mechanism. It is especially useful for visualizing and debriding palmar tears of the lunotriquetral ligament. It also aids in the repair or debridement of dorsally located tears of the triangular fibrocartilage (TFC) since the proximity of the 4–5 and 6R portals makes triangulation of the instruments difficult.

Two dorsal distal radioulnar (DRUJ) portals have been described [5]. The dorsal DRUJ portals may be used to assess the status of the articular cartilage of the ulnar head and sigmoid notch. This information may be useful in cases of DRUJ instability or when there is the suspicion of early osteoarthritis in which case arthroscopy may differentiate between the need for DRUJ stabilization vs. ulnar head excision/arthroplasty. With inflammatory disorders such as rheumatoid arthritis DRUJ, an arthroscopic synovectomy may obviate the need for a capsular incision. The dorsal DRUJ portals are infrequently used as an adjunct to arthroscopic wafer resections of the ulnar head. The volar aspect of the distal radioulnar joint can be visualized through the VU portal to assess the foveal attachment of the triangular fibrocartilage in cases of suspected peripheral detachment of the TFC.

Contraindications

Contraindications to the use of dorsal or volar portals would include any cause of marked swelling which distorts the topographic anatomy, large capsular tears which might lead to extravasation of irrigation fluid, neurovascular compromise, bleeding disorders, or infection. Unfamiliarity with the regional anatomy is a relative contraindication.

Relevant Anatomy

The standard portals for wrist arthroscopy are mostly dorsal (Fig. 4.1a–d). This is in part due to the relative lack of neurovascular structures on the dorsum of the wrist as well as the initial emphasis on assessing the volar wrist ligaments. The dorsal portals are named in relation to the extensor compartments. One anatomical study determined that branches of the superficial radial nerve (SRN) pass within 3 mm (range 1–6 mm) of the 1–2 portal [1]. The radial artery was found at an average of 3 mm radial to the portal (range 1–5 mm). Either partial or complete overlap of the lateral antebrachial cutaneous nerve (LABCN) with the SRN occurs up to 75 % of the time. Steinberg et al. recommended placing this portal no more than 4.5 mm dorsal to the first extensor compartment and within 4.5 mm of the radial styloid [19]. Branches of the SRN that were radial to the 3–4 portal were located at a mean distance of 16 mm and were generally

Fig. 4.1 *Dorsal portal anatomy*. (**a**) Cadaver dissection of the dorsal aspect of a left wrist demonstrating the relative positions of the dorsoradial portals. *EDC* extensor digitorum communis, *EPL* extensor pollicis longus, *SRN* superficial radial nerve, *MCR* midcarpal radial portal Lister's tubercle=(*). (**b**) Relative positions of the dorsoulnar portals. *EDM* extensor digiti minimi, *DCBUN* dorsal cutaneous branch of the ulnar nerve. *MCU* midcarpal ulnar portal. (**c**) Radial side of the wrist illustration the superficial radial nerve branches relative to the 1–2 portal *APL* abductor pollicus longus, SR1-3 sensory radial nerve branches 1,2,3 (*blue circle*). (**d**) Ulnar view highlighting the triquetrohamate (*T-H*) and *6U* portal and surrounding structures. *ECU* extensor carpi ulnaris, *DCBUN* dorsal cutaneous branch of ulnar nerve, *FCU* flexor carpi ulnaris, *UN* ulnar nerve (© David Slutsky 2012 – All Rights Reserved)

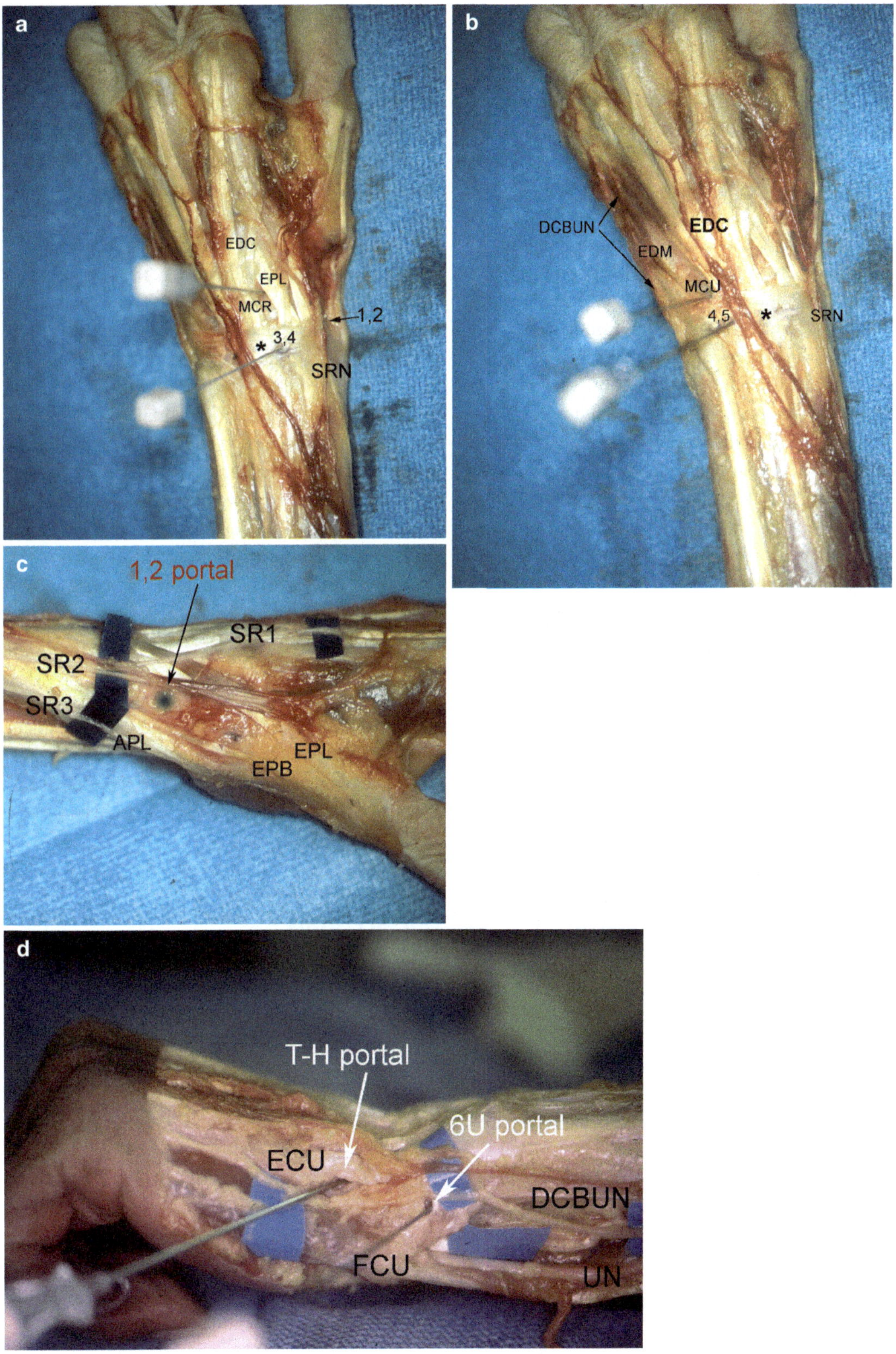
a
EDC
EPL
MCR
1,2
3,4
*
SRN
b
DCBUN
EDC
EDM
MCU
4,5
*
SRN
c
1,2 portal
SR1
SR2
SR3
APL
EPB
EPL
d
T-H portal
6U portal
ECU
DCBUN
FCU
UN

remote from the 4–5 portal. Branches of the SRN were found radial to the midcarpal radial portal at a mean of 7.2 mm. The dorsal cutaneous branch of the ulnar nerve (DCBUN) passes within 2.5 mm of the 6R portal and 17.5 mm from the dorsal distal radioulnar portal.

In an anatomic study performed by the author, a volar radial (VR) portal was established by introducing a blunt trochar through the floor of the flexor carpi radialis (FCR) tendon sheath at the level of the proximal wrist crease. The trochar was noted to enter the radiocarpal joint between the radioscaphocapitate ligament and the long radiolunate ligament in 4 of 5 specimens. The palmar cutaneous branch was closest in proximity but always lay to the ulnar side of the FCR. The palmar radiocarpal arch, which corresponds to the distal border of the pronator quadratus, was at least 1 cm proximal to the portal. There was a safe zone comprising the width of the flexor carpi radialis (FCR) tendon plus at least 3 mm or more in all directions at the level of the proximal wrist crease, that was free of any neurovascular structures [13, 14]. In a companion study, a volar ulnar (VU) portal was made by making a 2-cm incision in the proximal wrist crease overlying the ulnar edge of the finger flexor tendons. The ulnar styloid marked the proximal point of the VU portal, approximately 2 cm distal to the pronator quadratus. The portal was in the same sagittal plane as the ECU subsheath and penetrated the ulnolunate ligament (ULL) adjacent to the radial insertion of the triangular fibrocartilage. The ulnar nerve and artery were generally more than 5 mm from the trochar, provided the capsular entry point was deep to the ulnar edge of the profundus tendons. The palmar cutaneous branch of the ulnar nerve (nerve of Henlé) was highly variable and not present in every specimen. This inconstant branch provides sensory fibers to the skin in the distal ulnar and volar part of the forearm to a level 3 cm distal to the wrist crease. Its territory may extend radially beyond the palmaris longus tendon. There is no true internervous plane due to the presence of multiple ulnar-based cutaneous nerves to the palm, which puts them at risk with any ulnar incision; hence, careful dissection and wound spread technique should be observed.

Methodology

The patient is positioned supine under general anesthesia with the arm abducted under tourniquet control. A 2.7-mm 30°-angled scope along with a camera attachment is used along with some method of overhead traction. The structures that should be visualized as a part of a standard exam include the radius articular surface, the proximal scaphoid and lunate, the volar carpal ligaments, the scapholunate (SLIL) and lunotriquetral (LTIL) interosseous ligaments, and the triangular fibrocartilaginous complex (TFCC). In the patient with wrist pain, the scope is inserted in the 3–4 portal followed by various combinations of the 4–5 portal and 6R portal. The 6U portal is mostly used for outflow but it may be used for instrumentation when debriding palmar LTIL tears. Midcarpal arthroscopy is performed to assess the stability of the intercarpal ligaments and to inspect for chondral lesions or loose bodies in the midcarpal joint. When there is a history of radial-sided pain, the VR portal can be used to visualize the palmar SLIL and the dorsal radiocarpal ligament (DRCL). If the patient has ulnar-sided wrist pain, the VU portal can be established to assess the palmar LTIL and dorsal radioulnar ligament (DRUL), the extensor carpi ulnaris (ECU) subsheath, and radial TFCC attachment. The dorsal and volar DRUJ portals are used in suspected cases of a foveal TFCC detachment.

Dorsal Portals

3–4 Portal

The surgeon is initially seated facing the dorsal surface of the wrist. The concavity overlying the lunate between the EPL (extensor pollicis longus) and the extensor digitorum communis (EDC) is located just distal to Lister's tubercle, in line with the second webspace. The radiocarpal joint is identified with a 22-gauge needle that is sloped 10° palmar to account for the volar inclination of the radius. The joint is injected with 5 cc of saline. A shallow skin incision is made to avoid injuring small branches of the SRN or superficial veins. Tenotomy scissors or blunt forceps are then used to spread the soft tissue and pierce the dorsal capsule. This technique is repeated for each portal. The vascular tuft of the radioscapholunate ligament (RSL) is directly in line with this portal. Superior to the RSL is the membranous portion of the SLIL. The insertion of the dorsal capsular attachment can often be visualized by rotating the scope dorsally while looking ulnarward. The radioscapholunate (RSL) and long radiolunate ligaments (LRL) are radial to the portal and can be probed with a hook in the 4–5 portal. The LTIL, TFCC, ulnolunate (ULL), and ulnotriquetral (ULT) ligaments are ulnar to the portal.

4–5 Portal

The interval for the 4–5 portal is identified with a 22-gauge needle inserted between the extensor digitorum communis (EDC) tendons and the extensor digiti minimi (EDM), in line with the ring metacarpal. Due to the normal radial inclination of the distal radius, this portal lies slightly proximal and about 1 cm ulnar to the 3–4 portal. Views of the ulnar half of the lunate are obtained by moving the scope radially, whereas the triquetrum is seen by angling the scope in a superior and ulnar direction. The LTIL is often difficult to differentiate from the carpal bones without probing. The ULL and ULT can be seen on the far end of the joint. Proximally, the radial insertion of the TFCC blends imperceptibly with the sigmoid notch of the radius, but it can be palpated with a hook probe in either the 3–4 or 6R portal. The peripheral insertion of the TFCC slopes upward into the ulnar capsule. The volar and dorsal radioulnar ligaments can be probed for laxity/tears but they are not seen as distinct structures seen since they blend with the TFCC. The pisotriquetral orifice (PTO) is just distal and anterior to the prestyloid recess and is found within the substance of the ULT just anterior to the proximal articular surface of the triquetrum (Fig. 4.2).

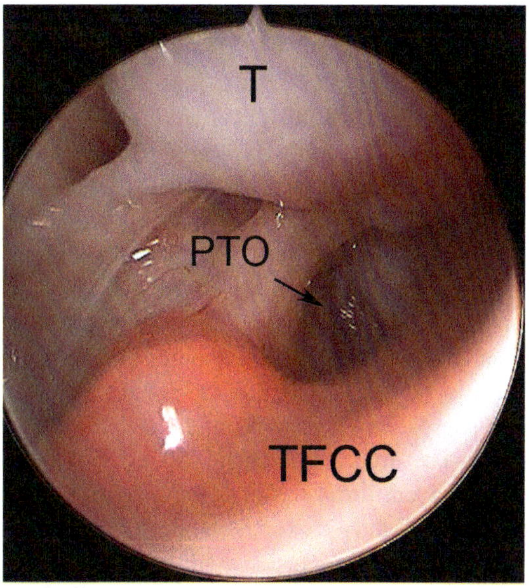

Fig. 4.2 *Pisotriquetral orifice*. View of the pisotriquetral orifice (*PTO*) (*arrow*) from the 6R portal. *T* triquetrum, *TFCC* triangular fibrocartilaginous complex (© David Slutsky 2012 – All Rights Reserved)

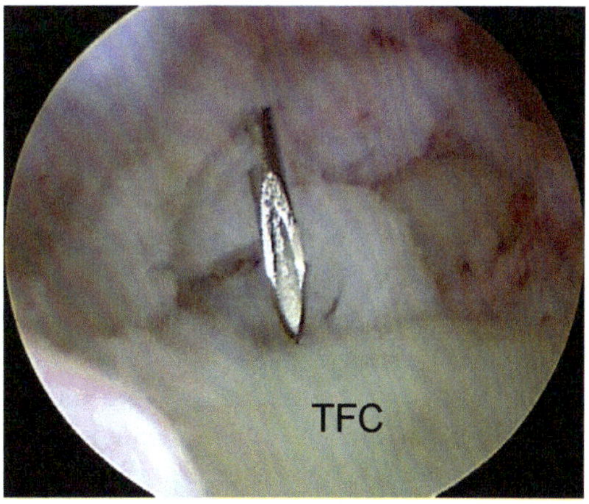

Fig. 4.3 View from the 3–4 portal of a needle in the accessory 6 R portal. *TFC* triangular fibrocartilage (© David Slutsky 2012 – All Rights Reserved)

6R and 6U Portals

The 6R portal is identified on the radial side of the ECU tendon, just distal to the ulnar head. The scope should be angled 10° proximally to avoid hitting the triquetrum. The TFCC is immediately below the entry site. The LTIL is located radially and superiorly, whereas the ulnar capsule is immediately adjacent to the scope. The 6U portal is located ulnar to the ECU tendon. This portal can be used to view the dorsal rim of the TFCC or for instrumentation when debriding the palmar LTIL. Geissler has recently described an accessory 6R portal that is made approximately 1.5 cm distally in line with the traditional 6R portal [9]. He uses it for an all-arthroscopic knotless foveal reattachment of the TFCC using a push lock anchor. This portal is located with an 18-gauge needle inserted through the skin and aimed at the fovea of the ulnar head (Fig. 4.3).

Midcarpal Portals

Dorsal Midcarpal Portals

The midcarpal radial (MCR) portal is found 1 cm distal to the 3–4 portal. The scaphotrapezial-trapezoidal (STT) joint lies radially and can be seen by rotating the scope dorsally. The scapholunate (SL) articulation which is proximal to this portal can be probed for instability or step-off. By moving the scope in an ulnar direction, the lunotriquetral (LT) articulation comes into view. Superiorly, the proximal surface of the capitate, the interosseous ligament, and the hamate are seen. The midcarpal ulnar (MCU) portal is located 1 cm distal to the 4–5 portal or 1.5 cm ulnar and slightly proximal to the MCR portal, in line with the ring metacarpal axis. Normally, there is very little step-off between the distal articular surfaces. When there is any doubt, the traction should be released and the SL joint should be viewed with the scope in the MCU, whereas the LT joint should be viewed with the scope in the MCR.

Triquetro-Hamate (TH) Portal

This portal was originally described by Viegas et al. [21]. It enters the midcarpal joint at the level of the triquetro-hamate joint ulnar to the ECU tendon. The entry site is both ulnar and distal to the MCU. It is also approximately 1 cm distal to the accessory 6R portal described previously and provides access to the triquetro-hamate joint. It is useful for proximal hamate resection when there is OA of the proximal pole and for arthroscopic-guided internal fixation of displaced intra-articular fractures of the triquetrum (Fig. 4.4a, b). It can also be used for outflow. Branches of the DCBUN are most at risk.

Scaphotrapezial Portals

STT-U Portal

Bowers and Whipple have described a scaphotrapezial joint (STT-U) portal (Fig. 4.5a) which they used to facilitate arthroscopic resections of the distal scaphoid with scaphotrapezial osteoarthritis [5]. They used this portal in conjunction with the MCR for evaluation and treatment of disorders of the STT joint. The STT-U portal is located in line with the midshaft axis of the index metacarpal, just ulnar to the EPL. Entry into this portal requires traction on the index finger. Leaving the EPL to the radial side of the STT portal protects the radial artery in the snuffbox from injury. The portal is also useful for arthroscopic-guided fixation and bone grafting of scaphoid nonunions [22].

STT-R Portal

A radial portal for STT arthroscopy (STT-R) has been reported [6]. This portal is radial to the abductor pollicus longus (APL) tendon at the level of the STT joint (Fig. 4.5b). Access to the joint is facilitated by use of a 1.9-mm 30°-angled arthroscope. Cadaver dissections demonstrated that maintaining a position palmar and radial to the APL tendon at the STT joint level avoids the radial artery by a mean of 8.8 mm (range 6–10 mm). The angle between the two portals is 130° which facilitates triangulation of the instrumentation. As with the 1–2 portal, branches of the superficial radial nerve virtually surround the arthroscopic field; hence, blunt dissection of the capsule and knowledge of the regional anatomy is essential.

STT-P Portal

Baré and coworkers also described another accessory palmar portal (STT-P) based on a dissection of ten cadaver arms [4]. They identified a safe portal of entry that was midway between the radial styloid and the base of the first metacarpal, 3 mm ulnar to the APL tendon and 6 mm radial to the scaphoid tubercle (Fig. 4.4b). The trocar is inserted into the STT joint aiming toward the base of the fifth metacarpal while holding the thumb in extension and adduction. This portal lays 7.6 mm (5–11 mm) from the radial artery, 6.5 mm (4–11 mm) from the superficial branch of the radial artery, and 11.6 mm (3–20 mm) from the closest radial sensory nerve branch. Ashwood et al. used a portal that was radial to the EPL tendon (STT-R) along with the RMC for arthroscopic debridement of isolated STT OA [2]. They recommended a 1.5-cm skin incision to enable safe blunt dissection.

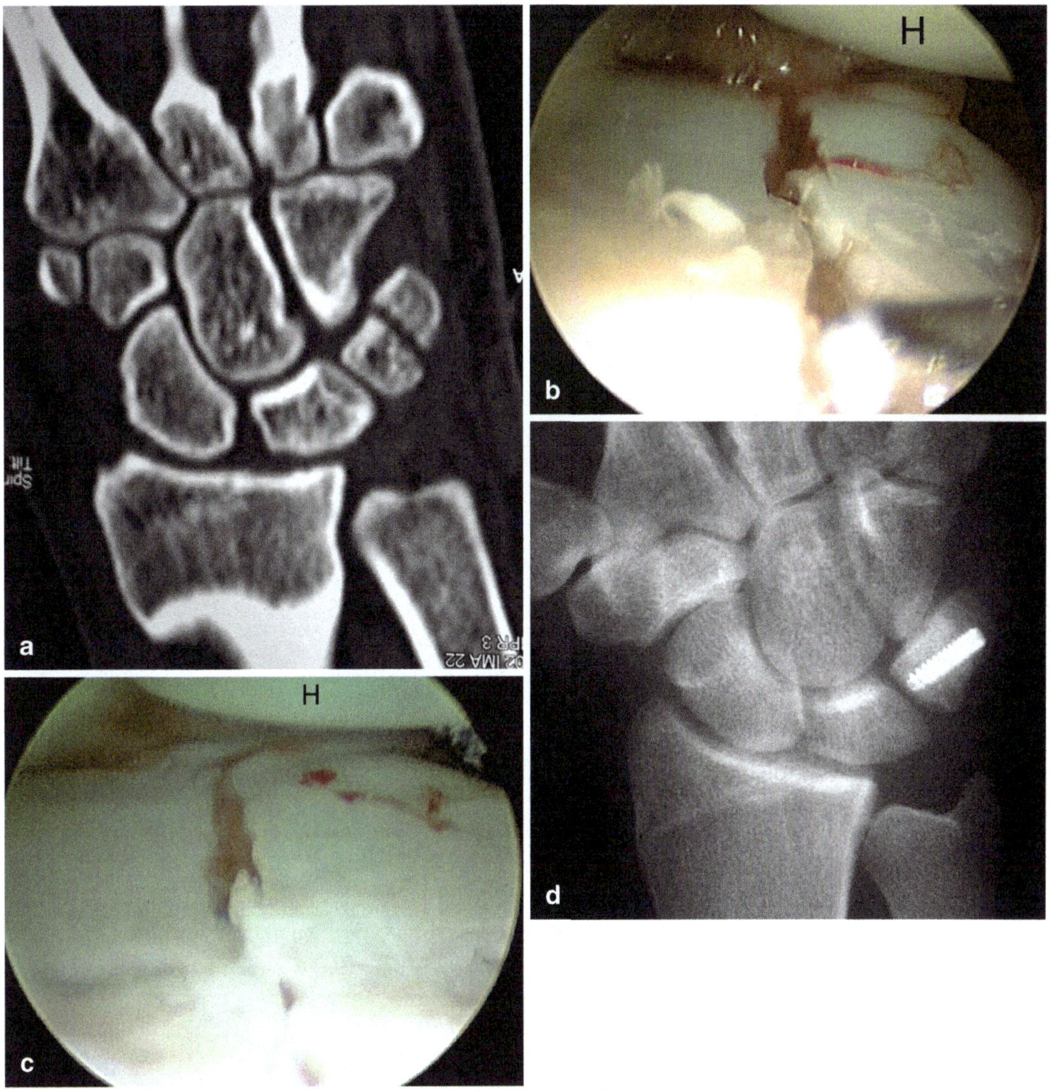

Fig. 4.4 Triquetro-hamate portal. (**a**) CT scan of a displaced intra-articular fracture of the triquetrum. (**b**) View of the articular surface from the T-H portal. *H* hamate. (**c**) Following reduction and percutaneous screw fixation. (**d**) Final x-ray appearance (© David Slutsky 2012 – All Rights Reserved)

Volar Portals

Volar Radial Portal

To establish the VR radial portal, the surgeon is seated facing the volar aspect of the wrist. A 2-cm transverse or longitudinal incision is made in the proximal wrist crease overlying the flexor carpi radialis (FCR) tendon (Fig. 4.6). It is not necessary to specifically identify the adjacent neurovascular structures, provided that the anatomical landmarks are adhered to. The tendon sheath is divided, and the FCR tendon is retracted ulnarly. The radiocarpal joint space is identified with a 22-gauge needle and distended with 5 cc of saline. Tenotomy scissors or forceps are used to pierce the volar capsule. A blunt obturator and trocar are then introduced followed by the arthroscope. The midcarpal joint can be accessed through the same skin incision by angling the trocar 1 cm distally and approximately 5° ulnarward. A hook probe

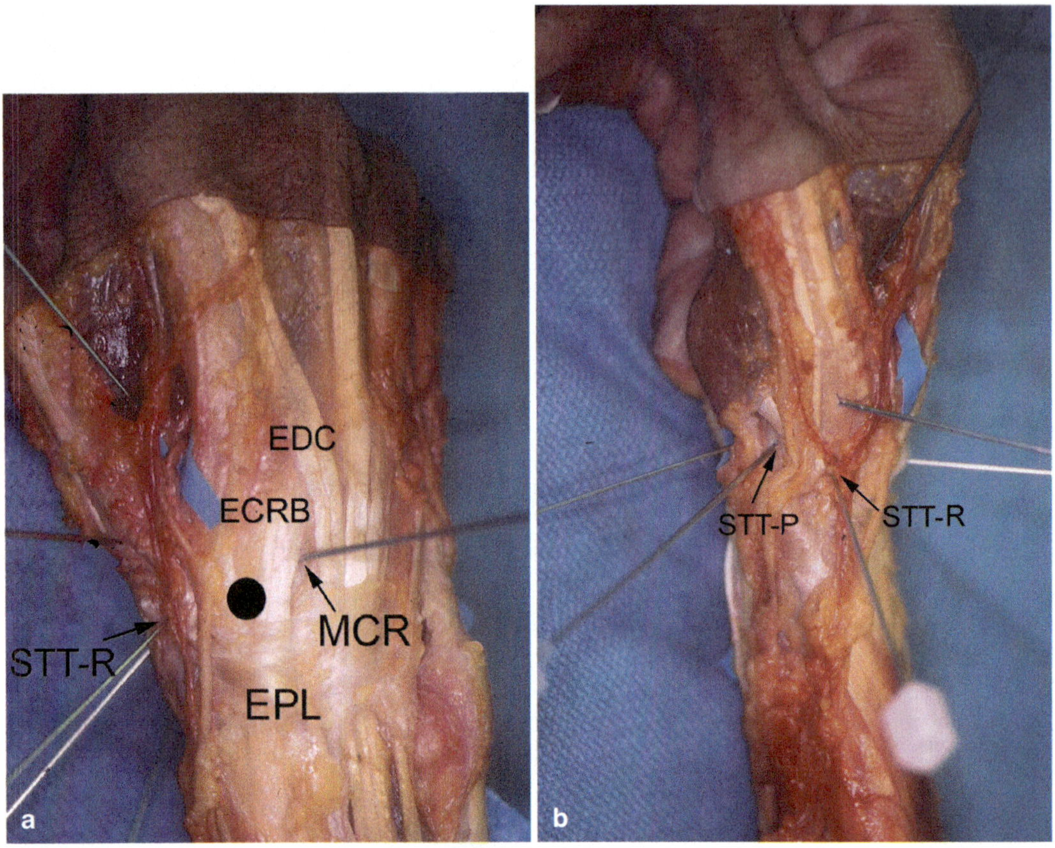

Fig. 4.5 *Scaphotrapezial portals*. (**a**) Relative position of the STT-U portal (*black circle*) in relation to the dorsal wrist tendons. *EDC* extensor digitorum communis, *EPL* extensor pollicis longus, *ECRB* extensor carpi radialis brevis *MCR* midcarpal radial portal. (**b**) Radial side of the wrist showing relative position of the STT-P portal (© David Slutsky 2012 – All Rights Reserved)

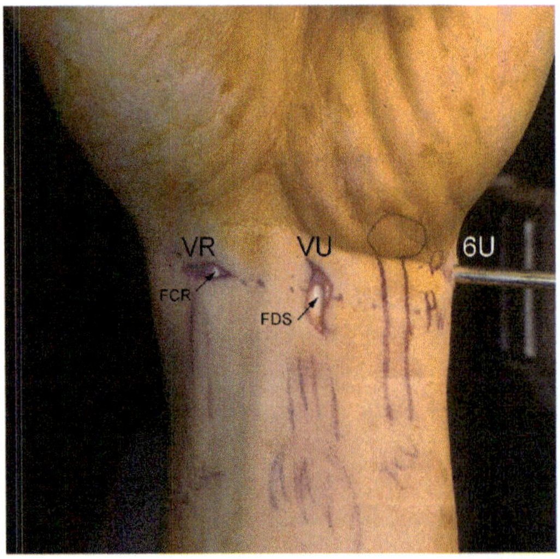

Fig. 4.6 Surface anatomy for the volar portals showing the VR and VU portals. *FCR* flexor carpi radialis, *FDS* flexor digitorum superficialis (© David Slutsky 2012 – All Rights Reserved)

is inserted through the 3–4 portal, and it is used to assess the palmar aspect of the SLIL and the DRCL. A useful landmark when viewing from the VR portal is the intersulcal ridge between the scaphoid and lunate fossae. The origin of the DRCL is seen immediately ulnar to this ridge, just proximal to the lunate.

Volar Radial Midcarpal (VRM) Portal

The volar aspect of the midcarpal joint is identified with a 22-gauge needle through the same skin incision, and a blunt trochar is inserted. It is necessary to angle the trochar in a distal and ulnar direction (approximately 5°) in order to access the midcarpal joint through the same skin incision. The trochar passes deep to the superficial palmar branch of the radial artery, which courses more superficially over the scaphoid tuberosity at this level. The distance between the volar radiocarpal and volar midcarpal entry sites averages 11 mm (7–12 mm).

Volar Ulnar Portal

The volar ulnar portal is established via a 2-cm longitudinal incision centered over the proximal wrist crease along the ulnar edge of the finger flexor tendons. The tendons are retracted to the radial side, and the radiocarpal joint space is identified with a 22-gauge needle. Blunt tenotomy scissors or forceps are used to pierce the volar capsule, followed by insertion of a 2.7-mm 30° arthroscope. The ulnar nerve is protected by use of the cannula and a more radial entry site. The median nerve is protected by the interposed flexor tendons. The palmar region of the LTIL can usually be seen slightly distal and radial to the portal. A hook probe is inserted through the 6R or 6U portal.

Author's Experience

The volar radial portal has been used in over 100 patients since 1998. Additional pathology that could not be seen from a dorsal portal is often present and included avulsion of the radioscapholunate ligament, palmar tears of the SLIL, and DRCL tears [18].

The midcarpal joint was accessed from the volar radial portal in three cases. In one patient with Preiser's disease, the use of the volar radial midcarpal portal (VRM) allowed a more complete assessment of the distal articular surface of the scaphoid. Another patient had an unrecognized osteochondral fracture of the capitate head following a perilunate dislocation. The VRM portal admirably demonstrated the intact dorsal portion of the SLIL in the patient with the palmar tear. Using the dorsal midcarpal portals, one patient was found to have a chondral defect that was seen on the proximal hamate along with a midcarpal loose body.

DRUJ Arthroscopy

Anatomical and biomechanical studies have highlighted the importance of the deep attachment of the TFCC for maintaining stability of the distal radioulnar joint (DRUJ). The functional consequence of incompetent foveal fibers is DRUJ instability. In the absence of a quantifiable objective definition, however, the determination of DRUJ instability is largely dependent upon a subjective interpretation of the physical findings.

The standard arthroscopic assessment of the TFCC does not allow one to definitively determine if the deep fibers are indeed intact, and establishing the diagnosis of a foveal detachment remains an exacting challenge even for the experienced arthroscopist. Ruch first described the hook test as a means to test the foveal insertion of the TFCC during the arthroscopic treatment of distal radius fractures wherein if the TFCC can be pulled upward and radially, this is indicative of a foveal detachment [12]. Similarly, Tay et al. [20] as well as Atzei and coworkers [3] have written that if one can drag the TFCC dorsally with an arthroscopic hook probe, then that is indicative of a foveal detachment. In both methods, however, one must ultimately perform a DRUJ capsulotomy to directly observe the foveal fibers in order to definitively make the diagnosis.

Relevant Anatomy

TFCC Anatomy

The triangular fibrocartilaginous complex has been well described. It consists of the articular disc, the meniscus homologue, the palmar (PRUL) and dorsal radioulnar ligaments (DRUL), the ECUS, the ulnar capsule, and the ulnolunate and ulnotriquetral ligaments. The PRUL and DRUL contain a superficial and a deep portion which are conjoined at the radius attachment. The superficial portion surrounds the articular disc but has no clear definable insertion into the ulnar styloid. The fibers of the deep portion of the DRUL and the PRUL interdigitate to form a conjoined tendon as they converge toward their insertion into the fovea at the base of the ulnar styloid. The foveal insertion has a greater effect on stability than the styloid insertion. Recent work suggests that DRUJ instability may be caused by ulnar detachment. The ligamentum subcruentum is an inconstant region of vascularized connective tissue which lies between the foveal attachment and the ulnar styloid but by itself provides little mechanical support.

When viewed in the axial plane, the ulnar styloid lies relatively dorsally on the end of the ulnar head. The DRUL drapes over the dorsal aspect of the ulnar head as it converges toward the fovea. These factors limit the field of view and make it difficult to insert anything larger than a 1.9-mm scope through a dorsal DRUJ portal. There is more room on the volar ulnar aspect of the DRUJ for insertion of an arthroscope with relatively unimpeded views of the proximal articular disc and the foveal attachments. The dorsal DRUJ portals remain useful, however, for outflow and for instrumentation.

Surgical Technique

Volar Distal Radioulnar (VDRU) Portal

The topographical landmarks and establishment of the VDRU portal are identical to those of the VU portal. The capsular entry point lies 5–10 mm proximally (Fig. 4.7a, b). The VDRU portal is accessed through the VU skin incision. A 1.9-mm small joint arthroscope can be used since gaining access to the DRUJ can be difficult, especially in a small wrist but I have found that a standard 2.7-mm scope provides a better field of view. The ulnocarpal joint is first identified as described above. It is useful to leave a needle or cannula in the ulnocarpal joint for reference during this step. The DRUJ is then located by angling a 22-gauge needle 45° proximally and then injecting the DRUJ with saline. Alternatively, the skin incision can be extended proximally for 1 cm so that it lies at the same level as the VDRU capsular entry point. Once the correct plane is identified, the volar DRUJ capsule is pierced with tenotomy scissors followed by a cannula with a blunt trocar and then the arthroscope. Alternatively, a probe can be placed in the distal dorsal radioulnar joint portal and advanced through the palmar incision to help locate the joint space. It can then be used as a switching stick over which the cannula is introduced. Initially, the DRUJ space appears quite confined, but over the course of 3–5 min, the fluid irrigation expands the joint space, which improves visibility. A burr or thermal probe can be substituted for the 3-mm hook probe through the dorsal DRUJ portal as necessary.

Atzei et al. described a direct foveal portal [3]. This portal is 1 cm proximal to the 6U portal (Fig. 4.8). The scope is inserted with the wrist in full supination since the ulnar styloid and the ECU tendon displace dorsally and the fovea and the ulnar-most area of the distal ulna become subcutaneous.

Dorsal DRUJ Portals

The dorsal radioulnar joint can be accessed through a proximal and distal portal (Fig. 4.8a, b). The proximal portal (PDRUJ) is located in the axilla of the joint, just proximal to the sigmoid notch and the flare of the ulnar metaphysis. This portal is easier to penetrate and should be used initially to prevent chondral injury from insertion of the trochar. The forearm is held in supination to relax the dorsal capsule and to move the ulnar head volarly. This also lifts the central disc distally from the head of the ulna. Reducing the traction to 1–2 lb permits better views between the ulna and the sigmoid

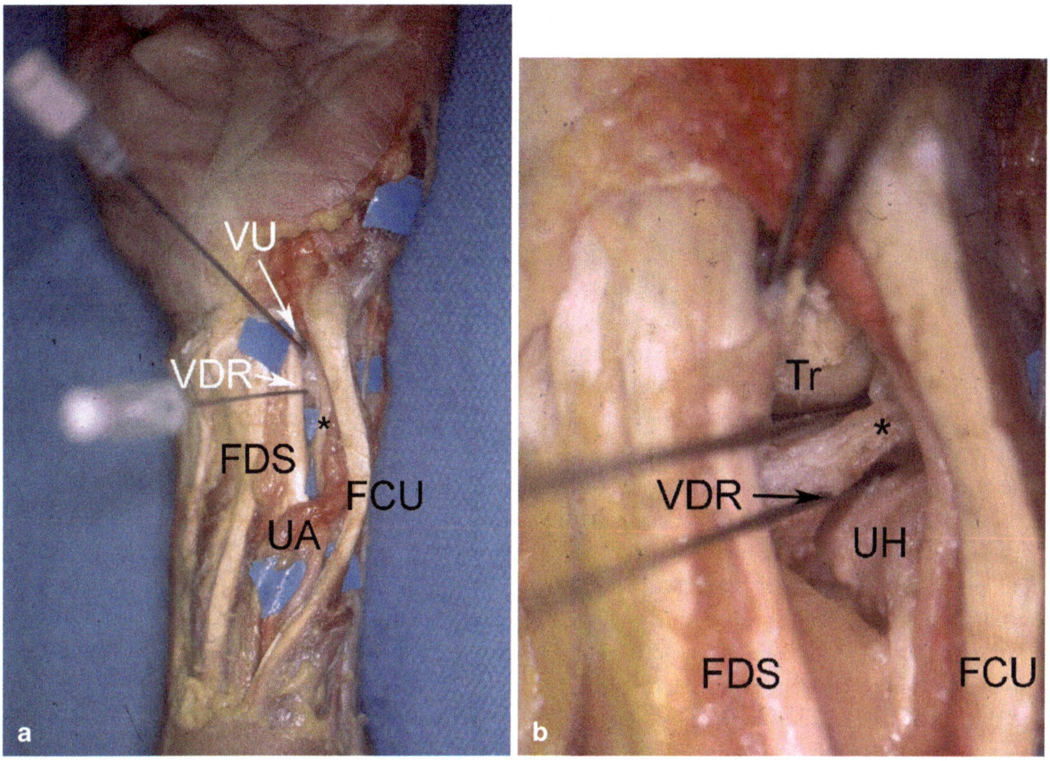

Fig. 4.7 *VDRU portal*. (**a**) Relative positions of the VU and VDRU portals. *FDS* flexor digitorum sublimis, *FCU* flexor carpi ulnaris *UA* ulnar artery, * ulnar nerve. (**b**) Close-up view of the VDRU portal. Note the foveal attachment of the deep fibers (*) of the palmar radioulnar ligament (*PRUL*). *UH* ulnar head, *Tr* triquetrum (© David Slutsky 2012 – All Rights Reserved)

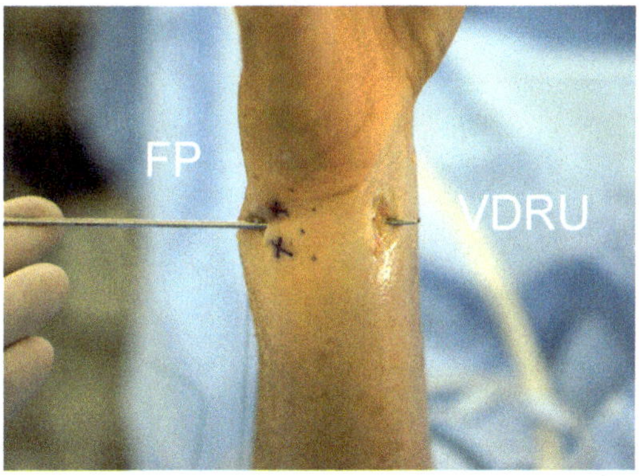

Fig. 4.8 Relative positions of the foveal portal (*FP*) and the *VDRU* portal (© David Slutsky 2012 – All Rights Reserved)

notch by reducing the compressive force caused by axial traction. The joint space is identified by first inserting a 22-gauge needle horizontally at the neck of the distal ulna. Fluoroscopy facilitates the needle placement. The joint is infiltrated with saline, and the capsule is spread with tenotomy scissors through a small incision. A small cannula and trochar for the 1.9-mm scope are introduced followed by insertion of a 1.9-mm 30°-angled scope. Entry into this portal provides views of the proximal sigmoid notch cartilage and the articular surface of the neck of the ulna. One should systematically look for loose bodies or synovial hypertrophy.

The distal portal (DDRUJ) is identified 6–8 mm distally with the 22-gauge needle and just proximal to the 6R portal. This portal can be used for outflow drainage or for instrumentation. It lies on top of the ulnar head but underneath the TFCC; hence, it cannot be used in the presence of a positive ulnar variance. The TFCC has the least tension in neutral rotation of the forearm which is the optimal position for visualizing the articular dome of the ulnar head, the undersurface of the TFCC, and the foveal insertion of the PRUL. Because of the dorsal entry of the arthroscope, the course of the dorsal radioulnar ligament is not visible until its attachment into the fovea is encountered (Fig. 4.9).

Author's Experience

The volar ulnar portal has been used in 68 patients since 1998. The volar aspect of the distal radioulnar joint was accessed in 14 of these patients to rule out a tear of the deep foveal attachment of the TFCC [16]. A preoperative MRI in each patient could not definitively determine whether the foveal fibers were indeed intact. The foveal attachment of the TFC was seen to be intact in 8 out of14 patients and directly contributed to the decision making as to the type of surgical treatment (Fig. 4.10a). In two patients, the attachment was poorly seen due to foveal scarring from an associated peripheral TFCC tear and the DRUJ portal was not helpful. In two cases, the TFCC and the foveal fibers were intact but the radioulnar ligaments were attenuated. These patients were treated with an open dorsal radioulnar imbrication and a tendon graft reconstruction of the DRUJ. In two patients, the foveal fibers were clearly torn or absent (Fig. 4.10b). These patients were treated with a tendon graft reconstruction of the DRUJ and a foveal reattachment of the TFCC.

Arthroscopy of the 4th/5th Carpometacarpal Joints

Arthroscopy of the first carpometacarpal (CMC) joint has become routine. The literature contains multiple reports of arthroscopic treatment of trapeziometacarpal OA and arthroscopic-guided percutaneous pin fixation of Bennett's fractures. The same techniques can be applied to articular disorders of the fourth and fifth CMC joints. Arthroscopy is especially useful in fracture dislocations involving the fifth CMC since the articular fracture fragment is often volar and difficult to visualize and reduce from a dorsal approach [16, 17].

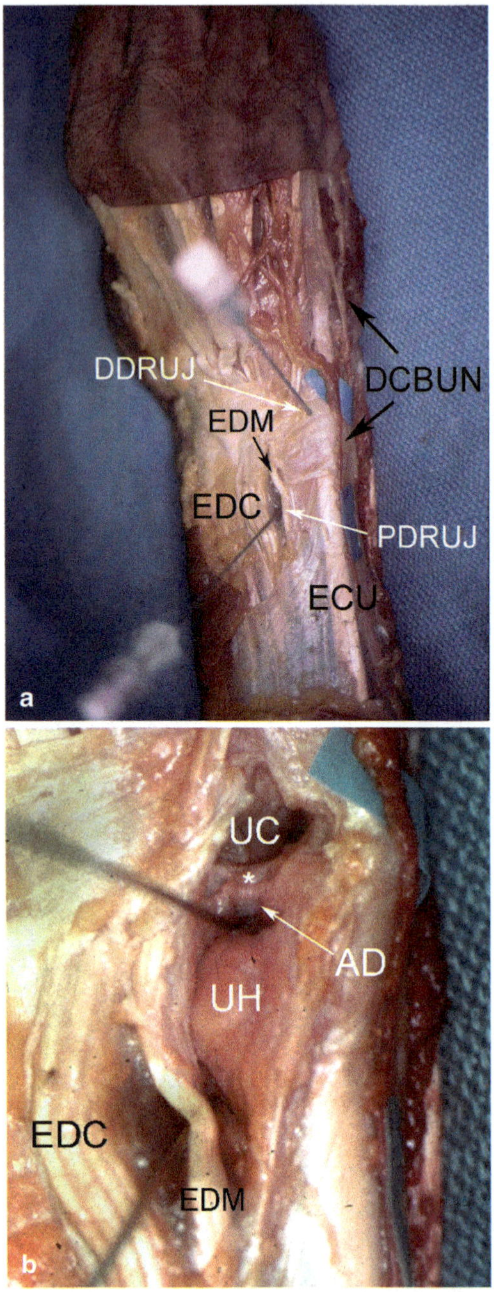

Fig. 4.9 *Dorsal DRUJ portals*. (**a**) Relative positions of the proximal (PDUJ – circle 1) and distal (DDRUJ – circle 2) portals in relation to the dorsal cutaneous branch of the ulnar nerve (*) *EDC* extensor digitorum communis, *DCBUN* dorsal cutaneous branch of the ulnar nerve, *PDRUJ* proximal distal radioulnar joint. (**b**) Close-up view of the portals with a needle in the ulnocarpal joint and dorsal DRUJ. *DRUL* dorsal radioulnar ligament, *UH* ulnar head, *EDM* extensor digiti minimi, *ECU* extensor carpi ulnaris *EDC* extensor digitorum communis, *AD* articular disc, *UC* ulnocarpal joint (© David Slutsky 2012 – All Rights Reserved)

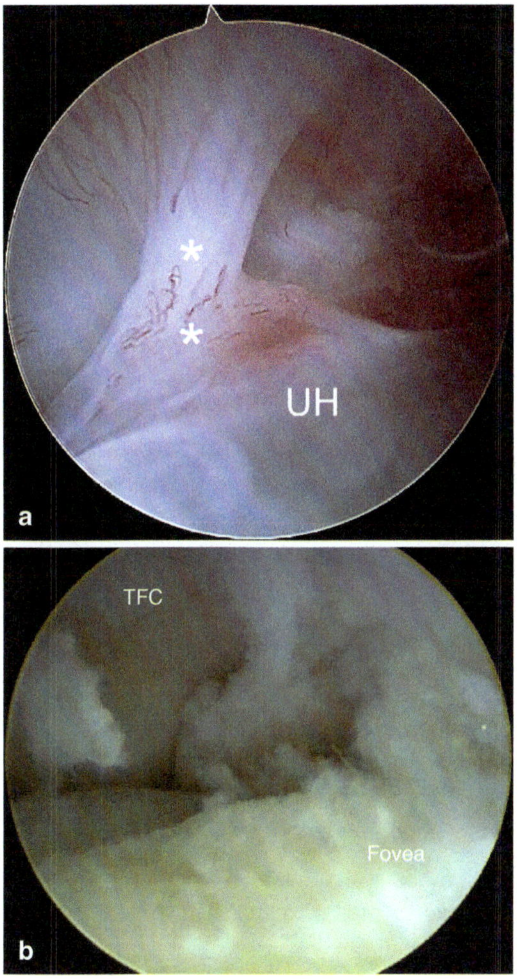

Fig. 4.10 *View from the VDRU portal.* (**a**) The foveal attachment (*) can be seen inserting on the ulnar head (*UH*). (**b**) There is an absence of the foveal fibers. *TFC* undersurface of triangular fibrocartilage (© David Slutsky 2012 – All Rights Reserved)

Relevant Anatomy

Nakamura et al. studied 80 cadaver arms and described the carpometacarpal joint detail [11]. Two distinct dorsal ligaments were identified that attached to the dorsal aspect of the fifth metacarpal (MC). One of these extended from the ulnar base of the fifth metacarpal to the hamate (fifth MC ulnar side base to hamate ligament) and the other from the radial base of the fifth metacarpal to the hamate and sometimes to the fourth metacarpal ulnar base (fourth MC ulnar side base to fifth MC radial side base ligament). There was an intermetacarpal ligament that attached the radial base of the fifth metacarpal to the ulnar base of the fourth metacarpal. There was one volar ligament that attached to the fifth MC base and extended either to the hook of the hamate or to the ulnar base of the fourth MC. There were no intra-articular ligaments except for one ligament which was located between the 3rd/4th MC and the capitate/hamate.

Dzwierzynski et al. also studied the intermetacarpal ligament anatomy [8]. They noted that the alignment of the interosseous ligaments between the fourth and fifth metacarpals differed from the ligament alignment between the second to third and third to fourth metacarpals, which allows a greater degree of motion in the fifth CMC joint (approximately 25° of flexion/extension) as compared to the fourth CMC joint (approximately 15°). They also observed that when these metacarpals flex at the CMC joints, as in grasping, the dorsal interosseous ligament tightens and the anterior interosseous ligament relaxes. When the metacarpals extend at the CMC joints, the anterior ligament tightens and the posterior ligament relaxes, which retains a rigid interconnection between the bones.

Equipment and Implants

In general, a 2.7-mm 30°-angled scope along with a camera attachment is used although a 1.9-mm scope can be substituted. A 3-mm hook probe is needed for palpation of intracarpal structures. At least 10–15 lb of traction is crucial to the success of the procedure, either with a traction tower or some other type of overhead traction. A motorized 2.9-mm full radius resector is needed for debridement of hematoma as well as small curettes and a dental hook for manipulation of the fracture fragments. A 2.9-mm arthroscopic burr is needed for any bony resection. Intraoperative fluoroscopy is often used.

Surgical Technique

The patient is positioned supine on the operating table with the arm extended on a hand table. The small and ring fingers are suspended by Chinese

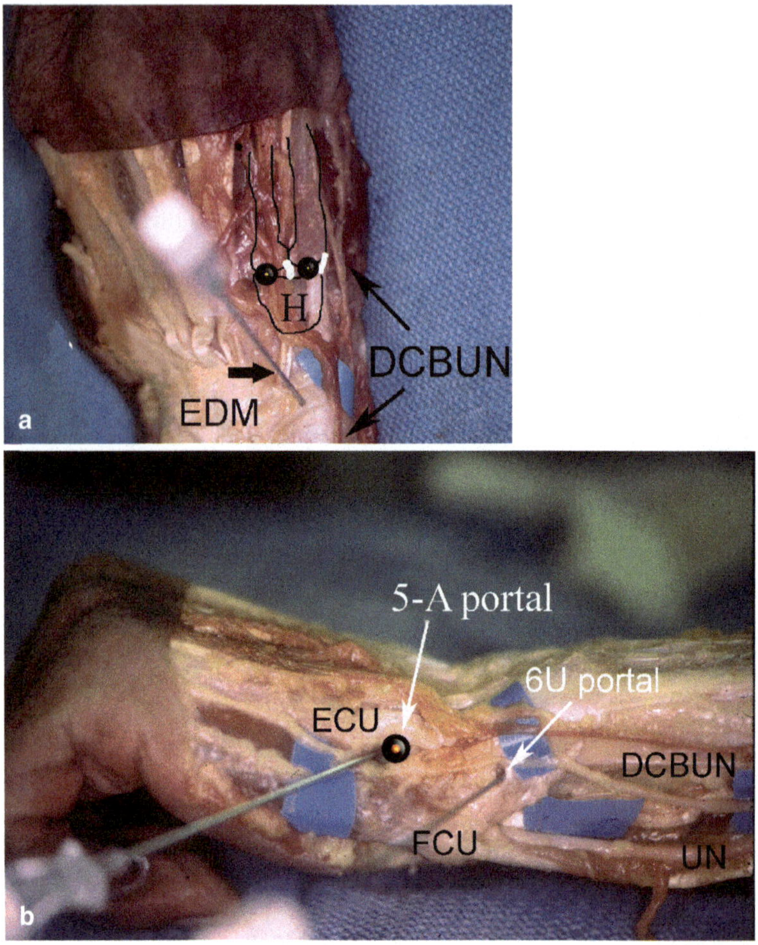

Fig. 4.11 *CMC portals*. (**a**) Cadaver dissection demonstrating the position of the two dorsal arthroscopy portals at the base of the fourth and fifth metacarpal bases (*radio buttons*) in relation to the metacarpo-hamate ligaments (*in white*). *EDM* extensor digiti minimi, *DCBUN* dorsal cutaneous branch of the ulnar nerve, *H* hamate. (**b**) Lateral view demonstrating the relative position of the 5-A (accessory) portal which is located at the level of the fifth CMC joint, volar to the extensor carpi ulnaris (*ECU*). *UN* ulnar nerve, *FCU* flexor carpi ulnaris (© David Slutsky 2012 – All Rights Reserved)

finger traps with 10–15 lb of countertraction. The relevant landmarks are outlined including the proximal and dorsal edge of the fifth metacarpal base, the extensor carpi ulnaris (ECU) tendon, and, if possible, the extensor tendons to the small and ring fingers. The procedure is performed with a tourniquet elevated to 250 mmHg. It is my preference to use a dry technique with intermittent saline irrigation through the scope using a 10-cc syringe and suction using the full radius resector, akin to the technique described by Del Piñal for wrist arthroscopy [7]. Two main portals are used (Fig. 4.11a, b). There is an ulnar portal or 5th metacarpo-hamate portal (5-MH) which is located between the 5th MC ulnar side base—Hamate ligament and the extensor digiti quinti tendon, at the level of CMC joint. The radial portal, or the 4th metacarpo-hamate portal (4-MH) is just radial to the 4th MC ulnar side base—Hamate ligament, just radial to the extensor tendon to the ring finger. Each joint is localized with a 22-gauge needle followed by injection of 2 cc of saline. This step may be facilitated by fluoroscopy. A small transverse skin incision is made followed by wound spread technique with tenotomy scissors. The capsule is pierced and a cannula and blunt trocar are inserted, followed by the arthroscope. The portals are interchangeably used to systematically inspect the joint, which is facilitated by judicious use of a 2.9-mm resector. An accessory portal (5-A) can facilitate triangulation and is located along the ulnar base of the fifth metacarpal just dorsal to the hypothenar muscles and approximately 1 cm distal to the 6U wrist arthroscopy portal. Although the skin incision may be similar to the T-H portal, the capsular entry point is distal to it since it provides access to the distal articular surface

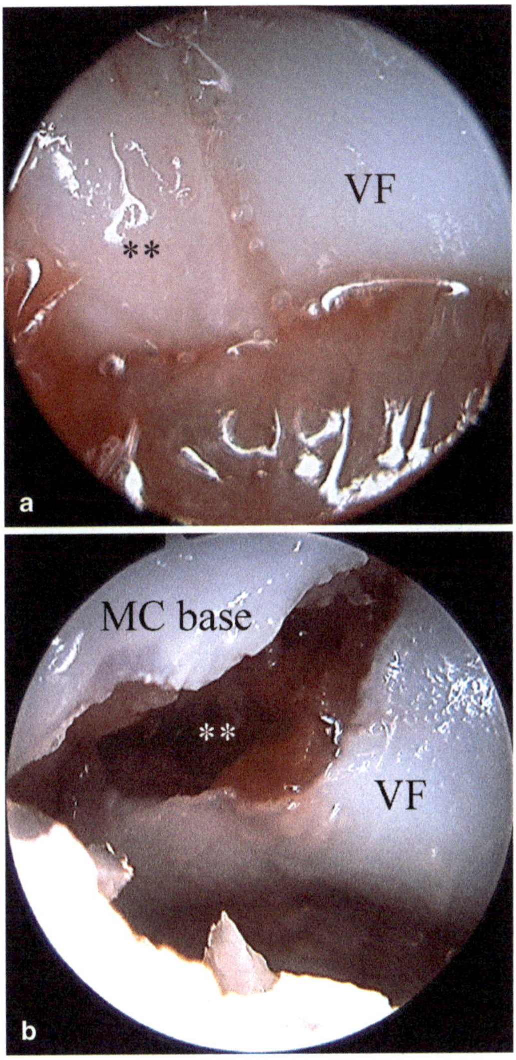

Fig. 4.12 *Fracture dislocation of fifth metacarpal base.* (**a**) View of the volar articular fragment (*VF*) of the fifth metacarpal base with the arthroscope in the 4-MH portal demonstrating the attached intermetacarpal ligament (*). (**b**) The fracture gap (*) is visualized by angling the scope dorsally and distally. *MC base* dorsal metacarpal base (© David Slutsky 2012 – All Rights Reserved)

of the hamate whereas the T-H portal provides access to the proximal hamate surface. Excellent views of the fourth and fifth metacarpal base and the attached volar intercarpal ligament can be obtained (Fig. 4.12a, b). There is no internervous plain and injury to the dorsal cutaneous branch of the ulnar nerve is a risk with all of these portals; hence, careful wound spread technique is mandatory.

References

1. Abrams RA, Petersen M et al (1994) Arthroscopic portals of the wrist: an anatomic study. J Hand Surg Am 19(6):940–944
2. Ashwood N, Bain GI et al (2003) Results of arthroscopic debridement for isolated scaphotrapeziotrapezoid arthritis. J Hand Surg Am 28(5):729–732
3. Atzei A, Rizzo A et al (2008) Arthroscopic foveal repair of triangular fibrocartilage complex peripheral lesion with distal radioulnar joint instability. Tech Hand Up Extrem Surg 12(4):226–235
4. Bare J, Graham AJ et al (2003) Scaphotrapezial joint arthroscopy: a palmar portal. J Hand Surg Am 28(4):605–609
5. Bowers WH, Whipple T (1991) Arthroscopic anatomy of the wrist. In: McGinty J (ed) Operative arthroscopy. Raven, New York, pp 613–623
6. Carro LP, Golano P et al (2003) The radial portal for scaphotrapeziotrapezoid arthroscopy. Arthroscopy 19(5):547–553
7. del Piñal F (2008) Dry arthroscopy of the wrist: its role in the management of articular distal radius fractures. Scand J Surg 97(4):298–304
8. Dzwierzynski WW, Matloub HS et al (1997) Anatomy of the intermetacarpal ligaments of the carpometacarpal joints of the fingers. J Hand Surg Am 22(5):931–934
9. Geissler WB (2011) Arthroscopic knotless peripheral ulnar-sided TFCC repair. Hand Clin 27(3):273–279
10. Geissler WB, Freeland AE et al (1996) Intracarpal soft-tissue lesions associated with an intra-articular fracture of the distal end of the radius. J Bone Joint Surg Am 78(3):357–365
11. Nakamura K, Patterson RM et al (2001) The ligament and skeletal anatomy of the second through fifth carpometacarpal joints and adjacent structures. J Hand Surg Am 26(6):1016–1029
12. Ruch DS, Vallee J et al (2004) Arthroscopic reduction versus fluoroscopic reduction in the management of intra-articular distal radius fractures. Arthroscopy 20(3):225–230
13. Slutsky DJ (2002) Volar portals in wrist arthroscopy. J Am Soc Surg Hand 2(4):225–232
14. Slutsky DJ (2002) Wrist arthroscopy through a volar radial portal. Arthroscopy 18(6):624–630
15. Slutsky DJ (2004) The use of a volar ulnar portal in wrist arthroscopy. Arthroscopy 20(2):158–163
16. Slutsky DJ (2011) Arthroscopic evaluation of the foveal attachment of the triangular fibrocartilage. Hand Clin 27(3):255–261
17. Slutsky DJ (2011) Arthroscopic reduction and percutaneous fixation of fifth carpometacarpal fracture dislocations. Hand Clin 27(3):361–367
18. Slutsky DJ, Nagle DJ (2008) Wrist arthroscopy: current concepts. J Hand Surg Am 33(7):1228–1244
19. Steinberg BD, Plancher KD et al (1995) Percutaneous kirschner wire fixation through the snuff box: an anatomic study. J Hand Surg Am 20(1):57–62

20. Tay SC, Tomita K et al (2007) The "ulnar fovea sign" for defining ulnar wrist pain: an analysis of sensitivity and specificity. J Hand Surg Am 32(4):438–444
21. Viegas SF (1994) Midcarpal arthroscopy: anatomy and portals. Hand Clin 10(4):577–587
22. Wong WY, Ho PC (2011) Minimal invasive management of scaphoid fractures: from fresh to non-union. Hand Clin 27(3):291–307

Ulnar Imaging for Arthroscopic Surgeons

5

Luis Cerezal and Faustino Abascal

Introduction

Ulnar wrist pain is a common and frequently disabling complaint that may be caused by a broad spectrum of osseous or soft tissue disorders. In an adequate clinical setting, conventional radiographic findings of anatomic variants or pathologic conditions of the ulnar wrist can suggest the diagnosis of a given entity. However, diagnosis remains difficult and often delayed because symptoms and clinical findings are usually nonspecific and similar among the different pathologic conditions in the ulnar wrist; moreover, significant disease and incapacitating pain may be present despite minimal evidence at conventional radiography.

Imaging evaluation in the ulnar-sided wrist disorders represents a major diagnostic challenge because of the complex anatomy and the small size of individual structures. Recent advances in noninvasive imaging techniques such as ultrasound, computed tomography (CT), and magnetic resonance (MR) have increased our diagnostic capabilities.

This chapter reviews the usefulness of imaging techniques in the evaluation of ulnar-sided wrist pain.

L. Cerezal (✉) • F. Abascal
Department of Radiology,
Diagnóstico Médico Cantabria (DMC),
Castilla 6-Bajo, 39002 Santander, Spain
e-mail: lcerezal@gmail.com

Imaging Methods

Radiography

For optimal evaluation of wrist pathology, standardized positioning and high-quality radiographs must be obtained (Fig. 5.1). The radiographic protocol in patients with ulnar-sided wrist pain always includes the acquisition of posteroanterior and lateral views. However, these views may not be sufficient, as superimposed bone may hide pathology [8, 48]. Therefore, in some cases, additional views are necessary for a more precise evaluation of ulnar-sided wrist injuries. The semisupinated oblique view highlights the pisiform bone and the pisotriquetral joint and shows the palmar portion of the hook of the hamate, and the semipronated oblique view allows evaluation of the dorsal ulnar wrist. The carpal tunnel view is useful to visualize the hook of hamate and possible pisotriquetral pathology. The lateral radiographic view with the hand radially deviated and the thumb abducted provides good depiction of fractures of the entire hook of the hamate, including the base [8].

Ultrasound

There is a wide spectrum of ultrasound equipments, from high level machines with all kinds of advanced applications to portable ones, specially designed for small offices, interventional or anesthetic procedures.

F. del Piñal et al. (eds.), *Arthroscopic Management of Ulnar Pain*,
DOI 10.1007/978-3-642-30544-3_5, © Springer-Verlag Berlin Heidelberg 2012

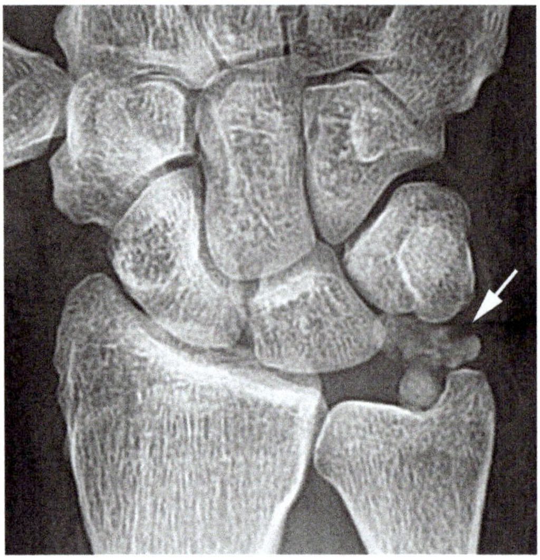

Fig. 5.1 Synovial osteochondromatosis. PA radiograph shows several nodular calcifications on the ulnar side of the wrist (*arrow*). No erosions could be identified radiographically

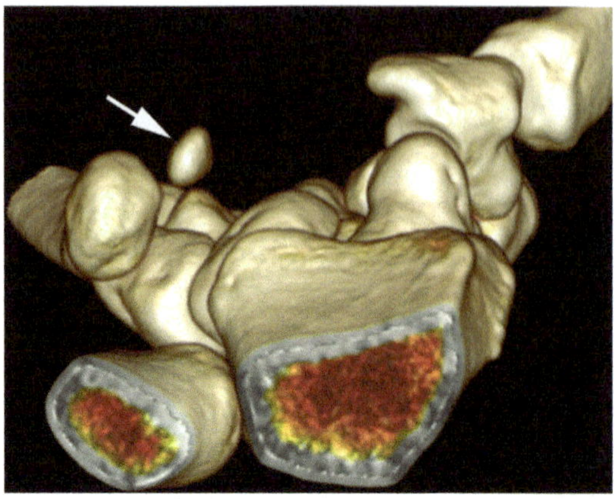

Fig. 5.2 Os hamuli proprium. 3D MDCT image shows an os hamuli proprium (*arrow*), unfused secondary ossification center of hook of hamate

Known advantages of ultrasound are its dynamic and real-time assessment, the facility to perform bilateral comparative study, and to analyze a long segment of the extremity, and Doppler imaging [6].

Ultrasound is the imaging technique of choice in tendinous injuries and neuropathies of the wrist and hand. The dynamic capabilities and high spatial resolution (higher than MR imaging) allow to identify the full spectrum of tendinous pathology, including instability (e.g., extensor carpi ulnaris tendon) [40]. This pathology is usually misdiagnosed in static studies like MR imaging. Ultrasound reveals nerve shape changes and possible extrinsic space-occupying lesions that may cause nerve compression within the tunnels [6].

The main disadvantage of this method is that it has important limitations in the evaluation of the TFCC injuries and ligaments [48].

Computed Tomography

CT is one of the imaging techniques with most important evolution in recent years. Multidetector helicoidal technology with a progressive increase of detectors allows obtaining an isotropic or volumetric image, which means that multiplanar reconstruction in each of the axes has the same resolution. Multidetector CT (MDCT) offers several diagnostic tools like multiplanar reconstructions (MPR), curved MPR, and 3D volume reformation (Fig. 5.2) [8, 26, 30]. MDCT studies (64 and higher) allow performing dynamic studies (4D studies, which mean 3D reformations in movement) flexo-extension, ulnar to radial deviation, forceful pronation clenched fist, or any other forceful position.

MDCT is especially useful in detecting or excluding occult fractures, the precise evaluation of fractures, [26, 48], the assessment of fracture consolidation (Fig. 5.3), evaluation of carpal dislocations and vascularized bone grafts, as well as malrotation of the radius and ulna [2]. CT allows performing a high-resolution angiography for an accurate and quick assessment of vascular injuries [8].

MR Imaging

There is a wide spectrum of MR equipments, from low-field magnets (0.2–0.35) to high-field magnets (1.5–3 T). Low-field magnets have an open bore that is friendly for the patients, but the images are of low quality, and usually not valid for an accurate diagnosis of most wrist and hand injuries. High-field MR imaging is required to

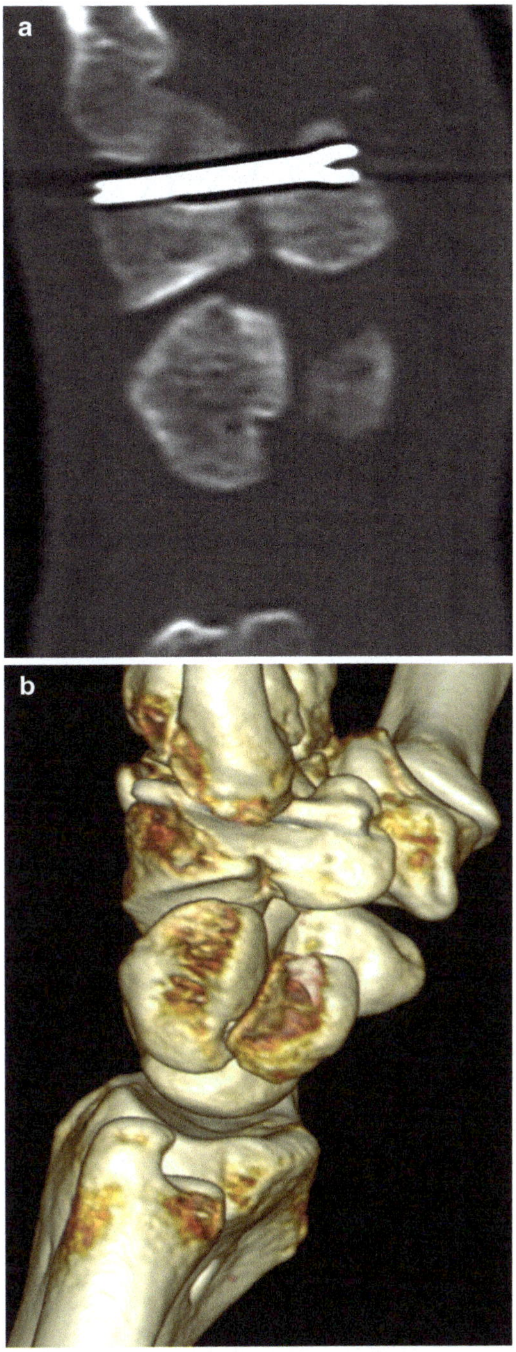

Fig. 5.3 (a, b) Sagittal reformatted and 3D MDCT images of a fracture of the hook of the hamate treated with screw osteosynthesis. Note the malplacement of the screw into the carpometacarpal joint

obtain high-resolution MR imaging, essential to evaluate normal and abnormal features of the hand and wrist. Recent studies demonstrate that 3 T MR improves diagnostic capability compared with 1.5 T MR related to injury to the TFCC and wrist ligaments [3].

In the near future, there will be ultrahigh-field magnets, 7 T and higher, now under investigation. The potential main advantage of 7 T will be the improvement of functional MR imaging to detect biochemical changes (loss of glycosaminoglycans) in cartilage damage and in the evaluation of cartilage repair techniques.

In general terms, MR imaging is the most valuable imaging tool in the diagnosis of injuries of the ulnar wrist. However, MR imaging has important limitations in two of the most common wrist pathology groups, like ulnar-sided TFCC tears (Palmer class 1B lesions) [25] and wrist instability.

CT Arthrography and MR Arthrography

CT arthrography and MR arthrography are especially useful for evaluating TFCC as well as wrist ligaments, solving the main limitations of the conventional MR imaging [7, 17, 19].

Palmer class 1B lesion is one of the principal indications of MR arthrography that can precisely detect partial and complete tears of the ulnar attachment of the TFC. Partial foveal injuries without communication with radiocarpal compartment are a challenging diagnosis. This type of injury is frequently misdiagnosed on conventional MR and in radiocarpal MR arthrography. Partial noncommunicating tears affecting the foveal ulnar attachment can be adequately diagnosed with distal radioulnar joint MR arthrography [37].

Recent advances in wrist arthroscopy, like recent del Piñal's works [20], have shown that there often exist TFCC injuries not included in the Palmer's classification. Usually, these lesions are not diagnosed on MR. MR arthrography can adequately evaluate these non-Palmer TFC complex injuries such as capsular detachments of the TFCC and carpal detachment or Nishikawa lesion [32]. MR arthrography gives a precise evaluation of intrinsic and extrinsic ligaments, allowing a proper diagnosis of early stage of carpal instability (predynamic form) with a better therapeutic outcome.

CT arthrography is an alternative to the MR arthrography in the evaluation of TFCC and ligament injuries [19].

Dynamic volume CT arthrography combines the advantages of the static CT arthrography, identifying anatomic structures, with the dynamic information of the wrist. CT arthrography dynamic study (4D MDCT) is the imaging technique of choice in the evaluation of wrist instability.

Differential Diagnosis

Intra-Articular Injuries

Triangular Fibrocartilage Complex (TFCC) Injuries

Injuries of the TFCC are a well-recognized cause of ulnar wrist pain.

Palmer devised a classification system to guide treatment of TFCC tears [34]. The main division is between traumatic (class I) and degenerative (class II) tears.

Traumatic Tears of TFCC

Traumatic injuries are subdivided into four types based on the site of injury (Fig. 5.4): Class IA (avascular disc central slit) (Figs. 5.5 and 5.6), class IB (tear of the ulnar insertion of TFCC) (Figs. 5.7, 5.8, and 5.9), class IC (avulsion of the ulnotriquetral and ulnolunate ligaments from the carpal attachment), and class ID (radial avulsion) (Fig. 5.10). Class IB and ID injuries have been recently subdivided according to the different structures that can be detached from the ulnar or radial insertion of the TFCC and its relationship to DRUJ instability [4, 31, 47]. Based in recent arthroscopic advances in knowledge, the complex myriad of injuries included as Palmer class IB has been described by del Piñal as a "constellation" of ligamentous, osseous, and capsular damage (Fig. 5.7 and

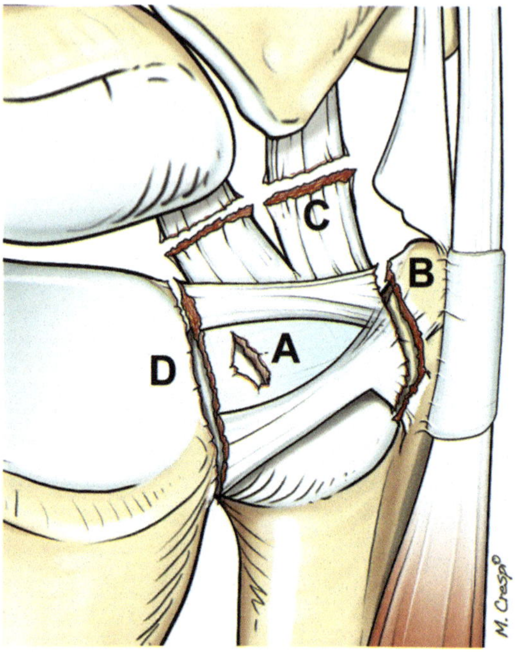

Fig. 5.4 Diagram illustrates the different types of TFCC Palmer class I injuries. Class IA, central slit. Class IB, ulnar tear. Class IC, ulnocarpal ligaments rupture. Class ID, radial tear

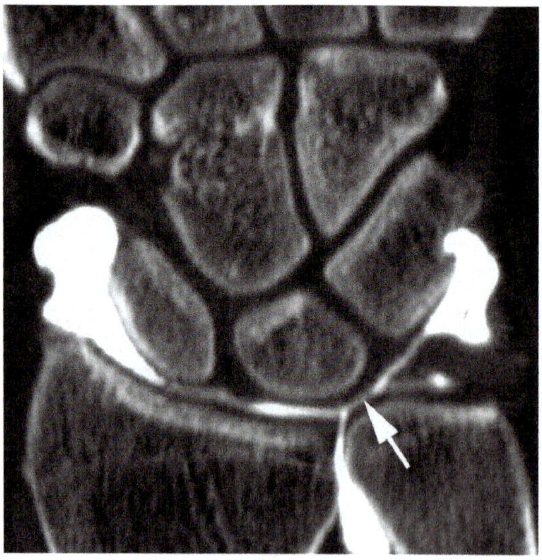

Fig. 5.5 Coronal CT arthrography image shows a Palmer class IA traumatic tear of the TFC (*arrow*)

Chap. 6). The variable combination of injuries of the TFCC ulnar insertion included partial

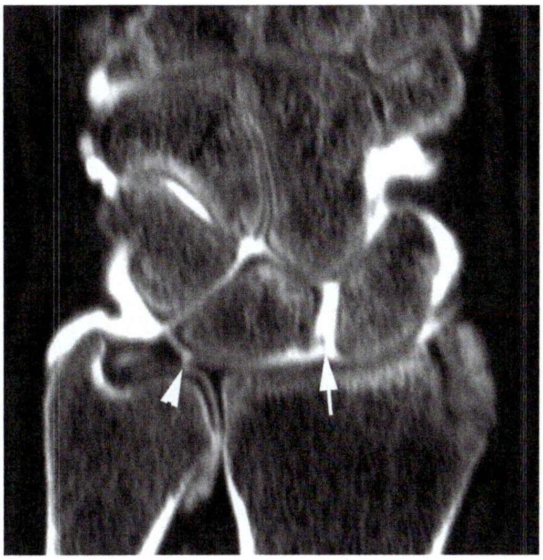

Fig. 5.6 Coronal CT arthrography image reveals a distal radius fracture associated with a complete scapholunate ligament tear (*arrow*) and Palmer class IA lesion (*arrowhead*)

tears (noncommunicating tears) affecting the foveal insertion (proximal lamina) [4, 5, 29, 39] (Figs. 5.7b and 5.8) or styloid insertion (distal lamina) of the TFCC (Fig. 5.7a) and complete tear of the ulnar insertion (Fig. 5.7c). Each of these injuries could be associated with US fracture (Fig. 5.7d, 5.7e, and 5.7f) and ligamentous injuries of the ulnar side of the wrist [5, 29, 39]. Peripheral partial noncommunicating tears with only styloid insertion involvement are not associated with DRUJ instability; nevertheless, in foveal noncommunicating detachment of TFCC, DRUJ instability is expected.

The connection from the hyaline cartilage of the radius to the TFC indicates a rather weaker connection than the peripheral ligament–bone connection. The radial tears of the TFCC include fibrocartilage central tear and dorsal or palmar radioulnar ligament tears (these tears could be associated to dorsal and palmar radial

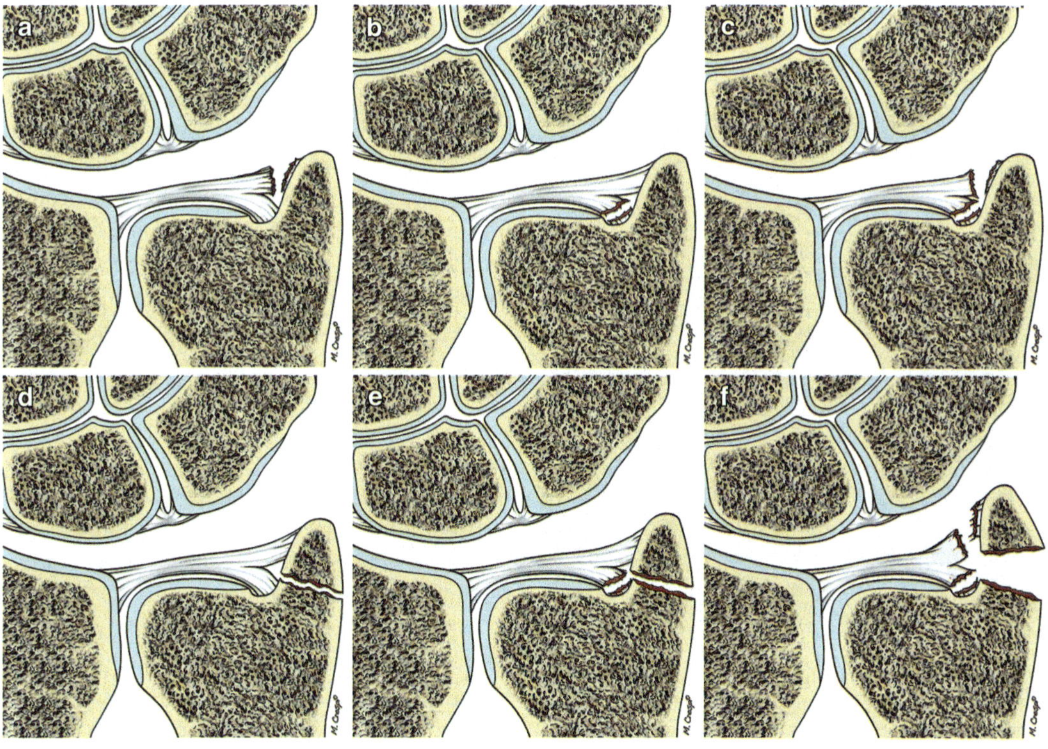

Fig. 5.7 There are a wide constellation of type 1B injuries. (**a**) Styloid insertion (distal lamina). (**b**) Foveal insertion (proximal lamina). (**c**) Complete ulnar insertion detachment. (**d**) US fracture with styloid insertion tear. (**e**) US fracture with foveal insertion tear. (**f**) US fracture with complete ulnar insertion detachment

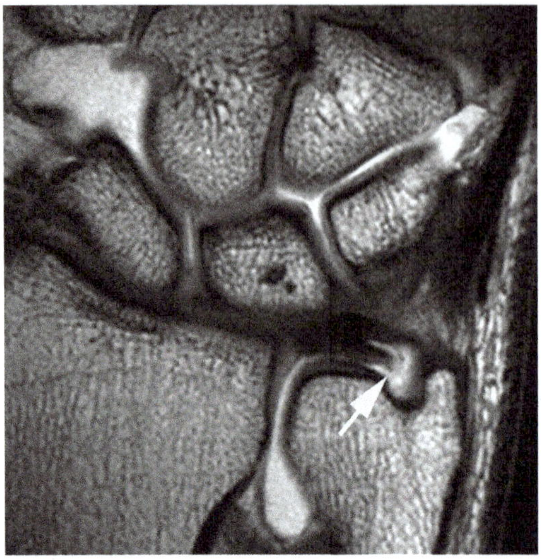

Fig. 5.8 Palmer class IB foveal tear (noncommunicating tear) in a patient with moderate DRUJ instability at clinical examination. Coronal T1-weighted DRUJ and midcarpal MR arthrogram image reveal a foveal tear (*arrow*) of the TFC and intact styloid insertion (*arrowhead*) without communication between DRUJ and radiocarpal compartments

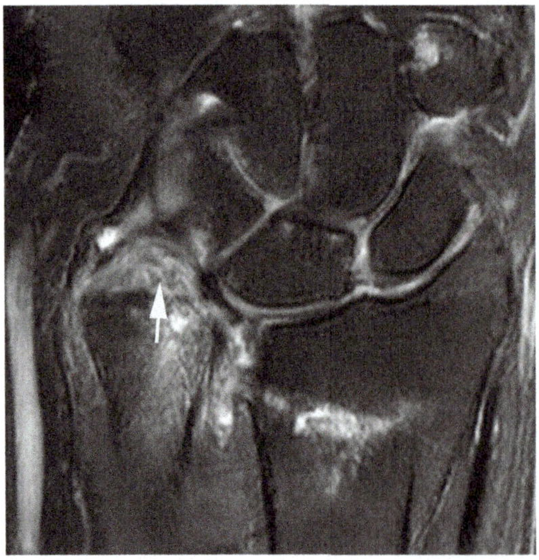

Fig. 5.9 Palmer class IB complete tear of the TFCC in a patient with severe DRUJ instability at clinical examination. Coronal proton density fat-suppressed MR image reveals a complete ulnar detachment of the TFCC (*arrow*). Note the secondary ulnocarpal synovitis

rim fractures, respectively); the latter two injuries may induce DRUJ instability [31, 47].

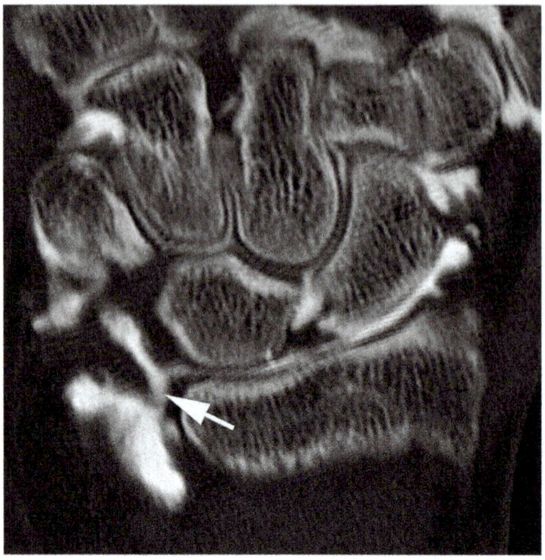

Fig. 5.10 Palmer class ID lesion in a patient with ulnar wrist pain and severe radioulnar joint instability. CT arthrogram image shows a radial detachment of the volar radioulnar ligament (*arrow*)

Palmer class IA and IB lesions are by far the most common types of TFC injuries. Class 1D injuries are much less frequent, and class 1C injuries are exceptional. Moreover, we must take into account the existence of traumatic TFCC lesions not included in the Palmer's classification (Fig. 5.11), as volar or dorsal radioulnar ligaments detachment from the capsule, and the avulsion of the dorsal capsule or meniscus homologue from the insertion in the dorsal aspect of the triquetrum, an injury called carpal detachment or Nishikawa lesion [11, 32], see Chap. 12 (Fig. 5.12).

Imaging Diagnosis

In traumatic injuries of the TFCC, radiographs may be normal but often show fractures of the US, and less frequently marginal fractures of the sigmoid cavity of the radius.

MR allows a reliable assessment of lesions of the central tears (class IA) and the radial insertion injuries (Class ID), with a diagnostic accuracy above 95 %. However, in the assessment of the spectrum of ulnar insertion lesions (Palmer class IB), MR provides a very low sensitivity and specificity (about 18 %) [25]. The low MR accuracy in the evaluation of Palmer class IB injuries could be related to the

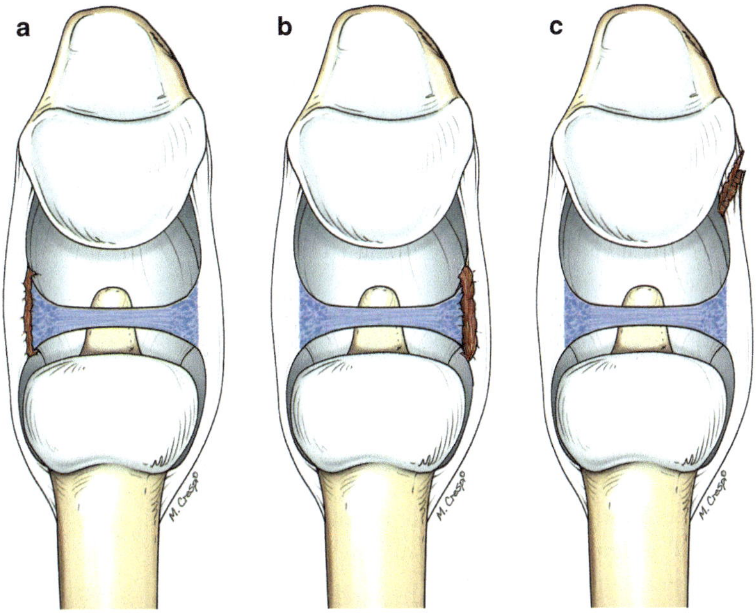

Fig. 5.11 Diagrams illustrate the most common injuries not included in Palmer classification (del Piñal): (**a**) Anterior capsular TFC detachment. (**b**) Posterior capsular TFC detachment. (**c**) Ulnar detachment or Nishikawa lesion

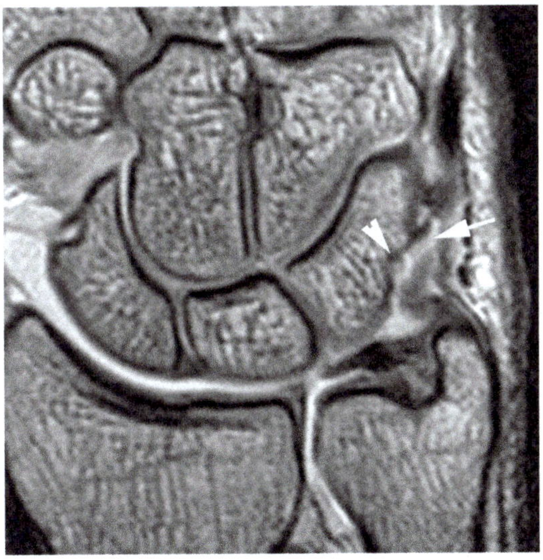

Fig. 5.12 Carpal detachment or Nishikawa lesion. Coronal T1-weighted MR arthrogram image shows a dorsal capsular (ulnomeniscal homologue) detachment from triquetral insertion (*arrow*) and cartilage delamination in the dorsal aspect of the triquetrum (*arrowhead*)

complex anatomy of the ulnar insertion of the TFCC [13]. Moreover, the existence of joint fluid or synovitis in the prestyloid recess can produce a misdiagnosis of ulnar insertion tear. In patients with acute fracture or nonunion of the US process, the evaluation of the TFCC ulnar insertion, mainly the foveal insertion, is very difficult, and MR imaging offers a low diagnostic accuracy [17].

Articular distention with contrast in CT arthrography and MR arthrography allows a precise evaluation of Palmer class IB injuries (Fig. 5.8). Due to the frequency and clinical relevance of foveal avulsion, it is recommended to start arthrographic studies with DRUJ injection of contrast. When there is detachment of both the foveal and styloid insertion of TFCC (complete tear), communication between DRUJ and radiocarpal joint is easily observed at CT/MR arthrography.

The very uncommon Palmer class IC injuries are usually not detected on MR imaging. Sagittal MR or CT arthrography images are the most suitable to assess ulnocarpal ligaments. It is important to determine if there is an associated lunotriquetral ligament tear.

Ulnar-Sided Wrist Impaction Syndromes

Ulnar-sided wrist impaction syndromes can be divided into four main categories: (1) ulnar impaction syndrome, (2) ulnar impingement syndrome, (3) ulnar styloid impaction syndrome, and (4) hamatolunate impaction syndrome [10, 15, 16].

Ulnar Impaction Syndrome

Chronic impaction between the ulnar head and the TFCC and ulnar carpus results in a continuum of pathologic changes described by Palmer as class II (degenerative) lesions of the TFCC (Fig. 5.13). Class IIA injuries represent TFCC wear. Class IIB injuries associate lunate or ulnar chondromalacia to TFCC wear. IIC injuries occur when complex perforation of the TFC is present together with lunate or ulnar chondromalacia. Class IID lesions are defined when lunotriquetral (LT) ligament perforation is associated (complex perforation of the TFC, lunate or ulnar chondromalacia, and LT ligament perforation). Class IIE injuries include a TFCC perforation, lunate or ulnar chondromalacia, LT ligament perforation, and additional ulnocarpal arthritis [22].

The pathologic changes that appear in ulnar impaction syndrome frequently occur with positive ulnar variance but can occasionally occur with neutral or negative ulnar variance. The most common predisposing factors are congenital positive ulnar variance, malunion of the distal radius, premature physeal closure of the distal radius, Essex-Lopresti fracture, and previous surgical resection of the radial head.

In the absence of obvious structural abnormalities, ulnar impaction syndrome may result from daily activities that cause excessive intermittent loading of the ulnar carpus. It also has been shown that asymptomatic changes in ulnar impaction syndrome develop over time so that this condition may be present even if symptoms are not evident [22].

Clinical manifestation of ulnar impaction syndrome generally consists of chronic or subacute ulnar wrist pain, often exacerbated by activity and relieved by rest. Anything that causes a relative increase in ulnar variance (e.g., firm grip, pronation, ulnar deviation of the wrist) evokes increased symptoms [10, 22].

Physical examination reveals swelling and tenderness that is usually localized to the region of the TFCC and LT joint. Limitation of forearm rotation and wrist motion usually is present [22].

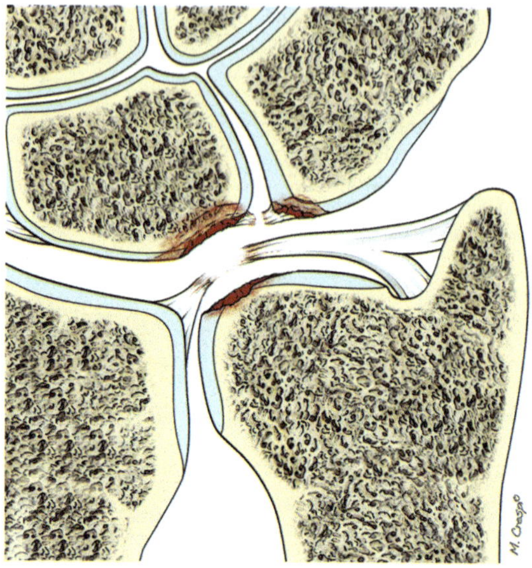

Fig. 5.13 Diagram illustrates the full spectrum of pathologic conditions in ulnar impaction syndrome, including chondromalacia of the ulnar head, and the ulnar side of the lunate bone, central perforation of the TFC, and LT ligament tear

Imaging Diagnosis

Radiographic findings in ulnar impaction syndrome usually show positive ulnar variance. Pronation grip radiographs are useful in determining the increase in ulnar variance and the impaction between ulnar carpus and the dome head with axial load. Underlying abnormalities, such as malunion of a distal radius fracture with residual radial shortening and abnormal dorsal tilt, may be present. Premature physeal arrest of the distal radius or previous Essex-Lopresti fracture or resection of the radial head may also be evident on conventional radiographs. Secondary changes in the ulnar carpus include subchondral sclerosis and cystic changes in the ulnar head, ulnar aspect of the proximal lunate bone, and proximal radial aspect of the triquetral bone. Although the radiographic changes may be striking, the features of ulnar impaction syndrome may be subtle in its early and late stages [15].

In the setting of negative or doubtful negative conventional radiographs and a strong clinical suspicion for ulnar impaction, MR

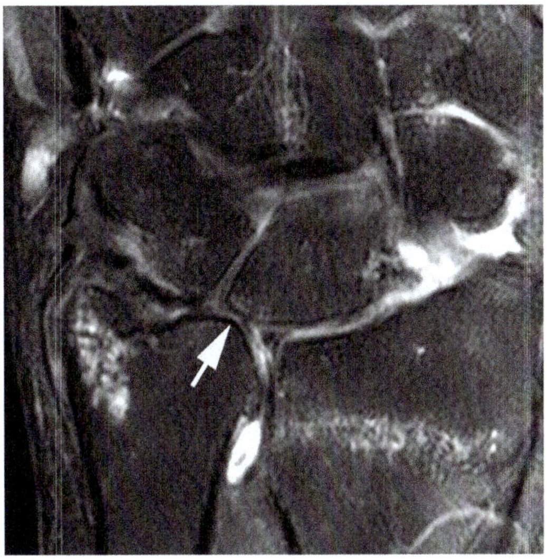

Fig. 5.14 Palmer class IIC lesion. Ulnocarpal impaction secondary to distal radius malunion shortening. Coronal proton density fat-suppressed MR image demonstrates an extensive central TFC perforation with communication between the radiocarpal and DRUJ compartments (*arrow*). Note the existence of small intraosseous cyst in the US

imaging is helpful in detecting radiologically occult lesions. Softening, fibrillation, or partial-thickness defects of articular cartilage in the wrist are detected inconsistently by MR imaging; however, the accuracy of MR imaging tends to be more favorable for high-grade or large cartilage defects. Indirect or secondary signs of chondromalacia manifested with subchondral bone marrow edema and synovitis are frequent findings in ulnar impaction syndrome. Bone marrow edema can even be seen in patients without cartilaginous degeneration revealed at arthroscopy, indicating that it is also a sensitive sign of ulnar impaction [15]. Progression of the syndrome results in sclerotic changes and subchondral cysts. These degenerative changes usually are appreciated much earlier in MR images than in conventional radiographs.

MR imaging is particularly helpful in the assessment of degenerative changes and partial tears involving the proximal ulnar dome aspect of the TFC that are arthroscopically occult (class IIA and IIB TFCC) [18]. Complete TFCC perforations are easily detected on MR imaging (Fig. 5.14).

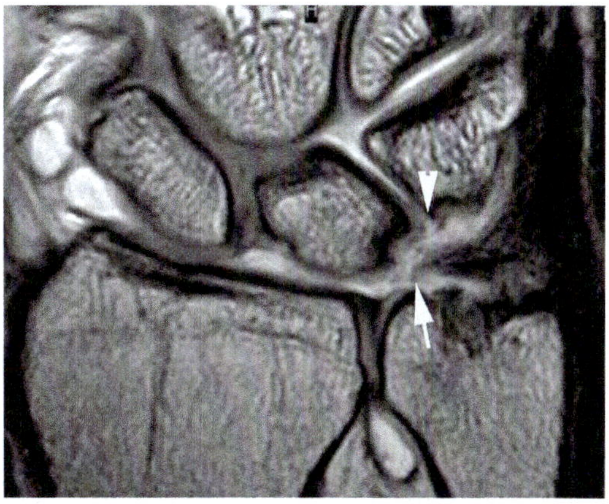

Fig. 5.15 Palmer class IID lesion (ulnar impaction syndrome). Coronal T1-weighted MR arthrogram image demonstrates a central TFC perforation (*arrow*) and a chronic tear of the LT ligament (*arrowhead*). The diagnostic reliability of conventional MR imaging is limited in the diagnosis of the LT ligament tears (stage 2D). MR arthrography allows an accurate diagnosis of these injuries

The LT ligament tears are inconsistently visible with MR imaging. MR arthrography may be necessary in selected cases for determining the status of the LT ligament, allowing to distinguish between Palmer class IIC and IID [17, 33] (Fig. 5.15).

Ulnar Impingement Syndrome

Ulnar impingement syndrome is painful condition caused by a shortened distal ulna that impinges on the distal radius proximal to the sigmoid notch.

Markedly shortened distal ulna results most frequently from any of the surgical procedures that involve resection of the distal ulna secondary to prior wrist trauma, rheumatoid arthritis, or correction of Madelung deformity (Fig. 5.16a). Less commonly, ulnar impingement may be present in patients with negative ulnar variance or premature fusion of the distal ulna secondary to prior trauma [48] (Fig. 5.16b).

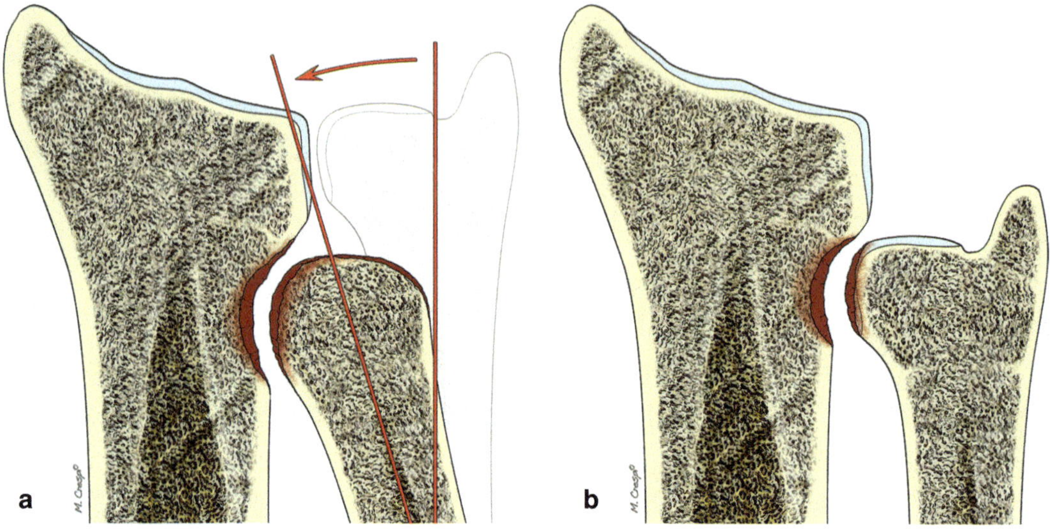

Fig. 5.16 Diagrams illustrate the cardinal features of ulnar impingement. (**a**) Ulnar impingement syndrome secondary to distal ulnar resection: a shortened ulna proximal to the sigmoid notch, scalloping of the distal radius, and radioulnar convergence (*red arrow*). (**b**) Ulnar impingement secondary to significant negative ulnar variance or premature fusion of the distal ulna. Note the scalloping of the distal radius proximal to the sigmoid notch

The clinical manifestation of ulnar impingement syndrome can be similar to that of ulnar impaction syndrome. Typically, the patients experience pain on pronation and supination of the forearm and weakness on lifting even light objects. Compression of the DRUJ on forearm rotation increases the symptoms or produces grating in affected patients and is useful in identifying incongruity of the DRUJ.

Imaging Diagnosis

Ulnar impingement can produce erosive and proliferative cortical changes along the ulnar margin of the distal radius proximal to the sigmoid notch level that appear as scalloping (Fig. 5.17a) and bone hypertrophy on conventional radiographs [15]. By the time such changes are seen, the condition has been present for many years. The stress-loaded radiologic view described by Lees and Scheker will confirm the diagnosis before erosive changes are visible showing the radioulnar convergence.

MR imaging is helpful in confirming the diagnosis before erosive changes are visible in the conventional radiographs, showing subtle sclerosis and bone edema at the corresponding level of the radius and on the distal ulna (Fig. 5.17b). In advanced stages, scalloping and sclerosis along the ulnar margin of the distal radius cephalad to the sigmoid notch, sclerosis in the ulnar seat, and bone spurs or osteophytes in both margins are clearly visualized on MR images [18].

Ulnar Styloid Impaction Syndrome

US (ulnar styloid) impaction syndrome is an under recognized etiology of ulnar wrist pain caused by impaction between the US and the triquetrum bone and the surrounding soft tissues [46] (Fig. 5.18). This group of pathologic entities more commonly develops in wrists with negative ulnar variance and result from repetitive or acute forced ulnar deviation and dorsal flexion of the wrist.

The presence of anatomic variations including supernumerary ossicles and morphological variations of the US is frequent. The US process is a continuation of the prominent subcutaneous ridge of the shaft of the ulna, which projects distally toward the triquetral bone for a variable distance (3–6 mm) and with medial angulation exceeding 15°. Garcia-Elias has developed a method of assessing the relative size of the US called the US

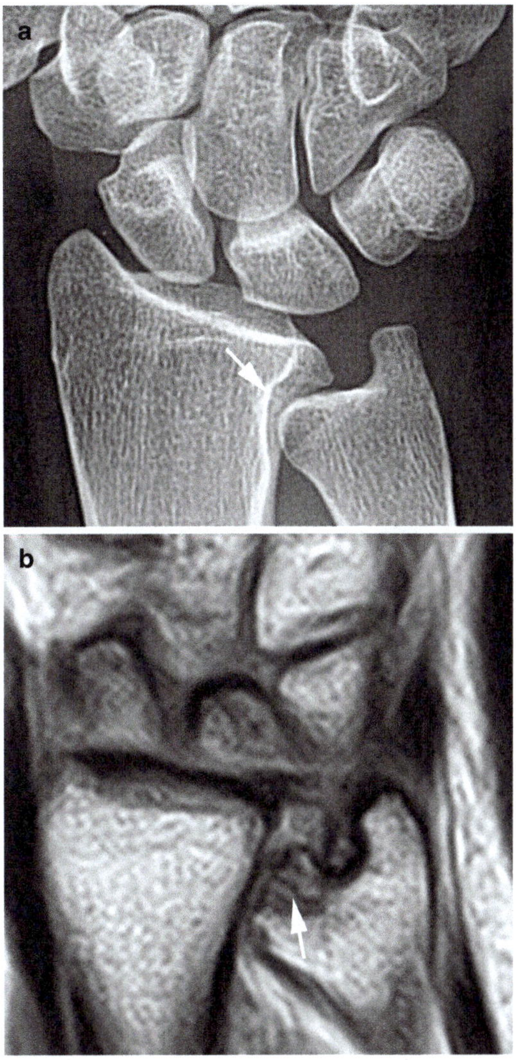

Fig. 5.17 Ulnar impingement. (**a**) PA radiograph of the left wrist shows prominent ulnar shortening, scalloping (*arrow*), and sclerosis along the ulnar margin of the distal radius proximal to the sigmoid notch. (**b**) Coronal T1-weighted MR image demonstrates negative ulnar variance, subtle radial remodeling, and chondromalacia in the ulnar seat (*arrow*)

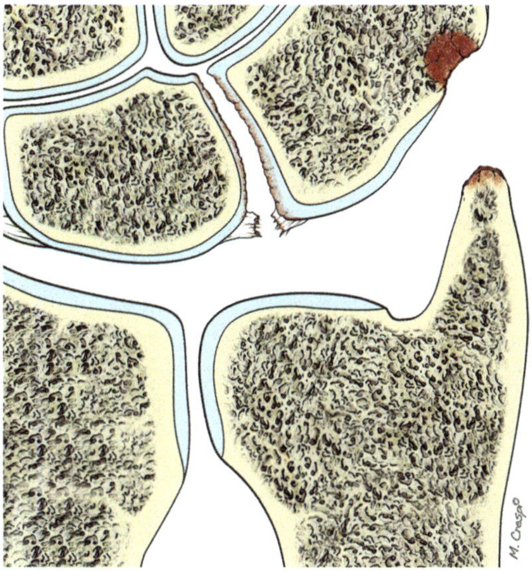

Fig. 5.18 Diagram illustrates the full spectrum of pathologic conditions in US impaction syndrome, including chondromalacia of the dorsal aspect of the triquetral bone and on the tip of the styloid process, and LT ligament tear

process index (USPI). An excessively long US has a USPI greater than 0.21 ± 0.07 or an overall length greater than 6 mm [16].

US impaction syndrome may occur secondary to morphological variations (elongated, radially deviated, or enlarged US process) or pathological conditions (nonunion, malunion, or hypertrophy) of the US process. US impaction syndromes have been classified by del Piñal in four subtypes based in different morphological or pathologic conditions of the US implicated in the etiology of this clinical entity [16] (Fig. 5.19). An elongated US is the commonest variant implicated in the development of US impaction syndrome. A pathologic sequence of events has been postulated in patients with US impaction syndrome with long or radially deviated US. One-time or repetitive impaction between the tip of the US process and the triquetral bone results in contusion, which leads to chondromalacia of the opposing articular surfaces, synovitis, and pain. If a single-event trauma is forceful enough, fracture of the dorsal triquetral bone (chip fracture) may occur.

US fractures occur commonly in association with distal radius fractures. Severely displaced basilar fractures of the US are commonly associated with DRUJ instability. However, these fractures could have a stable DRUJ if ulnar foveal insertion of the TFCC is respected. On the other hand, in "chip" fractures of the US, the DRUJ is usually stable but in cases can also be associated with instability if there is a concomitant TFCC injury [10].

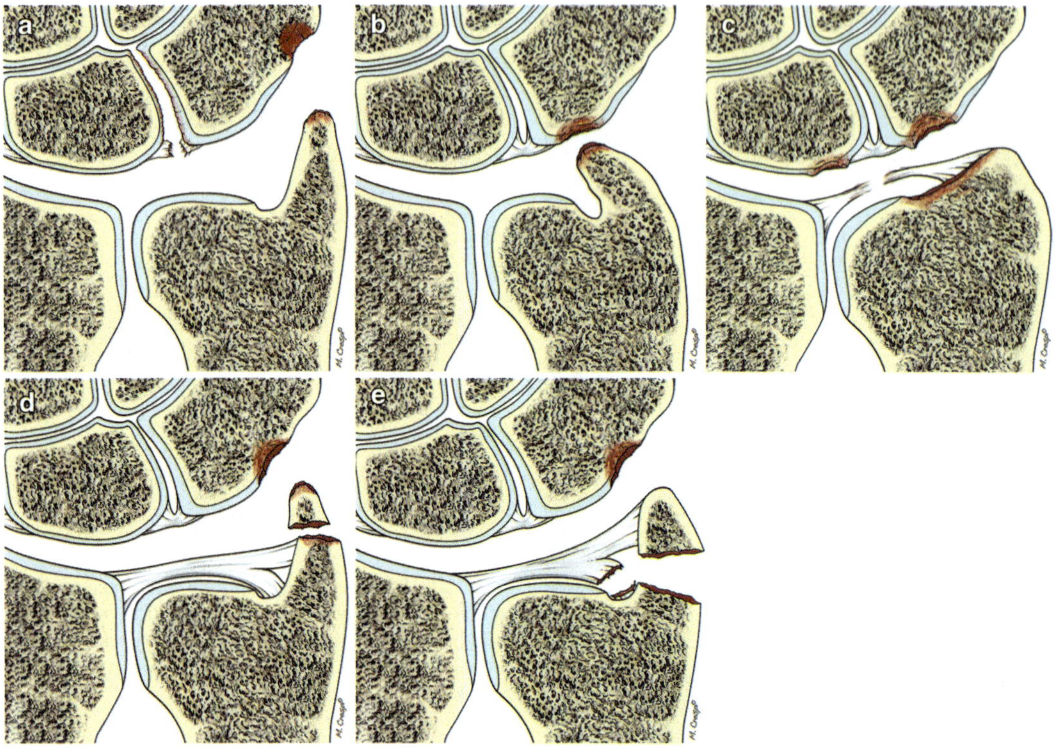

Fig. 5.19 Diagrams illustrate the different subtypes of US impaction syndrome according to Piñal. (**a**) Elongated US. (**b**) Radially deviated or parrot beaked US. (**c**) Enlarged US. (**d**) Nonunion of the US without DRUJ instability. (**e**) Nonunion of the US with DRUJ instability

A nonunion of the US may become symptomatic for different reasons. The nonunited fragment may act as an irritative loose body or abut the carpus. A malaligned fibrous nonunion may cause impingement of the ECU tendon sheath. The nonunion may also be symptomatic because of associated TFC complex for TFCC perforation or as stated as a result of complete rupture of the ulnar attachments of the TFC complex for TFCC and hence an unstable DRUJ [10, 36].

Imaging Diagnosis

The diagnosis of US impaction syndrome is based primarily on the patient's clinical history and physical examination and is supported by radiographic evidence of morphological variations or pathological conditions of the US [10].

The US architecture measurements (US length, angle, and width) and ulnar variance should be recorded in the neutral PA view of the wrist. In advanced stages, plain radiographs may reveal degenerative changes in the US and the triquetrum bone.

MR imaging is the most useful imaging method for detecting the osseous and soft tissue abnormalities present in this syndrome and ruling out other potential causes of chronic ulnar wrist pain [48]. In patients with US impaction syndrome, an early finding on MR imaging is the presence of synovitis in the dorsal aspect of the ulnocarpal joint. In more advanced stages, MR imaging may show chondromalacia on the tip of the US and focal chondral delamination at the dorsal aspect of the triquetrum. Secondary subchondral changes, including bone marrow edema, sclerosis, and cysts, in characteristic locations can be detected in MR imaging in patients without significant abnormalities in the routine plain films [48].

In patients with US impaction syndrome secondary to nonunion of the US, MR imaging is an excellent modality for visualizing the presence of ununited bone fragments and the associated chondromalacia and subchondral bone changes of the carpus (Fig. 5.20). Tenosynovitis or tendinosis of the ECU secondary to irritative loose body can also be detected in MR imaging. MR arthrography allows a precise assessment of the TFCC ulnar insertion in cases of US nonunion [17].

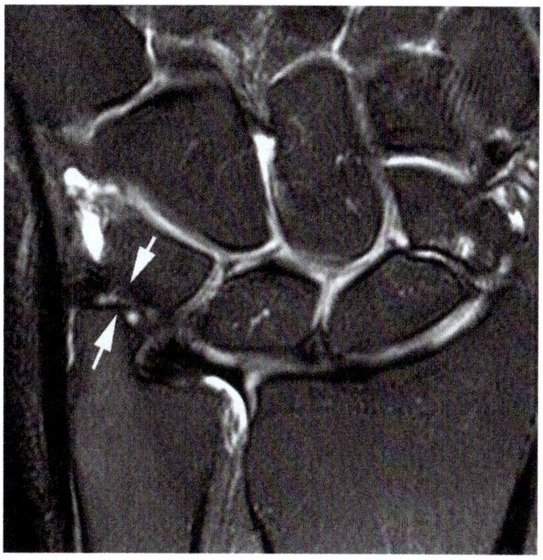

Fig. 5.20 US impaction syndrome in a patient with severe chronic ulnar-sided pain. Coronal proton density fat-suppressed MR image shows an excessively long US process, a chondromalacia of the dorsal aspect of the triquetral bone and tip of the US (*arrows*). Resection of the two most distal millimeters of the US process was performed, resulting in good recovery of function and relief of symptoms

Hamatolunate Impaction Syndrome

Hamatolunate impaction is an uncommon cause of ulnar-sided wrist pain secondary to chondromalacia of the proximal pole of the hamate bone in patients with lunate bones that have a medial articular facet on the distal surface for articulation with the hamate bone [27, 43] (Fig. 5.21).

The anatomic variation of an articulation between the hamate and the lunate described by Viegas et al. (type II lunate bone), which is present in between 57 and 73 % of wrists, produces an alteration of the normal uniform loading and focally altered mechanics that leads to a higher incidence of cartilage erosion with exposed subchondral bone on the proximal pole of the hamate bone than in those without this articulation (type I lunate bone) [27, 43].

The repeated impingement and abrasion of these two bones when the wrist is used in full ulnar deviation is the suggested mechanism for the development of the chondromalacia.

Patients experience pain in full ulnar deviation of the wrist, and it is by repeating this maneuver, especially when combined with first holding the distal carpal row in forced supination, that their pain can be reproduced [27, 43].

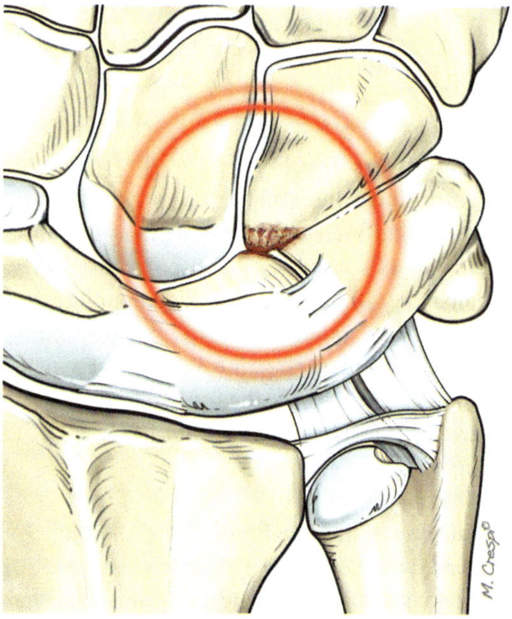

Fig. 5.21 Diagram illustrates hamatolunate impaction syndrome, with Viegas type II lunate bone, chondromalacia of the proximal pole of the hamate bone and secondary subchondral changes

Imaging Diagnosis

In the clinical setting of ulnar-sided wrist pain, the radiographic evidence of a type II lunate bone should raise the question of arthrosis at the proximal pole of the hamate as the most likely source of the complaint.

MR imaging has low sensitivity for early stages of chondromalacia but can detect bone edema, sclerosis, and subchondral cysts in the proximal pole of the hamate bone as secondary

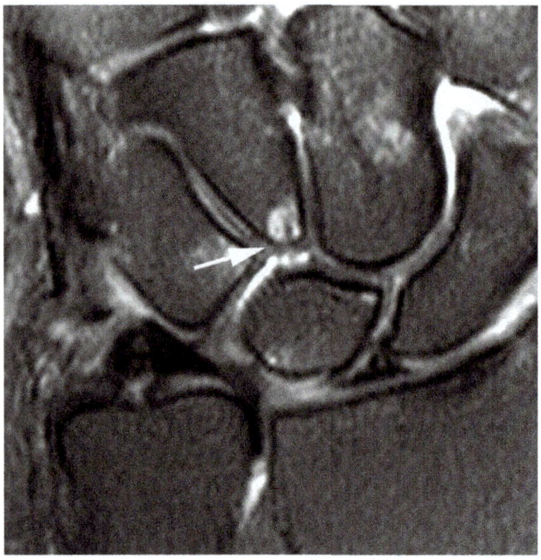

Fig. 5.22 Hamatolunate impaction syndrome. Coronal proton density fat-suppressed MR image shows type II lunate bone with advanced chondromalacia in the proximal pole of the hamate bone, and secondary subchondral bone marrow edema (*arrow*). Arthroscopic resection of the proximal pole of the hamate bone resulted in completely relief of symptoms

signs of chondromalacia and focal osteoarthritis [48] (Fig. 5.22). Midcarpal synovitis is a common indirect MR sign of hamatolunate impaction.

Ligamentous Injuries

Lunotriquetral Instability

LT dissociation is the second most common ligamentous cause of carpal instability. Compared with scapholunate ligament injuries, LT ligament injuries are quite uncommon. Frequently, either the injury is missed or is misdiagnosed as another ulnar-sided wrist lesion such as midcarpal instability or a TFCC injury [21].

Disruption of the LT ligament causes a dynamic or static instability of the LT joint. An increased frequency of LT ligament tears in association with degenerative tears of the TFCC has been reported [23].

Complete disruption of the LT ligament in combination with insufficiency of the secondary stabilizer, the dorsal radiocarpal ligament, will result in a pattern of volar intercalated segmental instability (VISI). In this setting, the scaphoid forces the lunate into palmar flexion with concomitant proximal translocation of the triquetrum. These patients will present with ulnar-sided wrist pain and demonstrate point tenderness over the LT interval [23].

Imaging Diagnosis

Isolated LT ligament tears usually show no radiographic abnormality. However, in more severe cases where there is an injury to the secondary restrains, the wrist will assume a VISI configuration with palmar angulation of the lunate (radiolunate angle 10° volar) with palmar displacement of the capitate in relation to the metacarpal axis. The longitudinal scapholunate axis will decrease and be less than 30° [48].

On conventional MR imaging, ligament disruption is inconstantly seen. Injuries of the dorsal and volar portions of the LT ligament are better assessed in the axial slices [41]. CT arthrography and MR arthrography are the imaging modalities of choice for visualizing the size, location, and morphology of LT ligament tears [7, 19, 38, 42] (Fig. 5.23).

Midcarpal Instability

Midcarpal instability (MCI) is a dynamic disorder associated with injury of the (volar) arcuate ligament. Palmar MCI is the most common type. The arcuate ligament has a broader and thicker ulnar arm (triquetrohamocapitate ligament), and its injury along with DRC involvement is associated with palmar MCI. Normally, the proximal carpal row smoothly transitions between a flexed and an extended position as the wrist moves from radial to ulnar deviation. During this motion, the arcuate ligament becomes taut and assists in pulling the proximal carpal row into extension. In dynamic palmar MCI, there is often tenderness over the triquetrohamate joint, and a symptomatic "clunk" is observed when moving the wrist into ulnar deviation and pronation because when the ulnar arm of arcuate ligament becomes deficient, the proximal carpal row remains in a flexed position until the triquetrum engages the hamate and the proximal row alignment abruptly changes from flexion to extension, resulting in a painful "clunk" [23, 48].

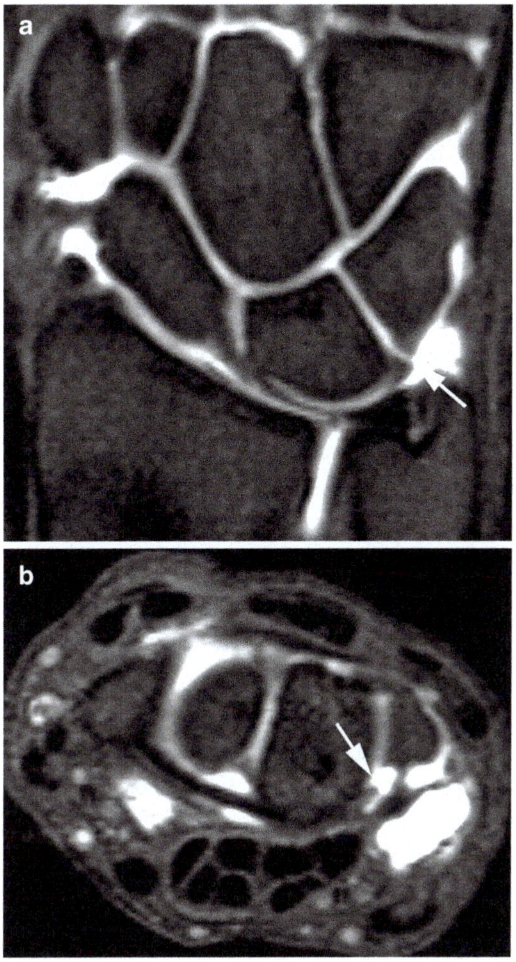

Fig. 5.23 Partial LT ligament tear (central and volar components). (**a**) Coronal fat-suppressed T1-weighted MR arthrogram image shows a central perforation of the LT ligament (*arrow*). (**b**) Axial fat-suppressed T1-weighted MR arthrogram image reveals a tear of the volar component of the LT ligament (*arrow*)

Imaging Diagnosis

These sudden changes in alignment serve as helpful diagnostic sign during videofluoroscopy. In static palmar MCI, the entire proximal carpal row appears abnormally flexed in the PA radiograph (the flexed scaphoid produces a ring sign). This nondissociative VISI pattern results in an increased capitolunate angle (>30°) on the lateral view: however, the scapholunate angle is within normal ranges (30–60°) [45].

Extrinsic carpal ligament injuries (volar and dorsal) are less commonly identified at MR imaging. Again, CT arthrography and MR arthrography are the preferred methods of evaluating these ligaments [42, 45, 48].

Osseous Injuries

Fractures

Stress Reactions and Stress Fractures

Stress reactions and stress fractures of the distal ulna and hook of the hamate are being increasingly recognized as a cause of ulnar wrist pain. These stress fractures most typically occur due to repetitive direct impaction or repetitive loading at tendon and ligament attachment sites.

Imaging Diagnosis

Radiographs may be normal or may show mild periostitis or a small cortical lucency at the site of the stress fracture. MR imaging is very sensitive to these injuries and will show marrow edema (stress reaction) with a small hypointense fracture line (if a stress fracture is present).

Ulnar Styloid Fracture

US fractures occur as isolated injuries or in association with distal radius and other wrist fractures. A great number of US fractures (65 %) go on to nonunion, causing ulnar wrist problems [48].

Hamate Fractures

A high index of suspicion is required to identify hamate fractures. Hamate fractures account for 1.7 % of all carpal fractures and are usually nondisplaced. More common fractures of the hamate are fractures of the hamate hook [24] (Fig. 5.24).

Diagnosing a fracture of the hook of the hamate is often delayed because the symptoms can be nonspecific. Typically, there is tenderness on deep palpation over the hook of the hamate and pain with resisted flexion of the fourth and fifth fingers with ulnar deviation of the wrist.

Much more infrequent than fractures of the hamate hook are fractures of the body of the hamate. These fractures may occur as a result of an axial force that is transmitted through the metacarpals or a direct blow to the ulnar aspect of the wrist and are commonly associated with dislocations of the fourth and fifth carpometacarpal joints, particularly the coronally oriented fractures [8, 35].

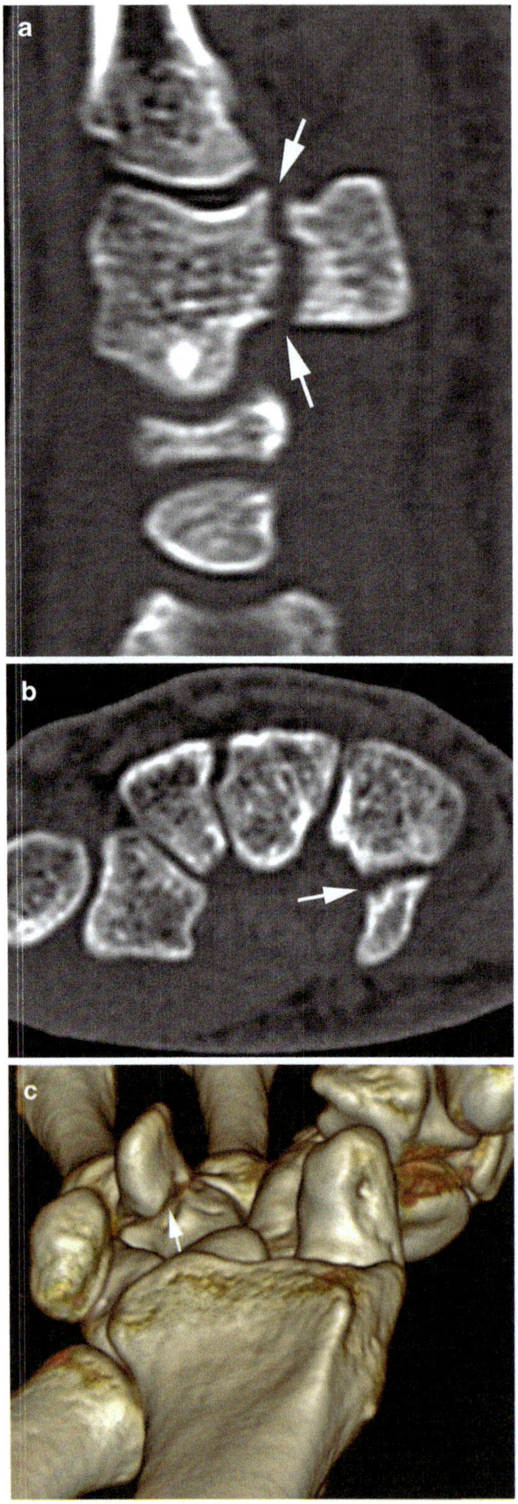

Fig. 5.24 Hook of the hamate fracture. (**a**–**c**) Sagittal, axial, and 3D CT images show an acute fracture of the hook of the hamate (*arrows*)

Pisiform Fracture

Fracture of the pisiform is uncommon (1–2 % of all carpal fractures), but when it does occur, it is frequently associated with other injuries to the carpus or distal radius [24, 35]. An acute pisiform fracture typically results from a direct impact or muscular avulsion. Avulsion fracture results when the flexor carpi ulnaris resists forcible hyperextension of the wrist. Delayed diagnosis of pisiform fractures may lead to long-term disability. Complications may include pisotriquetral joint arthrosis and ulnar nerve injury [8].

Fifth Metacarpal Base Fracture

Fracture of the base of fifth metacarpal can be oblique, horizontal, or vertical and may have an intra-articular component of the fracture that makes it prone to dislocation [48].

Imaging Diagnosis

Routine posteroanterior and lateral radiographs constitute the initial diagnostic imaging approach in the clinical context of a traumatic event. Fractures of the US and fifth metacarpal base fracture are usually adequately visualized on routine views. However, visualization of the pisiform and especially the hook of the hamate can be difficult due to complex carpal anatomy and overlapping of the carpal bones. Oblique supinated view, carpal tunnel view, and the lateral radiographic view with the hand radially deviated and the thumb abducted can be helpful [8].

CT offers a more detailed anatomical information and can help to determine the degree of fracture displacement, a critical point that aids therapeutic decision-making [8, 26] (Fig. 5.24).

MR is helpful in evaluating ligaments, tendons, and nondisplaced fractures [48] (Fig. 5.25). In cases of hook of the hamate pseudoarthrosis, contrast-enhanced MR may be beneficial in assessing the blood supply to the hamulus and may affect surgical decision-making.

Kienböck Disease

Necrosis of the lunate (Kienböck disease) is most commonly seen in the dominant hand of men, between the ages of 20 and 40 years. Kienböck disease is a disorder with an unknown

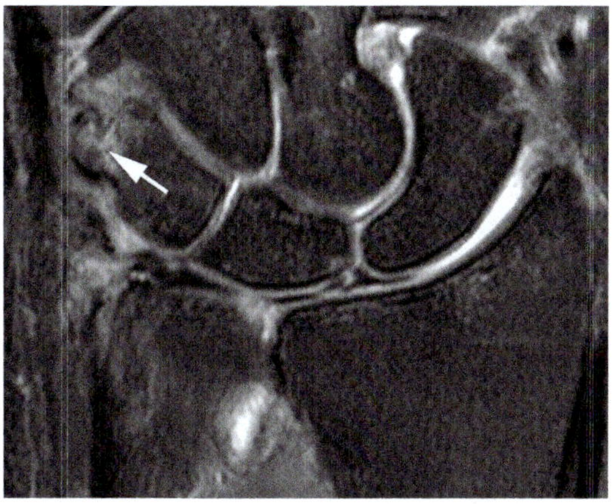

Fig. 5.25 Dorsal chip fracture of the triquetrum. Coronal proton density fat-suppressed MR image reveals a small fracture of the dorsum of the triquetrum (*arrow*) with overlying bone marrow and soft tissue edema

cause, probably multifactorial, an uncertain natural history [48].

Ulnar negative variance increases the shearing forces and stress on the lunate bone, which may be a contributing factor in the development of necrosis.

Symptoms typically have an insidious onset with a dull ache along the middorsal aspect of the affected wrist but can also manifest as ulnar-sided wrist pain.

Lichtman classified Kienbock disease into four stages to help to match the most appropriate treatment for each patient (Fig. 5.26). In 2010, Lichtman updated his classification and introduced a new stage IIIC, corresponding to the chronic coronal fracture.

Imaging Diagnosis

Radiographs are insensitive in the early stages of Kienböck disease, and the diagnosis is commonly delayed since the start of symptoms.

A CT is useful to demonstrate fracture or fragmentation of the lunate.

MR imaging can be helpful in the early detection of the disease. MR imaging can help to determine the Lichtman stage and facilitates ruling out other disorders (pseudo-Kienböck lesions) [48].

Contrast-enhanced MR imaging is important in order to determine the degree of necrotic tissue, which is important in choosing the most appropriate treatment option in stages II and IIIA (Fig. 5.27), and to assess the postoperative response to direct and indirect revascularization procedures.

Pseudo-Kienböck

A common occurrence is the misinterpretation of imaging findings of several lunate processes, mainly in MR imaging, as Kienböck disease.

The entities commonly confused with Kienböck disease are ulnocarpal impaction syndrome, intraosseous ganglia, bone contusion of the lunate, infantile and juvenile lunatomalacia, and arthritis.

The distribution of imaging changes within the lunate bone is the key to distinguishing Kienböck disease from ulnar impaction. MR imaging changes in Kienböck disease lesions affect the radial half of the lunate bone or are more diffuse compared with involvement of only the ulnar aspect in ulnar impaction syndrome [17] (Fig. 5.28a).

Intraosseous ganglia that communicate with the scapholunate joint are frequently symptomatic and show diffuse bone marrow edema on MR imaging, simulating Kienböck disease (Fig. 5.28b). The identification of the cyst and cortical break on MR imaging and correlation with conventional radiographs finding where cysts appear as a hyperlucent area within the radial aspect of the lunate bone that communicates with the LT joint space [17].

Lunotriquetral Coalition

A carpal coalition is an osseous, fibrous, or cartilaginous fusion between individual carpal bones. By far, the most frequent idiopathic coalition is LT coalition, the spectrum of which has been classified by Minnaar. The incidence in the general population is approximately 0.1 % [44]. Although coalitions are usually asymptomatic, fibrous or cartilaginous LT coalitions (Minnaar type 1) may produce ulnar wrist pain secondary to an acute traumatic or microtraumatic event.

Imaging Diagnosis

LT coalition Minnaar type 1 appears in plain films as a narrowing and irregularity of the proximal

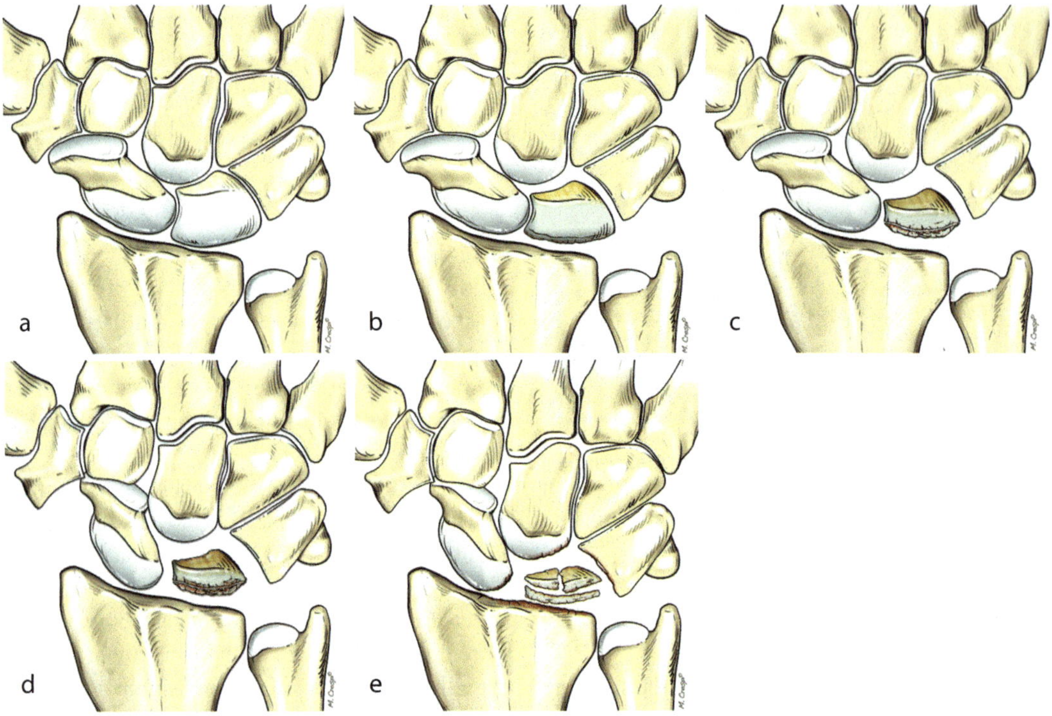

Fig. 5.26 Lichtman's classification of Kienböck disease. (**a**) Stage I. Normal radiographs. Characteristic focal or diffuse MR imaging abnormalities. (**b**) Stage II. Sclerosis of the lunate. Collapse of the lunate has not occurred. Multiple lunate fracture lines may be seen. (**c**) Stage IIIA. Collapse of the lunate without carpal instability. (**d**) Stage IIIB. Collapse of the lunate with carpal instability. (**e**) Stage IV. Carpal (radiocarpal and/or midcarpal) arthrosis

aspect of the LT joint. Symptomatic LT coalitions appear on MR imaging as bone marrow edema surrounding the fibrous or cartilaginous coalition and secondary synovitis (Fig. 5.29).

Pisotriquetral Joint

Primary osteoarthritis is the main cause of pisotriquetral joint osteoarthritis, which usually affects patients older than 50 years, especially women [8]. Secondary osteoarthritis is usually a sequela of a misdiagnosed fracture of the pisiform or triquetrum or subluxation of the pisiform bone. Osteoarthritis of the pisotriquetral joint may be associated with a synovial cyst, which most often communicates with the superior recess. Synovial cysts also may extend into the Guyon's canal and cause ulnar nerve compression.

Pisotriquetral osteoarthritis is associated with local pain and tenderness, which are exacerbated by grinding of the pisiform bone dorsally against the triquetrum. Instability is subtle, subjective, and therefore difficult to diagnose [8].

Imaging Diagnosis

Injection of a local anesthetic or corticosteroid, combined with the acquisition of a semisupinated oblique radiograph, enables the diagnosis of pisotriquetral joint dysfunction. Semisupinated oblique views clearly demonstrate loose bodies in the superior and inferior recesses of the pisotriquetral joint, often missed on other views [8].

MR imaging or CT arthrography may be indicated for a precise detection of all the loose bodies in the preoperative evaluation (Fig. 5.30).

Extra-articular Injuries

Tendinous Injuries

Extensor Carpi Ulnaris

ECU tendinopathy is common, second only to de Quervain's disease. The spectrum of injuries of this tendon includes tendinopathy, tenosynovitis, subluxation, dislocation, and rupture [1, 28] (Fig. 5.31).

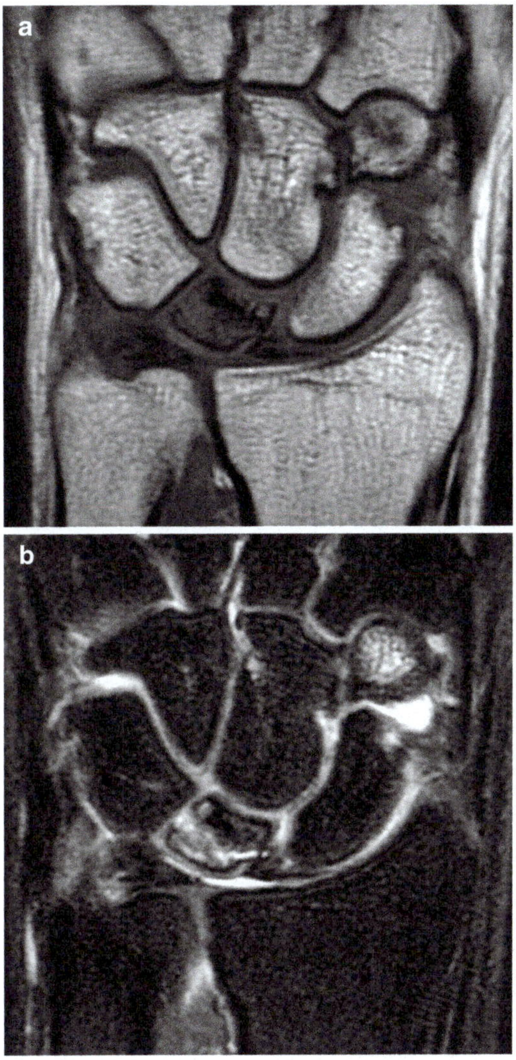

Fig. 5.27 Stage 2 Kienböck disease. (**a**) Coronal T1-weighted MR image demonstrates a lunate with a normal shape and diffuse low signal. (**b**) Coronal T1 fat-suppressed image after gadolinium administration shows a subchondral fracture and a complete absence of enhancement of the lunate that represents a necrotic bone

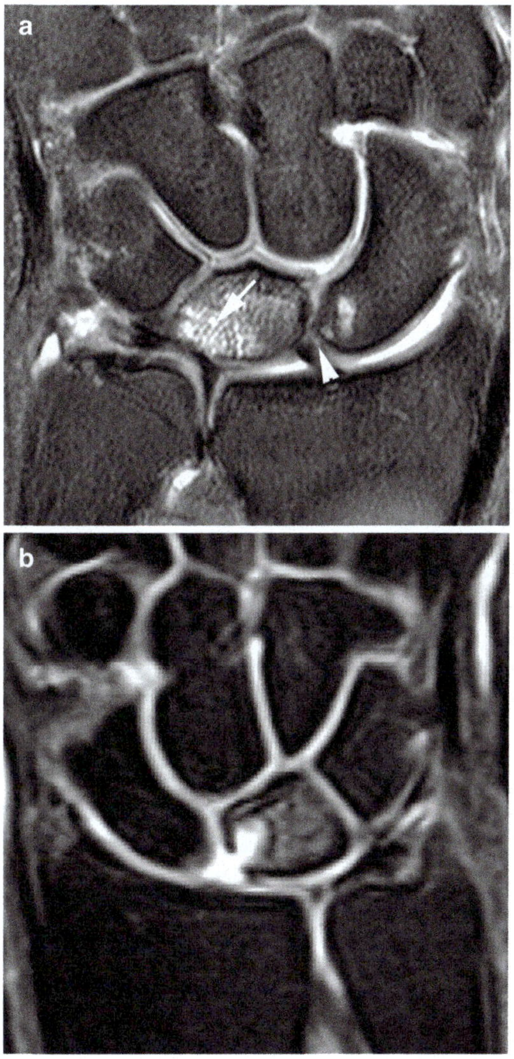

Fig. 5.28 Pseudo-Kienböck. (**a**) Ulnocarpal impaction. Coronal proton density fat-suppressed MR image reveals a central wear of the TFCC, and focal chondromalacia in the ulnar aspect of the lunate bone with secondary diffuse bone marrow edema of the lunate (*arrow*). Note the existence of a central tear of the scapholunate ligament (*arrowhead*). (**b**) Intraosseous cyst of the lunate. Coronal proton density fat-suppressed MR image shows an intraosseous cyst with small cortical rupture and extension into the scapholunate joint. Note the secondary diffuse bone marrow edema of the lunate

Isolated ECU lesions are rare, and associated TFCC tears, and LT ligament tears are frequently found, as are other pathologic processes, such as an anomalous tendon slip, an US nonunion, or a flat tendon groove [28].

Subluxation of the ECU results from rupture or attenuation of the subsheath, usually due to a sudden volar flexion ulnar deviation stress. ECU tendon instability is frequently associated with tenosynovitis. Dislocation of the ECU tendon may develop as a result of recurrent instability, distal radial fractures with disruption of the extensor retinaculum, and posttraumatic or rheumatoid arthritis-related distal radioulnar subluxation. When subluxation or dislocation is symptomatic, the patient usually complains of a painful snap

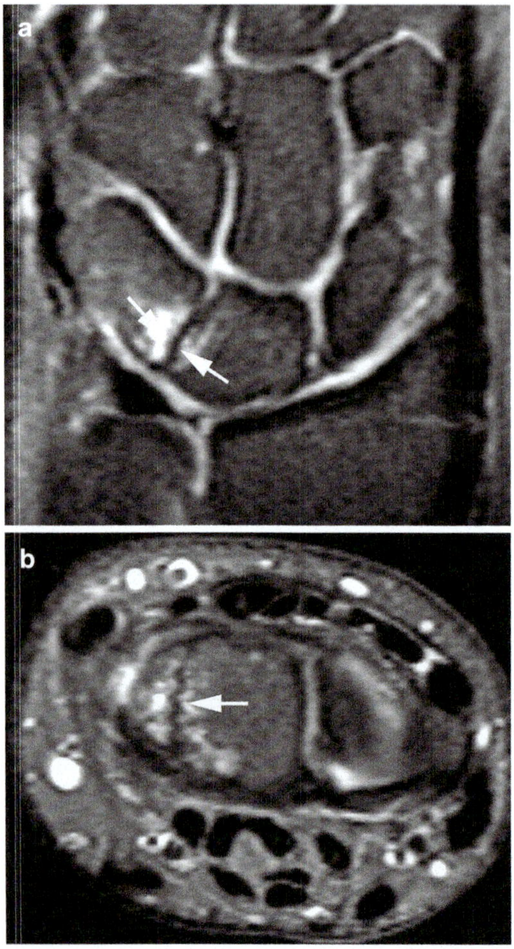

Fig. 5.29 Symptomatic LT coalition (Minnaar type 1). (**a**, **b**) Coronal and axial proton density fat-suppressed MR images show a fibrous LT coalition. The proximal LT joint is narrowed and with jagged margins. Note the subchondral bone marrow edema suggestive of active arthritis in a Minnaar type 1 LT coalition (*arrows*)

over the dorsoulnar aspect of the wrist when the forearm supinates and wrist ulnarly deviate, and the subluxation or luxation can be easily palpated and observed [14].

Closed, nonrheumatoid ruptures of the ECU tendon are rare. Partial tears are more frequent and result from chronic attrition of the tendon in patients with underlying instability or chronic stenosing tenosynovitis.

Imaging Diagnosis

Conventional radiography is usually normal. Ultrasound is the imaging method of choice in the diagnosis of the full spectrum of ECU tendon

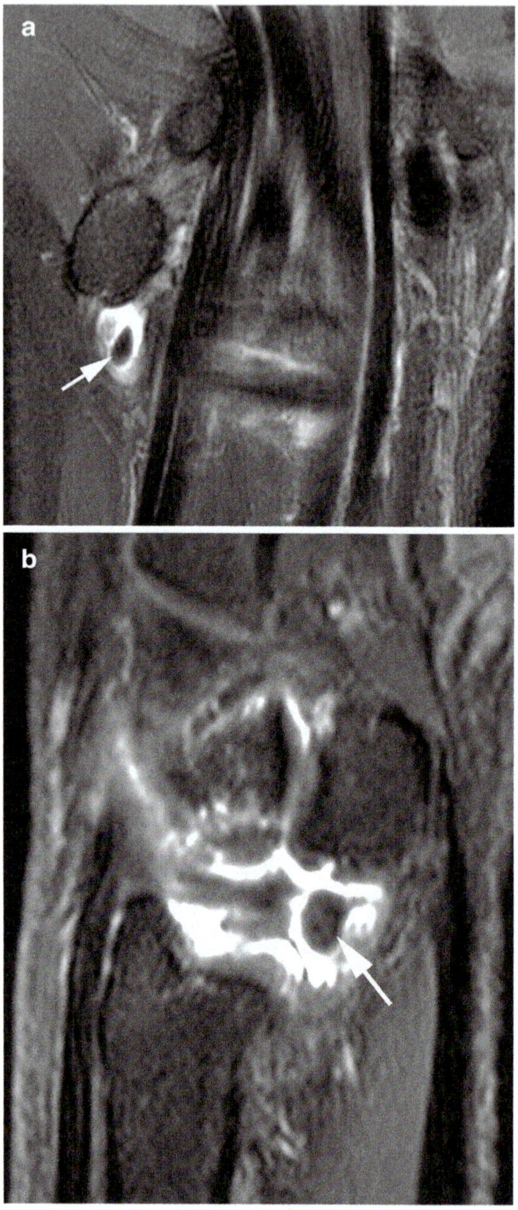

Fig. 5.30 Pisotriquetral joint arthrosis. (**a**) Coronal proton density fat-suppressed MR image shows a loose body in the proximal recess of the pisotriquetral joint (*arrow*). (**b**) Sagittal proton density fat-suppressed MR image demonstrates pisotriquetral joint osteoarthritis and secondary loose body in the proximal joint recess (*arrow*)

pathology. Dynamic ultrasound is an effective and noninvasive method of diagnosing ECU tendon subluxation or luxation [28, 40].

Tendinopathy, tenosynovitis, and tendon rupture are well evaluated by MR imaging (Figs. 5.32 and 5.33). However, both subluxation and dislocations

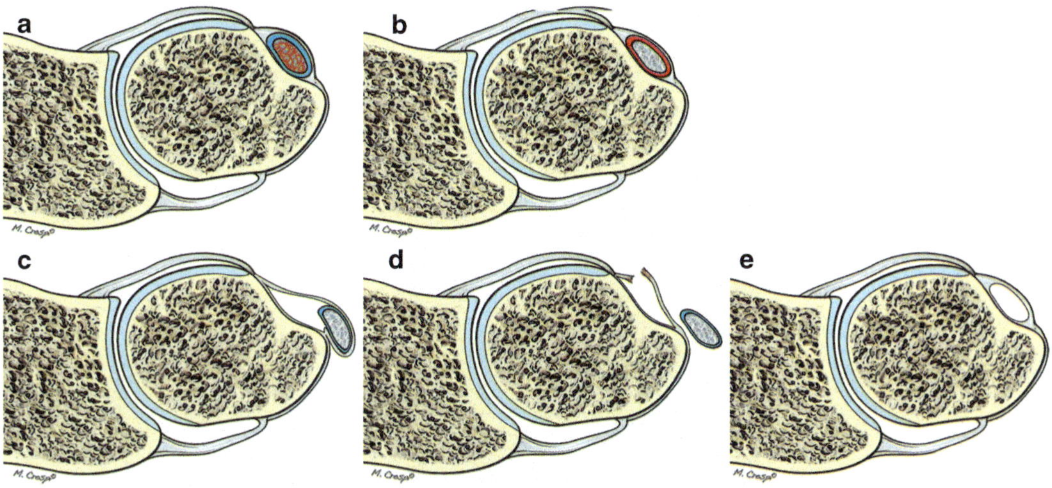

Fig. 5.31 Illustration of the spectrum of pathology of the ECU tendon. (**a**) Tendinosis. (**b**) Tenosynovitis. (**c**) Subluxation. (**d**) Luxation. (**e**) Tear

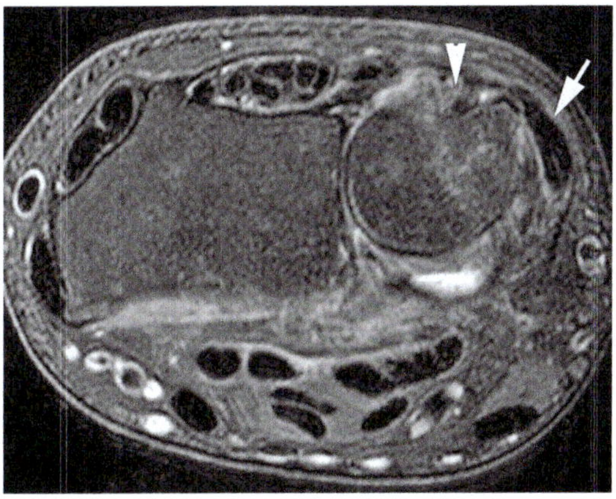

Fig. 5.32 Luxation of the ECU tendon. Axial fat-suppressed,T2-weighted MR image reveals rupture of the subsheath (*arrowhead*) and ulnar luxation of the ECU tendon (*arrow*)

are frequently missed on conventional MR imaging. Moreover, ECU subluxation is a common misdiagnosis on MR imaging performed with the new dedicated coils with the wrist in vertical position at the patient's side. The wrist is in supination and ECU adopted an anteromedial position on the groove.

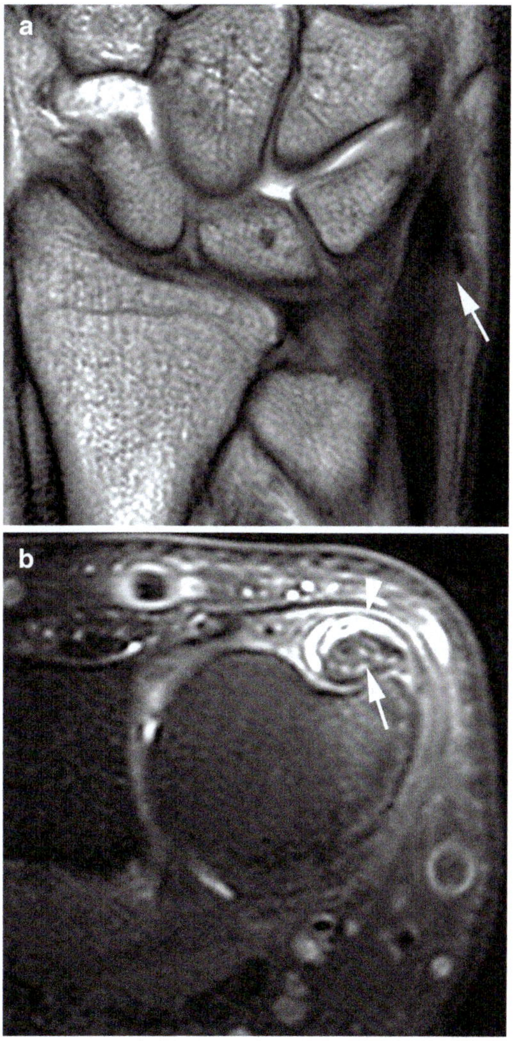

Fig. 5.33 Tenodinosis and partial tear of the ECU tendon. (**a**) Coronal T1-weighted MR image shows a tendon thickening and small superficial tear (*arrow*). (**b**) Axial fat-suppressed T2-weighted MR image reveals tendinosis (*arrow*) with associated tendon sheath distention (*arrowhead*)

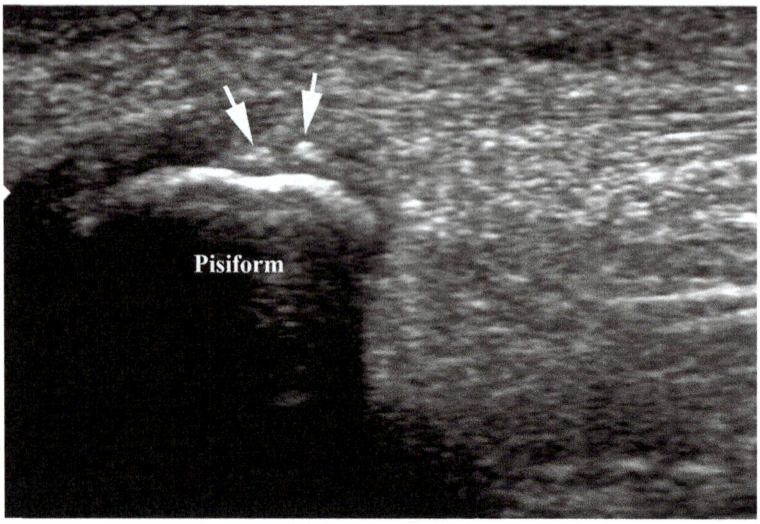

Fig. 5.34 FCU calcified tendinosis. Sagittal ultrasound image shows focal tendon thickening and small nodular intratendinous calcifications, next to pisiform insertion

Flexor Carpi Ulnaris

The spectrum of injuries of the flexor carpi ulnaris (FCU) includes tendinosis (most common calcified tendinosis) and rupture. Calcifications of the tendon sheath tend to occur most commonly close to the insertion of the FCU tendon into the pisiform [12].

Clinical findings include pain on palpation of this tendon or the pisiform and painful ulnar flexion against resistance [14].

Imaging Diagnosis

Ultrasound is the most useful imaging technique in the assessment of FCU lesions (Fig. 5.34). It permits an easy identification of tendinous changes and precise detection of small intratendinous calcifications [40]. These calcifications are usually missed on MR imaging.

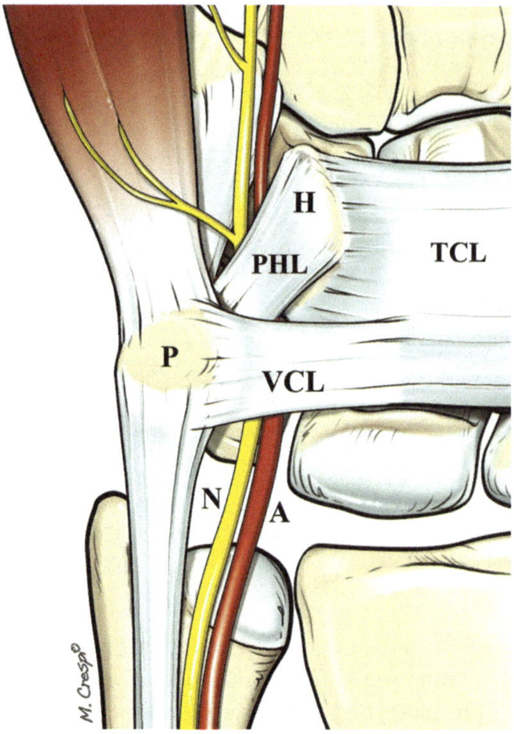

Fig. 5.35 Diagram illustrates the normal anatomy of the Guyon's canal. This tunnel is formed by two bones (the pisiform and hamate) and the ligament that connects them. *A* ulnar artery, *N* ulnar nerve, *H* hook of hamate, *PHL* pisohamate ligament, *P* pisiform, *VCL* volar carpal ligament, *TCL* transverse carpal ligament

Ulnar Nerve Neuropathy

Entrapment of the ulnar nerve in Guyon's canal (Fig. 5.35) (Guyon's canal syndrome) can be a cause of ulnar-sided wrist pain with the common causes of ulnar nerve compression, including carpal bone fractures, deformity of the carpal bone following osteoarthritis, ganglions, anomalous muscles, and ulnar artery aneurysms [8]. Symptoms include numbness and paresthesias in the distribution of the ulnar nerve: the fifth finger and the ulnar side of the fourth finger. Weakness of the abductor digiti quinti, hypothenar atrophy, intrinsic hand muscle atrophy, and/or claw hand may also be seen.

Imaging Diagnosis

Radiography and CT are useful for evaluating the abnormality of bones such as carpal bone fractures (especially the hook of the hamate) and the deformity of carpal bone following osteoarthritis. However, these techniques have a limited ability in visualizing soft tissue structures in Guyon's canal.

Dynamic and contralateral comparative ultrasound study of the Guyon's canal allows an accurate diagnosis of ulnar nerve entrapment in Guyon's canal [6].

MR imaging may identify the site of compression. Ulnar neuropathy findings on MR imaging include flattening of the nerve within Guyon's canal and proximal enlargement and edema of the ulnar nerve and its branches and muscle denervation (muscle edema in acute phase and atrophy in chronic stages) [9] (Fig. 5.36). MR imaging can show pathology that may be causing the compression such as a hamate fracture, ganglion, anomalous muscles, osteoarthritis of the pisotriquetral joint ulnar artery aneurysm, or neoplasm [9].

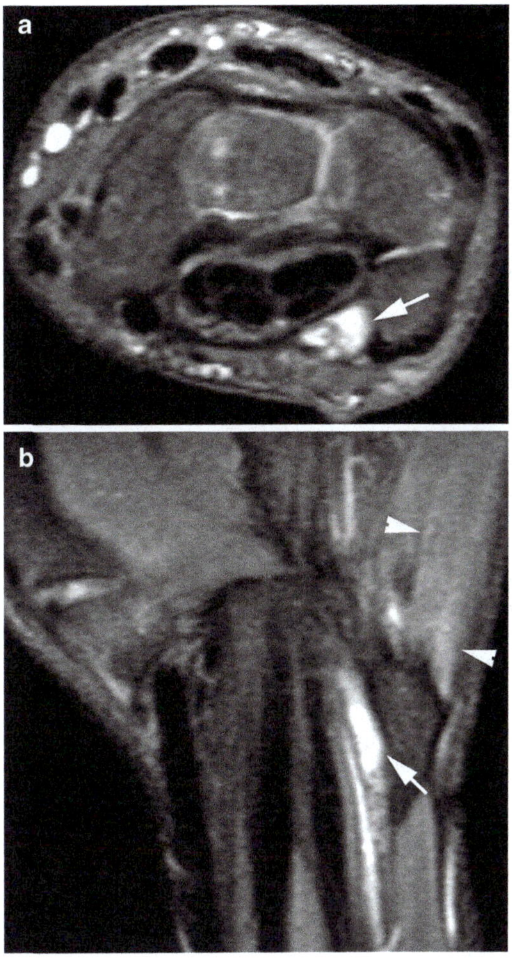

Fig. 5.36 Compressive ulnar nerve neuropathy. (**a**) Axial proton density image shows an enlarged ulnar in the Guyon's canal (*arrow*). (**b**) Coronal proton density reveals a fusiform nerve enlargement (*arrow*) and muscle edema in the hypothenar eminence (acute denervation) (*arrowheads*)

Vascular Injuries

Hypothenar Hammer Syndrome

The hypothenar hammer syndrome is caused by blunt repetitive injury to the ulnar artery and superficial palmar arch from impact against the hamulus. The ulnar artery is more prone to injury distally near the hook of the hamate because it is only covered by skin, subcutaneous fat, and the palmaris brevis muscle. Palmar arches and digital arteries also may be occluded. Typically, the resultant trauma to the hypothenar eminence is chronic, although severe acute episodes of the syndrome have been reported [8].

Intimal hyperplasia is almost invariably present in hypothenar hammer syndrome, along with duplication and fragmentation of the internal elastic lamina. Arterial wall damage may lead to aneurysm formation with or without vessel thrombosis and to microemboli formation and compression of the sensory branch of the ulnar nerve.

Patients may present with intolerance to cold, pain in the palm, numbness and ischemia in the fourth and fifth fingers, Raynaud syndrome, and a tender mass in the hypothenar eminence. Several studies suggest a high prevalence of subclinical disease among workers who use the hand as a hammer or who use vibrating tools.

Imaging Diagnosis

The diagnosis can be confirmed easily with Doppler ultrasound. However, conventional angiography, CT angiography, or MR angiography is required to determine the most appropriate treatment. MDCT angiography is the examination of choice for the detection of lesions and for

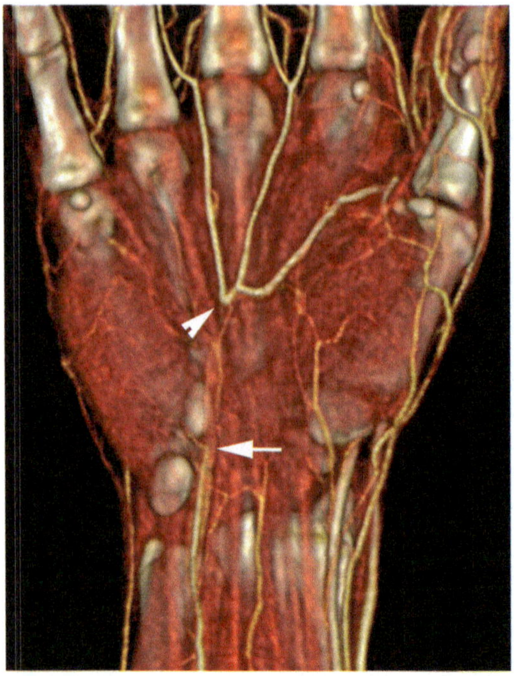

Fig. 5.37 Hypothenar hammer syndrome in a patient with acute pain in the hypothenar eminence and with paresthesia of the fourth and fifth fingers. Coronal 3D CT image shows a segmental occlusion of the ulnar artery (*arrow*). Note the normal superficial palmar arch (*arrowhead*)

precise vascular mapping (Fig. 5.37). Moreover, it can be used to rule out a hamate fracture and to show the relationship between the ulnar artery and the hamulus [8].

Conclusion

Most of the diagnosis of ulnar-sided wrist pain relies on clinical findings supported by conventional radiology. When a particular disease is suspected, it may be useful to carry out specific radiographic projections. Ultrasound is the most useful tool for the diagnosis of tendon pathology and compressive neuropathies. Ultrasound facilitates guidance of infiltrations and interventional procedures. MDCT's role is the diagnosis of occult fractures and three-dimensional evaluation of fractures, especially in articular fractures. MR imaging is a useful tool for the diagnosis of most intra-articular and extra-articular pathologies of the wrist. However, MR imaging still have two major limitations, diagnosis of lesions of TFCC Palmer class 1B and carpal instability. Arthrographic sectional techniques (CT arthrography and MR arthrography) may overcome these limitations of conventional MR imaging, allowing a precise diagnosis of TFCC lesions, LT ligament injuries, and midcarpal instability.

Acknowledgment I would like to thank my friend, Paco Piñal, whose encouragement, guidance, and support for many years have enabled me to develop an understanding of the subject.

References

1. Allende C, Le Viet D (2005) Extensor carpi ulnaris problems at the wrist: classification, surgical treatment and results. J Hand Surg Br 30:265–272
2. Amrami KK, Moran SL, Berger RA et al (2010) Imaging the distal radioulnar joint. Hand Clin 26:467–475
3. Anderson ML, Skinner JA, Felmlee JP et al (2008) Diagnostic comparison of 1.5 Tesla and 3.0 Tesla preoperative MRI of the wrist in patients with ulnar-sided wrist pain. J Hand Surg Am 33(7):1153–1159
4. Atzei A (2010) Arthroscopic management of DRUJ instability following TFCC ulnar tears. In: Del Piñal F, Mathoulin C, Luchetti R (eds) Arthroscopic management of distal radius fractures. Springer, Berlin
5. Atzei A, Luchetti R (2011) Foveal TFCC tear classification and treatment. Hand Clin 27:263–272
6. Bianchi S, Montet X, Martinoli C et al (2004) High-resolution sonography of compressive neuropathies of the wrist. J Clin Ultrasound 32(9):451–461
7. Bille B, Harley B, Cohen H (2007) A comparison of CT arthrography of the wrist to findings during wrist arthroscopy. J Hand Surg Am 32(6):834–841
8. Blum AG, Zabel JP, Kohlmann R et al (2006) Pathologic conditions of the hypothenar eminence: evaluation with multidetector CT and MR imaging. Radiographics 26:1021–1044
9. Bordalo-Rodrigues M, Amin P, Rosenberg ZS (2004) MR imaging of common entrapment neuropathies at the wrist. Magn Reson Imaging Clin N Am 12(2):265–279
10. Borelli P, Luchetti R (2010) Treatment of the associated ulnar-sided problems. In: Del Piñal F, Mathoulin C, Luchetti R (eds) Arthroscopic management of distal radius fractures. Springer, Berlin
11. Buck FM, Gheno R, Nico MAC et al (2009) Ulnomeniscal homologue of the wrist: correlation of anatomic and MR imaging findings. Radiology 253(3):771–779
12. Budoff JE, Kraushaar BS, Ayala G (2005) Flexor carpi ulnaris tendinopathy. J Hand Surg Am 30(1):125–129
13. Burns J, Tanaka T, Ueno T et al (2011) Pitfalls that may mimic injuries of the triangular fibrocartilage and

proximal intrinsic wrist ligaments at MR imaging. Radiographics 31:63–78
14. Buterbaugh GA, Brown TR, Horn PC (1998) Ulnar-sided wrist pain in athletes. Clin Sports Med 17(3): 567–583
15. Cerezal L, Del Piñal F, Abascal F et al (2002) Imaging findings in ulnar-sided wrist impaction syndromes. Radiographics 22:105–121
16. Cerezal L, Del Piñal F, Abascal F (2004) MR imaging findings in ulnar-sided wrist impaction syndromes. Magn Reson Imaging Clin N Am 12:281–299
17. Cerezal L, Abascal F, García-Valtuille R, Del Piñal F (2005) Wrist MR arthrography: how, why, when. Radiol Clin North Am 43:709–731
18. Coggins CA (2006) Imaging of ulnar-sided wrist pain. Clin Sports Med 25:505–526
19. De Filippo M, Pogliacomi F, Bertellini A et al (2010) MDCT arthrography of the wrist: diagnostic accuracy and indications. Eur J Radiol 74(1):221–225
20. del Piñal F (2009) The 1B constellation. Presented at the FESSH Congress in Poznan, Poland. Book of abstracts
21. Fontés D (2010) Lunotriquetral and extrinsic ligaments lesions associated with distal radius fractures. In: Del Piñal F, Mathoulin C, Luchetti R (eds) Arthroscopic management of distal radius fractures. Springer, Berlin
22. Friedman SL, Palmer AK (1991) The ulnar impaction syndrome. Hand Clin 7(2):295–310
23. Garcia-Elias M, Geissler WB (2005) Carpal instability. In: Green DP, Hotchkiss RN, Pederson WC, Wolfe SW (eds) Green's operative hand surgery. Elsevier Churchill Livingstone, Philadelphia
24. Goldfarb CA, Yin Y, Gilula LA, et al (2001) Wrist fractures: what the clinician wants to know. Radiology 219(1):1–18
25. Haims AH, Schweitzer ME, Morrison WB et al (2002) Limitations of MR imaging in the diagnosis of peripheral tears of the triangular fibrocartilage of the wrist. AJR Am J Roentgenol 178(2):419–422
26. Kaewlai R, Avery LL, Asrani AV et al (2008) Multidetector CT of carpal injuries: anatomy, fractures, and fracture-dislocations. Radiographics 28: 1771–1784
27. Malik AM, Schweitzer ME, Culp RW et al (1999) MR imaging of the type II lunate bone: frequency, extent, and associated findings. AJR Am J Roentgenol 173:335–338
28. MacLennan AJ, Nemechek NM, Waitayawinyu T, Trumble TE (2008) Diagnosis and anatomic reconstruction of extensor carpi ulnaris subluxation. J Hand Surg Am 33(1):59–64
29. Moritomo H, Masatomi T, Murase T et al (2010) Open repair of foveal avulsion of the triangular fibrocartilage complex and comparison by types of injury mechanism. J Hand Surg 35(12):1955–1963
30. Moser T, Dosch JC, Moussaoui A et al (2008) Multidetector CT arthrography of the wrist joint: how to do it. Radiographics 28(3):787–800
31. Nakamura T (2010) Radial side tear of the triangular fibrocartilage complex. In: Del Piñal F, Mathoulin C, Luchetti R (eds) Arthroscopic management of distal radius fractures. Springer, Berlin
32. Nishikawa S, Toh S, Miura H, Arai K (2002) The carpal detachment injury of the triangular fibrocartilage complex. J Hand Surg Br 27(1):86–89
33. Omlor G, Jung M, Grieser T, Ludwig K (2008) Depiction of the triangular fibro-cartilage in patients with ulnar-sided wrist pain: comparison of direct multi-slice CT arthrography and direct MR arthrography. Eur Radiol 19(1):147–151
34. Palmer AK (1989) Triangular fibrocartilage complex lesions: a classification. J Hand Surg Am 14:594–606
35. Papp S (2007) Carpal bone fractures. Orthop Clin North Am 38(2):251–260
36. Protopsaltis TS, Ruch DS (2010) Triangular fibrocartilage complex tears associated with symptomatic ulnar styloid nonunions. J Hand Surg 35(8): 1251–1255
37. Rüegger C, Schmid M, Pfirrmann C et al (2007) Peripheral tear of the triangular fibrocartilage: depiction with MR arthrography of the distal radioulnar joint. AJR Am J Roentgenol 188:187–192
38. Schmid MR, Schertler T, Pfirrmann CW et al (2005) Interosseous ligament tears of the wrist: comparison of multi-detector row CT arthrography and MR imaging. Radiology 237(3):1008–1013
39. Slutsky D (2011) Arthroscopic evaluation of the foveal attachment of the triangular fibrocartilage. Hand Clin 27:255–261
40. Tagliafico A, Rubino M, Autuori A et al (2007) Wrist and hand ultrasound. Semin Musculoskelet Radiol 11(2):95–104
41. Tanaka T, Ogino S, Yoshioka H (2008) Ligamentous injuries of the wrist. Semin Musculoskelet Radiol 12:359–378
42. Theumann N, Etechami G, Duvoisin B et al (2006) Association between extrinsic and intrinsic carpal ligament injuries at MR arthrography and carpal instability at radiography: initial observations. Radiology 238:950–957
43. Thurston AJ, Stanley JK (2000) Hamato-lunate impingement: an uncommon cause of ulnar-sided wrist pain. Arthroscopy 16(5):540–544
44. Timins ME (1999) Osseous anatomic variants of the wrist: findings on MR imaging. AJR Am J Roentgenol 173:339–344
45. Toms A, Chojnowski A, Cahir J (2011) Midcarpal instability: a radiological perspective. Skeletal Radiol 40:533–541
46. Topper SM, Wood MB, Ruby LK (1997) Ulnar styloid impaction syndrome. J Hand Surg Am 22:699–704
47. Trumble T (2011) Radial side (1D) tears. Hand Clin 27:243–254
48. Watanabe A, Souza F, Vezeridis PS et al (2010) Ulnar-sided wrist pain. II. Clinical imaging and treatment. Skeletal Radiol 39:837–857

6 The 1B Constellation: An Attempt to Classify Palmer 1B Class

Francisco del Piñal

In the landmark paper of Palmer [8], class 1B already revealed the difficulties inherent in any "simple" classification. A subdivision was already required (with and without styloid fracture) in an attempt to include all possible variants.

During those early years, some confusion existed as to the best way of managing the 1B tears. While arthroscopists [3] favored capsular reattachment, others preconized an open repair [7]. Furthermore, at that time, a policy of aggressive ulnar styloid fixation was in vogue. The said confusion resulted in some patients doing very well. Others, however, did not, despite a well-executed operation.

After heated (but constructive) discussions with some of the authors of this book and many other EWAS members, it dawned on me that the subdivision of type 1B into two types was too simplistic: there were three anatomic structures (TFC, capsule, and the ulnar styloid) interacting in less than 1 cm^2 (Fig. 6.1).

Each of these structures (alone or in combination) could cause pain, sense of instability, true instability, impingement symptoms, etc. To sum up, rather than a type 1B with two subtypes, there were many more possibilities, and I came up with what I named the "1B constellation" [4] (Fig. 6.2). In this classification, each of the structures (TFC, ulnar styloid, and capsule) is responsible for its own set of problems. However, although pure forms of the classification exist, structures are so close together that it is rare to find single injuries. The norm (rather than the exception) is combined forms.

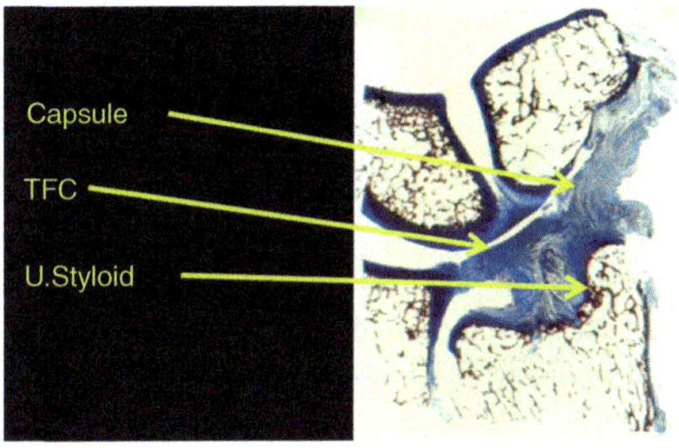

Fig. 6.1 The proximity of the TFCC, the ulnar styloid and the capsule (ECU subsheath, meniscus-collateral ligament, and ulno-carpal ligaments) are evident in this anatomic specimen borrowed from Dr. Nakamura (Fig. 2.5)

TFCC

In my present understanding of the three different pathological forms of the rupture of the TFC, the credit belongs entirely to Atzei and Luchetti [2]. They realized that a distal rupture could cause pain but no instability and that a proximal (foveal) disinsertion could cause instability despite the

F. del Piñal, M.D., Dr. Med.
Hand-wrist and Plastic Surgery,
Private Practice and Mutua Montañesa,
Paseo de Pereda 20-1°,
E-39004 Santander, Spain
e-mail: drpinal@drpinal.com, pacopinal@gmail.com

F. del Piñal et al. (eds.), *Arthroscopic Management of Ulnar Pain*,
DOI 10.1007/978-3-642-30544-3_6, © Springer-Verlag Berlin Heidelberg 2012

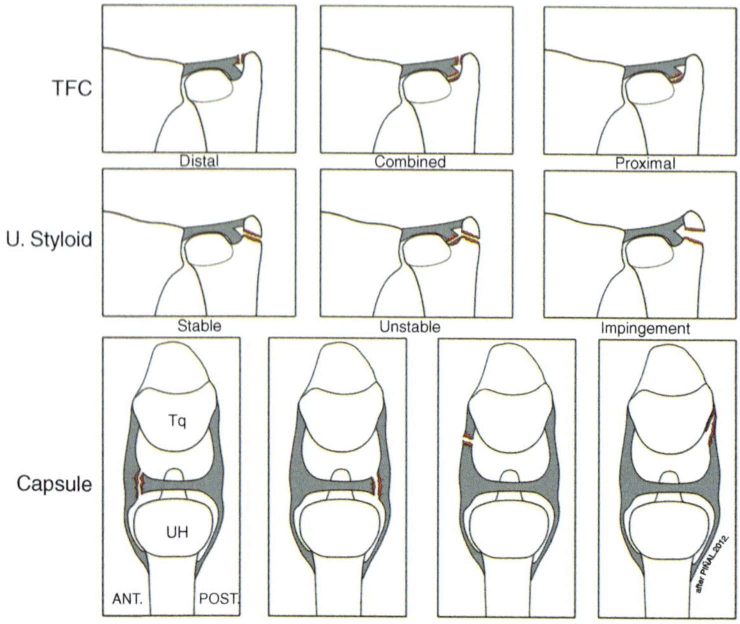

Fig. 6.2 The 1B constellation (Copyright Dr. Piñal 2012)

fact that at radiocarpal arthroscopy, the ulnar compartment could be normal. A clue for diagnosis of the different forms was the refinement of the hook test previously described by Ruch et al. [9] for distal radius fractures.

Dr. Haerle describes all this in detail in the next chapter of this book, and I send the reader there for better illustration.

Ulnar Styloid

A non-united ulnar styloid may also be an important source of pain, instability, or both. By the same token, an ulnar styloid non-union may just be a finding unrelated to the patient's complaints. The main point is that radiologically symptomatic and asymptomatic ununited ulnar styloid can look quite similar, despite the implications being quite different. Thus, the surgeon has to assess the role of each non-united styloid on the clinical picture when a patient complains about ulnar pain.

I have divided this type into three groups:

Stable: The ulnar styloid is fractured in about 50 % of distal radius fractures and remains non-united in about half of those. It rarely causes symptoms, however. This first type, which I would say is quite a common scenario, complicates the picture for the surgeon. It is paramount to discard its role on the clinical picture by exploring the wrist: maneuvers of ulnar styloid impaction (Ruby's test) and to test of DRUJ instability preoperatively are paramount. Arthroscopically, few clues will be given in this "stable-asymptomatic" type.

Unstable: It is now well known that a fracture of the styloid will not cause DRUJ instability unless the fovea itself is either also included in the fractured fragment (Fig. 6.3) or the foveal attachments to the fovea are torn concomitantly [1]. However, the acute setting does not pose so many diagnostic difficulties and purposely are left out of this classification (see also Chap. 22).

In this class, what I want to include are patients who, already having an ulnar styloid non-union, develop instability after a second traumatic event. Quite often, the energy required is rather small. The typical history is a patient who had had an old fracture in infancy with occasional or no pain at all. After a recent incident, this patient then presents with an increase in pain and a bothering sense that their wrist gives way during pronation-supination activities.

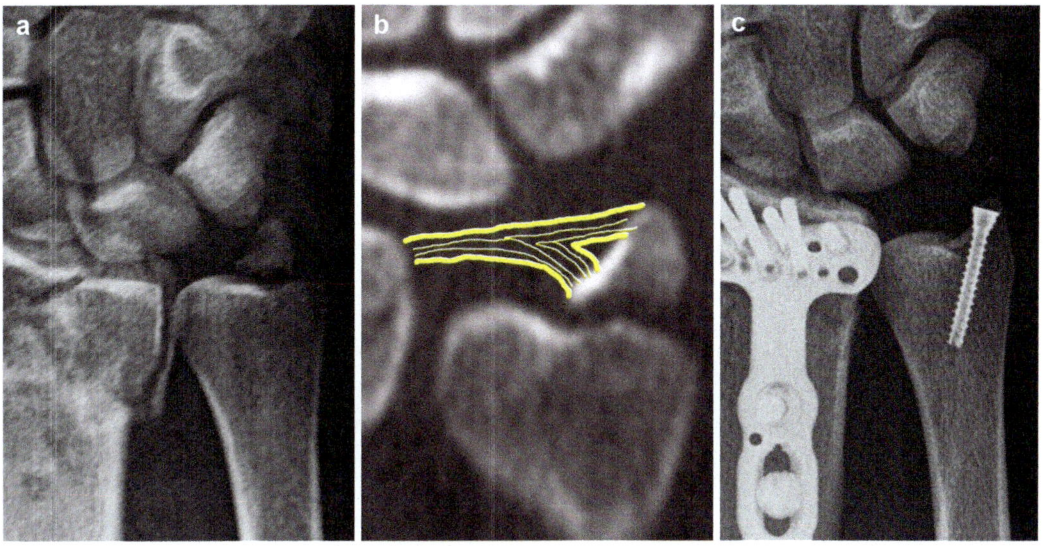

Fig. 6.3 (**a**) When the ulnar styloid fragments includes also the fovea (**a**), instability should be suspected as the deep TFC attachments will also be torn (**b**), (**c**) a screw is my preferred fixation method as it is sufficient rigid as to allow immediate mobilization (Courtesy of Dr. Piñal in [1]. Copyright by Springer-Verlag (2010))

Management includes not only reinsertion of the TFC but in my view resection of the non-united fragment. The latter acts in one way or another as a foreign body, contributing in many cases to residual ill-defined pain if not addressed (Fig. 6.4).

Impingement: In this last group, the symptoms are mechanical. The ulnar styloid fragment acts as a foreign body in the ulnar recess and progressively erodes the ulnar aspect of the triquetrum. The clinical picture is indistinguishable from the one due to a long ulnar styloid (see Chap. 14). The pathogenesis of why asymptomatic non-united styloid ceases to be so has two explanations. In one group, mostly young who sustained a benign fracture in their infancy, the styloid fragment enlarges progressively to the point of becoming a foreign body in the ulnar recess (Fig. 6.5). In the older population, ununited styloid is usually symptomatic since the day of injury. Typically, however, despite the patient's complaints, no attention had been given due to the relative minor importance in comparison to the radius fracture itself. The hope that many of those ill-defined complaints will go away, but did not, makes the patients seek a second opinion. Even minor elongations will cause symptoms! One has to understand that even if the radius is minimally shortened, it will have a detrimental effect on any relative "lengthening" of the styloid, impinging on the triquetrum even in apparently minor cases (Fig. 6.6).

Capsule

In Nakamura's hammock concept (see Chap. 2), what I call the "capsule" is formed by all peripheral and distal attachments. Admittedly, this is a wide group composed of heterogeneous structures. However, I have found it very useful for treatment and for understanding purposes to group all them together. Capsular problems are divided into four types: anterior and dorsal TFC detachments (from the capsule) and anterior and dorsal capsular detachments (from the bones).

Anterior detachments of the TFCC are very rare. I personally have seen only one case. Although now I will put a volar stitch with the technique I am using for the volar scapholunate ligament rupture [5] at the time I saw the patient, I did not have that technical recourse

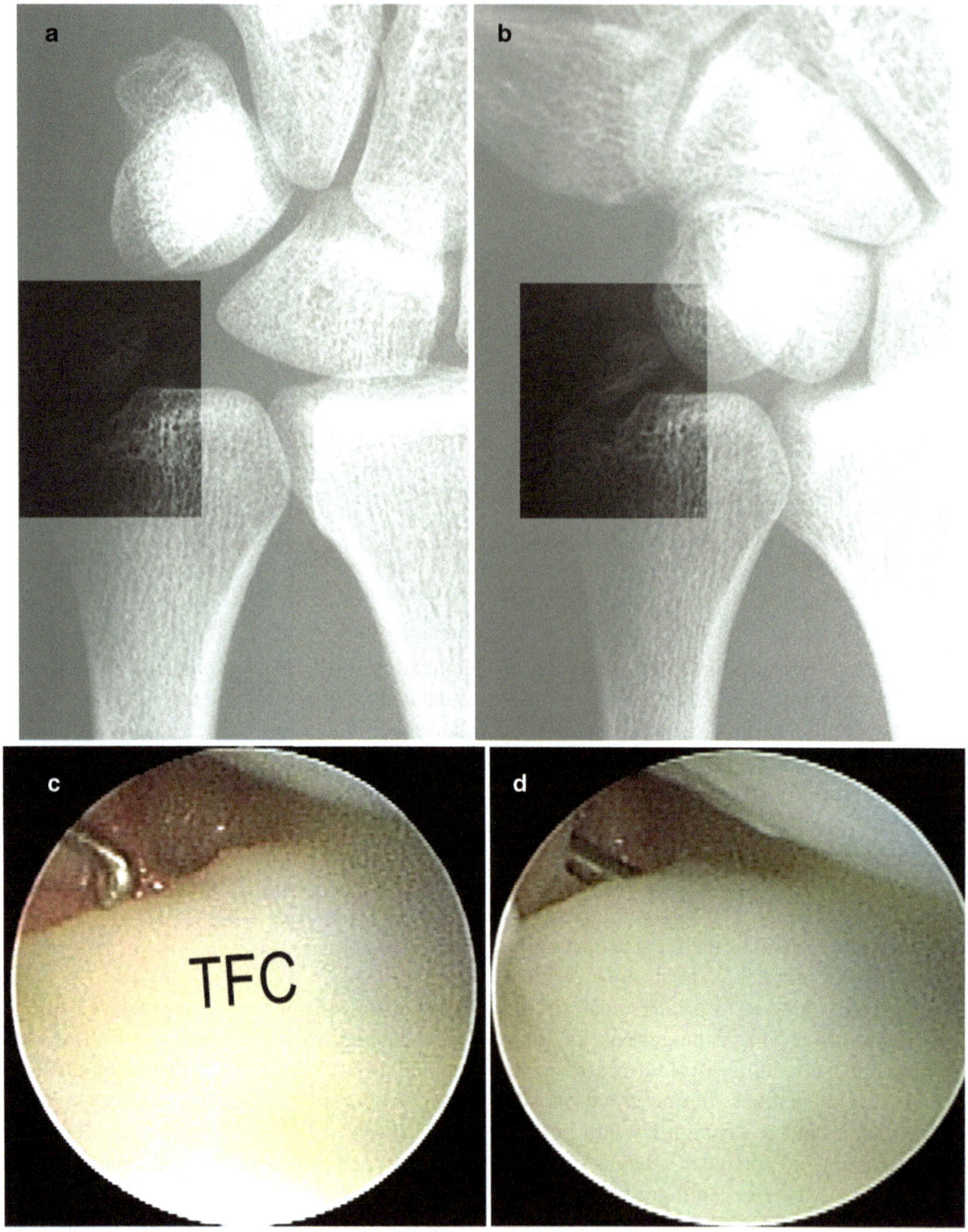

Fig. 6.4 This motocross racer had a long history of falls, including an extraarticular distal radius fracture treated conservatively 3 years previously. After a fall 3 months earlier, he noticed persistent DRUJ instability. (**a**, **b**) Subtle instability on the ulnar non-united fragment can be seen in forced ulnar deviation. (**c**, **d**) At arthroscopy, the TFC could be lifted from the foveal insertion, confirming the diagnosis of non-united styloid and foveal detachment. Treatment consisted of excision of the large non-united fragment through a 1.5-cm ulnar incision (**e**), insertion of a bone anchor in the fovea (**f**) and placement of a mattress suture under arthroscopic guidance (**g**). After 3 weeks, prono-supination was permitted. Despite our advice to wait 4 months, he resumed his competitive activity at 2.5 months (**h**) (Copyright Dr. Piñal 2012)

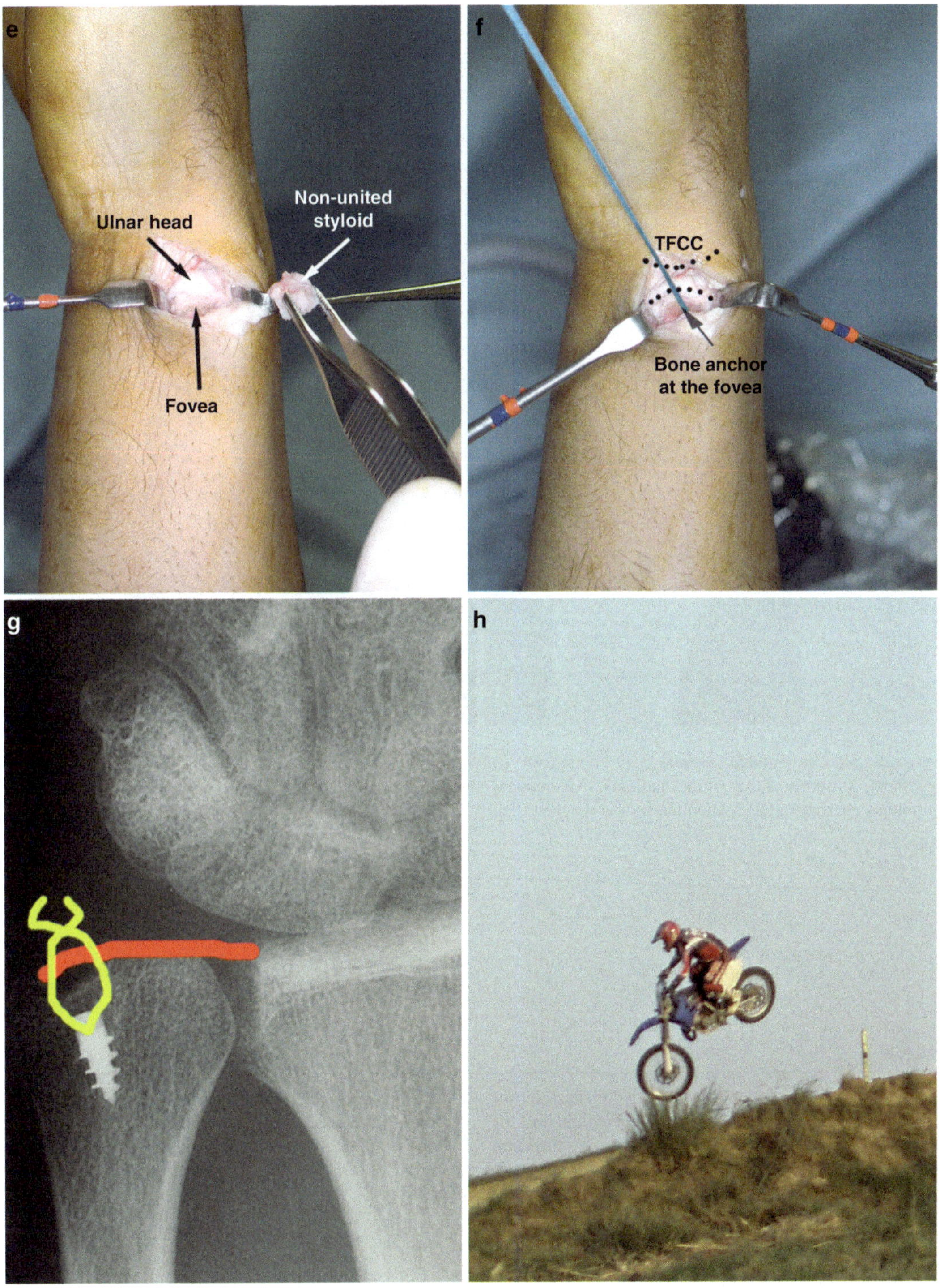

Fig. 6.4 (continued)

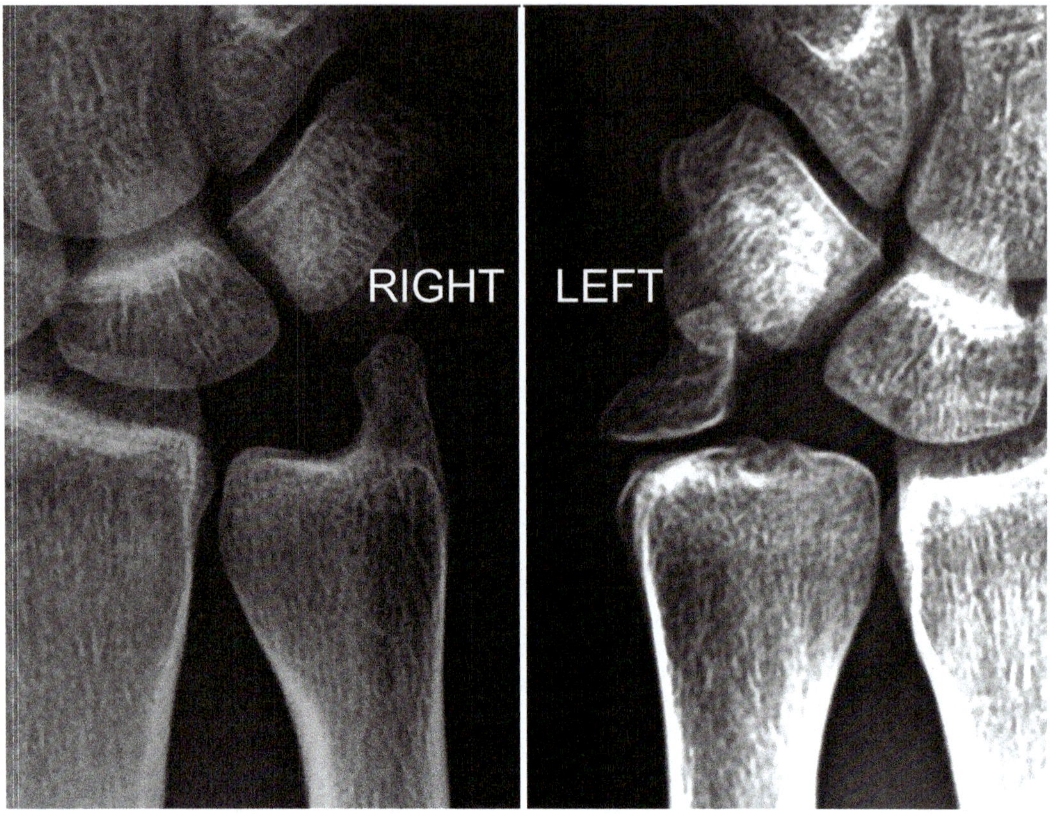

Fig. 6.5 The non-united styloid can overgrow to "gigantic" proportions in some patients. Mechanical symptoms are unavoidable when the styloid reaches such proportions. Compare the non-united with the healthy side (Copyright Dr. Piñal 2012)

Fig. 6.6 (**a**) This 65-year-old lady sustained an extraarticular fracture. Despite her bitter complaints of ulnar pain, no attention was given as the fracture had healed in a very well-aligned position. (**b**) Florid synovitis is evident in the dorsal recess of the radiocarpal joint (scope in 3–4 portal). (**c**) After the synovitis was cleared, the arthroscope could be advanced showing a large ulcer on the ulnar aspect of the triquetrum (*encircled*), caused by the (intraarticular) ulnar styloid (*US*). (**d**) Arthroscopic resection of the non-united ulnar styloid was curative (Copyright Dr. Piñal 2012)

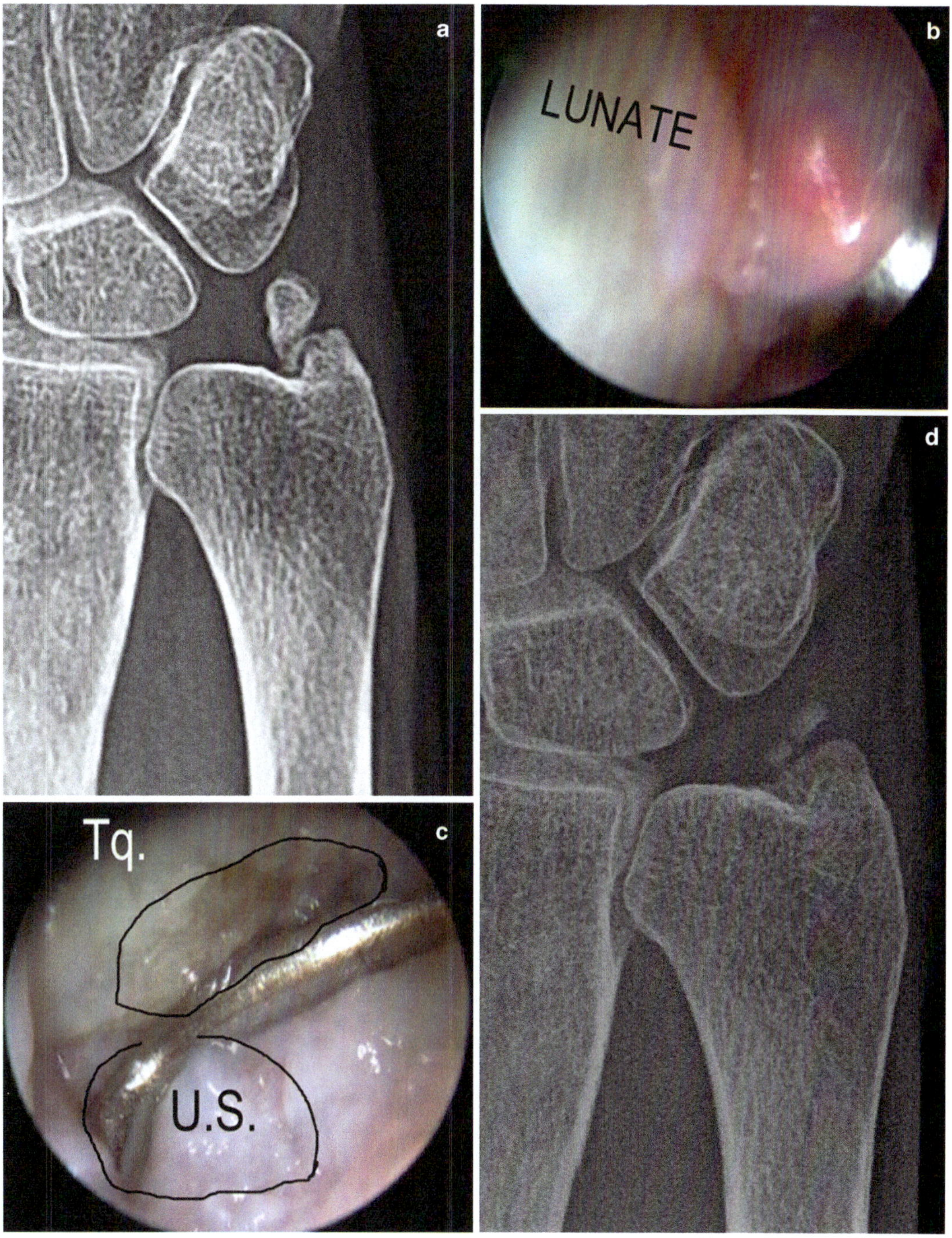
a
b
LUNATE
c
Tq.
U.S.
d

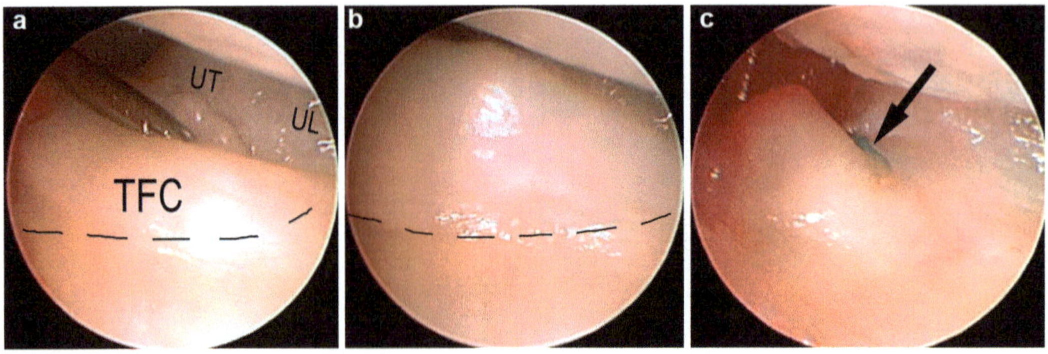

Fig. 6.7 Anterior TFCC detachment. (**a**) The probe can be seen sinking anteriorly between the TFC and the ulno-carpal ligaments (*UT* Ulno-triquetrum, *UL* Ulno-lunate). (**b**) The TFC can be seen being lifted radially with the probe. (**c**) Reinsertion to the fovea by a mattress suture (*arrow*) (Copyright Dr. Piñal 2012)

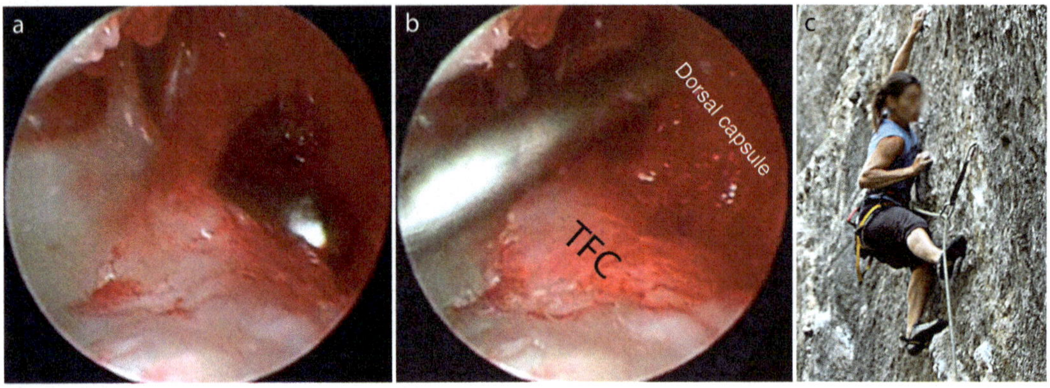

Fig. 6.8 This professional climber complained of sudden ulnar pain during a forceful motion. Conservative treatment and immobilization failed to resolve her symptoms. At arthroscopy, a partial detachment of the TFC from the capsule was seen and treated by a suture. (**a**) Notice that the probe cannot pass under the TFC (as in a total rupture), but that the smooth transition between the dorsal capsule and the disc has been lost (**b**). (**c**) Suturing the partial detached TFC to the dorsal capsule allowed her to resume her athletic activity to a professional level (Copyright Dr. Piñal 2012)

and I directly attached the TFC to the fovea with a bone anchor (Fig. 6.7).

Posterior TFC detachments, conversely, are among the most common causes of ulnar pain. The typical injury corresponds to a complete separation of the TFCC from the dorsal capsule. This entity will not be covered here as they are extensively discussed in Chap. 8. Less recognized are partial detachments that surprisingly can be very symptomatic. I have seen such partial injuries frequently in professional athletes. In my experience, partial tears respond just as well to suturing and sugar-tong splint for 3 weeks (to block the pronation-supination) as the complete tears counterparts (Fig. 6.8).

The third type of the "1B constellation" corresponds to detachments of the anterior ulno-carpal ligaments, which in fact are equivalent to the so-called 1C tears. They are extremely uncommon in my experience (as well as in the experience of other members of the EWAS). Apart from debridement, there is not much we can do arthroscopically speaking at this moment (Fig. 6.9).

Finally, I have a wide group of patients who, having sustained a fall (with the hand in supination if they recall it), a twisting injury, or a hyperflexion injury, refer chronic, unremitting pain in the dorso-ulnar region. The pain is exacerbated when pressure is applied on the dorsal

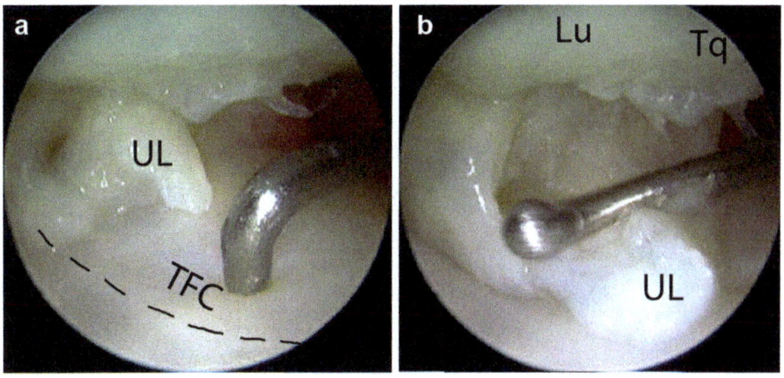

Fig. 6.9 (**a**) The distal stump of the ulno-lunate (UL) ligament can be seen "floating" freely in the joint. (**b**) When "sweeping" with the probe the ligament can still be seen connected proximally (*Lu* lunate, *Tq* triquetrum) (Copyright Dr. Piñal 2012)

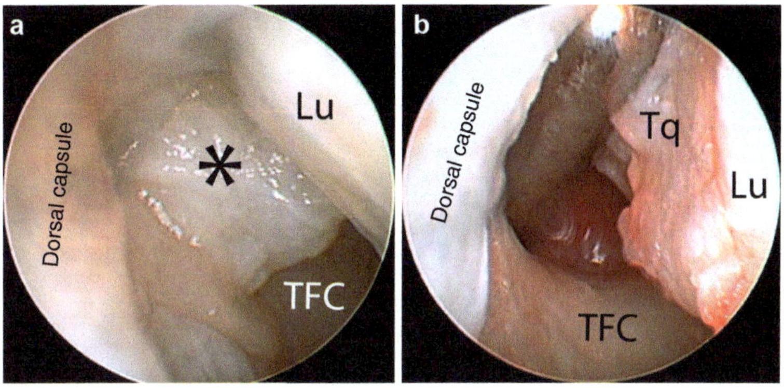

Fig. 6.10 (**a**) Hypertrophic synovium and scarred tissue (*asterisk*) is occupying the dorsal recess in this patient with dorso-ulnar pain. (**b**) Resection was curative. Notice the area of bare bone on the dorsum of the triquetrum (scope in 3–4, synoviotome in 6R, *left wrist*) (Copyright Dr. Piñal 2012)

aspect of the triquetrum by the surgeon's thumb. Typically, Ruby's maneuver (see Chap. 3) is also painful, although at times many of the ulnar maneuvers are also painful. At arthroscopy, what I have found is hypertrophic synovitis and scar tissue filling the dorso-ulnar recess. When removing this tissue, the dorsal bony surface of the triquetrum frequently becomes exposed with bare bone (Fig. 6.10).

Whether this condition is the same as the one described in Chap. 11 by Nishikawa and Toh, a form of acute impaction of the ulnar styloid while hyperextending the wrist in supination [6] or a variant of the TILT syndrome [10] is unknown. What is clear from my experience is that these patients respond very well to debridement and immediate mobilization. A word of caution should be given, as dorso-ulnar synovitis might also be present in other conditions that cause ulnar pain and are just a finding. The diagnosis of ulno-dorsal detachment can only be made by exclusion after a thorough assessment of the ulnar compartment of the wrist.

Conclusions and Limitations

Soon after I came up with this classification, I realized how incomplete it was and the difficulties one has trying to encase any medical knowledge into simple niches. Coronal and horizontal tears are among the most important subtypes that were left out of this "1B constellation." The former will be dealt with in Chap. 16, but the latter also deserves a comment, as they are not so rare.

Horizontal tears are seen after an unspecific trauma that leaves the patient with ulnar soreness and, as in one of my patients, clicking. Physical examination in the cases I have seen is unhelpful. MRI is also quite unspecific. The positive aspect about these puzzling patients is that the diagnosis is evident once the surgeon inserts the scope in 3–4 portal, and treatment takes 5 min. Resection of the "root" and removal of the piece of fibrocartilage is curative (Fig. 6.11).

In *conclusion*, I believe that it is helpful to bear several classifications in mind when trying

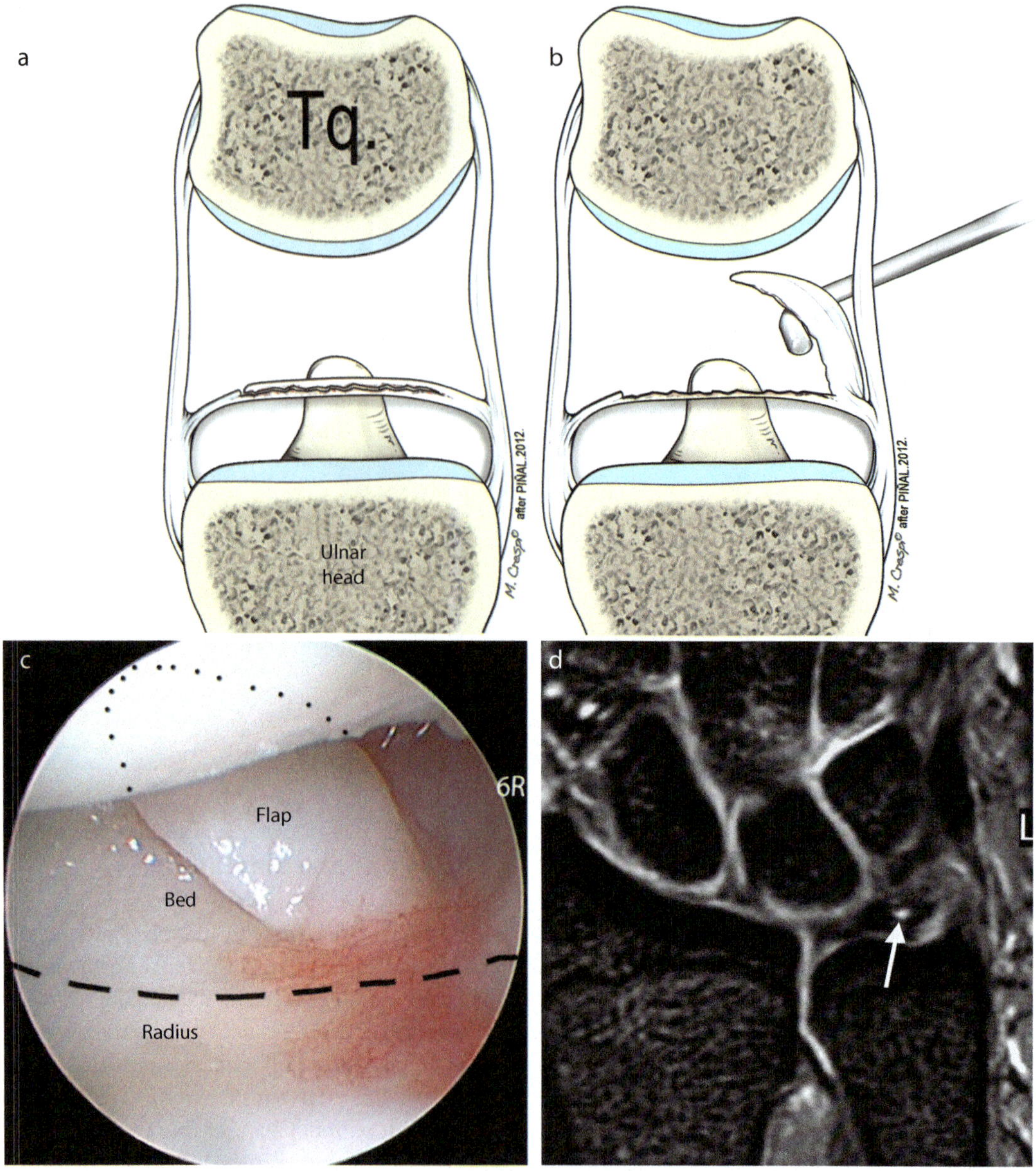

Fig. 6.11 Horizontal tear. (**a**, **b**) Schematic representation of the intraoperative findings (the probe is inserted from 6R). (**c**) Despite a confusing physical examination, the diagnosis was evident at arthroscopy. (**d**) Only in retrospect were the importance of the cystic changes at the disc (*arrow*) brought into attention (Copyright Dr. Piñal 2012)

to assign a condition to a patient without a diagnosis. Nevertheless, just as important as this is to know that the patient may not fit in any of the established groups, simply because there is still very much for us to learn.

References

1. Atzei A (2010) Arthroscopic management of DRUJ instability following TFCC ulnar tears. In: del Piñal F, Mathoulin C, Luchetti C (eds) Arthroscopic management of distal radius fractures. Springer, Berlin, pp 73–88
2. Atzei A, Garcia LR, Elias M (2007) Lesioni capsulo-legamentose Della radio-ulnare distale e fibrocartilagine triangolare. In: Landi A, Catalano F, Luchetti R (eds) Trattato di chirurgia Della mano. Verduci Editore, Roma, pp 159–187
3. de Araujo W, Poehling GG, Kuzma GR (1996) New Tuohy needle technique for triangular fibrocartilage complex repair: preliminary studies. Arthroscopy 12:699–703
4. del Piñal F (2009) The 1B constellation. Presented at the FESSH Congress in Poznan, Poland. Book of abstracts
5. del Piñal F, Studer A, Thams C, Glasberg A (2011) An all-inside technique arthroscopic suturing of the volar scapholunate ligament. J Hand Surg Am 36:2044–2046
6. Garcia-Elias M (1987) Dorsal fractures of the triquetrum-avulsion or compression fractures? J Hand Surg Am 12:266–268
7. Hermansdorfer JD, Kleinman WB (1991) Management of chronic peripheral tears of the triangular fibrocartilage complex. J Hand Surg Am 16:340–346
8. Palmer AK (1989) Triangular fibrocartilage complex lesion: a classification. J Hand Surg Am 14A: 494–606
9. Ruch DS, Yang CC, Smith BP (2003) Results of acute arthroscopically repaired triangular fibrocartilage complex injuries associated with intra-articular distal radius fractures. Arthroscopy 19:511–516
10. Weinzweig J, Watson HK (1999) Triquetral impaction ligament tear (TILT). J Hand Surg 24B:321–324

7 Central TFCC Debridement: Technique and Indication in the Twenty-First Century

Terry L. Whipple

Introduction

As described in Chaps. 1 and 2, the anatomy of the triangular fibrocartilage complex (TFCC) is complex, including an important prestyloid synovial recess at the volar, ulnar margin of the disc. The ulnar styloid process is the hub of rotation for the radio-carpal and ulno-carpal joints through pronation and supination of the forearm. The prestyloid recess accommodates the head of the ulna in positions of forearm supination as the TFCC sweeps dorsally across the seat of the ulna. Alternatively, the recess is covered by the volar and central portions of the TFCC in varying degrees of pronation [12] (Fig. 7.1).

Biomechanically, greatest strain is applied along the volar margin of the disc in full forearm supination and along the dorsal margin during full pronation. Along these margins, the TFCC is thickened and blends with fibrous connective tissue known as the volar and dorsal radio-ulnar ligaments.

The thinner central disc is composed of fibrocartilage containing both type 1 and type 2 collagen for flexibility, as well as abundant fibrous tissue for toughness. The central disc of the TFCC is interposed between the prominent seat of the ulna and the ulnar aspect of the proximal pole of the lunate as well as the proximal pole of the triquetrum. With applications of axial loading forces, the central TFCC disc becomes compressed between those bony structures.

On its radial edge, the central disc blends into the hyaline cartilage of the distal radius sigmoid notch (Fig. 7.2). At this juncture, there is a loss of fibrous composition and a reduced number of cellular lacunae, constituting a weaker area of the central disc and increased susceptibility to injury.

Obviously, the greater the length of the ulna, the greater is the compression load on the TFCC central disc. The ulna is relatively longer than the radius in cases of positive ulnar variance [5] or in increasing degrees of pronation as the diaphysis of the radius rotates around the ulna. During forearm rotation, the radius passes from a parallel alignment relative to the ulna in supination to an oblique alignment in pronation, the radius thus being relatively shorter than the ulna at the wrist in full pronation.

Mechanism of Injury

Mechanisms of injury to the central disc of the TFCC are essentially functions of excessive traumatic compression or chronic shear between the seat of the ulna and the proximal carpal row

T.L. Whipple, M.D.
Chief of Orthopaedics, American Self, PLC, Richmond, VA, USA

Associate Professor of Orthopaedic Surgery, Virginia Commonwealth University, Richmond, VA, USA

Director, Orthopaedic Research of Virginia, Richmond, VA, USA
e-mail: whipple@americanself.com

F. del Piñal et al. (eds.), *Arthroscopic Management of Ulnar Pain*,
DOI 10.1007/978-3-642-30544-3_7, © Springer-Verlag Berlin Heidelberg 2012

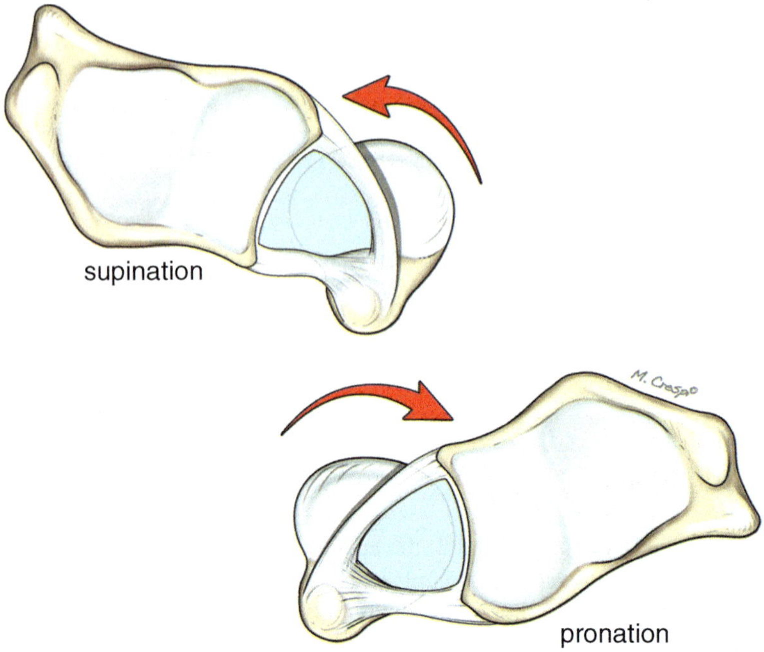

Fig. 7.1 Rotational relationship between the prestyloid recess and the TFCC

(Palmer 2C and Palmer 1A) [6]. Compression loads are most common during falls in which an individual absorbs the force of the fall with an outstretched hand.

When an individual falls forward onto the hands, axial load is applied to the wrist in forearm pronation. The radius being in a shortened position relative to the ulna, central disc compression is unavoidable (Figs. 7.3 and 7.4). Backward falls onto the hands usually occur with the forearm supinated and with the central TFCC disc less exposed, although simultaneous ulnar deviation of the wrist increases compression on the disc somewhat.

Thus, the central TFCC disc is in greatest jeopardy during forearm pronation combined with axial load, although that is not the only circumstance in which it can be injured. In wrists with positive ulnar variance, chronic shearing forces are applied to the central disc through years of repeated forearm rotation and may create wear attrition to the central disc cartilage (Fig. 7.5) [5, 12]. It should be taken into account that superimposed traumatic tears on degenerative tears are often seen (Fig. 7.6).

Indications for Surgery

The central disc is essentially avascular (Fig. 7.7). As such, it possesses little potential to heal if torn or ruptured. When degenerative or traumatic disruption of the central TFCC disc results in painful symptoms, treatment is directed at removal of any loose flaps or shards of cartilage to avoid additional compression between the lunate and the ulnar seat as, during wrist motion, this can produce sensitive traction applied to the peripheral aspects of the TFCC attachments [2].

Debridement or excision of the central disc poses no loss to the stabilizing function of the TFCC for the distal radio-ulnar joint [4, 7]. The central disc plays a lesser role than the thicker dorsal and volar TFCC ligaments in stabilizing the distal radio-ulnar joint. In cases of positive ulnar variance, however, removal of the central disc may result in increased shear contact between the hyaline cartilage of the lunate and the prominent ulna seat.

As in the case of the medial and lateral menisci of the knee, preserved thick peripheral rims of the disc help to share axial load and shear forces

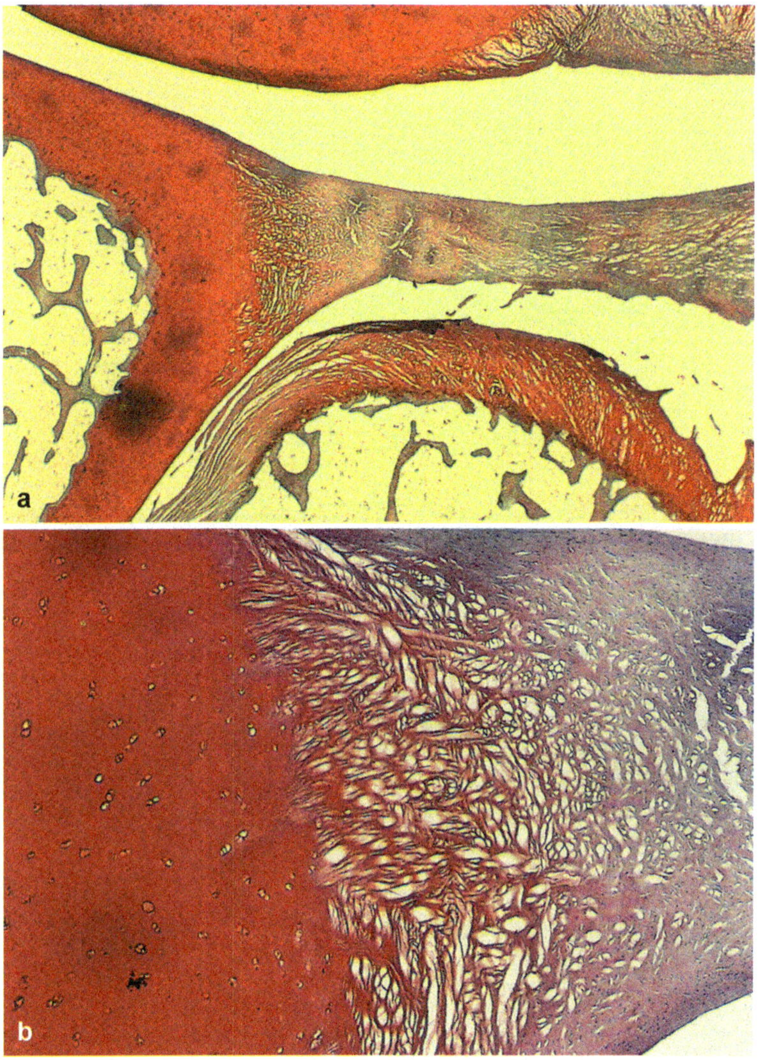

Fig. 7.2 Photomicrograph showing triangular fibrocartilage complex central disc attachment to the radius. (**a**) Fibers of the central disc are attached to the distal ulnar corner of the sigmoid notch distal to the head of the ulna. (**b**) Fibrocartilage fibers merge with hyaline cartilage of the articular surfaces of the radius. Safanin-O stain (Courtesy of B. Mandelbaum, M.D., Santa Monica, CA. Reproduced with permission from Lippincott, Philadelphia)

between the adjacent articular cartilage surfaces. Thus, repair or reconstruction of peripheral injuries to the TFCC is essential in the wrist whereas the central disc may be removed without loss of wrist function except in cases of positive ulnar variance.

Should a tear of the central TFCC disc extend to the marginal vascular elements at its periphery, there is some potential for reconstitution of the central defect from remodeling of a fibrous clot formed from those small vessels over time. Tatebe et al. reported observation of such reconstitution in 50 % of patients who had TFCC central disruptions and underwent ulnar shortening osteotomies [9]. Unglaub et al. have documented the presence of vascular elements at the periphery of central TFCC tears in 43 % of patients biopsied at the time of central disc debridement [11].

Surgical Technique

Here, it should be noted that without the use of preoperative wrist arthrography or MRI (which is less sensitive), some tears of the central TFCC disc are not evident until the time of arthroscopic examination. A hook probe should

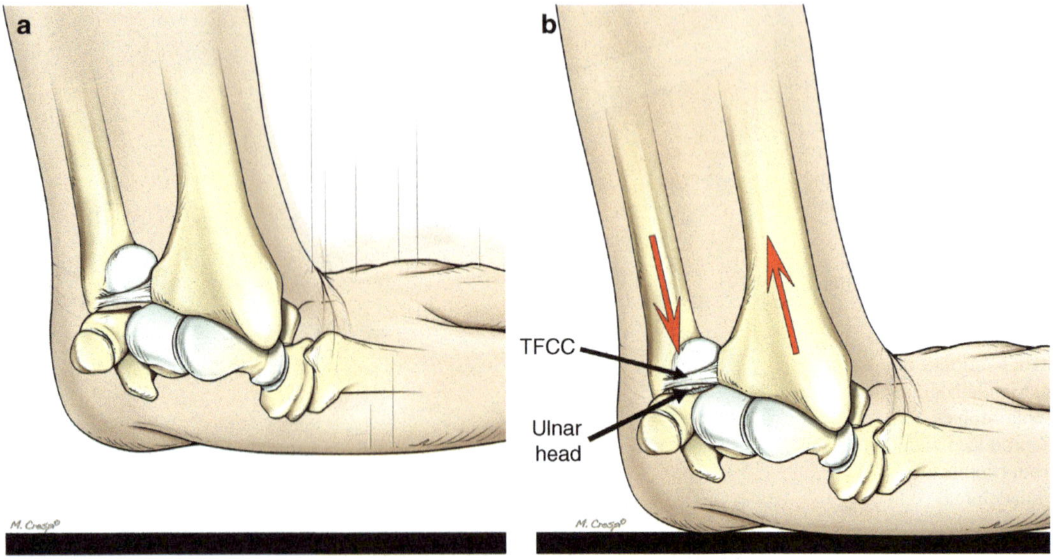

Fig. 7.3 Forward fall onto left hand in forearm pronation. (**a**) Radius is foreshortened in pronation. (**b**) Axial load transfers force to radius as the ulna tears through the TFCC central disc

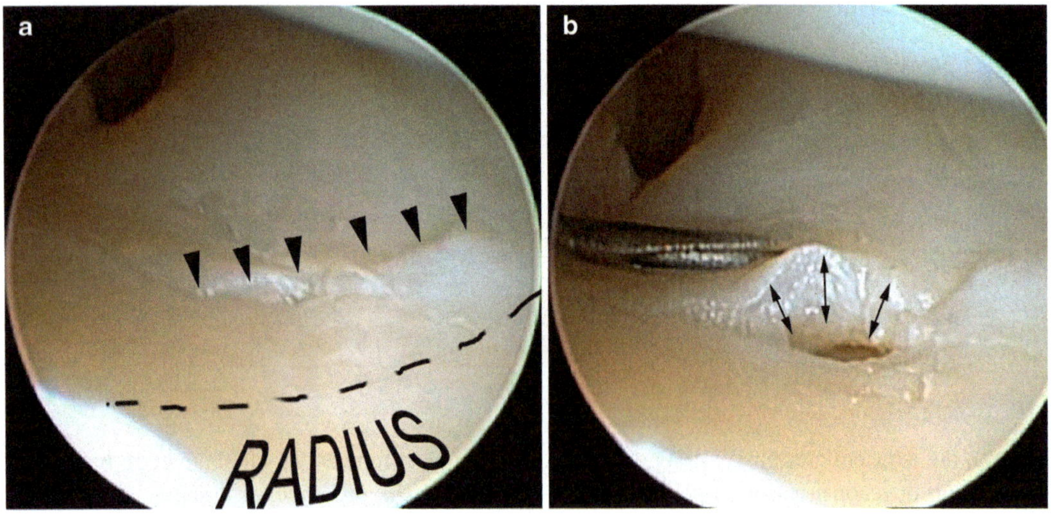

Fig. 7.4 (**a**) Traumatic central tear (Palmer IA) in a left wrist as viewed from 3–4 portal. *Arrowheads* point to the tear. The *dashed line* marks the junction of the TFC and the lunate fossa. (**b**) The ulnar flap is being lifted with a needle inserted from 6R. Notice the thickness of the TFC and that the tear involves the full thickness (*double arrows*) (Courtesy of Dr. Piñal © 2011)

always be employed to explore the integrity of the central disc. This will permit the demonstration of unstable flap tears of the disc that may cause impingement pain as opposed to simple longitudinal tears or perforations that are otherwise stable lesions (Fig. 7.8).

Similarly, certain examination techniques are advisable. Compressing or pinching the patient's distal radio-ulnar joint (DRUJ) when the radiocarpal joint is inflated with saline will cause synovium to protrude from the DRUJ through an obscure tear in the disc (Fig. 7.9). The author has

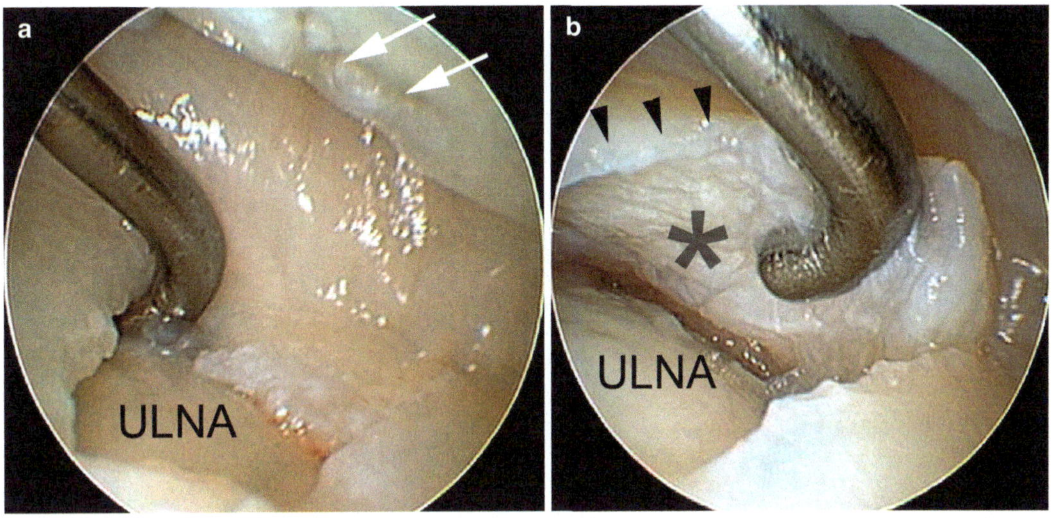

Fig. 7.5 (**a**) Large central perforation of the TFC disc due to degenerative, chronic shear forces (Palmer type 2C). Note chondromalacia on the lunate (*white arrows*), (**b**) Notice that contrary to a traumatic tear (Palmer type 1A), the edges of the disc are extremely thinned, (*arrowheads*) and the undersurface is worn down (*asterisk*). Viewed through the 3–4 portal with hook probe through the 6R portal (Courtesy of Dr. Piñal © 2011)

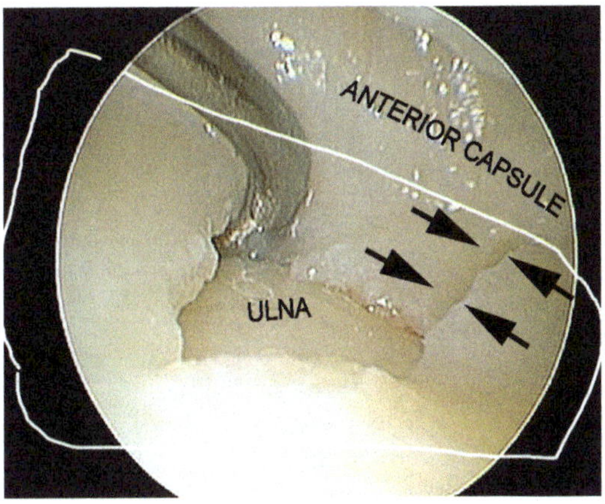

Fig. 7.6 Traumatic tear (Palmer type 1A) superimposed on a degenerative tear (Palmer type 1C). This positive ulnar variance patient suffered a twisting injury and referred pain and clicks afterward. Notice the traumatic tear (limited by *arrows*) going all the way to the volar capsular attachments (the outline of the disc in *white*) (Courtesy of Dr. Piñal © 2011)

dubbed this a "poor man's arthrogram" as no radiographs or contrast material are necessary.

A variety of approaches are recommended for removal of the central TFCC disc [12]. Surgical access approaches are similar, regardless of the method used. The author prefers vertical traction of 4–5 kg applied to the wrist through soft finger traps on the index and long fingers using a traction tower (Figs. 7.10 and 7.11). Optimal visualization is obtained with the arthroscope placed through the 3–4 portal. The 6R portal is the best working portal for accessory cutting instruments (Fig. 7.12). The edges of the tear are resected as necessary to prevent their painful entrapment, but utmost care should be taken to preserve the palmar and dorsal radio-ulnar ligaments. In most cases, a suction punch or a straight and 30° angled basket forceps are sufficient to debride the tear. Scant loose shards can be debrided with a 2.0 or 2.9 mm full radius resector blade on a powered shaver or with a similar sized radiofrequency ablator (Fig. 7.13) [12].

Variations, depending on preference of access, employ the 6U or the 4–5 working portal. Often, it is necessary to exchange the arthroscope to the 6R and the cutting instruments to the 3–4 portal to access the most ulnar part of the disc. With a suction punch or basket through the 6R portal, the volar and radial portions of central disc can be excised, protecting the volar radioulnar ligament. Then switching arthroscope to the 6R portal and the punch to the 3–4 or the 6U portal, the dorsal portion of the disc can be excised, still protecting the dorsal radioulnar ligament (Fig. 7.14).

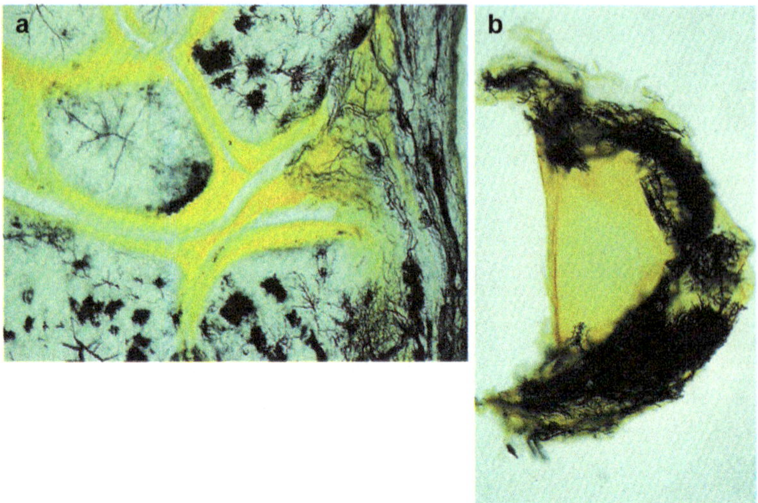

Fig. 7.7 Photomicrograph (whole mount) showing the vascular supply to the triangular fibrocartilage complex central disc. India ink injection demonstrates the capillary network in the peripheral one-third of the articular disc. The central two-thirds are avascular. (**a**) Coronal section. (**b**) Transverse section (Courtesy of S. Arnoczky, DVM, East Lansing, MI. Reproduced with permission from Lippincott, Philadelphia)

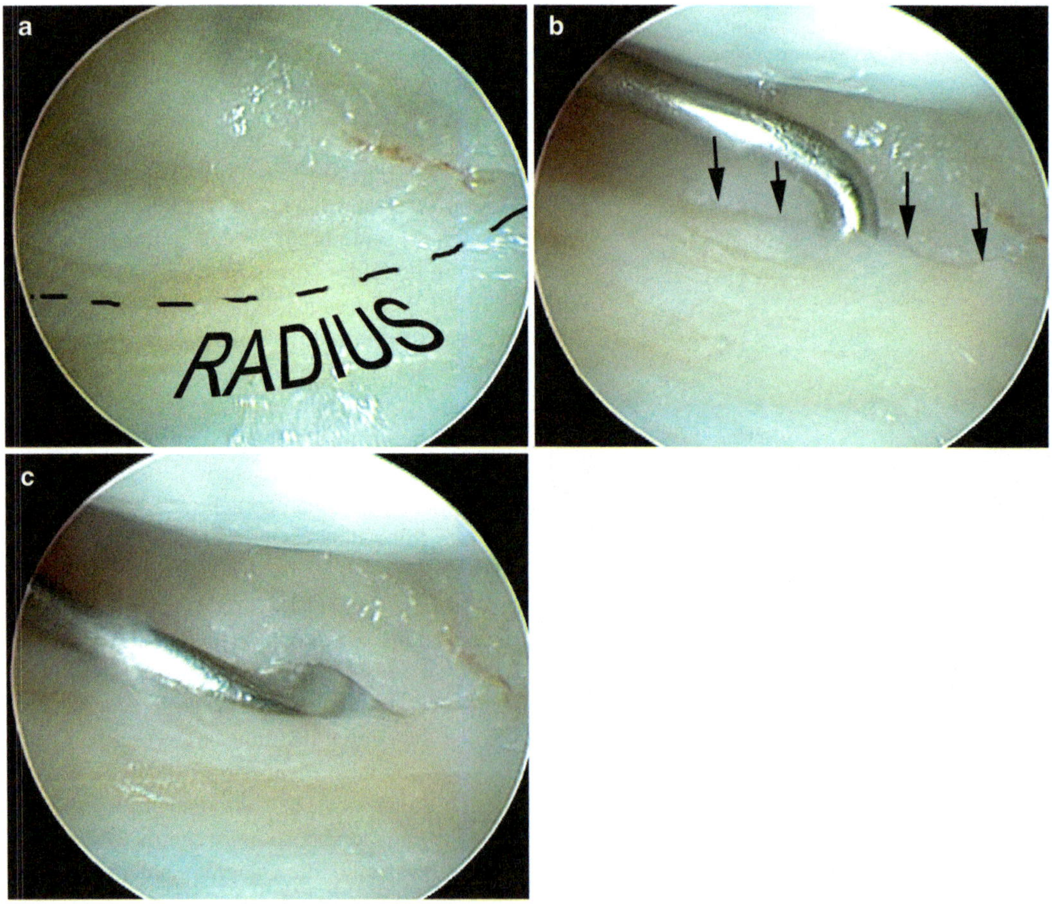

Fig. 7.8 Ulnar view of the left wrist from 3–4 portal. (**a**) The TFC is apparently normal, but during probing, the tear is identified (*arrows*) (**b**) and its instability is shown. (**c**) As the tear does not reach the DRUJ ligaments, simple debridement will be sufficient (Courtesy of Dr. Piñal © 2011)

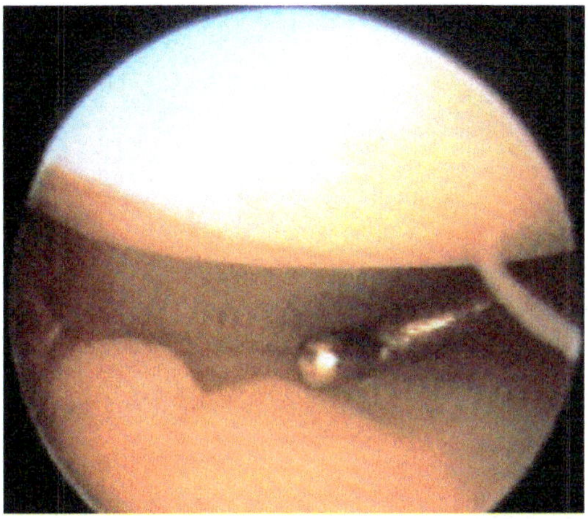

Fig. 7.9 Right wrist with occult tear of the TFCC central disc evidenced by protrusion of DRUJ synovium through an obscure defect in the fibrocartilage in response to anterior-posterior pressure applied to the distal radio-ulnar joint. Viewed through the 3–4 portal (Reproduced with permission from Lippincott, Philadelphia)

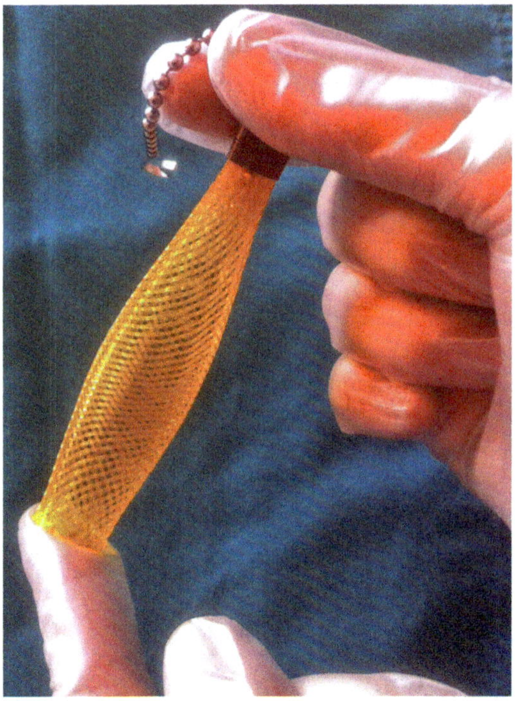

Fig. 7.10 Nylon finger trap is disposable, soft, and flexible (Linvatec, Largo, FL) (Reproduced with permission from Lippincott, Philadelphia)

Alternatively, a "banana" blade can be inserted through the 6R portal. By rotating the blade to cut first the volar and ulnar attachments,

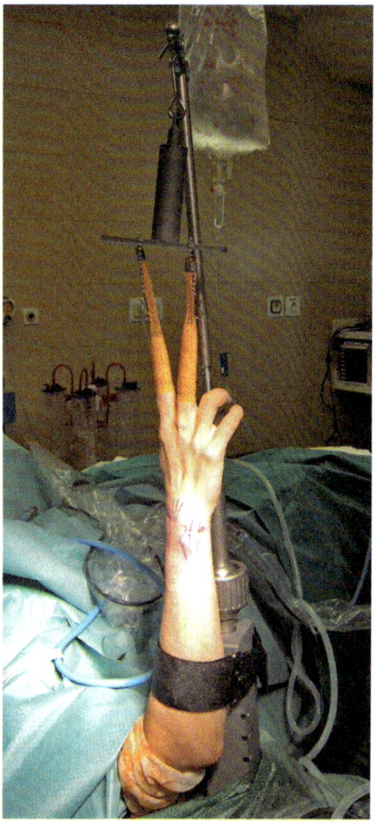

Fig. 7.11 Traction applied through finger traps on index and long fingers using Traction Tower™ (Linvatec, Largo, FL) (Reproduced with permission from Lippincott, Philadelphia)

then rotating in the opposite direction to cut the volar and radial attachments, all but the dorsal side of the TFCC disc can be incised. The leading tip of the blade then can be swept lateral to medial to incise the remaining dorsal attachment. Exchange the "banana" blade for a mosquito grasping forceps to remove the large free fragment from the joint. Then, any irregularities can be debrided smooth with a full radius resector blade (Fig. 7.15).

It has been reported that a bipolar radiofrequency ablator probe [5] or specific laser wave lengths introduced arthroscopically through rod lenses [3] can also be used safely and effectively to debride the entire central articular disc of the TFCC or to trim smooth the remaining edges of a mechanically excised disc. The author's experience with these modalities is limited, but caution should be exercised to avoid inadvertent damage

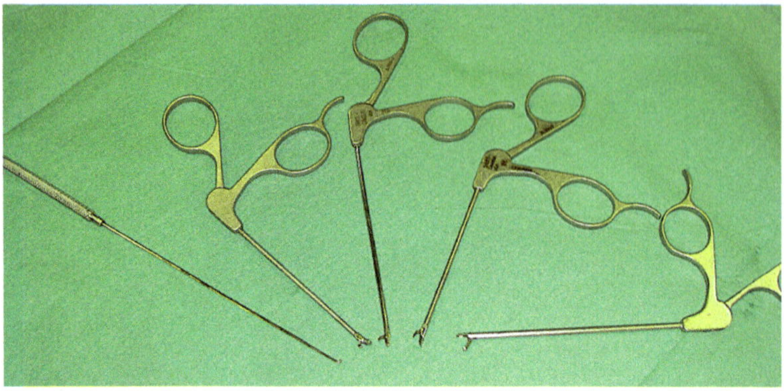

Fig. 7.12 Miniature suction punch (Linvatec, Largo, FL) connects to wall suction to aspirate tissue fragments excised by the punch-and-die design jaws. Different angle basket forceps

to the underlying articular cartilage on the seat of the ulna head when employing either laser energy or radiofrequency to vaporize the centrum of the TFCC disc.

Concurrent Ulnar Shortening

Safar has documented well the impact of an excessively longer ulna bone on the TFCC [8]. Normally, the seat of the ulna does not extend beyond the level of the medial edge of the lunate fossa of the radius bone. When it does, a condition described as "positive ulnar variance," the TFCC central disc is compressed between the seat of the ulna and the proximal carpal row, especially in positions of forearm pronation.

In cases of positive ulnar variance, a "wafer" procedure should be performed to shorten the prominent ulna by resection of the most distal 2–3 mm of the seat of the ulna [1, 10] (see Chap. 13 for technical details). In those instances after the tourniquet is deflated, postoperative bleeding from the exposed cancellous bone at the distal ulna will produce a blood clot in the ulnar aspect of the wrist. By immobilizing the wrist in forearm supination with a long arm cast for 2 weeks, the clot will adhere to the cut surface of the remaining peripheral rim of the TFCC. Over time, in approximately three postoperative months, the clot will begin to remodel into fibrous tissue with the influx of stem cells from the bone marrow that ultimately mature into spindle cells and fibrocytes. Production of new collagen results in a fibrous clot that will remodel over time into fibrocartilage to fill the defect in the TFCC. In the author's experience, this process will often reconstitute the central disc of the TFCC, as observed during second-look arthroscopic examinations, the eventual advantage being to protect the proximal pole of the lunate from the irregular cut surface of the resected seat of the ulna.

In cases of negative ulnar variance where a wafer procedure or ulna shortening is unnecessary, still an attempt can be made to reconstitute the TFCC central disc after excision by injecting into the wrist joint 2 cc of autologous blood, which also contains stem cells, at the conclusion of the surgical procedure. The wrist is then immobilized in a position of supination for 2 weeks.

Alternatively, without the effort to reconstitute the central disc after excision, and in the absence of other concurrent injury or procedure in the extremity, postoperative care would consist of immediate mobilization of the wrist and forearm. However, axial or impact loading should be avoided, as well as extremes of pronation, supination, and ulnar deviation of the wrist for approximately 4 weeks.

Discussion

Excision of the central disc of the TFCC has proven inconsequential for subsequent wrist mobility and function [4]. Whereas the dorsal and volar radio ulnar ligaments of the TFCC contribute extensively to the stability of the distal radio ulnar joint and prevent dorsal subluxation

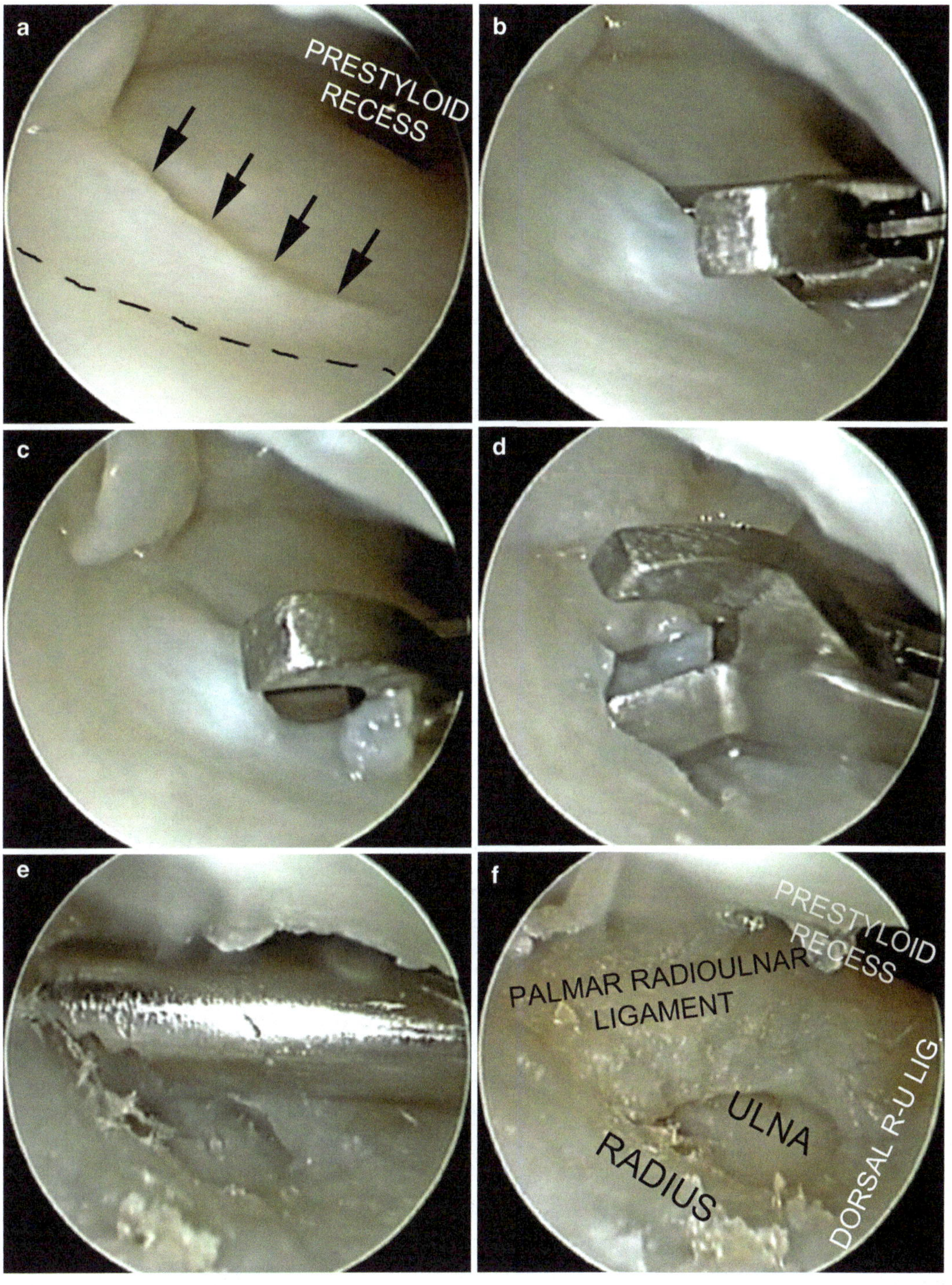

Fig. 7.13 (**a–d**) The unstable tear flaps (*arrows*) are resected with a different angle basket forceps taking care not to violate the palmar and dorsal radio-ulnar ligaments. (**e**) With a 2.9-mm shaver, the debris are aspirated and the edges of the flaps are smoothed. (**f**) Final appearance. Notice that the most anterior and dorsal parts of the TFC have been untouched. (Right wrist, scope in the 3–4, instruments in the 6R) (Courtesy of Dr. Piñal © 2011)

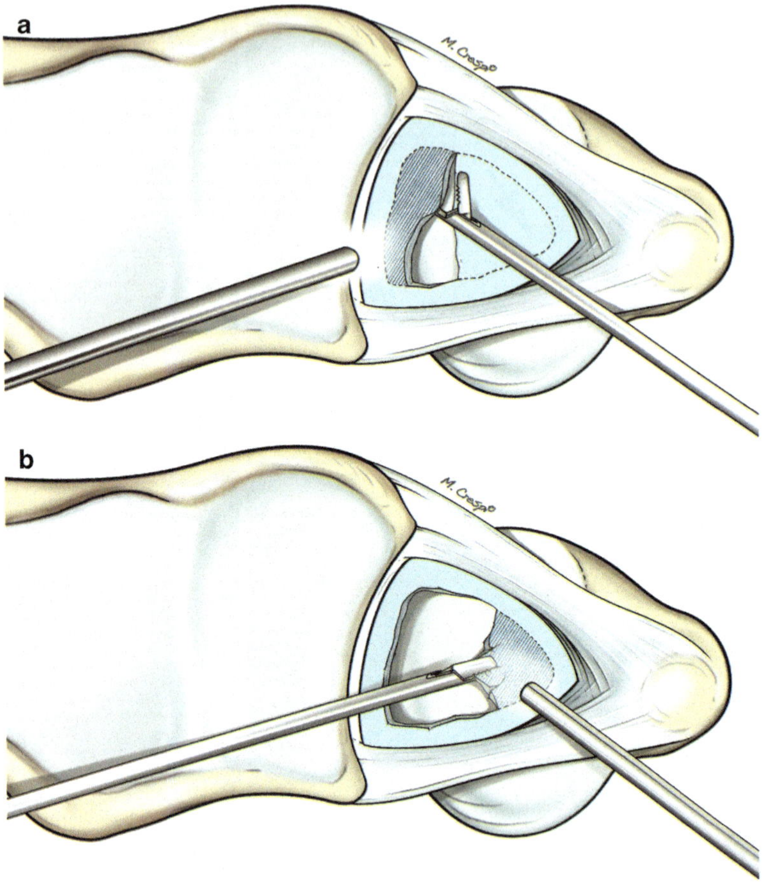

Fig. 7.14 Switching portals is often necessary to access to the most ulnar aspect of the tear. (**a**) From 6R only the radial part of the tear can be debrided with the basket forceps (*shaded area*). (**b**) Swapping instrument portals is frequently necessary to debride the ulnar part of the tear (striped)

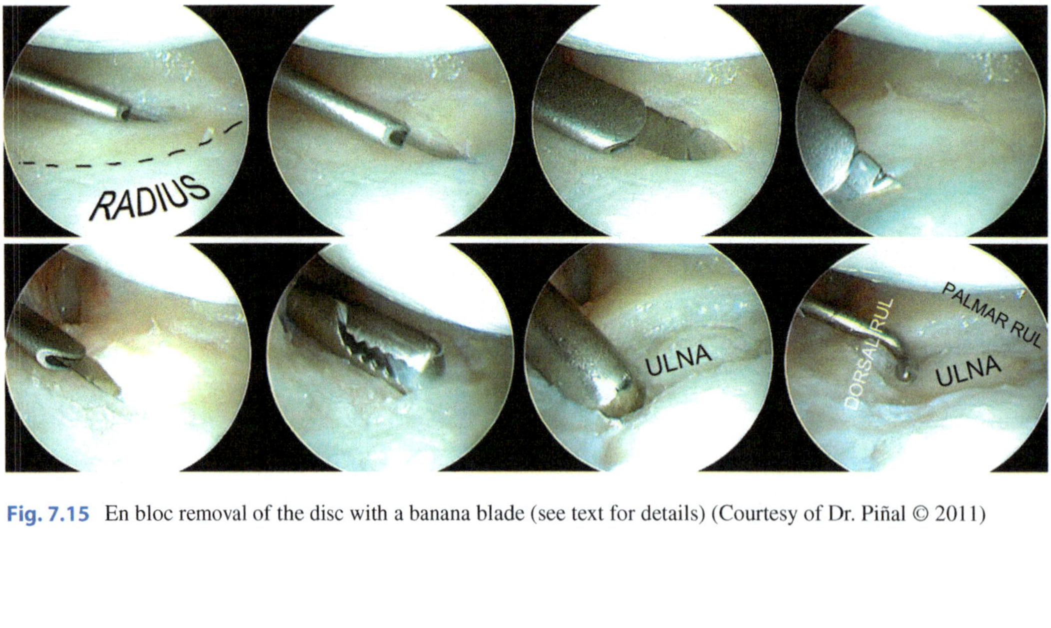

Fig. 7.15 En bloc removal of the disc with a banana blade (see text for details) (Courtesy of Dr. Piñal © 2011)

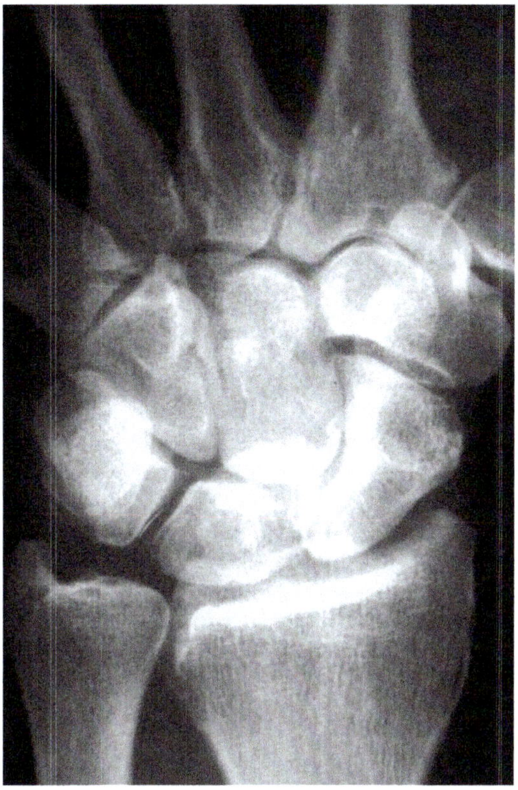

Fig. 7.16 PA radiograph of left wrist in forearm pronation showing relative positive ulnar variance (Reproduced with permission from Lippincott, Philadelphia)

of the ulna in pronation, the central disc is nonessential for this purpose [7].

Similarly, it is the dorsal and volar radio-ulnar ligaments that provide support to the ulnar side of the proximal carpal row in axial loading of the wrist and power grip. Except in cases of positive ulnar variance where shear forces between the ulna and proximal carpal row produce an ulnar impaction syndrome with increased shear forces, the central disc provides little functional role. It is recommended that preoperative posteroanterior x-rays of the wrist be obtained in full forearm pronation to assess the functional length of the ulna (Fig. 7.16). Excision of the disc, rather than attempts at repair of this avascular fibrocartilage, is therefore expedient for relieving ulnar wrist pain due to degenerative or traumatic disruption and usually permits immediate return to one's premorbid activities.

Arthroscopic surgical access obviates the surgical trauma of wrist arthrotomy and provides excellent visualization and illumination of the central TFCC disc for evaluation and precise, delicate excision.

References

1. Bernstein MA et al (2004) A comparison of combined arthroscopic triangular fibrocartilage complex debridement and arthroscopic wafer distal ulna resection versus arthroscopic triangular fibrocartilage complex debridement and ulna shortening osteotomy for ulnocarpal abutment syndrome. Arthroscopy 20(4):392–401
2. Chloros GD et al (2008) Current concepts in wrist arthroscopy. Arthroscopy 24(3):343–354
3. Darlis NA et al (2005) Arthroscopic triangular fibrocartilage complex debridement using radiofrequency probes. J Hand Surg Br 30(6):638–642
4. Husby T, Hangsvelt JR (2001) Long term results after arthroscopic resection of lesions of the triangular fibrocartilage complex. Scand J Plast Reconstr Surg Hand Surg 35(1):79–83
5. Intanger M, Grimm D (2009) Meniscus and discus lesions of the TFCC: treatment by laser-assisted wrist arthroscopy. J Plast Reconstr Aesthet Surg 62(4): 466–471
6. Palmer A (1989) Triangular fibrocartilage complex lesions: a classification. J Hand Surg Am 14A:594–605
7. Palmer AK, Werner FW (1981) The triangular fibrocartilage complex of the wrist – anatomy and function. J Hand Surg Am 6A:151–162
8. Saffar P (2007) The pathology of the long ulna: anatomy and treatment. J Hand Surg Eur 32(6):608–619
9. Tatebe M et al (2000) Repair of the triangular fibrocartilage complex after ulna-shortening osteotomy: second-look arthroscopy. J Hand Surg 32(4):445–449
10. Tomaino MM, Elfar J (2005) Ulnar impaction syndrome. Hand Clin 21(4):567–575
11. Unglaub F et al (2009) Incidence and distribution of blood vessels in punch biopsies of palmer 1A disc lesions in the wrist. Arch Orthop Trauma Surg 129(5):631–634
12. Whipple T (1992) Arthroscopic surgery: the wrist. Lippincott, Philadelphia

8 Treatment of Stable Peripheral TFC Tears

Max Haerle

Introduction

Open and arthroscopic surgery has, in the past, helped in understanding the biomechanics and type of injuries of the TFC complex. As described in the preceding chapters of this book, the evolution of this knowledge is still ongoing. One of the starting points was the classification of Palmer [6], which was orientated to a more topographic type of classification. The more recent biomechanically orientated classification of Atzei et al. [1] takes into account the damaged anatomic structure, the distal radial ulnar joint stability (DRUJ), and the healing potential of the lesion (Table 8.1). He distinguishes three basic relevant types of lesions at the ulnar side of the TFCC: Class 1 corresponds to a distal capsular detachment, class 3 corresponds to a proximal foveal detachment, and class 2 corresponds to a complete lesion which is a combination of the two.

In this chapter, we will focus on the distal capsular detachment of the TFCC, which will not lead to clinical relevant instability in the distal radial ulnar joint.

M. Haerle
Department of Hand and Plastic Surgery,
Orthopedic Clinic Markgröningen,
Kurt-Lindemann-Weg 10,
D-71706 Markgröningen, Germany
e-mail: m.haerle@okm.de

Diagnosis and Indications

Ulnar-sided wrist pain has many potential origins, and the differential diagnosis has been already highlighted. We are focusing in this chapter on patients with a distal class 1 TFCC tear following the Atzei classification (Table 8.1). These patients suffer from a persisting typical pain for TFCC lesions, without demonstrating a major DRUJ instability. This persisting typical ulnar wrist pain is located in correspondence to the 6U portal. It can be provoked by pressure applied just palmarly to the ulnar styloid (6U) and dorsally just radially to the extensor carpi ulnaris tendon (6R portal). Often, these patients experience pain in hyperpronation and hypersupination, while the ulnar compression test and the ballottement test are mostly negative.

The difficulty in clinical assessment is the degree of (in)stability. For accurate and relevant testing, the wrist must be in neutral position and the patient has to relax completely. Stability is then tested in neutral wrist position and in radial and ulnar abduction. For comparison, the contralateral side must be tested. Unfortunately, not all patients are able to relax at the time of the clinical investigation. Also, individually variable degrees of joint laxity may interfere. In cases of chronic instability (traumatic or constitutional), the secondary stabilizers such as the pronator quadratus muscle try to react by hypertrophy through hyperactivity. Their basic muscle tonus is much higher than in the normal wrists. These patients are almost unable to relax to a point where this

F. del Piñal et al. (eds.), *Arthroscopic Management of Ulnar Pain*,
DOI 10.1007/978-3-642-30544-3_8, © Springer-Verlag Berlin Heidelberg 2012

Table 8.1 Atzei's classification based on arthroscopic findings

		Clinical DRUJ instability	Involved TFCC component proximal	distal	TFCC healing potential	Status of DRUJ cartilage	Treatment
Class 1: Repairable distal tear	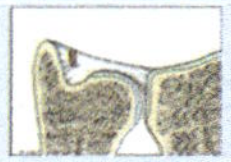	None or slight	Torn	Intact	Good	Good	Suture (ligament to capsule)
Class 2: Repairable proximal tear	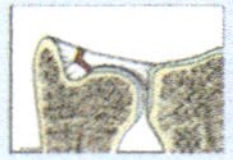	Mild or severe	Torn	Torn	Good	Good	Foveal reinsertion
Class 3: Repairable complete tear	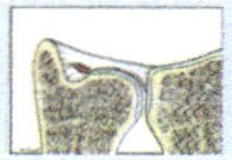	Mild or severe	Intact	Torn	Good	Good	Foveal reinsertion
Class 4: Non-repairable	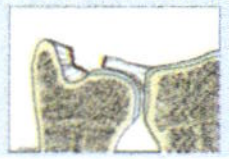	Severe	Torn	Torn	Poor	Good	Reconstruction (tendon graft)
Class 5: Arthritic DRUJ	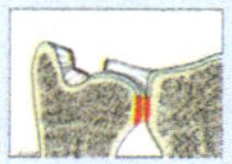	Mild or severe	Indifferent	Indifferent	Indifferent	Poor	Salvage procedure

From Atzei et al. [1]

The first column reports findings of clinical instability of DRUJ. Class 1 are repairable tears that should be treated by suture. Classes 2 and 3 are repairable tears associated with DRUJ instability that require foveal reattachment. Class 4 are non-repairable lesions that should undergo reconstruction by tendon graft. Class 5, associated with DRUJ cartilage degeneration, is suitable for salvage procedures instability is tested correctly. Therefore, this exam is subjective and should be repeated preoperatively under anesthesia.

Besides the standard X-rays, MRI studies are mandatory, primarily to exclude all other concurrent pathologies. These partial TFCC injuries can be identified by MRIs with high resolution, and oedema is frequently found at the capsular level. Unfortunately, many false-positive and false-negative MRI results have led to low probability of diagnosing these partial ruptures by MRI.

If these lesions are to be considered post-traumatic lesions, immobilization and conservative therapy is the first approach especially in recent lesions.

Diagnostic Arthroscopy

Diagnostic arthroscopy is indicated in patients with ulnar wrist pain refractory to conservative therapy. Diagnostic arthroscopy may then reveal the capsular lesion of the TFCC.

Once inside the ulnar compartment, generally, the TFCC demonstrates a slightly lowered trampoline test and a more or less marked pathological hook test. A small part of the TFCC can be elevated from the capsule (Fig. 8.1). At that point, we must differentiate between acute and chronic lesions and between complete and partial lesions.

In acute lesions, generally, the arthroscopic probe can be inserted into the ulnar recess and the TFC can be elevated from its capsular attachments but cannot be completely retracted (as it is possible in class 2 complete tears with foveal avulsion). The lesions correspond to a local circumscript detachment of the TFC from the capsule. These lesions may be found located more toward the dorsal or palmar side, depending upon whether the detachment involves the dorsal or the palmar triangular radioulnar ligament.

In chronic lesions, generally, these areas are covered by exuberant synovium. After shaving these areas and resection of the synovium, the lesions become evident. The shaving at this point has the advantages of freshening the lesion site and stimulating new scar formation.

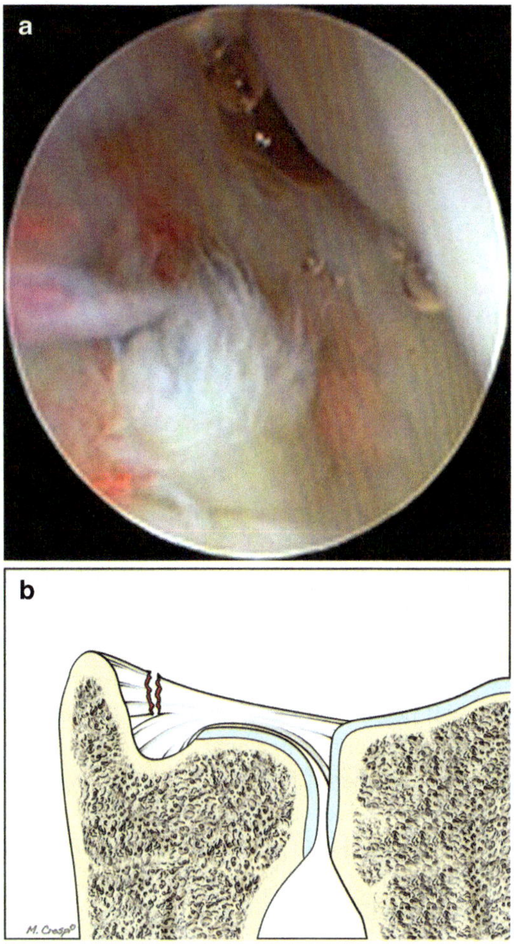

Fig. 8.1 (**a**, **b**) A small flap of the TCC can be elevated from the ulnar capsule in class 1 lesions

For acute and chronic lesions, the repair strategy is a capsular reattachment (suture) of the TFC. As conservative therapy was not able to produce spontaneous healing, these sutures should permit the reattachment of the TFC to its physiological insertions.

Arthroscopic Suture Technique

The arthroscopic technique of suturing the ligament to the capsule has multiple variations. All inside sutures are used with success [2]. The most frequent technique is ulnar reattachment by outside-in technique from the 6U or 6R portal.

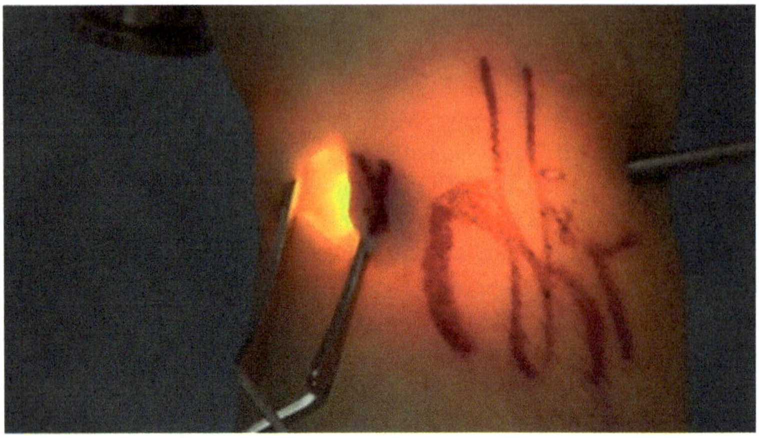

Fig. 8.2 A small self-retaining retractor is placed in the 6U portal, and the light source of the arthroscope leads directly to the ulnocarpal joint

Generally, the arthroscope is positioned in the 3/4 portal, and the decision must be made through which portal the suture has to be performed. Suturing the TFC to the capsule through the bed of the sixth extensor compartment is a well-known technique. This technique has the advantage of positioning the suture of the dorsal triangular radioulnar ligament close to the dorsal capsular insertion. This technique leaves a knot within the bed of the extensor compartment, which can irritate the extensor tendon secondarily. Moreover, the TFCC is suspended like a hammock in the ulnocarpal compartment, where the apical ulnar insertions correspond more to the 6U portal.

Therefore, many prefer to perform the suture through the 6U portal. The wrist is kept in supination for an easier approach to the 6U portal, which can easily be palpated just distal and palmar to the ulnar styloid and always palmar to the ECU tendon. A small longitudinal incision of about 1 cm is made in order not to damage the dorsal branch of the ulnar nerve. The soft tissue and the extensor retinaculum is retracted, and the ulnar styloid is palpated. A small self-retaining retractor is placed, and the light source of the arthroscope leads directly to the ulnocarpal joint (Fig. 8.2). At that point, a needle is armed with the suture (generally 3-0 monofilament). This suture is directed from proximal to distal at the tip of the ulnar styloid and introduced into the ulnar recess. Once the needle tip is seen, the needle is slightly retracted and then brought under the TFC and then perforates the TFC about 3 mm from its insertion (Fig. 8.3). The needle is then slightly retracted, so that the suture is forming a loop.

A second needle is then introduced parallel to the former suture and perforates the TFC about 2–3 mm more palmarly (Fig. 8.4). Many surgeons prefer a 3-0 resorbable suture, but due to knot irritation, we prefer a more soft and flexible multifilament (braided) suture. This second needle with its suture is then directed through the loop (Fig. 8.5), the loop is retracted, and the monofilament suture is pulled outside (Fig. 8.6). The exact perforating points of the needles depend on where the major instability of the TFC is found and in consequence to whether there is a more palmar or more dorsal capsular detachment. If it is more dorsal, greater tension will be placed on the dorsal ligament: If it is more palmar, greater tension will be placed on the palmar ligament.

Once the suture is correctly positioned, the distraction weight is released and the suture is tied tightly in supination (Fig. 8.7). If the extensor retinaculum was divided, it is sutured using a 4-0 PDS suture. The same suture technique is adapted for sutures in the bed of the sixth extensor compartment.

In the post-operative protocol, a 3–6-week period of splinting is employed to avoid supination and pronation in order to improve stable ligament scarring. Forceful loading should be avoided for up to 3 months.

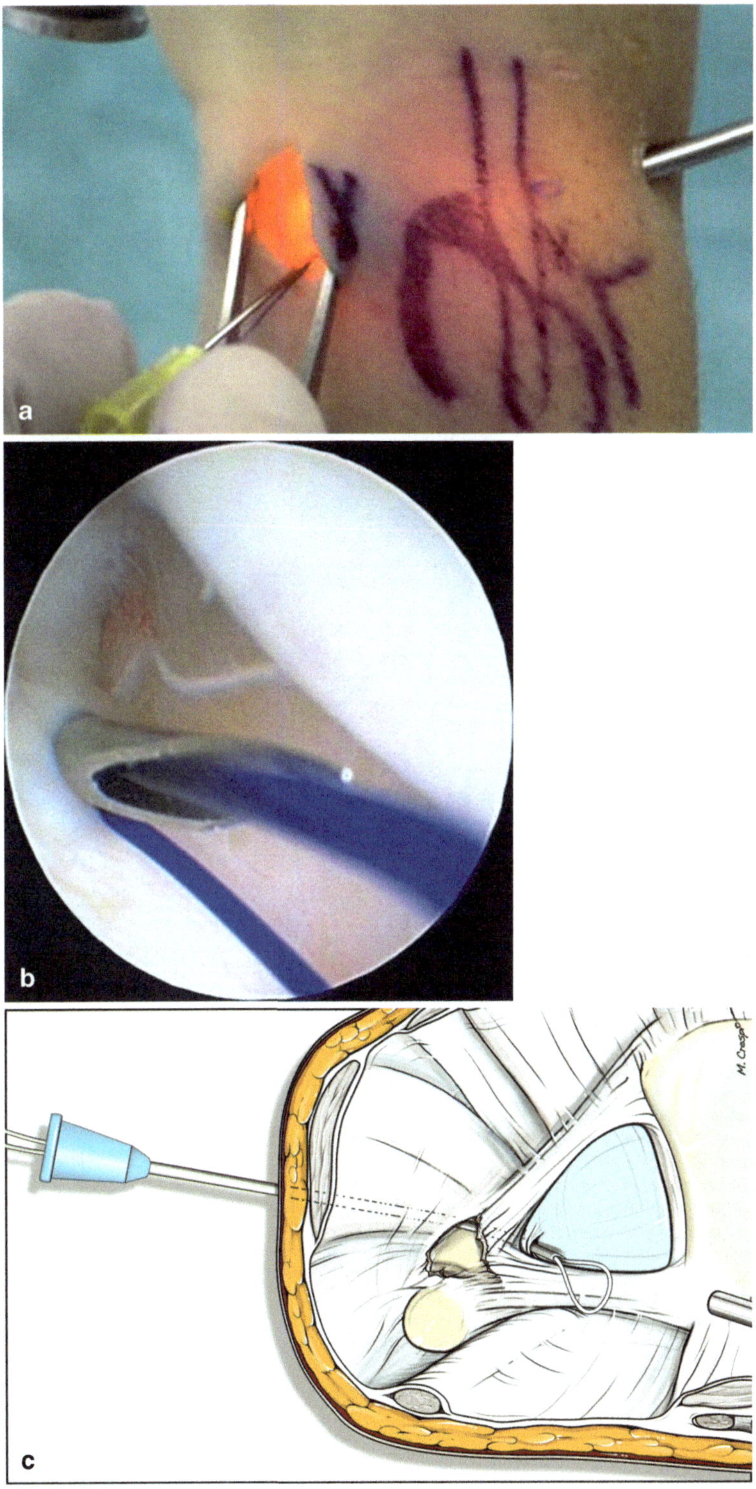

Fig. 8.3 (**a**, **b**, **c**) The needle perforates the TFC about 3 mm from its insertion. The needle is retracted slightly, and the loop is formed

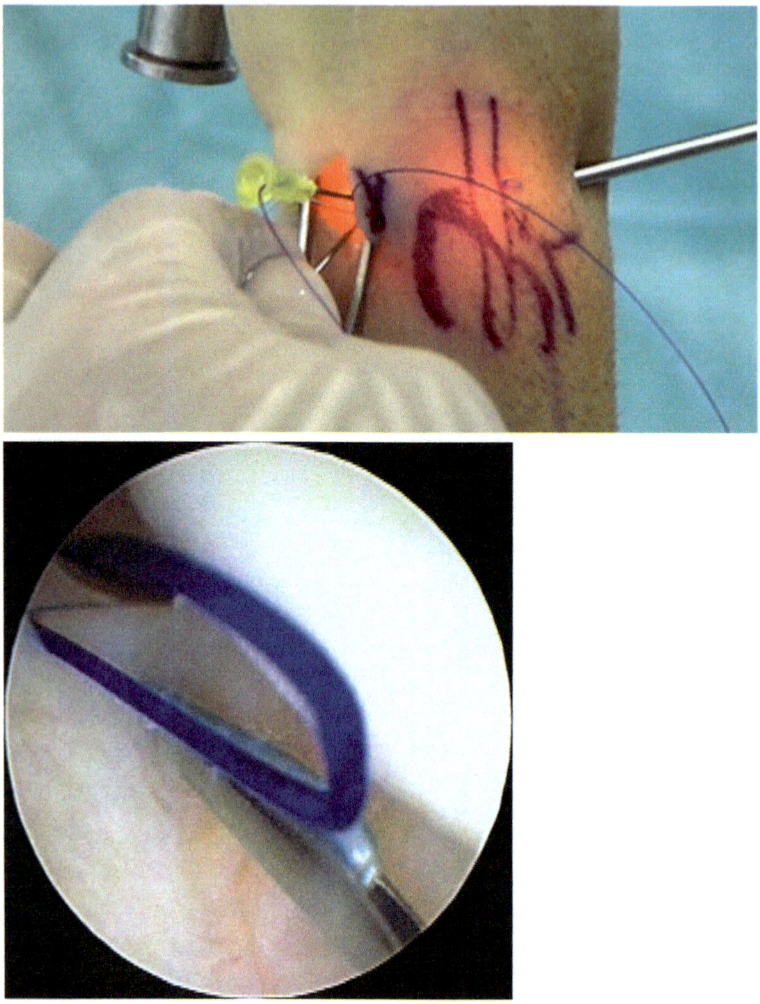

Fig. 8.4 The needle perforates the TFC about 3 mm from its insertion. The needle is retracted slightly, and the loop is formed

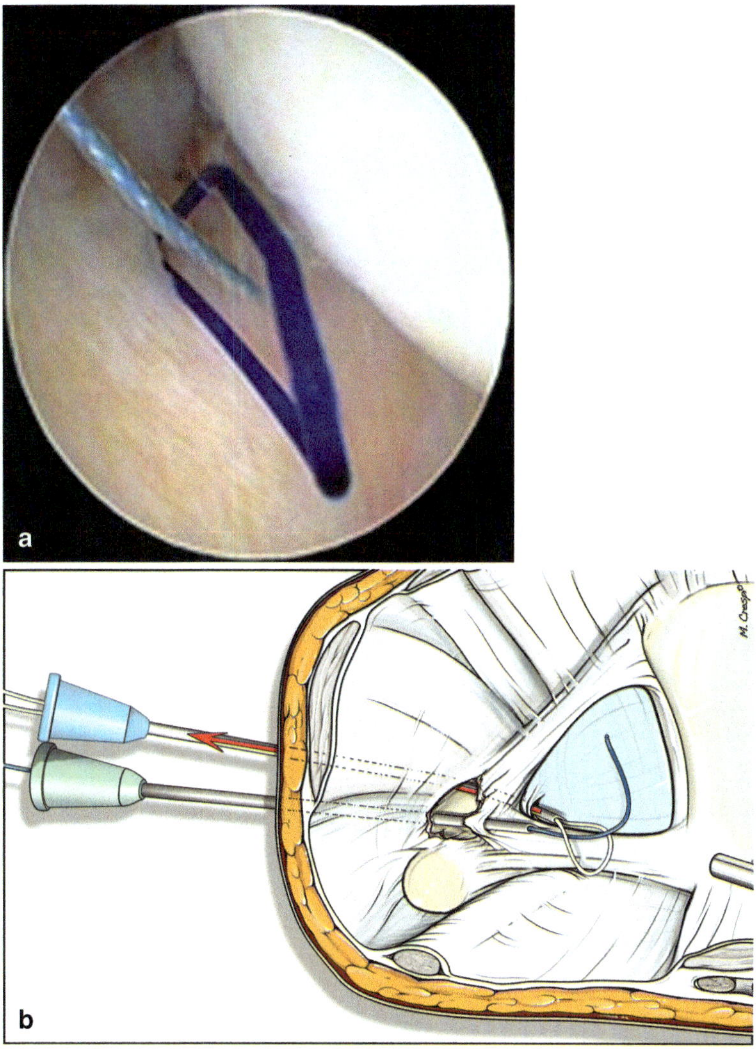

Fig. 8.5 (**a**, **b**) The multifilamentary suture is passed through the loop. *Red arrow*: Pulling direction

Fig. 8.6 The multifilamentary suture pulled out by the loop

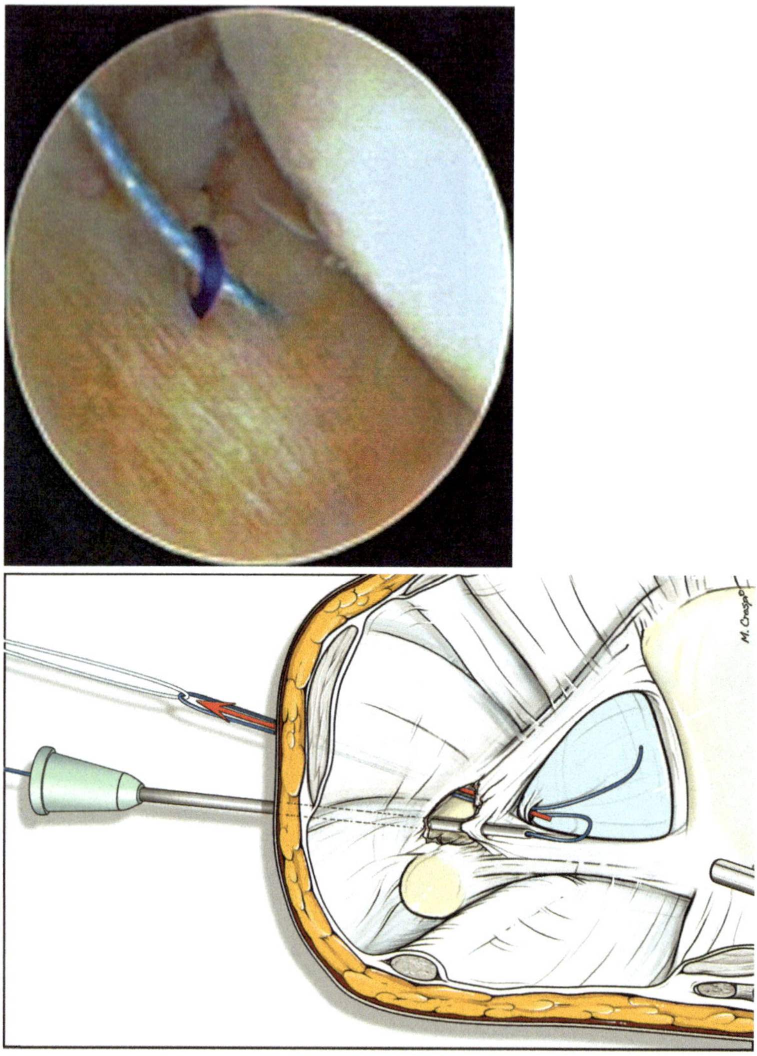

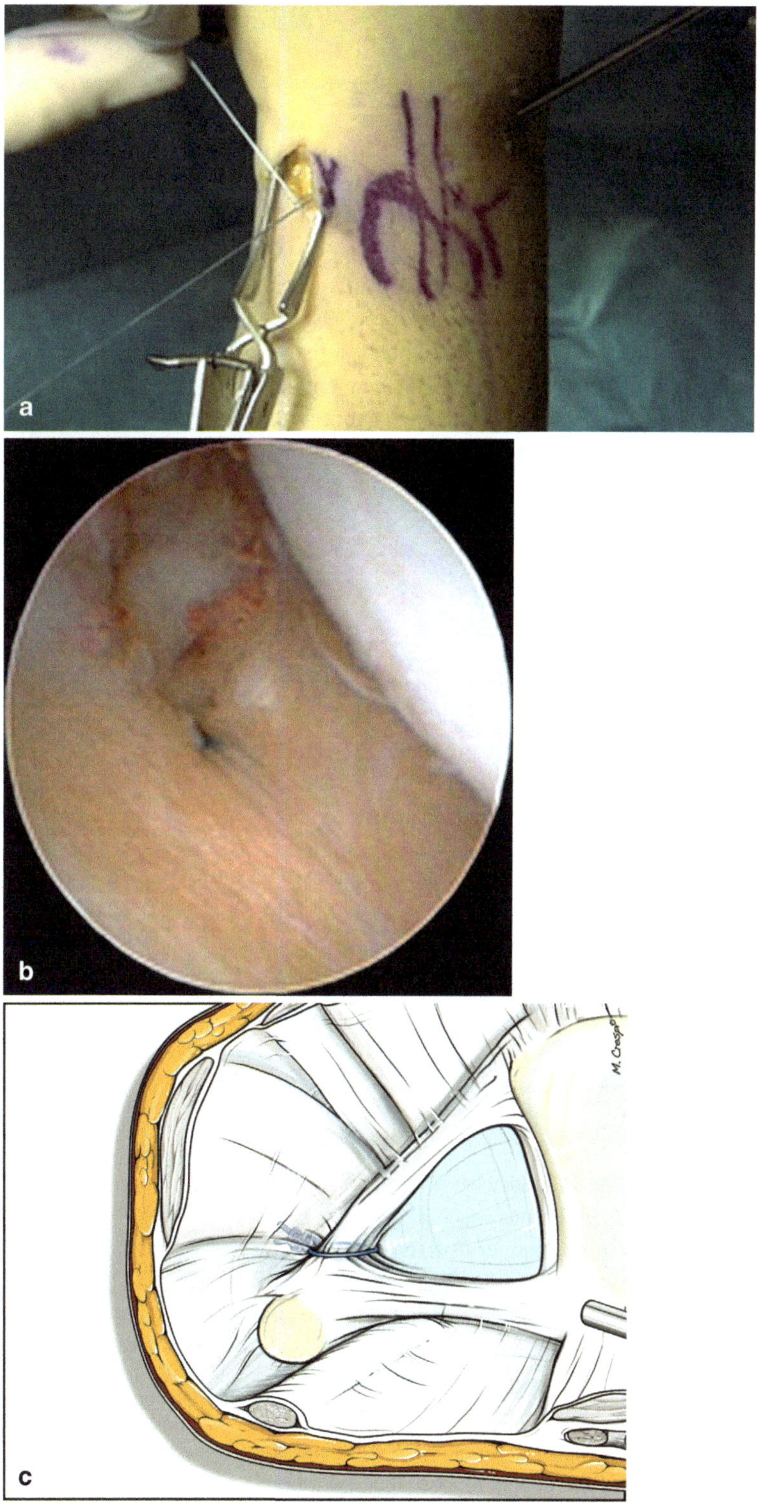

Fig. 8.7 (**a**, **b**, **c**) The knot is tightened and the TFCC reattached to the ulnar capsule

Results

The debate on stability of these sutures is ongoing [4]. Some of the capsular sutures have shown to give initially excellent results, but to be insufficient in the medium term. As stated previously, more precise knowledge about peripheral, proximal or the combination of these lesions has been only recently recognized. Therefore, the results are all short-term. Many unhappy results of the past can, in our view, be avoided by a more precise distinction of the different lesion types. But even with the new procedure, it remains debatable if a more solid fixation in all lesions would resolve definitively the underlying problem.

Preferred Procedure

Before the diagnostic arthroscopy, I purposefully remain undecided regarding my operative plan. If I am in doubt about instability and the extent of the lesion, bony reattachment is my preferred solution. In isolated capsular lesions, especially in younger patients, I always suture through the 6U portal. I avoid the monofilament sutures due to irritation from the large knot. I have not seen notable differences in sparing the extensor retinaculum within this technique. I immobilize generally for 6 weeks in a special splint (Fig. 8.8), which allows elbow flexion/extension but inhibits supination and pronation.

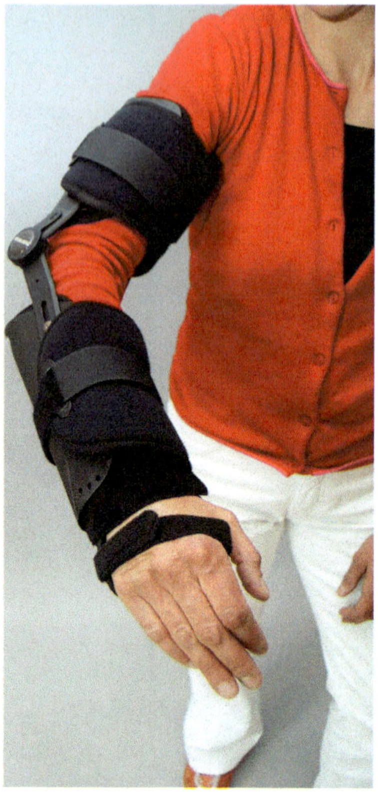

Fig. 8.8 An orthesis inhibiting pronation and supination is applied for 3–6 weeks

Discussion

As in the past, the difference between peripheral and proximal TFCC [5] lesions was not so evident to the majority of us, may many of us fixed all lesions by capsular sutures. Ignoring that we have tried to fix by this technique also the more complex lesions, the post-operative result was sometimes deceiving [3]. We have learned that the transosseous reinsertions of the TFCC give a more stable fixation, and the results have been improved. Therefore, the diagnostic arthroscopy and the distinction between peripheral and proximal lesions, with or without instability, are crucial, and this forms the basis for the decision between a pure capsular or bony reattachment.

References

1. Atzei A, Rizzo A, Luchetti R (2008) Arthroscopic foveal repair of triangular fibrocartilage complex peripheral lesion with distal radioulnar joint instability. Tech Hand Up Extrem Surg 12(4):226–235
2. Del Piñal F, Garcia-Bernal FJ, Cagigal L, Studer A, Regalado J, Thams C (2010) A technique for arthroscopic all-inside suturing in the wrist. J Hand Surg Eur 35(6):475–479
3. Kleinman WB (2007) Stability of the distal radioulnar joint: biomechanics, pathophysiology, physical diagnosis and restoration of function. What we have learned in 25 years. J Hand Surg Am 32:1087–1106
4. Millants P, De Smet L, Van Ransbeeck H (2002) Outcome study of arthroscopic suturing of ulnar avulsions of the triangular fibrocartilage complex of the wrist. Chir Main 21(5):298–300
5. Nakamura T, Makita A (2000) The proximal ligamentous component of the triangular fibrocartilage complex. J Hand Surg Br 25:479–486
6. Palmer AK (1989) Triangular fibrocartilage complex lesion: a classification. J Hand Surg Am 14A:494–606

TFCC: A DRUJ Perspective

9

Mark Henry

Introduction

The triangular fibrocartilage complex (TFCC) is a group of anatomically distinct but functionally related structures in the ulnar wrist. The scope of this chapter is limited to the evaluation and treatment of pathology from the perspective of the distal radioulnar joint (DRUJ). There are two specific pathologies to be addressed. Toward the ulnar side of the DRUJ, acute traumatic rupture of the radioulnar ligament (RUL) from the fovea of the ulna can be evaluated and treated with arthroscopic repair. Toward the radial side of the DRUJ, chronic attrition of the proximal surface of the fibrocartilage disc against the ulnar head initiates the pattern of degenerative tearing of the disc that is distinct from acute traumatic tears. An intact fibrocartilage disc that suffers a high-energy singular trauma will split along natural planes of structural weakness in the vertical, sagittal plane, full thickness from proximal to distal. Chronic lower energy repeated trauma to the fibrocartilage disc causes it to shear and breakdown in the transverse, horizontal plane, separating first between more proximal and more distal layers and then eventually propagating into complex multiplanar patterns of disruption. Categorizing the pathology for the purpose of treatment should be dictated by the anatomic pattern of the lesion rather than by the temporal occurrence of the symptoms as treatment outcomes are directly related to the anatomic pattern [14].

Surgical Technique

The more difficult the operation, the more precise must be the technique. Large joint arthroscopy affords the surgeon considerable freedom in establishing portal locations, manipulating instruments, and a tolerance to plunging and withdrawing instruments in and out of the joint cavity. Small joint arthroscopy affords no such privileges. Some find very small joint arthroscopy too difficult to be practical, but that perception is often driven by the experience of struggling through a poor strategy from the outset rather than any inherent difficulty in working within small joints.

Setup for DRUJ Arthroscopy

Although one can see into a joint (arthroscopy) by inserting a camera into the joint cavity and rotating the angled lens, one cannot successfully operate in a joint without a practical spatial relationship between the viewing instrument and the surgical instruments. Core hand surgery textbooks, when addressing wrist arthroscopy, will often mention the DRUJ and show line drawings of dorsal portals

M. Henry, M.D.
Hand and Wrist Center of Houston,
1200 Binz Street, 13th Floor, Houston, TX 77004, USA
e-mail: mhenry@houstonhand.com

F. del Piñal et al. (eds.), *Arthroscopic Management of Ulnar Pain*,
DOI 10.1007/978-3-642-30544-3_9, © Springer-Verlag Berlin Heidelberg 2012

separated from each other by not more than 15–20 mm. Curiously, that is about where the discussion ends, with no further information on actually conducting any sort of manipulative surgery through those portals depicted in two dimensions. The obvious reason is that it is impossible to carry out meaningful surgery when the arthroscope, held in one of the surgeon's hands, is trying to enter the joint from the same direction with nearly the same orientation as the surgical instrument held in the surgeon's other hand. Arthroscopic surgery is best performed when the viewing instrument enters the joint as far away as possible from the operating instrument. This allows the maximum opportunity to watch what the operating instrument is doing without getting in the way of the operating instrument.

Accomplishing this goal in the DRUJ requires that one primary portal be located dorsally and the other located volarly (Fig. 9.1). Advancing the practice of arthroscopy in the DRUJ has been hampered by the fact that volar to the joint lie the ulnar nerve and ulnar artery. Iatrogenic injury to the ulnar nerve is a very serious complication, one that most surgeons hope to never inflict in the course of their careers. However, proper understanding of the spatial anatomy combined with careful technique permits safe creation and utilization of a volar ulnar portal that opposes a dorsal radial portal and achieves the ideal of maximum separation of the arthroscope from the surgical instruments. Skilled arthroscopists have already proven their ability to do so safely. Through a 2–2.5-cm longitudinal incision extending proximally from the 6-U portal, access is gained to the fovea for a combined open/arthroscopic repair technique. The authors called this open approach the direct foveal portal [2]. Another method of safely protecting the ulnar nerve is to use a 2-cm longitudinal open approach between the digital flexor tendons and the ulnar neurovascular bundle where this versatile strategy provides capsular entry to either the ulnocarpal joint or the DRUJ ([22, 23], see Chap. 3).

The choice of arthroscope is a balance between the surgeon's perceived field of view and mechanical injury to the joint. With technological advances such as higher quality optics and multichip designs, the surgeon's perceived field of view is not as different between the lens sizes as it used to be. Possible sizes for the radiocarpal joint and DRUJ include 2.7, 2.3 and 1.9 mm. Although, I previously used the 2.3-mm arthroscope for the radiocarpal joint and the 1.9-mm arthroscope for the DRUJ, I now prefer the 1.9-mm arthroscope for both (Fig. 9.2). The best arthroscope to use for a given case is the one that allows that surgeon to accomplish all tasks necessary to the case while inflicting the least amount of iatrogenic damage to the joint. The other surgical instruments should also be appropriately sized to fit the small joint: 2.5-mm shaver, 2.0-mm suction burr, and the smallest size thermal cautery probe available.

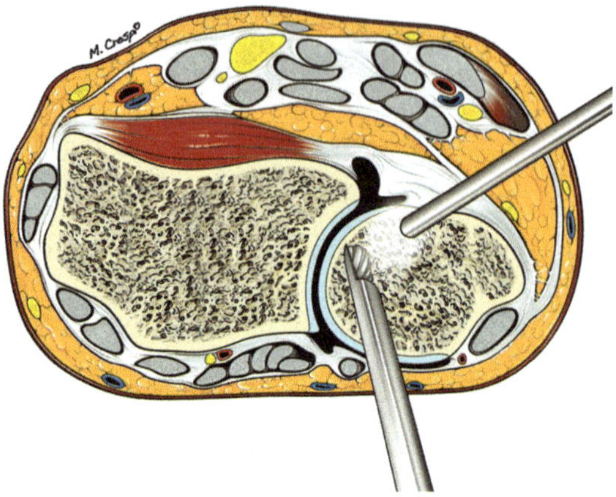

Fig. 9.1 Axial section of the DRUJ: 1.9-mm arthroscope enters ulnar to the FCU tendon but radial to the dorsal cutaneous branch of the ulnar nerve; 2.0–2.5-mm operative instrument (burr or shaver) enters dorsally

Portals for DRUJ Arthroscopy

The dorsal radial portal is marked just at the point where the ulnar head begins to curve proximally to meet the sigmoid notch such that the portal will pass proximal and ulnar to the fibers of the dorsal limb of the radioulnar ligament as it inserts on the radial margin of the sigmoid notch (Fig. 9.3). The volar ulnar portal is marked at the corresponding level of the joint along the proximal to distal axis, coincident with the ulnar border of the flexor carpi ulnaris (FCU) tendon.

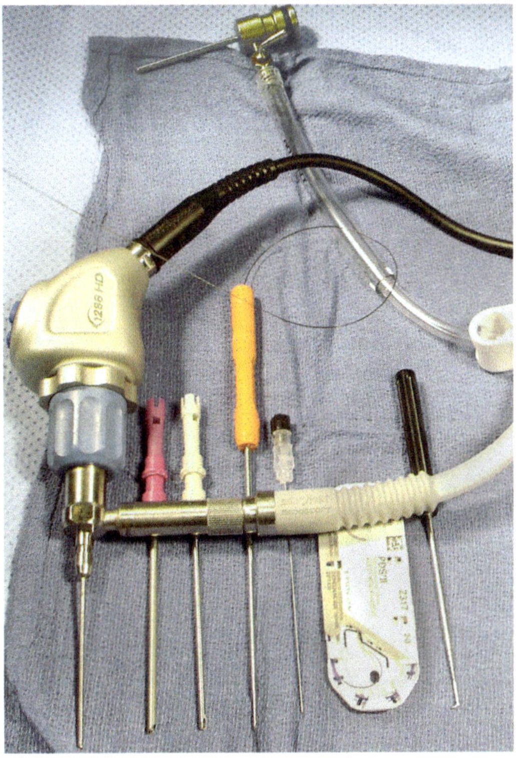

Fig. 9.2 Instruments used for DRUJ arthroscopy: 1.9-mm 30° arthroscope, 2.0-mm burr, 2.5-mm shaver, radiofrequency probe (not shown), retractable arthroscopic suture snare, 22-G spinal needle, 2-0 PDS suture, and small hook probe

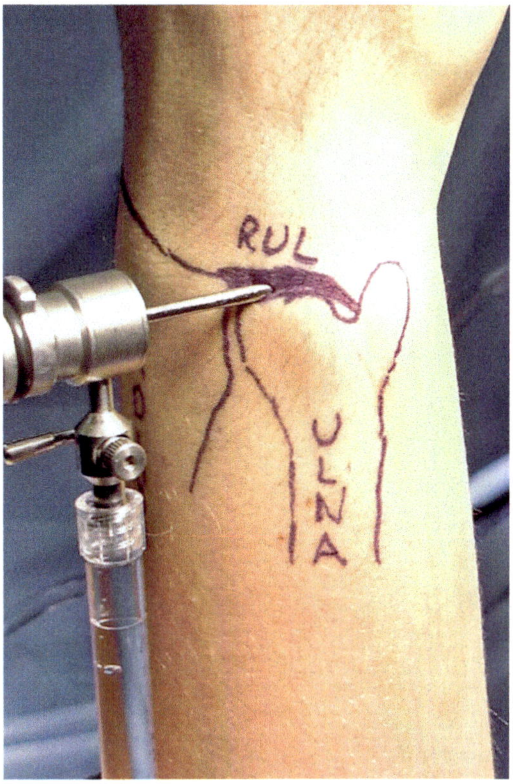

Fig. 9.3 Dorsal portal marking for DRUJ arthroscopy: portal will pass proximal and ulnar to the fibers of the dorsal limb of the radioulnar ligament as it inserts on the radial margin of the sigmoid notch

Historical texts on arthroscopy describe such maneuvers as first inflating the joint with saline and dissecting down to the joint capsule with a hemostat. Such procedures are totally unnecessary, and the hemostat dissection can actually increase the likelihood of nerve injury. The subcutaneous tissue plane in which the small caliber cutaneous nerves run is composed of a three-dimensional architecture of fine fascial fibers that form a matrix linking all the local tissues to one another. If that matrix remains as undisturbed as possible, then the local tissues will assist the cutaneous nerve branches in shifting away from the smooth passage of an instrument gently twisting and rotating its way from the surface down to the joint capsule. If the surgeon dissects the fine fascial matrix with a hemostat before trocar placement, he/she is more likely to isolate the nerve branch from its environment and leave it stranded alone in the path of the trocar, increasing the chances of nerve injury.

The dorsal radial portal provides for the initial joint inspection and confirmation of the ability to view all aspects of the joint from the sigmoid notch radially to the foveal insertion of the radioulnar ligament ulnarly. The volar ulnar portal is then established by passing the arthroscope across the surface of the ulnar head to reach the volar ulnar joint capsule at the previously marked location. The previous skin marking will fall directly in the center of the circle formed on the skin by the glow of the arthroscope's light coming from within the joint (Fig. 9.4). The arthroscope is then withdrawn and replaced by the trocar which is gently rotated back and forth to emerge ulnar to the FCU tendon exactly at the marking where a small nick is made in the dermis (Fig. 9.5). The cannula is inserted from the skin

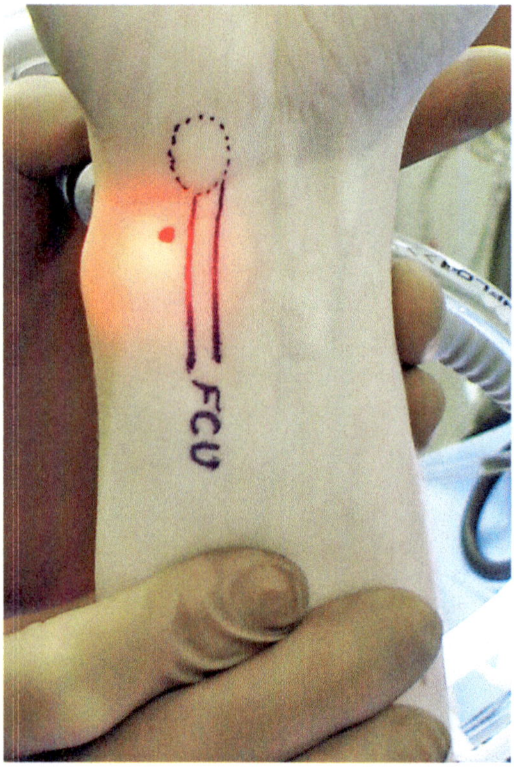

Fig. 9.4 Volar portal marking for DRUJ arthroscopy: when the arthroscope is in the dorsal radial portal, its light projection should be centered exactly on the volar ulnar portal marking

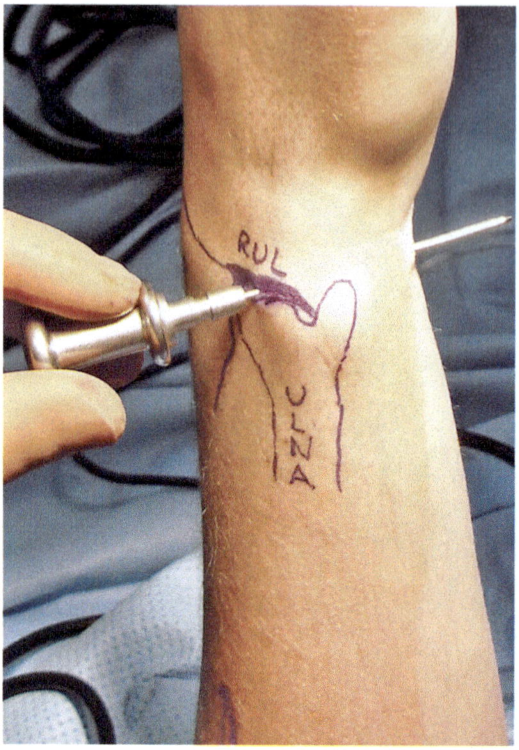

Fig. 9.5 After viewing the DRUJ from the dorsal portal, the switching trocar is reinserted from the dorsal portal to exit the joint capsule and pass ulnar to the FCU tendon but radial to the dorsal cutaneous branch of the ulnar nerve

surface volarly over the trocar as a guide with the same gentle rotating motion to ease its way through the tissues (Fig. 9.6). Notably, the dorsal cutaneous branch of the ulnar nerve lies just dorsal or ulnar to the path of the portal, and it is this nerve branch that is at risk, far more than the main ulnar nerve. The main ulnar nerve is protected by adherence to proper anatomic landmarks. The protection of the dorsal cutaneous branch is accomplished by precise and gentle technique as the branch may be located within a millimeter or two of the portal tract. The arthroscope is then placed through the cannula to establish the volar ulnar portal as the primary viewing portal and the dorsal radial portal becomes the primary operative portal (Fig. 9.7). The goal is to avoid slipping in and out of the joint, as each instance of needing to reestablish the portal poses some degree of risk to the nerves. Owing to the small size of the DRUJ, the surgeon only has a few millimeters of available range to insert and withdraw instruments. This "depth control" of the instruments must be under the command of the most precise muscles in the surgeon's body possible. That is not the upper arm and shoulder muscles that usually drive an object forward or pull it back, but rather the intrinsic muscles of the hand. By keeping the long finger of each hand on the surface of the patient's body, the surgeon can dial in very precise depth control of the arthroscope and other instruments, preventing inadvertent plunging and withdrawal and the need to reestablish the portals (Fig. 9.8).

Initial Joint Assessment

Before proceeding with the intended surgical procedure, a brief joint survey should be conducted to note any hyaline cartilage lesions, loose bodies, or other unexpected abnormalities.

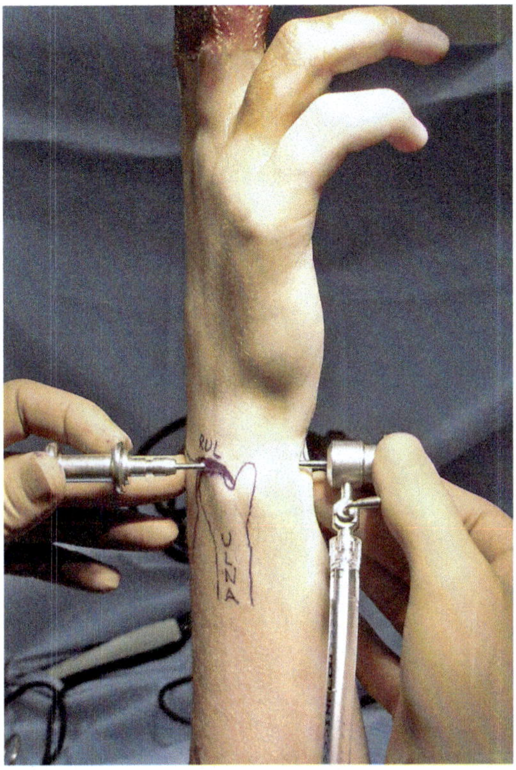

Fig. 9.6 The cannula for the 1.9-mm arthroscope is then lightly introduced over the surface of the switching trocar with a gentle twisting motion

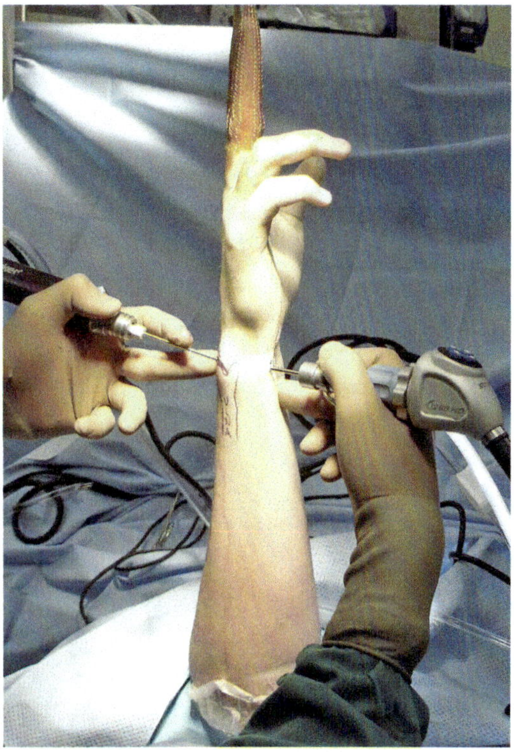

Fig. 9.7 The working configuration for DRUJ arthroscopy: arthroscope in volar ulnar portal and operating instrument in dorsal radial portal. While working in this configuration, note that the surgeon's long fingers must maintain contact with the patient's body surface for precise depth control to avoid repeated penetration and withdrawal events through the joint capsule

For chronic impaction pathology, one expects to find a frayed undersurface of the TFCC, frank perforations through to the ulnocarpal joint space, and synovitis of the sigmoid notch. For acute avulsions of the foveal attachment of the radioulnar ligament, one expects to find evidence of bleeding into the joint and the free detached tissue edge. For subacute traumatic avulsions, one expects to find additional signs of synovial reaction to the trauma. Regardless of the original diagnosis, all of these items should be checked in each case. Arthroscopy of the DRUJ is usually combined with arthroscopy of the ulnocarpal joint space for a complete evaluation of the patient with ulnar wrist pain.

Fibrocartilage Debridement

For chronic degeneration of the fibrocartilage disc in its early stages, the undersurface of the disc will have loose fibers hanging down into the DRUJ joint cavity, "crabmeat," and a synovial reaction to the local friction against the ulnar head created by those loose fibers (Fig. 9.9). The DRUJ will usually mount a synovial response to the frictional relationship between the ulnar head and the fibrocartilage disc (Fig. 9.10). This synovitis is most concentrated at the three-way interface between the ulnar head, the fibrocartilage disc, and the sigmoid notch. Viewing from the volar ulnar portal, the 2.5-mm suction shaver entering the dorsal radial portal effectively removes all the synovitis from the sigmoid notch (Fig. 9.11).

In more advanced stages of chronic degeneration or when additional acute tearing of an already degenerated fibrocartilage has occurred, then more dramatic fissures that pass from the DRUJ

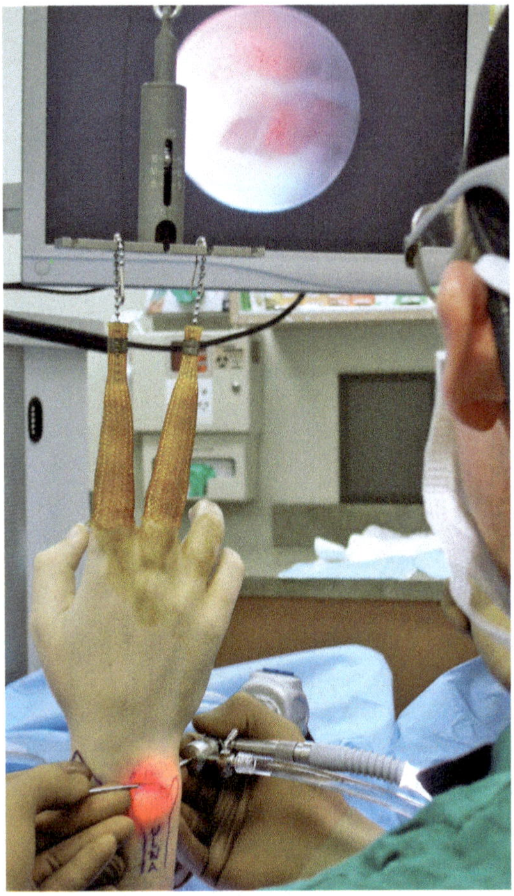

Fig. 9.8 While assuming a comfortable view of the monitor, the surgeon can also control supination and pronation of the forearm with the ulnar digits if needed. Use of strictly overhead traction from a boom allows circumferential access and more complicated procedures to be performed that would otherwise be obstructed by the typical on-table traction towers

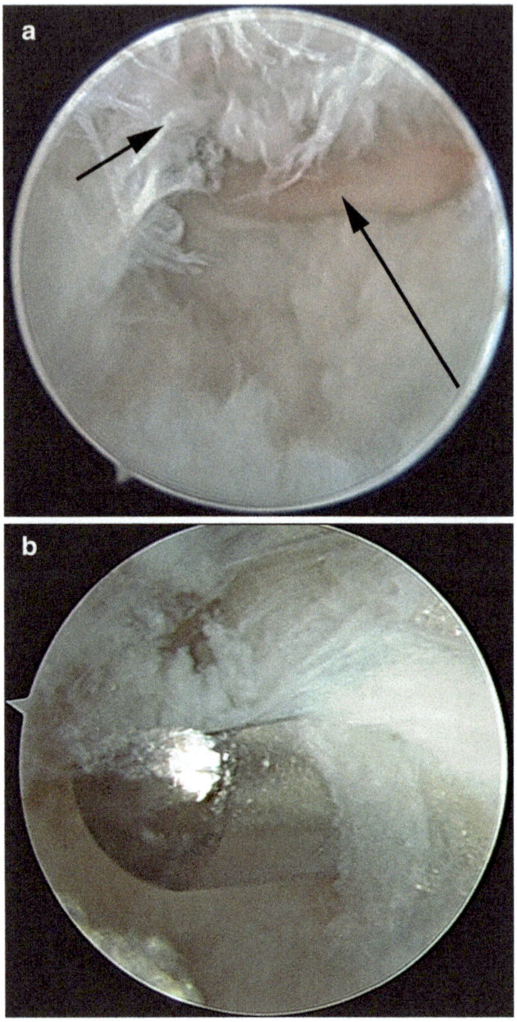

Fig. 9.9 (**a**) Appearance from the DRUJ of the frayed proximal surface of the fibrocartilage disc (*short arrow*) and synovitis (*long arrow*). (**b**) Debridement of the loose fibers by the 2.5-mm shaver through the dorsal portal, viewing from the volar portal

all the way through to the ulnocarpal joint can be found. In this case, it is not just thin fibers fraying from the surface that need to be debrided but actual segments of loose fibrocartilage substance. A radiofrequency ablation probe is needed for this work as fibrocartilage tissue is not effectively debrided by the suction shaver. Removal of the central substance of the fibrocartilage can be aggressive as no functional loss occurs, and the patient is more likely to be symptomatic from impingement of retained unstable fragments. In the more advanced stages of ulnocarpal impaction syndrome, the hyaline cartilage of the ulnar head will be eburnated. At this stage, ulnar shortening osteotomy is usually indicated.

Wafer Resection Confined to the DRUJ

The decision of whether or not to perform a bony modification of the ulna at all is a complex decision. The decision to shorten the ulna is usually straightforward when the degree of impaction is so great as to have caused bony reaction in the

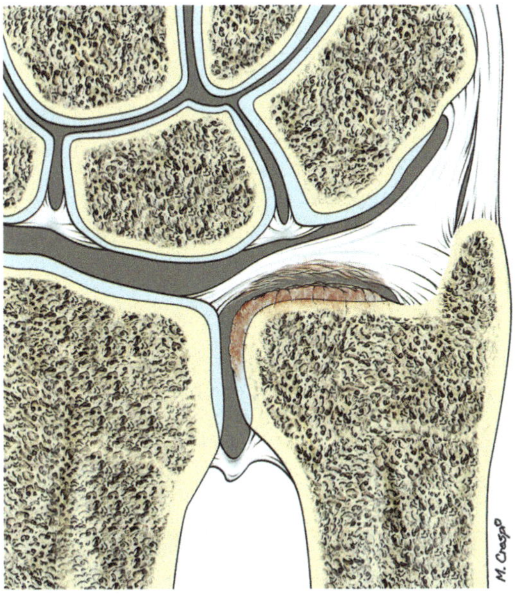

Fig. 9.10 Chronic proximal surface fraying and tearing of the fibrocartilage disc from repeated friction over the prominence of the ulnar head, accompanied by synovitis trapped in the sigmoid notch

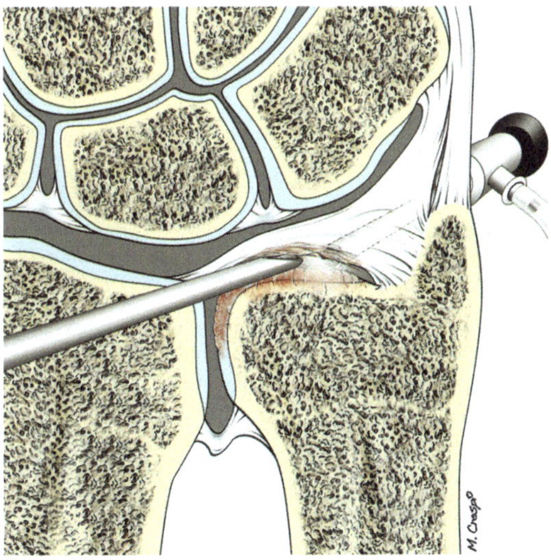

Fig. 9.11 Chronic proximal degenerative tearing of the fibrocartilage disc is debrided with the 2.5-mm shaver from the dorsal DRUJ portal under observation by the 1.9-mm arthroscope from the volar DRUJ portal

proximal ulnar corner of the lunate on magnetic resonance image (Fig. 9.12) or plain radiograph (Fig. 9.13). Absent these features, the decision becomes more difficult. If the patient and surgeon

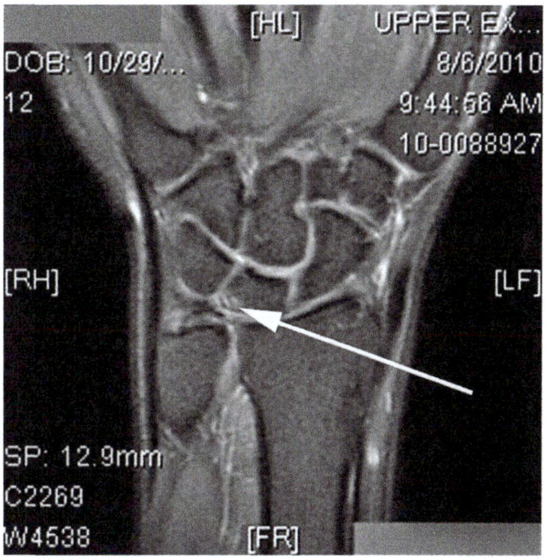

Fig. 9.12 Coronal MRI: ulnocarpal impaction demonstrates focal bony edema in the proximal ulnar corner of the lunate

together decide upon bony modification of the ulna, there are the choices of extra-articular and intra-articular to consider [4]. A complex analysis must take into consideration the exact conformation of the fit between the ulnar head and sigmoid notch and any signs of concomitant stylocarpal impaction. Some patients will be best served by an extra-articular osteotomy [10]. Most will do well with a wafer resection even if that means a concomitant mini-open resection of the ulnar styloid for those with true stylocarpal impaction as well. Alternatively, it is technically possible to resect the ulnar joint capsule and thus reach the extra-articular structure of the ulnar styloid and use arthroscopic instruments to resect the styloid, but the operation, at that point, has ceased to be arthroscopy and has become endoscopy of the tissue space adjacent to the joint. The primary detractor for the distal wafer resection is the prolonged duration of joint soreness and stiffness that appears to come from the raw bone surface of the distal ulna exposed to the joint environment. As long as patients are counseled in advance to expect this, they will tolerate the 4–6 months that it takes to eventually be rid of those symptoms. The intra-articular distal wafer shortening of the ulna was originally described as

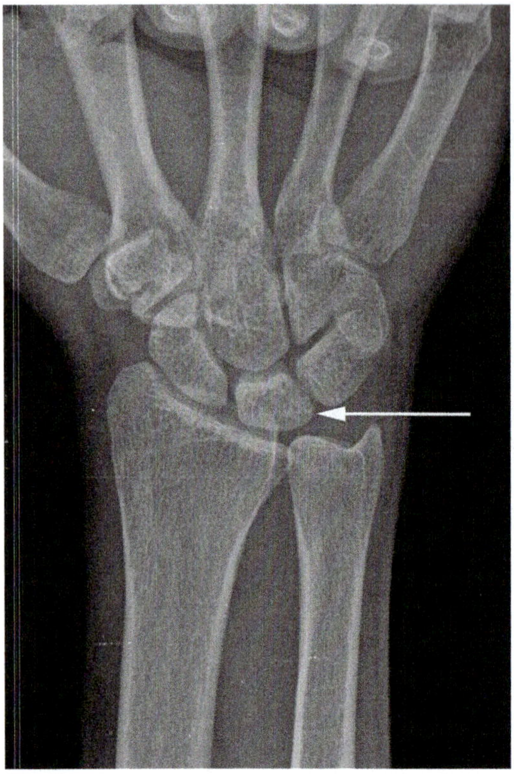

Fig. 9.13 PA radiograph: prominent distal ulna causing the radiographic lucent lesion in proximal ulnar corner of the lunate, "lunate impaction lesion," and clinical ulnocarpal impaction

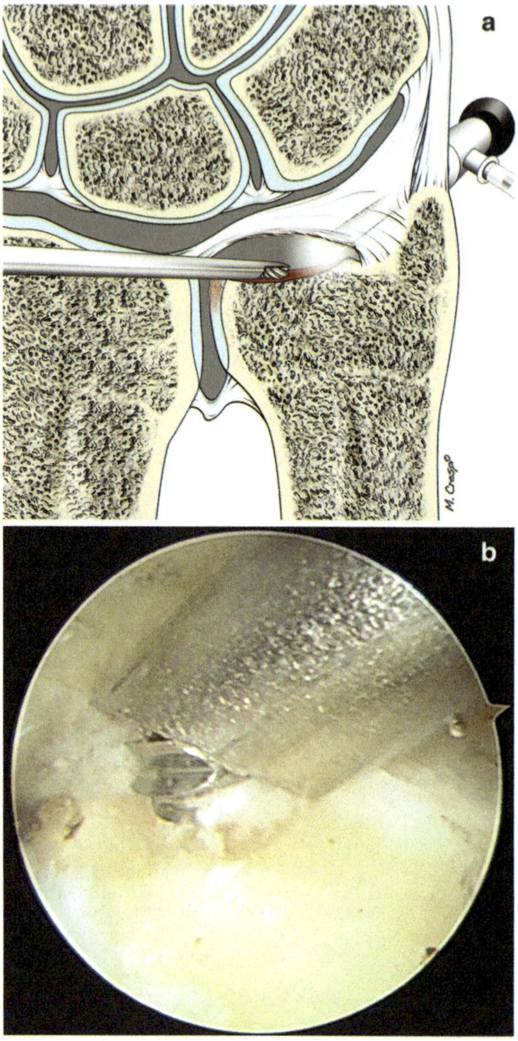

Fig. 9.14 Ulnocarpal impaction is decompressed by (**a**) removal of 2–3 mm of bone from the distal ulnar head with the 2.0-mm burr from the dorsal DRUJ portal while (**b**) viewing from the volar DRUJ portal

an open procedure but was subsequently modified with an option to perform the resection arthroscopically via the central window in the fibrocartilage disc created by debridement during an ulnocarpal joint arthroscopy [3]. The challenge when performing the resection by this method is gaining access to the breadth of the ulnar head via the central defect which requires rotating the forearm back and forth to the extremes of motion to deliver the volar and dorsal margins of the ulnar head into the operative "window" of the defect. This is not terribly hard to do once one has sufficient experience. However, not every case of clinical ulnocarpal impaction necessarily has a large defect in the fibrocartilage through which to work. These difficulties can be overcome by operating entirely through the joint space that contains the ulnar head, the DRUJ (Fig. 9.14). The configuration is the same as for all DRUJ arthroscopy: view from the volar ulnar portal and operate from the dorsal radial portal. The ulnar head is resected across its width with the 2.0-mm suction burr, stopping radially at the sigmoid notch and ulnarly at the origin of the RUL (Fig. 9.15). When using this method, the surgeon no longer needs to rotate the forearm into supination and pronation to have full access to performing a complete resection. Note that the ulnar

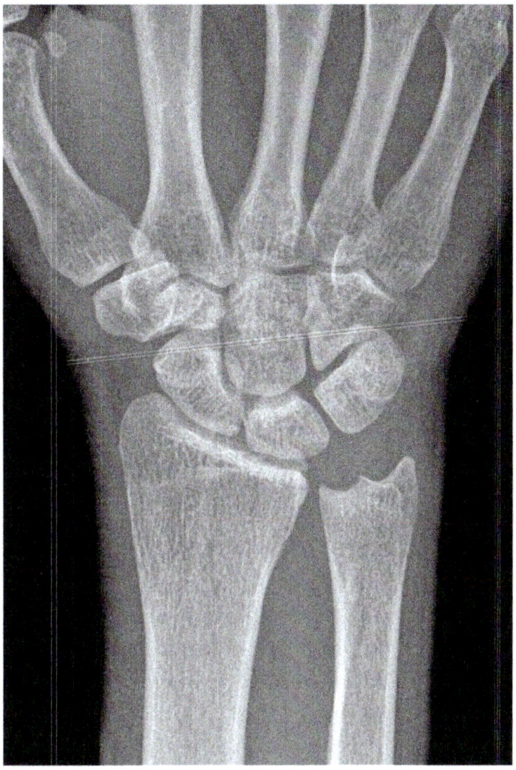

Fig. 9.15 PA radiograph: of distal ulnar head following resection of the prominent bone between sigmoid notch and fovea, decompressing ulnocarpal impaction

extent of the resection where one meets the fibers of the RUL is located far more radially than one would expect.

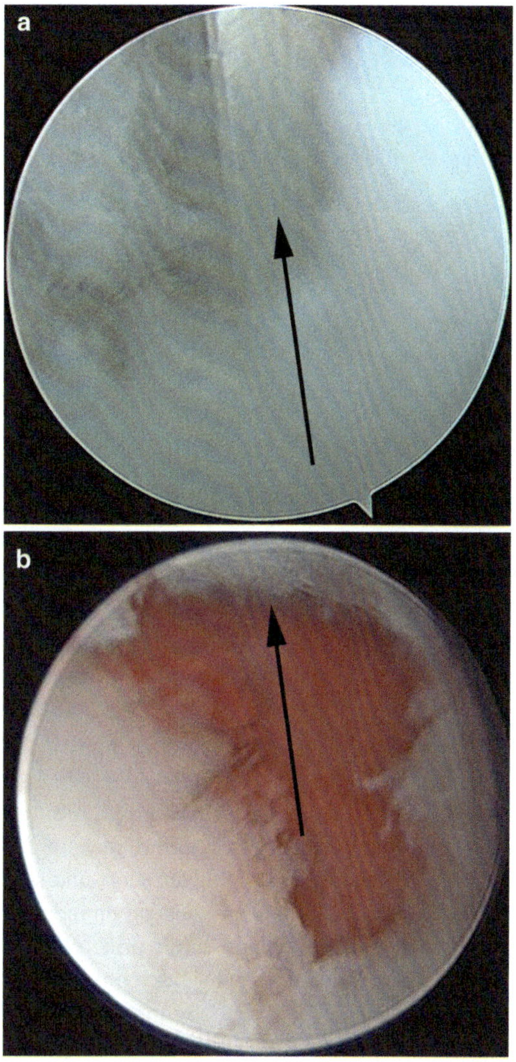

Fig. 9.16 The arthroscopic appearance of an (**a**) intact foveal insertion of the radioulnar ligament demonstrates vertically arising fibers from the fovea arching to extend radially and blend with the undersurface of the fibrocartilage disc whereas (**b**) a rupture at the fovea shows the loose fibers of the torn ligament displaced distally with lack of tissue continuity to the fovea

Anatomic Repair of Proximal Avulsion from Fovea

The primary determinant of DRUJ instability requiring surgical repair is the comprehensive clinical evaluation of the patient with the centerpiece being the manual stress exam to demonstrate true instability [6, 8, 11, 13, 25]. Nevertheless, the final confirmatory evaluation of the torn RUL occurs at the time of surgery through direct arthroscopic confirmation of the "vacant fovea" sign. A normal RUL demonstrates solid fibers arising vertically out of the fovea to arch radially and split into the volar and dorsal limbs of the RUL, passing on over to the margins of the sigmoid notch [17]. Arthroscopy of the torn RUL should show both the ruptured fibers displaced distally and radially from the normal location with a free edge of torn tissue as well as the absence of the normal stout fibers in the fovea, "vacant fovea" (Fig. 9.16). An important question

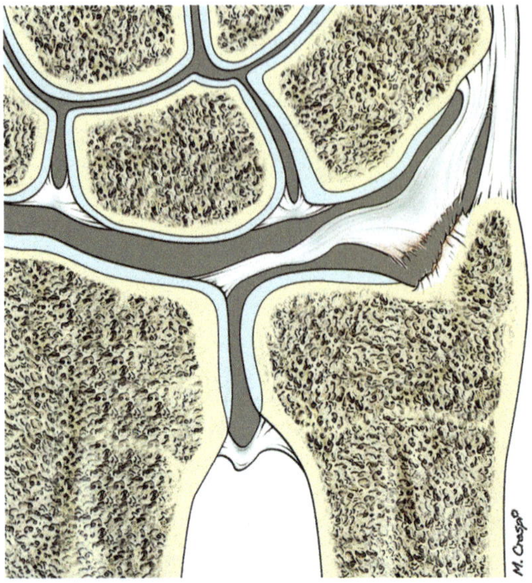

Fig. 9.17 Acute or subacute proximal detachment of the radioulnar ligament of the TFCC occurs consistently from the foveal insertion (unless accompanied by fracture)

remains unanswered regarding how long since original injury can a meaningful repair be achieved before such time as the patient requires a full free tendon graft reconstruction to achieve meaningful stability. No study answers this question, and surgeons will have to continue to depend on individual clinical experience and basic principles of injured tissues to make case by case clinical decisions. Points to keep in mind are that the RUL is not like the anterior cruciate ligament (ACL) of the knee. The ACL is a purely fibrous cable of an intra-articular ligament that experiences microscopic failure along the length of the ligament before reaching ultimate failure after which it consists of nothing more than shredded fibers. Even in acute injuries, only reconstruction is ever considered. The RUL is supported by its blending with the fibrocartilage disc and does not fail in the same manner. Detachment occurs right at the fovea of the ulna, but the detached ligament then changes little in length or quality (Fig. 9.17). It is in this instance where the blending and tissue connections of the TFC "complex" do indeed come into play [18]. The ruptured RUL neither retracts nor degenerates to the same degree as other intra-articular ligaments, but instead behaves more like other capsular-based ligaments that have proven their ability to be successfully repaired at later dates. I have found that most RUL ruptures can be repaired up to 3 months after injury [9]. Cases after 3 months would have to be very carefully considered for delayed repair as opposed to free tendon graft reconstruction.

After performing the complete joint inspection and evaluation, the fovea is "freshened" to stimulate a healing response with the 2.0-mm burr, exposing raw bone at the apex of the fovea (Fig. 9.18). Similarly, the torn edge of the RUL is lightly debrided with the 2.5-mm shaver to remove any scar tissue covering the true edges of the torn ligament that is expected to heal back to bone at the fovea. Four drill holes are created with 1.4-mm K-wires obliquely from the ulnar cortex to enter the fovea (Fig. 9.19). The holes are configured as one pair of more radial holes and one pair of more ulnar holes. Each pair will be used for a separate suture repair of the RUL pulling it back down into the fovea (Fig. 9.20). Once the correct path of the wires is confirmed, a small 1-cm skin incision is made to gain direct access to the ulnar cortex and a small recess in the cortex is created with a 3.5-mm drill bit to prevent the knots that will later be tied there from being prominent. Through the volar hole of each pair is inserted a 22-gauge spinal needle. The needle passes upward into the fovea and onward through the RUL and the ulnar margin of the disc to appear in the ulnocarpal joint space. At this time, arthroscopy is switched to the viewing through the 3–4 portal. The skin cut for the dorsal radial DRUJ portal can be shifted distally for reuse as the 4–5 portal where the small hook probe is needed to manipulate the suture. Through the dorsal hole of each pair is placed a suture snare. The probe through the 4–5 portal is used to depress the disc and provide counter pressure as the needle and the snare are pushed through (Fig. 9.21). A 2-0 PDS suture is threaded through the 22-gauge spinal needle to appear in the ulnocarpal joint, where it is captured by the suture

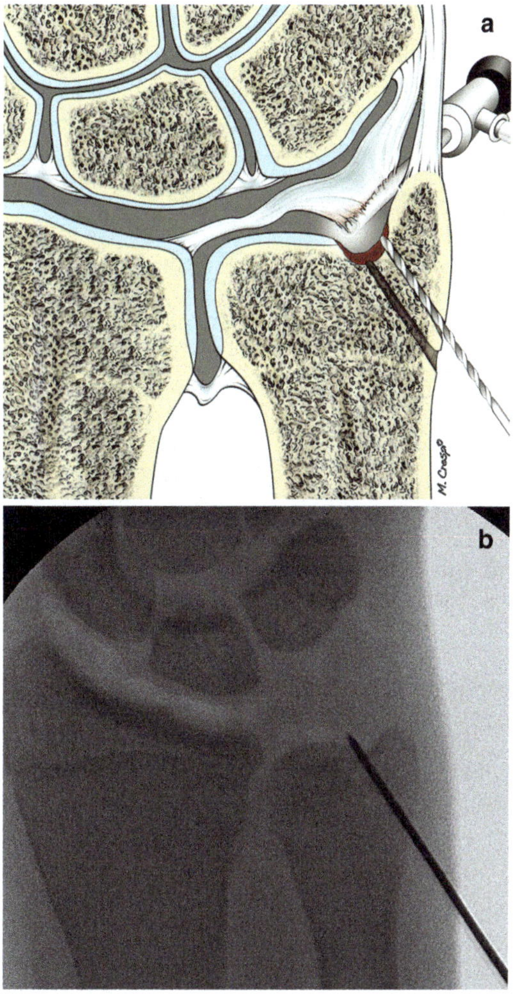

Fig. 9.19 (**a**, **b**) Four drill holes are created from the proximal ulnar cortex to form a square box configuration entering at the base of the fovea

snare and drawn back out to the ulnar cortex (Fig. 9.22). This is repeated for each pair of holes. The RUL is then sequentially tightened down into the fovea by alternating traction on each pair of suture strands until firmly seated

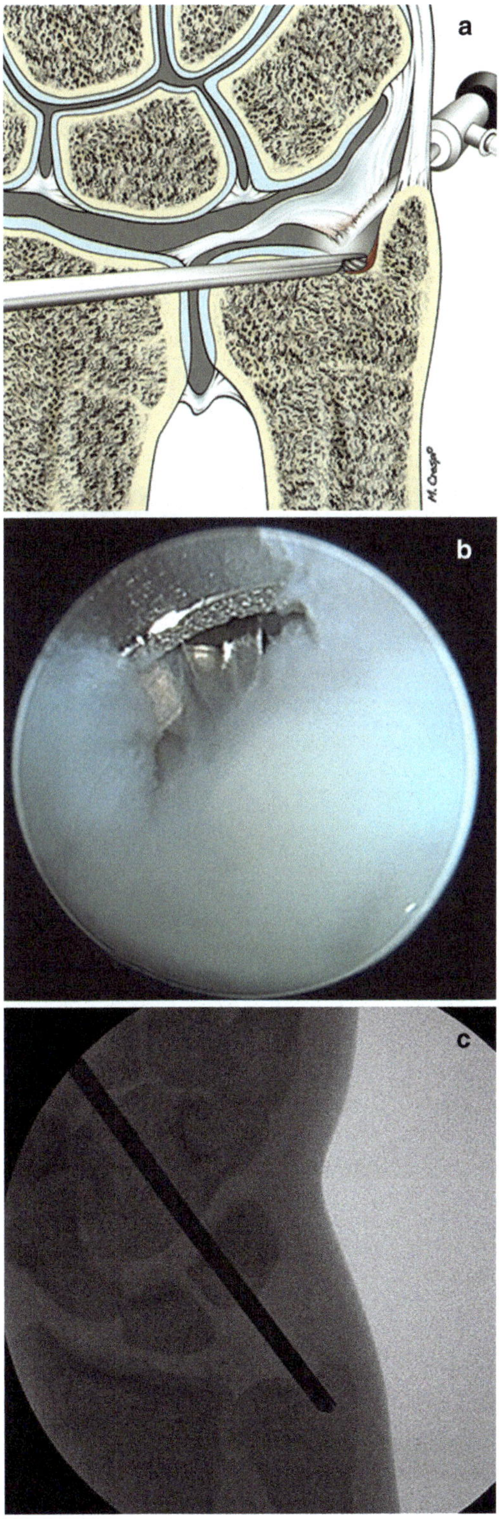

Fig. 9.18 (**a**, **b**) Especially in subacute proximal radioulnar foveal avulsions, the fovea should be burred to bleeding bone to stimulate the fibroblastic healing response to the reapproximated ligament fibers. (**c**) The 2.0-mm suction burr is demonstrated to be accurately located precisely to the concavity of the fovea

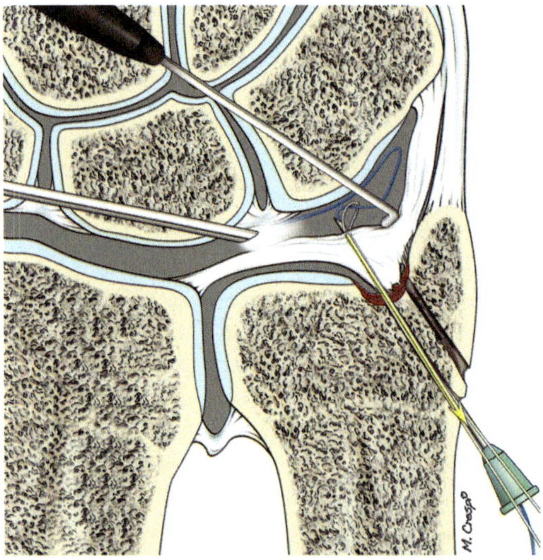

Fig. 9.20 Repair sutures of 2-0 PDS are passed from the volar hole to the dorsal hole for each pair of holes

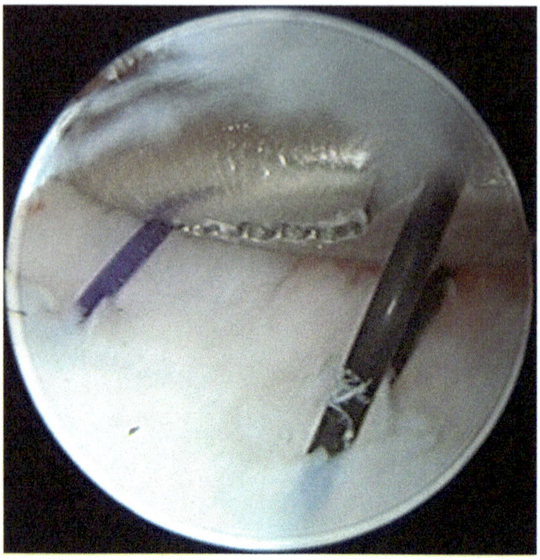

Fig. 9.22 A grasper reaches through the snare loop and captures the tail of the 2-0 PDS

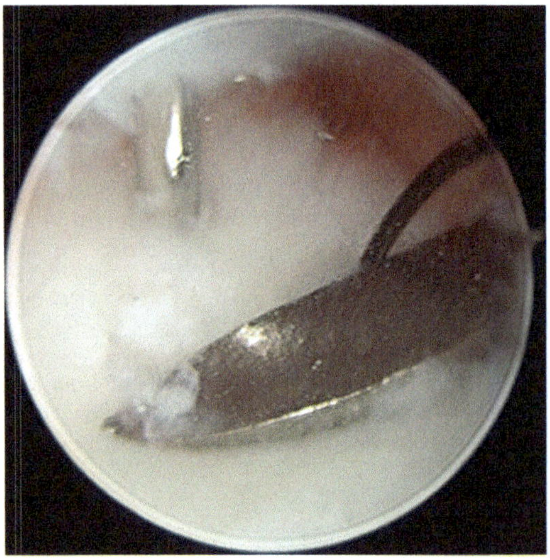

Fig. 9.21 A 2-0 PDS suture is passed by a 22-G spinal needle through the volar hole. A probe pushes down and assists the suture snare to penetrate through the fibrocartilage disc from the dorsal hole

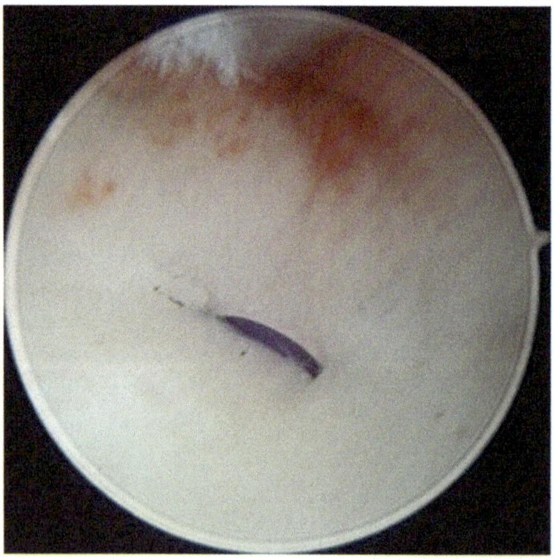

Fig. 9.23 As the sutures are tightened, the origin of the radioulnar ligament is drawn down to meet the prepared bone at the fovea

(Fig. 9.23). Before final seating of the repair and tying of the two knots in the recess at the ulnar cortex, the DRUJ relationship is congruently reduced and pinned in slight supination using two 1.6-mm K-wires proximal to the DRUJ, extra-articular (Fig. 9.24). The knots are then tied in the recess at the ulnar cortex, completing the repair (Fig. 9.25).

The patient is kept in a sugar-tong splint for 4 weeks, at which time the 1.6-mm K-wires are removed in the office and the splint is changed to a below-elbow orthoplast clamshell. Wrist flexion

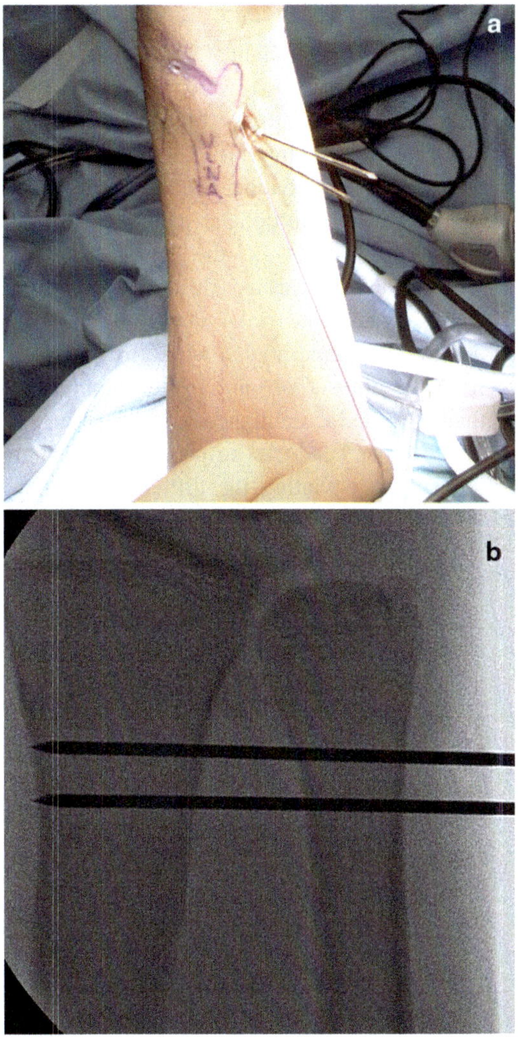

Fig. 9.24 (**a**, **b**) Before tightening and tying the two sutures, the DRUJ is congruently reduced and the ulna pinned to the radius with two transverse 1.6-mm Kirschner wires in neutral to slight supination

and extension are begun at 4 weeks in addition to full hand motion that has been encouraged since surgery. Forearm rotation is not formally included in the therapy plan until 6 weeks. The patient should use the orthoplast splint when up and active for at least 8 weeks following surgery. Grip strengthening with the wrist in neutral can begin at 8 weeks. More complex and heavier weight strengthening that stresses the DRUJ should not begin until 3 months postoperatively.

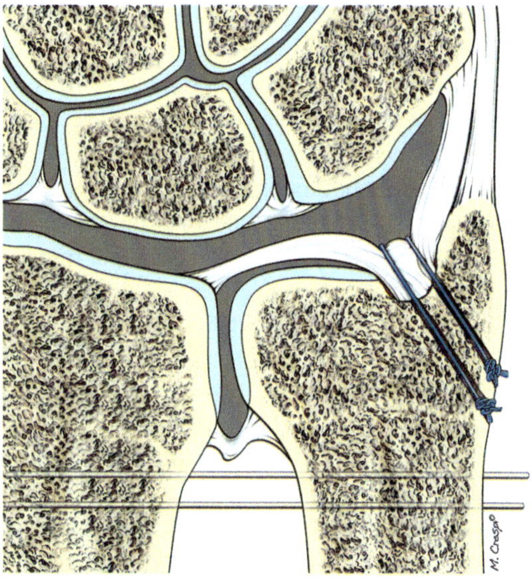

Fig. 9.25 After pinning the DRUJ, the two sutures are then sequentially tightened back and forth to work the ligament tightly down into the fovea and eventually tied with the knots in the planned cortical recess

Discussion

The earliest arthroscopic management of fibrocartilage substance tears consisted of debridement alone [14]. Given that surgeons recognized a tearing of tissue, there developed an enthusiasm for performing repairs. Both open and arthroscopic techniques evolved [7, 12, 15, 16, 24, 26]. Ongoing advancements in skill and technique have led to a very elegant all-arthroscopic technique that is versatile enough to be applied to different patterns of tears [5]. A 75-patient, nonrandomized comparison of open and arthroscopic repairs failed to identify significant differences in outcome, noting a higher incidence of dorsal ulnar nerve branch pain in the open group [1]. Another smaller study found that the chief factor affecting outcome was age [20]. No study has yet conclusively proven that any type of repair is needed unless the RUL is ruptured and the DRUJ is demonstrably unstable [2]. Some have wondered if patients with ulnar positive variance should automatically have an ulnar shortening osteotomy at the time of repair. A retrospective, nonrandomized study found no difference in outcomes for 51 patients when comparing arthroscopic repair with or without concomitant ulnar shortening [19]. It is not the existence of ulnar positive variance that creates the need for an ulnar shortening osteotomy, but rather the anatomic pattern of degenerative tearing seen at the time of arthroscopy as well as the clinical findings of ulnocarpal impaction syndrome preoperatively.

Multiple variables should be taken into account when determining which type of osteotomy to perform: extra-articular vs. intra-articular. These include the slope of the DRUJ, the shape of the ulnar head, the length of the ulnar styloid, and the existence of clinical patterns of ulnocarpal impaction, stylocarpal impaction, or DRUJ arthritis. The two most classic forms are the mid-diaphyseal ulnar extra-articular osteotomy with a large incision and 3.5-mm plate fixation and the intra-articular wafer resection of the distal portion of the ulnar head leaving a broad surface of cancellous bone exposed. But, there are many variations such as an open approach intra-articular osteotomy of the ulnar head that alters the congruent relationship of the ulnar head with the sigmoid notch and fixes the osteotomy with headless screws drilled through the articular surface [21]. Specific combinations of findings unique to each case may bias the preference toward one method of osteotomy or another. Overall comparisons indicate an equivalent outcome between the two classic forms but a higher complication rate for extra-articular osteotomy in terms of delayed union, nonunion, and the need for hardware removal [3, 4]. The complications of the extra-articular osteotomy may be mitigated by moving the site into the distal cancellous bone of the sub-capital region and using modern plate technology [10]. Eliminating the need to achieve bony union, the lack of hardware, and an all-arthroscopic procedure are features that appeal to patients considering the intra-articular resection of the distal ulnar head. Counterbalancing this appeal is the fact that contact pressures at the DRUJ are concentrated and increased, and the raw bone surface exposed to the intra-articular environment continues to irritate the joint for months after the procedure.

Conclusion

There are two fundamental TFCC pathologies that affect the DRUJ. Toward the radial side of the DRUJ, chronic attrition of the fibrocartilage disc begins at the interface between its proximal surface and the ulnar head, progressing to horizontal and multiplanar cleavage tears as well as synovitis of the sigmoid notch. Arthroscopy performed through the DRUJ allows for accurate evaluation as well as treatment of this pattern even when findings seen from the ulnocarpal joint are less impressive than expected. Simultaneous wafer resection of the ulnar head can be performed through the DRUJ, obviating the difficulties in performing a complete resection from the ulnocarpal joint through the fibrocartilage defect. In cases of clinical ulnocarpal impaction syndrome where the disc lacks a substantial full-thickness tear, shortening can be performed through DRUJ arthroscopy without having to iatrogenically create a large defect in the disc just to perform the wafer procedure.

Toward the ulnar side of the DRUJ, acute rupture of the RUL from the fovea can be confirmed by DRUJ arthroscopy. The fovea is prepared with a burr and the torn edge of the ligament with a shaver. An arthroscopic repair can be performed through the DRUJ. Alternating tension back and forth with the two sutures allows the ligament to be progressively drawn very firmly down into the fovea for a secure repair.

References

1. Anderson ML, Larson AN, Moran SL et al (2008) Clinical comparison of arthroscopic versus open repair of triangular fibrocartilage complex tears. J Hand Surg 33:675–682
2. Atzei A, Rizzo A, Luchetti R et al (2008) Arthroscopic foveal repair of triangular fibrocartilage complex peripheral lesion with distal radioulnar joint instability. Tech Hand Up Extrem Surg 12:226–235
3. Bernstein MA, Nagle DJ, Martinez A et al (2004) A comparison of combined arthroscopic triangular fibrocartilage complex debridement and arthroscopic wafer distal ulna resection versus arthroscopic triangu-

lar fibrocartilage complex debridement and ulnar shortening osteotomy for ulnocarpal abutment syndrome. Arthroscopy 20:392–401
4. Constantine KJ, Tomaino MM, Herndon JH et al (2000) Comparison of ulnar shortening osteotomy and the wafer resection procedure as treatment for ulnar impaction syndrome. J Hand Surg 25:55–60
5. Del Pinal T, Garcia-Bernal FJ, Cagigal L et al (2010) A technique for arthroscopic all-inside suturing in the wrist. J Hand Surg 35E:475–479
6. DiTano O, Trumble TE, Tencer AF (2003) Biomechanical function of the distal radioulnar and ulnocarpal wrist ligaments. J Hand Surg 28:622–627
7. Estrella EP, Hung LK, Ho PC et al (2007) Arthroscopic repair of triangular fibrocartilage complex tears. Arthroscopy 23:729–737
8. Haugstvedt JR, Berger RA, Nakamura T et al (2006) Relative contributions of the ulnar attachments of the triangular fibrocartilage complex to the dynamic stability of the distal radioulnar joint. J Hand Surg 31: 445–451
9. Henry MH (2008) Management of acute triangular fibrocartilage complex injury of the wrist. J Am Acad Orthop Surg 16:320–329
10. Henry MH (2009) Sub-capital ulnar shortening osteotomy. J Hand Microsurg 1:103–107
11. Henry MH, Smith DW, Masson MV (2004) Reconstruction of distal radioulnar joint instability. J Am Soc Surg Hand 4:35–41
12. Iwasaki N, Nishida K, Motomiya M et al (2011) Arthroscopic-assisted repair of avulsed triangular fibrocartilage complex to the fovea of the ulnar head: a 2 to 4 year follow-up study. Arthroscopy 27: 1371–1378
13. Kihara H, Short WH, Werner FW et al (1995) The stabilizing mechanism of the distal radioulnar joint during pronation and supination. J Hand Surg 20: 930–936
14. Minami A, Ishikawa J, Suenaga N et al (1996) Clinical results of treatment of triangular fibrocartilage complex tears by arthroscopic debridement. J Hand Surg 21:406–411
15. Moritomo H, Masatomi T, Murase T et al (2010) Open repair of foveal avulsion of the triangular fibrocartilage complex and comparison by types of injury mechanism. J Hand Surg 35:1955–1963
16. Nakamura T, Nakao Y, Ikegami H et al (2004) Open repair of the ulnar disruption of the triangular fibrocartilage complex with double three-dimensional mattress suturing technique. Tech Hand Up Extrem Surg 8:116–123
17. Nakamura T, Takayama S, Horiuchi Y et al (2001) Origins and insertions of the triangular fibrocartilage complex: a histological study. J Hand Surg 26B:446–454
18. Nishikawa S, Toh S (2002) Anatomical study of the carpal attachment of the triangular fibrocartilage complex. J Bone Joint Surg 84B:1062–1065
19. Papapetropoulos PA, Wartinbee DA, Richard MJ et al (2010) Management of peripheral triangular fibrocartilage complex tears in the ulnar positive patient: arthroscopic repair versus ulnar shortening osteotomy. J Hand Surg 35:1607–1613
20. Ruch DS, Papadonikolakis A (2005) Arthroscopically assisted repair of peripheral triangular fibrocartilage complex tears: factors affecting outcome. Arthroscopy 21:1126–1130
21. Slade JF 3rd, Gillon TJ (2007) Osteochondral shortening osteotomy for the treatment of ulnar impaction syndrome: a new technique. Tech Hand Up Extrem Surg 11:74–82
22. Slutsky DJ (2007) Distal radioulnar joint arthroscopy and the volar ulnar portal. Tech Hand Up Extrem Surg 11:38–44
23. Slutsky DJ (2011) Arthroscopic evaluation of the foveal attachment of the triangular fibrocartilage. Hand Clin 27:255–261
24. Smith DW, Henry MH (2002) Comprehensive management of associated soft tissue injuries in distal radius fractures. J Am Soc Surg Hand 2:153–164
25. Stuart PR, Berger RA, Linscheid RL et al (2000) The dorsopalmar stability of the distal radioulnar joint. J Hand Surg 25:689–699
26. Yao J, Lee AT (2011) All-arthroscopic repair of palmer 1B triangular fibrocartilage complex tears using the Fas T-Fix device. J Hand Surg 36:836–842

10 DRUJ Instability: Arthroscopic Repair of the Detached TFCC to the Fovea of the Ulna

Toshiyasu Nakamura

Introduction: Pathology of Foveal Detachment of the TFCC

The TFCC functions as a stabilizer between the radius and ulna as well as a stabilizer between the ulna and ulnar carpus, a load distributor between ulna and ulnar carpus, and allows smooth rotation of the forearm [13, 16]. The RULs (distal radioulnar ligaments) attach at the very dorsal and palmar edge of the sigmoid notch and at the fovea and base of the ulnar styloid process [12, 15] (see Fig. 2.1). Histological examination revealed the fovea is the largest attaching area of the RUL on the ulna [12, 15] (Fig. 2.5). As the RUL is the main stabilizer of the DRUJ, RUL tear at the fovea can result in DRUJ instability readily [3].

Palmer 1B tears [17] are defined with peripheral ulnar tears of the TFCC which may be associated with an ulnar styloid fracture because the TFCC had been considered to attach only to the ulnar styloid in the 1980s and 1990s. As the TFCC is anchored to the DRUJ via the RUL which attaches to the ulnar fovea and base of the ulnar styloid, a hyper rotation force or dislocation force applied to the RUL from the ulnar head, such as in fall, may disrupt the RUL not only from the ulnar styloid but also from the fovea.

T. Nakamura, M.D., Ph.D.
Department of Orthopaedic Surgery, School of Medicine, Keio University, 35 Shinanomachi, Shinjuku-ku, Tokyo 160-8582, Japan
e-mail: tosiyasu@sc.itc.keio.ac.jp

A foveal detachment of the TFCC is clearly evident in clinical practice [10, 11]. Atzei recently subclassified the Palmer 1B tear into a distal component, a proximal component, or both (complete) [1]. An isolated foveal detachment is equivalent to a proximal component tear.

Diagnosis of the Foveal TFCC Tear

There are several physical testing maneuvers including ulnocarpal stress test, fovea sign, and DRUJ instability test. Ulnocarpal stress test is effective for assessment of TFCC tear. Fovea sign, tenderness on the palmar side of the base of the ulnar styloid, suggests foveal tear [18]. Tenderness of dorsal aspect of the fovea may also indicate foveal detachment. Most reliable physical test is DRUJ instability test, including ballottement test, in which dorsopalmar stability between the ulna and radius is examined in the neutral, pronated, and supinated positions, respectively [8, 11]. When the "end point," which comes from ligamentous restraint, can be felt, there may not be foveal tear, while the complete foveal detachment induces no "end point" situation that may demonstrate multidirectional instability of the DRUJ. If the "end point" was noted either in dorsal or palmar direction, partial tear of the RUL may exist. Piano key sign, indicating the floating ulnar head in the pronation position, may also be helpful to diagnose the fovea avulsion.

F. del Piñal et al. (eds.), *Arthroscopic Management of Ulnar Pain*,
DOI 10.1007/978-3-642-30544-3_10, © Springer-Verlag Berlin Heidelberg 2012

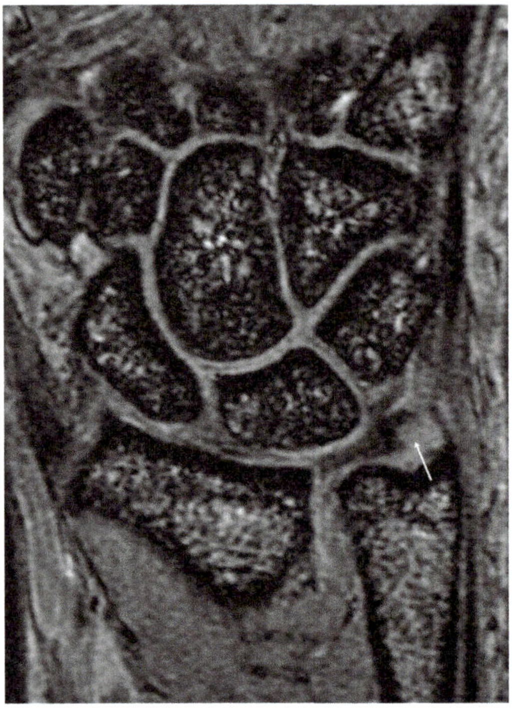

Fig. 10.1 Typical MRI of foveal detachment of the TFCC. Note high-signal-intensity area at the fovea without low-signal ligament structure (*arrow*)

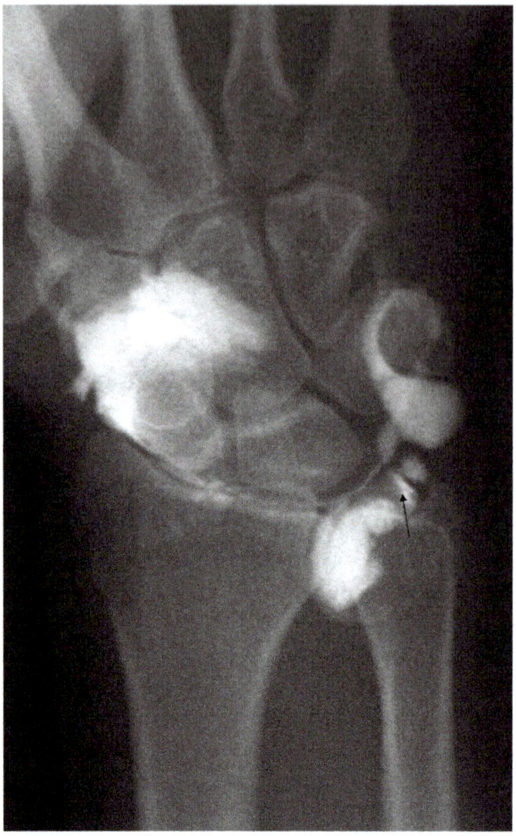

Fig. 10.2 Arthrogram of foveal tear. Dye infiltrates to the foveal lesion of the TFCC which indicates a foveal avulsion (*white arrow*)

MRI can demonstrate TFCC tear including foveal detachment clearly (Fig. 10.1). Gradient echo sequence T2*-weighted image indicates high delineation ability for TFCC structure [14]. In foveal detachment of the TFCC, arthrogram also shows pooling of the dye at the fovea, inclusion of the dye between the TFCC and ulnar fovea (Fig. 10.2), or dye infiltration into the proximal side of the TFCC.

DRUJ Arthroscopy Findings: A Classification of Foveal Tear

The wrist is suspended in vertical position by finger trap using overhead traction tower. General anesthesia is recommended. Counterweight of 2–3 kg is necessary to open the radiocarpal joint.

The wrist is systematically evaluated by normal radiocarpal arthroscopy using 1.9–2.7-mm arthroscope. The 3–4 portal is used for arthroscope and 4–5 or 6R portal for the probe. Associated soft tissue injury, such as intercarpal ligament tears, can be detected through radiocarpal arthroscopy. The TFCC is observed via radiocarpal arthroscopy. Radiocarpal arthroscope sometimes demonstrated intact TFC (no tear) or just the radial or central slit tear on the TFC. The slit tear of the TFC can be debrided arthroscopically. In DRUJ instability patients, radiocarpal arthroscopy can only demonstrate loss of trampoline effect as well as loss of peripheral tension (positive hook test) [1] in the disc in the patients with foveal disruption since the TFCC is not continuously connected to the ulna.

After radiocarpal arthroscopy is completed, the author recommends DRUJ arthroscopy, which can directly visualize the complete foveal rupture of the TFCC (Fig. 10.3). DRUJ (distal)

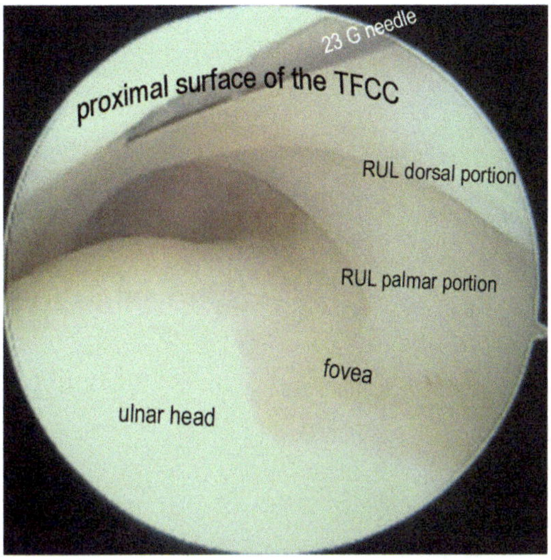

Fig. 10.3 DRUJ arthroscopy offers direct vision of the ulnar head, radial sigmoid notch, proximal surface of the TFCC, fovea, and RUL. This case shows an absence of the palmar portion of the radioulnar ligament (*RUL*) which is replaced by scar tissue. The dorsal portion of the RUL is intact

portal is just 5 mm proximal to 6R portal, just ulnar to the extensor digiti quinti tendon and just distal to the ulnar head. The saline is injected through 23-G needle to the DRUJ by 1 ml to expand the joint, and a longitudinal 5-mm incision is set just on the injected needle pinhole. Soft tissue is divided by mosquito forceps, then the tip of the mosquito can hit the ulnar head, and then it gradually divides and penetrates the upper side of the DRUJ joint capsule to go into the joint. The mosquito guides the 1.9-mm scope to the DRUJ.

In case of foveal detachment, joint space of the DRUJ including the fovea area can easily be seen because the DRUJ is loose [11]. When the TFCC is attached completely to the ulna without any DRUJ instability, the fovea area is difficult to be visualized with DRUJ arthroscopy, although the joint surface of ulnar head and sigmoid notch of the radius can be seen easily. There are several findings of the RUL in DRUJ instability patients through DRUJ arthroscopy: (1) the complete foveal detachment, which includes the empty RUL that is vacant ligament tissue surrounded by synovial tissue and fragile scaring; (2) partial avulsion either on the dorsal or palmar portion of the RUL, which indicates moderate DRUJ instability that has either palmar or dorsal endpoint; and (3) relaxation of the ligament which corresponds to partial healing of partial tear of the RUL, indicating mild DRUJ instability where the endpoint is obvious in both palmar and dorsal direction, but the DRUJ is looser than contralateral side [11] (Fig. 10.4).

Indication

We reserve arthroscopic repair technique for a relatively fresh (up to 6 months to 1 year after the initial injury), complete or partial ulnar disruption of the TFCC at the fovea [11]. The technique described is suited for wrists with the neutral or minus variance. In the wrists with positive ulnar variance, a certain shearing stress is expected to be present between the ulnar head and sutured site of the TFCC, which may induce subsequent rupture of sutures.

Technique

Option 1: Arthroscopic-Assisted Repair of Avulsed TFCC at the Fovea Using Suture Anchor

Concept of this technique is a modification of Atzei's [1, 2] mini-open repair technique using suture anchor. After the foveal detachment of the TFCC is confirmed by DRUJ arthroscopy, a small shaver is inserted to the DRUJ through the small incision just ulnar to the DRUJ distal portal. This is named the DRUJ ulnar portal. Debridement of the avulsed or torn RUL at the fovea area including removing adherent clot can be done by shaver for repair of the TFCC.

An approximately 2.5-cm small incision is made just proximal to the 6-U portal (Fig. 10.5). The forearm is in supinated position; then the fovea area becomes subcutaneous and can easily be exposed after sectioning the extensor retinaculum. The dorsal sensory branches of the ulnar nerve are identified and protected palmary by retractor before sectioning the extensor retinaculum. Open refresh of the fovea can be done in this step.

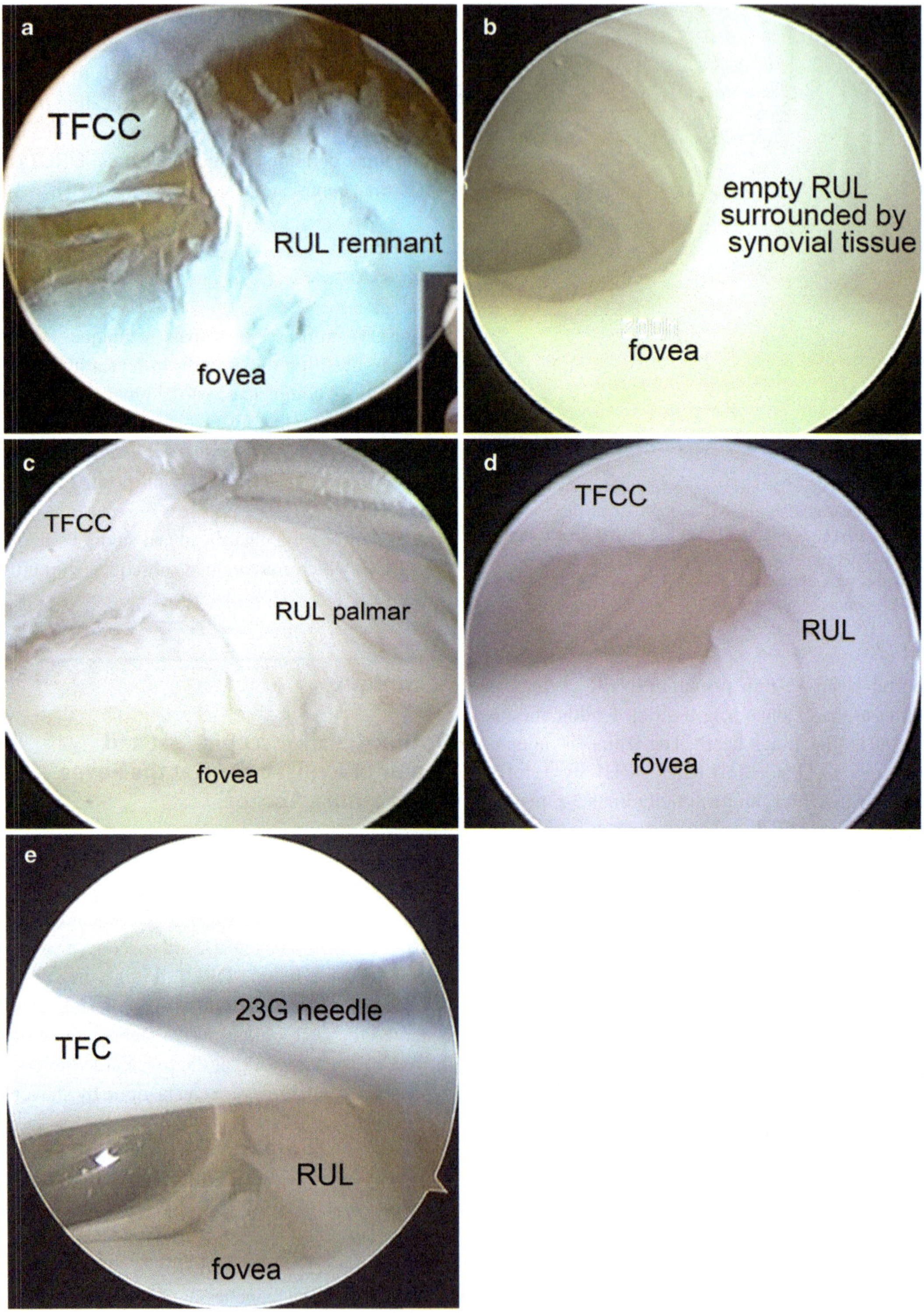
a
TFCC
RUL remnant
fovea
b
empty RUL surrounded by synovial tissue
fovea
c
TFCC
RUL palmar
fovea
d
TFCC
RUL
fovea
e
23G needle
TFC
RUL
fovea

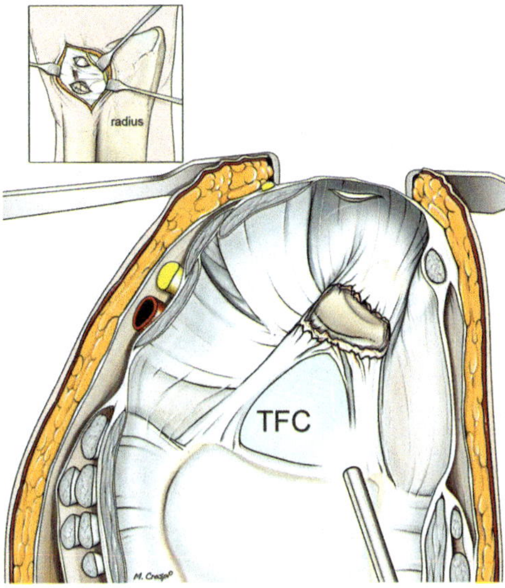

Fig. 10.5 In supinated position, a small 2.5-cm incision is made just proximal to the 6-U portal to access the palmar aspect of the fovea. Note that the superficial branch of the ulnar nerve must be retracted

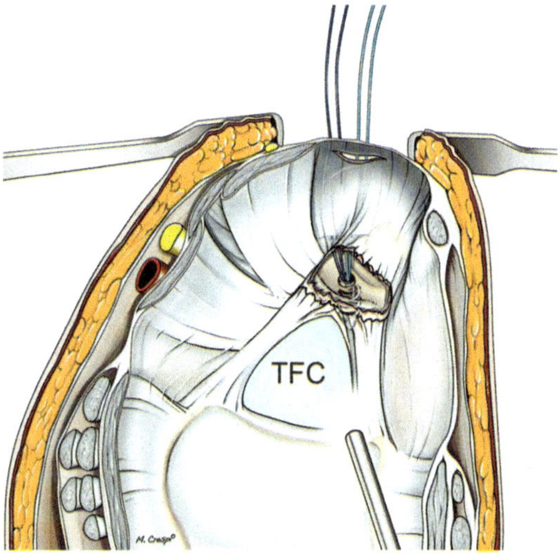

Fig. 10.6 The suture screw is inserted to center of the fovea from palmar aspect of the ulna. When the forearm is replaced in the neutral position, the sutures exit under the TFCC

To reconstitute the avulsed RUL to the fovea, care must be taken to insert a suture anchor or suture screw to the center of the fovea, where the rotation axis passes and is the isometric point during forearm rotation [9]. The author prefers to use Mitek microsuture anchor (DePuy Mitek, Raynham, MA) or Twinfix suture screw (Smith and Nephew, Andover, MA), in which the former has one nonabsorbable 3-0 polyester suture, while the latter is with two nonabsorbable 2-0 braided sutures.

After the suture anchor or screw is inserted to the fovea, the forearm is replaced in the neutral position. In this position, the TFC overlies the fovea, and the sutures exit under the TFCC (Fig. 10.6). Under the 3–4 portal view on the radiocarpal joint, one side of the suture is inserted into the radiocarpal joint through the RUL and ulnar-half area of the TFC using the suture loop technique [1, 4], where the suture end is inserted into the tip of a 21-G needle which is bended so that it creates a loop inside the joint (Fig. 10.7). The other 21-G injection needle, in which the 4-0 nylon loop suture was set, is passed through the RUL and TFC just dorsal to the first suture penetrated (Fig. 10.8). A grasper or mosquito inserted from 4 to 5 or 6R portal grasps the nearest loop and the suture end and introduces both sutures once outside the radiocarpal joint. The suture end is set into the 4-0 nylon loop (Fig. 10.8). Pulling the 4-0 nylon loop introduces the suture end through the TFC to RUL backward to the fovea area. When using the Twinfix, the other suture

Fig. 10.4 Classification of radioulnar ligament tear through DRUJ arthroscopy. Complete foveal detachment (**a**), which includes the empty RUL that is vacant ligament tissue surrounded by synovial tissue and fragile scaring (**b**); partial avulsion either on the dorsal or palmar portion of the RUL, which indicates moderate DRUJ instability that has either palmar or dorsal end point (**c**); relaxation of the ligament which corresponds to partial healing of partial tear of the RUL, indicating mild DRUJ instability where the end point is obvious in both palmar and dorsal direction, but the DRUJ is looser than contralateral side (**d**). Normal RUL, which indicates very narrow space between the proximal side of the TFCC and ulnar head (**e**)

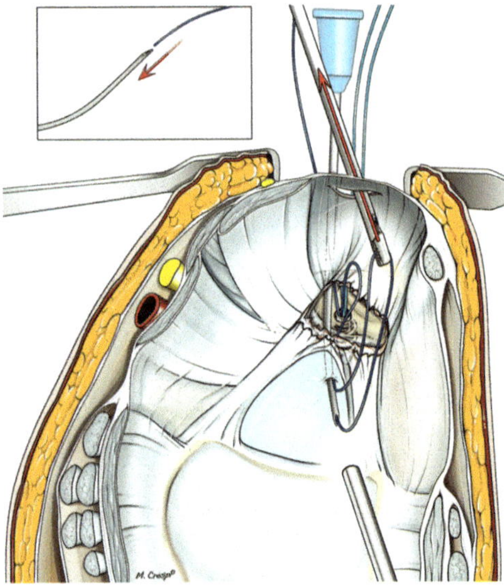

Fig. 10.7 Suture end is inserted into the tip of a 21-G needle which is bended. The needle penetrates from the RUL through the TFCC, and the suture creates a loop inside the joint

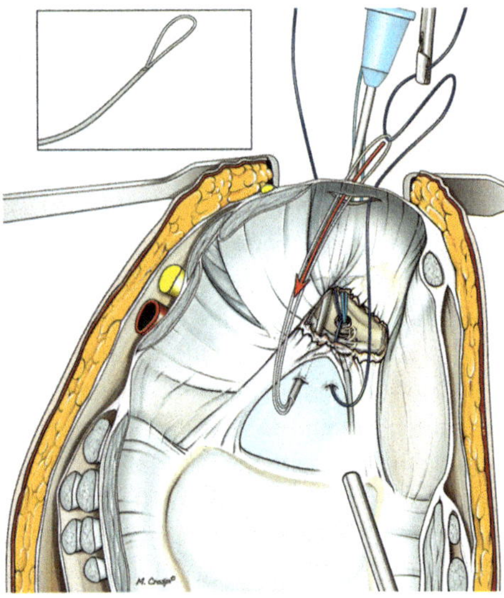

Fig. 10.8 The 21-G injection needle, in which the 4-0 nylon loop suture was set, is passed through the RUL and TFC just dorsal to the first suture penetrated. A mosquito inserted from 4 to 5 or 6R portal grasps the loop and the suture end, once introduces both sutures outside the radiocarpal joint. The suture end is set into the 4-0 nylon loop. The *red arrow* indicates the pull back direction of the nylon loop to introduce the suture

end again passes through the RUL and TFC in a slightly different area on the TFC. The sutures are tied, and knots are just close to the suture screw or anchor (Fig. 10.9).

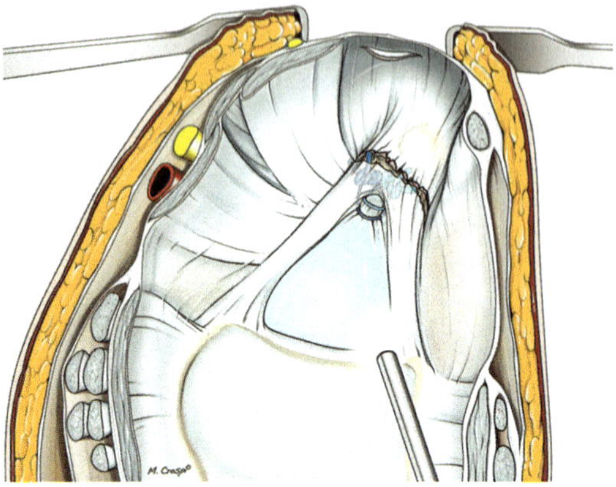

Fig. 10.9 Pulling the 4-0 nylon loop introduces the suture end through the TFC to RUL back to the fovea area. The sutures are tied, and knots are just close to the suture screw

Option 2: Arthroscopic Transosseous Repair of the TFCC

Concept of option 2 technique is based on the anatomical characteristics of the TFCC, in which the line between the ulnar-half area including apex of the TFC and 10–15-mm proximal point from the ulnar styloid (corresponding to just proximal to the ulnar prominent of the ulna) must pass through the center of the fovea, the isometric point of the forearm rotation [9] (Fig. 10.10). After the foveal detachment of the TFCC is confirmed by DRUJ arthroscopy, the fovea area is debrided by a small shaver inserted from DRUJ ulnar portal. An original target device (Fig. 10.11; Nakashima Medical, Okayama, Japan) was set through 4–5 or 6R portal, and approximately 1-cm longitudinal incision was made on the ulnar side of the ulnar cortex, 10–15 mm proximal from the tip of the ulnar styloid, with the periosteum elevated. Small spike on the target device is set on the ulnar half of the TFC. Two separate small holes are made from the ulnar cortex of the ulna with 1.2-mm K-wire to the ulnar-half portion of the TFC (Fig. 10.12). The 21-G injection needle, in which the loop nylon 4-0 stitch was set, is passed through one tunnel from the outside to the radiocarpal joint, then is repeated through the other bone tunnel. From 4-5 or 6R portal, both two loop stitches are once pulled out by mosquito nonhook forceps, then two nonabsorbable 3-0

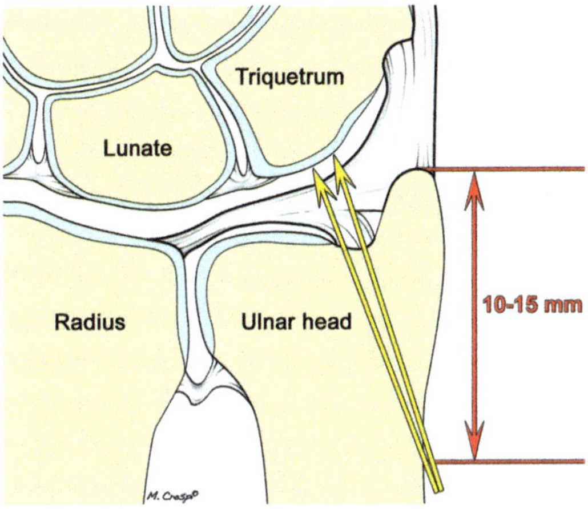

Fig. 10.10 Basic concept of the arthroscopic transosseous repair of the TFCC. The line between the point on the ulnar cortex of the ulnar shaft 10–15 mm proximal from the tip of the ulnar styloid (corresponding to small ulnar prominence just proximal to the ulnar head) and ulnar half of the TFC passes through the foveal lesion theoretically. If the stitches are induced into this area, theoretically the TFCC can be sutured to the fovea with outside-in pullout technique

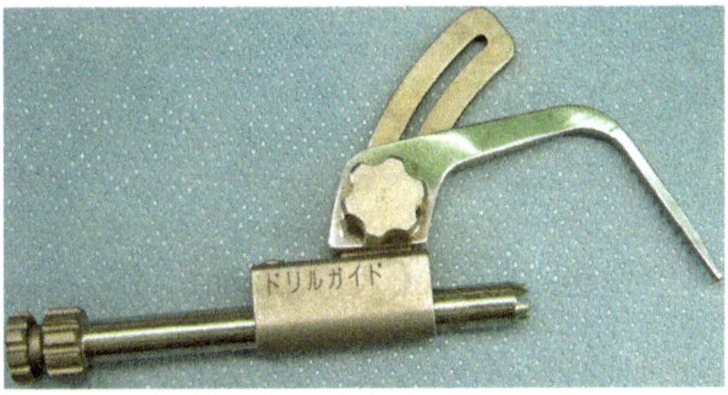

Fig. 10.11 Original targeting device

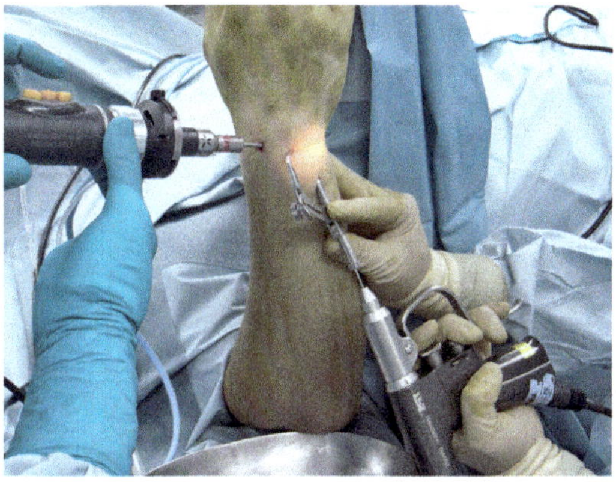

Fig. 10.12 A 1.2-mm K-wire is drilled from ulnar side of the ulnar to the ulnocarpal joint using target device

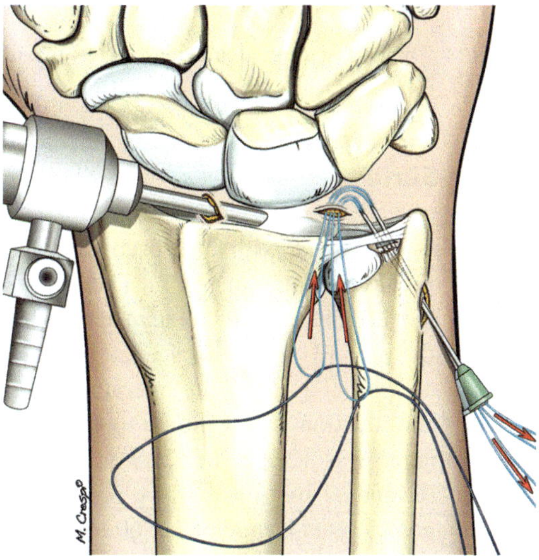

Fig. 10.13 A 21-G needle with loop nylon 4-0 stitch is passed from the ulnar cortex to the ulnar-half area of the TFC. This drawing indicates that one nonabsorbable 3-0 polyester stitch is introduced from the RC joint to the ulnar cortex of the ulna by loop stitches (*red arrows* indicate direction of introducing the nonabsorbable 3-0 polyester stitch)

polyester sutures (Ticron, Covidien, Mansfield, MA) are introduced from the RC joint to the ulnar cortex of the ulna by loop stitches (Fig. 10.13) to make outside-in pullout suture of the TFCC to the fovea. The TFCC is tightly sutured to the ulnar fovea with this technique, which restabilizes the DRUJ (Fig. 10.14).

Postoperative Course

Two weeks of long-arm casting and subsequent 3 weeks of short-arm casting are necessary. After removal of the cast at 5 weeks after the surgery, active ROM exercise started. Seven weeks after the operation, passive ROM exercise by an occupational therapist may be needed, if there is loss of forearm rotation. Usually, at 8–9 weeks after the operation, full pronation-supination range can be achieved, followed by isometric muscle power exercise with up to 3-kg weight. Three months after the operation, the weight may increase to 5 kg. The patient may be back to normal sports activity level 6 months after the surgery.

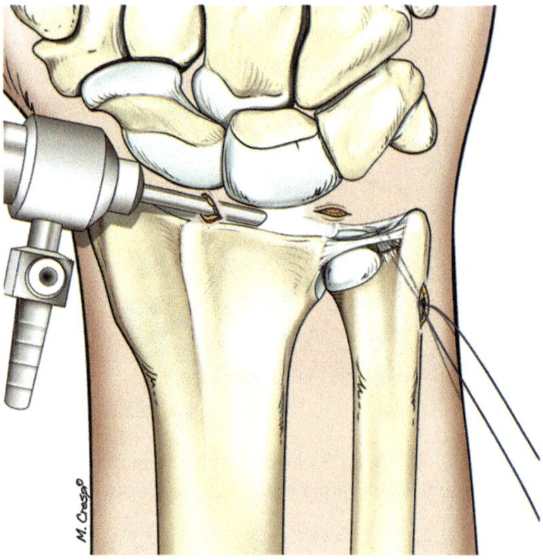

Fig. 10.14 Diagram of arthroscopic transosseous repair of the TFCC

Table 10.1 DRUJ evaluating system

	Point
Pain	
Severe (always painful)	0
Moderate (pain in motion or twisting)	1
Mild (occasionally painful)	2
No pain	4
Range of pronation/supination	
<100°	0
100–119°	1
120–139°	2
140–159°	3
>159°	4
DRUJ instability	
++ (No end point in any direction)	0
+ (At least one end point either in dorsal or palmar)	1
± (Loose than intact contralateral side)	2
– (Stable DRUJ)	4

Points of each category were added and evaluated as follows: excellent, 11–12 points; good, 9–10 points; fair, 6–8 points; poor, 0–5 points

Patient Series

We treated 26 wrists with arthroscopic transosseous repair technique (option 2). There were 14 males and 12 females, with a mean age of 28. Injured side was 13 right and 13 left. Period between the initial injury and operation was average 8 months (range of 1 month to 4 years). Ulnar variance was +2 mm in 5, +1 mm in 1, 0 mm in 18, and –1 mm in 2 wrists. Follow up was average 3.5 years (range of 12–60 months). All cases indicated ulnar detachment at the fovea. Pain, range of forearm pronation-supination, and DRUJ instability were examined in all cases. DRUJ evaluating system including relief of pain, range of pronation/supination, and DRUJ instability was used for clinical evaluation (Table 10.1) [11].

After the arthroscopic transosseous repair of the foveal detachment of the TFCC, 17 wrists among 26 wrists indicated no pain. Severe pain remained in two wrists. Recurrence of pain was found 8–12 months after the surgery in four wrists. Mild pain was noted in three wrists. There was no loss of range of rotation preoperatively, and 25 wrists indicated full range of pronosupination postoperatively, but one wrist indicated 45° of loss of supination postoperatively, which needed open release of the DRUJ. Instability at the DRUJ was found in all wrists preoperatively. There was no postoperative DRUJ instability in 19 wrists. Moderate to severe DRUJ instability was noted in seven wrists. Final clinical results obtained were 15 excellent, 3 good, 4 fair, and 4 poor results.

Discussion

Recent anatomical and biomechanical studies have advanced our knowledge on repair methods for a foveal disruption of the TFCC [9, 12, 15]. The TFCC can be thought of as a hammock, which surrounds and supports the carpus, with two tight anchors to the fovea corresponding to the dorsal and palmar portion of the RUL. Once both anchors are disrupted, the hammock is unsteady and unstable (Fig. 2.12). DRUJ stability can be restored by reanchoring the RUL [11]. The direction of the sutures had better to be parallel to direction of the vertical RUL fibers. Because of the isometricity of the RUL [9], the fibers must be attached to the center of the fovea [11].

Avulsion of the TFCC from the fovea may induce DRUJ instability [3], but the conventional arthroscopic capsular repair technique of the TFCC to the dorsal or ulnar joint capsule [4, 6, 7] does not reconstitute the foveal origin, where the RUL mainly arises. There are several papers on arthroscopic-assisted transosseous repair techniques of the TFCC. Atzei et al. explored the foveal lesion arthroscopically and used a mini-incision to insert a bone anchor at the fovea (option 1 in this chapter) [1, 2]. Iwasaki and Minami [5] used 2.9-mm drill hole made from the proximal ulnar cortex to the fovea under fluoroscopic control with a radiocarpal arthroscopically assisted suture of the TFCC to the ulnar periosteum. We also obtained excellent clinical results with arthroscopic transosseous repair technique (option 2 in this chapter) [11], which reattaches the TFCC into the fovea directly.

References

1. Atzei A (2010) Arthroscopic management of DRUJ instability following TFCC ulnar tears. In: Del Pinal F, Mathoulin C, Luchetti R (eds) Arthroscopic management of distal radius fractures. Springer, Berlin/Heidelberg, pp 73–88
2. Atzei A, Rizzo A, Luchetti R et al (2008) Arthroscopic foveal repair of triangular fibrocartilage complex peripheral lesion with distal radioulnar joint instability. Tech Hand Up Extrem Surg 12:226–235
3. Haugstvedt JR, Berger RA, Nakamura T et al (2006) Relative contributions of the ulnar attachment of the triangular fibrocartilage complex to the dynamic stability of the distal radioulnar joint. J Hand Surg 26A:445–451
4. Haugstvedt JR, Husby T (1999) Results of repair of peripheral tears in the triangular fibrocartilage complex using an arthroscopic suture technique. Scand J Plast Reconstr Surg 33:439–447
5. Iwasaki N, Minami A (2009) Arthroscopically assisted reattachment of avulsed triangular fibrocartilage complex to the fovea of the ulnar head. J Hand Surg Am 34:1323–1326
6. Lindau T, Adlercreutz C, Aspenberg P (2000) Peripheral tears of the triangular fibrocartilage complex cause distal radioulnar joint instability after distal radius fractures. J Hand Surg Am 25:464–468
7. Millants P, De Smet L, Van Ransbeeck H (2002) Outcome study of arthroscopic suturing of ulnar avulsion of the triangular fibrocartilage complex of the wrist. Chir Main 21:298–300
8. Moriya T, Aoki M, Iba K et al (2009) Effect of triangular ligament tears on distal radioulnar joint instability and evaluation of three clinical tests: a biomechanical study. J Hand Surg Eur 34:219–223
9. Nakamura T, Makita A (2000) The proximal ligamentous component of the triangular fibrocartilage complex: functional anatomy and three-dimensional changes in length of the radioulnar ligament during pronation-supination. J Hand Surg Br 25:479–486
10. Nakamura T, Nakao Y, Ikegami H et al (2004) Open repair of the ulnar disruption of the triangular fibrocartilage complex with double 3D-mattress suturing technique. Tech Up Extrem Surg 8:116–123
11. Nakamura T, Sato K, Okazaki M et al (2011) Repair of foveal detachment of the triangular fibrocartilage complex: open and arthroscopic transosseous techniques. Hand Clin 27:281–290
12. Nakamura T, Yabe Y (2000) Histological anatomy of the triangular fibrocartilage complex of the human wrist. Ann Anat 182:567–572
13. Nakamura T, Yabe Y, Horiuchi Y (1996) Functional anatomy of the triangular fibrocartilage complex. J Hand Surg Br 21:581–586
14. Nakamura T, Yabe Y, Horiuchi Y (1999) Fat-suppression magnetic resonance imaging of the triangular fibrocartilage complex – comparison with spin echo, gradient echo pulse sequence and histology. J Hand Surg Br 24:22–26
15. Nakamura T, Yabe Y, Horiuchi Y et al (2001) Origins and insertions of the triangular fibrocartilage complex – a histological study. J Hand Surg Br 26:446–454
16. Palmer AK, Werner FW (1981) The triangular fibrocartilage complex of the wrist -anatomy and function. J Hand Surg 6:153–162
17. Palmer AK (1989) Triangular fibrocartilage complex lesions: a classification. J Hand Surg Am 14:594–606
18. Tay SC, Tomita K, Berger RA (2007) The "ulnar fovea sign" for defining ulnar wrist pain: an analysis of sensitivity and specificity. J Hand Surg Am 32: 438–444

DRUJ Instability: Arthroscopic Ligament Reconstruction

11

Andrea Atzei

Introduction

The triangular fibrocartilage complex (TFCC) is a specialized tridimensional structure interposed between the distal radius, ulna, and carpus. From an anatomical and functional standpoint, the TFCC is composed by a "distal component (dc-TFCC)" and a "proximal component of the TFCC (pc-TFCC)" [19, 20]. The pc-TFCC is responsible for the stability of the distal radioulnar joint (DRUJ) and should be considered as the true DRUJ ligament. The pc-TFCC originates from the ulnar corners of the distal radius with two branches, palmar and dorsal, and attaches to the fovea ulnaris. The fovea is considered as the isometric area of the DRUJ ligament. Since the axis of rotation of the forearm passes through the fovea [15, 23], the foveal fibers of the pc-TFCC present an isometric behavior during pronosupination [19]. Though frequently overlooked, the foveal area is also of outmost importance for the stability of the ulnar carpus since this matches the area where the fibers of the ulnocarpal (UC) ligaments converge with the DRUJ ligament [17]. Therefore, following complete detachment of the TFCC from the fovea not only is DRUJ stability affected, but also UC instability may be present.

A fall on the outstretched hand or a violent traction and twisting injury of the wrist or forearm may cause a rupture of the TFCC at its periphery and produce the typical type 1-B TFCC tear according to Palmer's classification. Recent advances in arthroscopic evaluation of TFCC disorders have improved the definition of the peripheral tears, allowing for a new treatment-oriented classification [2] that considers different classes of type 1-B tears according to the involvement of the dc-TFCC and pc-TFCC either separately (classes 1 and 3, respectively) or together (class 2). Not only does the new classification (Table 11.1) provide treatment guidelines for the different conditions, so that class 1 tears should be repaired by arthroscopic suture [9] and classes 2 and 3 by refixation [5, 21], but also it introduces the new concept of nonrepairable tears (class 4).

Only arthroscopic inspection may give a hint on the healing capacity of the edges of a TFCC tear, even after extensive debridement. When arthroscopic appearance is suggestive of a poor healing potential of TFCC margins, the tear is classified as class 4 and is candidate to ligamentous reconstruction.

A number of procedures have been proposed in order to restore DRUJ stability through a nonanatomical reconstruction, either by the means of an extra-articular ulnocarpal sling or a direct radioulnar tether extrinsic to the joint [6, 7, 10, 13, 25], or a dynamic muscle transfer using the pronator quadratus [14]. These techniques are less effective

A. Atzei
Fenice Hand Surgery and Rehabilitation Team, Centro di Medicina, Treviso - Italy; Policlinico "San Giorgio", Pordenone - Italy
e-mail: andreatzei@email.it

F. del Piñal et al. (eds.), *Arthroscopic Management of Ulnar Pain*,
DOI 10.1007/978-3-642-30544-3_11, © Springer-Verlag Berlin Heidelberg 2012

Table 11.1 Classification of TFCC peripheral tears

	Class 1: Repairable distal tear	Class 2: Repairable complete tear	Class 3: Repairable proximal tear	Class 4: Non-repairable tear	Class 5: Arthritic DRUJ
	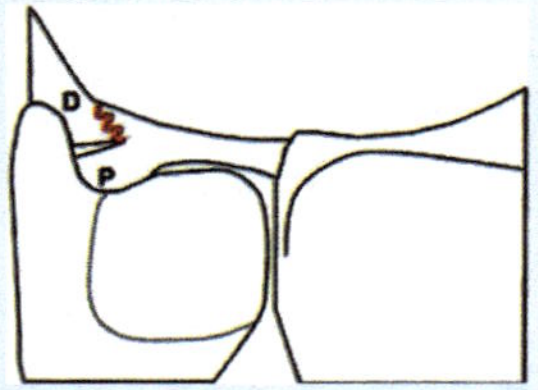	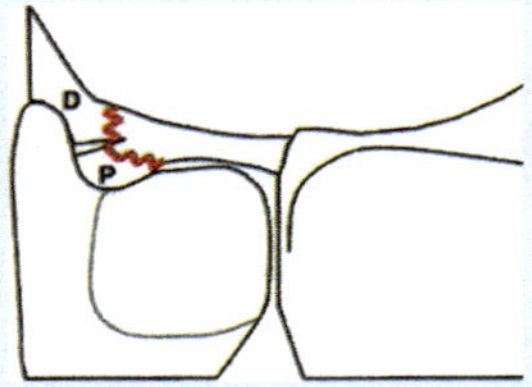	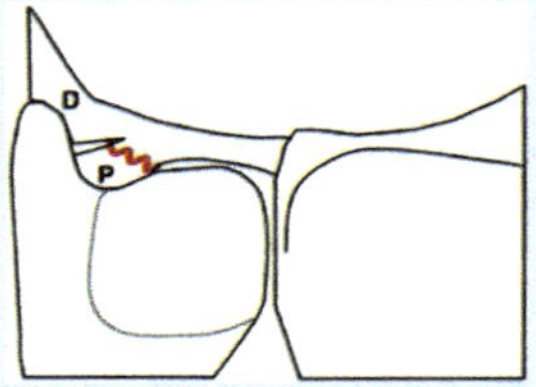	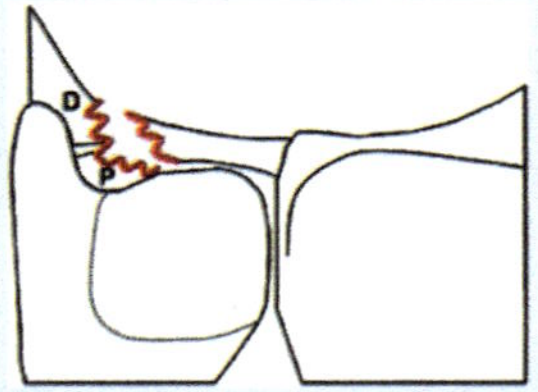	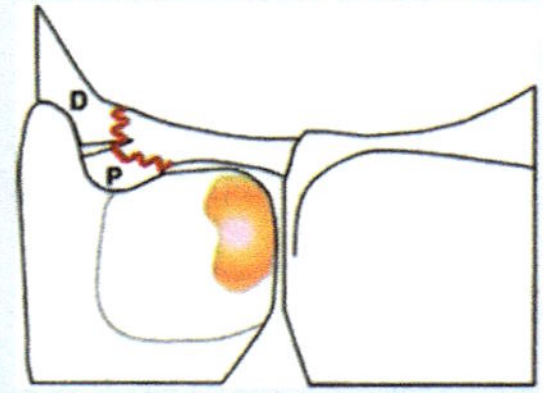
Clinical DRUJ instability	None/slight	Mild/severe		Severe	Mild/severe
Appearance of TFCC distal component (RC arthroscopy)	Torn	Torn	Intact	Torn	Variable
Status of TFCC proximal component (hook test/ DRUJ arthroscopy)	Intact	Torn	Torn	Torn	
Healing potential of TFCC tear's margins	Good	Good	Good	Poor	
Status of DRUJ cartilage	Good	Good	Good	Good	Poor
Treatment	*Repair* Suture (lig-to-capsule)	*Repair* Foveal refixation		*Reconstruction* Tendon graft	*Salvage* Arthroplasty or joint replacement

Modified from Atzei [2]

The classification system considers clinical and arthroscopic findings. Clinical assessment of DRUJ instability is performed by the ballottement test. Arthroscopy evaluates the TFCC by radiocarpal inspection and with the hook test. DRU-arthroscopy evaluates the cartilage of the sigmoid notch and ulnar head. Class 5 may show variable TFCC findings. Treatment is suggested according to the different classes in comparison to the anatomical reconstruction of the DRUJ ligaments using a tendon graft. In the early 1980s, Mansat et al. [16] preconized a technique using a palmaris longus graft passed through transosseous tunnels in the distal radius and ulna for anatomical DRUJ ligament reconstruction. Recently, the technique was refined and popularized by Adams et al. [1] so that it is currently considered the standard procedure for reconstruction of posttraumatic DRUJ instability.

During the last decade, arthroscopy has confirmed its role as the golden standard for diagnosis and treatment of many disorders of the wrist. Superior intra-articular visualization and reduced morbidity are the major advantages of arthroscopy over the open procedures, and this is especially true when operating in the ulnar compartment of the wrist.

An arthroscopically assisted technique for reconstruction of nonrepairable peripheral TFCC tears is meant not only to minimize surgical trauma in order to reduce postoperative pain and facilitate rehabilitation but also to allow greater accuracy in order to enhance the quality of the reconstruction and to improve the functional outcome.

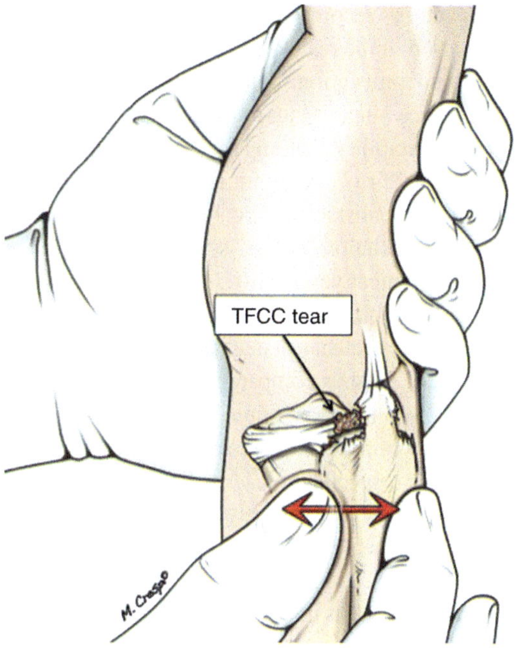

Fig. 11.1 The "ballottement test" evaluates DRUJ stability. The radius is hold firmly by the examiner's fingers, and the distal ulna is moved in dorsal and palmar directions with respect to the radius (*double side arrow*). In case of TFCC avulsion from the foveal attachment, the ulna shows an increased translation associated to a "soft" end-point resistance

Clinical Presentation

The patient seeks consultation complaining for a chronic pain on the ulnar side of the wrist, usually associated to intra-articular clicking and episodes of "giving way." Nonrepairable TFCC tear usually results from a severe or multiple and/or long-standing wrist injury. A fall on the outstretched pronated hand or a violent traction and twisting injury are the most common traumatic mechanisms. While taking patient's history, one should search for a severe trauma of the wrist or forearm that may have occurred in the past, even many years before the consultation, since it is quite usual that the patient only remembers a recent trivial injury or eventually a series of those minor wrist injuries. Concomitant systemic disorders, such as rheumatoid arthritis or chondrocalcinosis, should also be ruled out.

On a systematic examination of the painful wrist, special provocative maneuvers and diagnostic tests are performed to confirm the diagnosis of peripheral TFCC tear and/or achieve a differential diagnosis [3]. The most reliable clinical sign of peripheral TFCC tear is the ulnar fovea sign [24]; i.e., the patient has point tenderness over the ulnar capsule just palmar to the ECU tendon. Pain is exacerbated by passive forearm rotation and is usually associated to the presence of a "click" or "crepitus" or an intra-articular grinding sensation. Resisted rotational movements are often weak and reproduce patient's complaints.

A simple and reliable test to assess DRUJ laxity is the ballottement test [18]. This test consists of the passive anteroposterior and posteroanterior translation of the ulna on the radius in neutral rotation, in supination, and in pronation. Abnormal translation of the ulna head is present with the forearm in full supination and pronation and suggests complete TFCC disruption (Fig. 11.1).

Attempts can be made to assess the amount of radioulnar translation and provide a grading of DRUJ laxity [2], but these methods suffer from subjectivity and lack of interobserver validity.

The author recommends special care during evaluation of the resistance at the end point of the increased translation. This finding is of utmost importance since its loss correlates with clinical DRUJ instability. Though hyperlax, the DRUJ showing a "firm" end point is unlikely to cause a symptomatic instability. Conversely, an increased passive translation with a "soft" end-point resistance is indicative of DRUJ clinical instability, i.e., responsible for patient's complaint.

The ballottement test may show greater laxity of the painful wrist as compared to the opposite side, but only when forearm muscles are relaxed since protective contraction of the muscular stabilizers of the DRUJ (especially ECU and pronator quadratus) may cause false-negative findings. According to this fact, the author recommends that instability tests should be confirmed just before the operation, when the patient is under regional anesthesia.

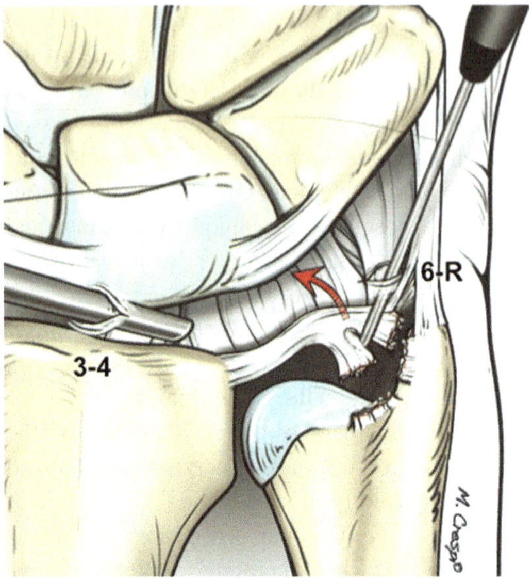

Fig. 11.2 The "hook test" evaluates the foveal attachment of the TFCC by applying traction to the ulnar part of the TFCC with a probe inserted through the 6-R portal. In case of DRUJ instability, when the ligamentous portion of the TFCC is ruptured or avulsed from the fovea, the TFCC can be elevated (*arrow*), and the test is positive

Diagnostic Imaging

Plain radiograms, arthrography, and magnetic resonance imaging (MRI) are of limited help in the diagnostic workout of a nonrepairable TFCC tear.

Their value is related to the possibility to rule out alternative causes of wrist pain, such as the presence of an associated ulnar styloid fracture or nonunion, lunotriquetral interosseous ligament disruption, chondrocalcinosis, or a concomitant positive ulnar variance or dysplastic ulnar head.

Conventional or MRI arthrograms may diagnose a tear but cannot accurately assess the size and location of the tear [22, 26] and, most remarkably, cannot provide any information about the quality of tear's edges and their healing potential.

Evidence of osteoarthritic changes of the DRUJ when confirmed arthroscopically may contraindicate ligamentous reconstruction.

Arthroscopic Assessment

Arthroscopy is the gold standard for diagnosis of a TFCC tear [11, 22].

Radiocarpal arthroscopy through the 3–4 portal permits visualization of the tear in the dorsoulnar corner of the TFCC that is probed through the 6-R portal. The trampoline test [12] and the hook test [2] are used to evaluate TFCC tension. The trampoline test assesses the TFCC tautness by applying a compressive load across it with the probe and is positive when the TFCC is soft and compliant. The hook test consists of applying traction to the ulnar-most border of the TFCC with the probe inserted through the 4–5 or 6-R portal (Fig. 11.2). The test is positive when the TFCC can be pulled distally and radially towards the center of the radiocarpal joint. Class 4 nonrepairable TFCC peripheral tears usually have a larger size, like in massive ruptures, or show gross degenerative changes of the margins, like in chronic mid-substance ligamentous tears. In the latter case, necrotic and retracted edges may show very limited, if any, healing capability, unless they are debrided back to a well-vascularized area (Fig. 11.3). An extensive debridement is needed, and it will result in a wide gap between tear's margins. Thus margin reapproximation may be impossible or may require such undue tension that direct repair is unlikely to be successful.

Poor healing can also be expected after chronic repetitive injury of the peripheral TFCC or after a

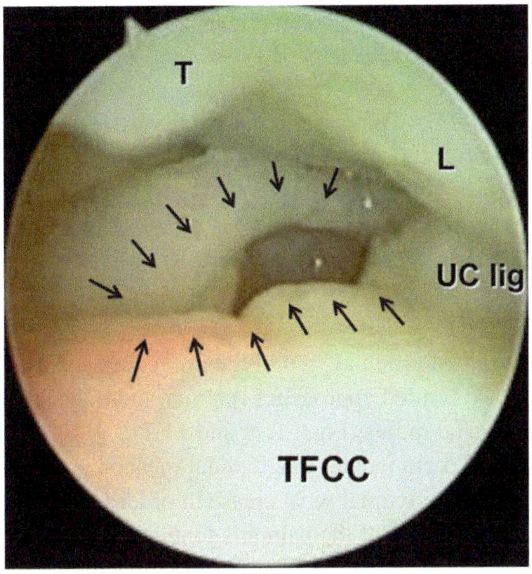

Fig. 11.3 Chronic massive peripheral tear of the TFCC. The large gap (*arrows*) between the sclerotic margins would become even larger after debridement, and it would be impossible to repair *T* Triquetum, *L* Lunate, *UC LIG* UlnoCarpal Ligaments

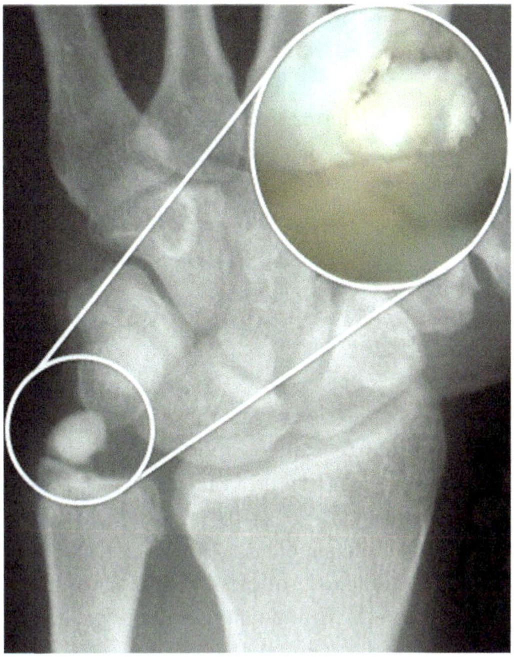

Fig. 11.4 Typical radiographic and arthroscopic picture of chronic calcium deposits causing degeneration of the peripheral TFCC. After debridement, degenerated tissues are unlikely to heal after direct repair

failed repair, causing ligament fraying and elongation. These conditions may be associated to calcium deposition as in chondrocalcinosis (Fig. 11.4) that shows poor outcome following direct repair.

Congenital hypoplasia of the styloid and foveal area with flattening of the ulnar head can also be associated with poor healing.

Indications for Arthroscopic TFCC Reconstruction

Patients with chronic symptomatic DRUJ instability, with positive ulnar fovea sign and ulnar ballottement that is not relieved by immobilization and conservative treatment for at least 3 months, should undergo arthroscopic inspection and treatment. Ligamentous reconstruction is indicated in patients in whom arthroscopic inspection shows the typical features of class 4 TFCC peripheral tears. These features can be summarized as (1) massive rupture of the TFCC or degenerated tear's margins, whose debridement may result in a large tissue loss that is impossible to repair by direct foveal refixation, or (2) frayed TFCC remnant or elongated scar after a failed suture that cannot hold the sutures.

Patients with contraindications to ligamentous reconstruction of DRUJ by tendon graft are those with chronic Essex-Lopresti injuries and axial forearm instability due to interosseous membrane insufficiency that can have very limited benefit from isolated DRUJ reconstruction.

Likewise, reconstruction is contraindicated in patients presenting significant degenerative changes of the DRUJ (class 5 type 1-B TFCC tear) and/or radiocarpal joint – in whom arthritic symptoms, more than DRUJ instability, should be addressed – and low physically demanding patients who are not healthy enough for surgery.

Relative contraindication is represented by cases with positive ulnar variance, in which accessory arthroscopic wafer procedure or ulnar shortening osteotomy is required according to the amount of variance.

The technique of TFCC reconstruction [4] is a modification of the open procedure that uses the palmaris longus (PL) or similar graft [1].

Surgical Technique of Arthroscopic Reconstruction of the TFCC

The operative setup is the same as for a standard wrist arthroscopy. After the wrist is suspended in a traction tower with 4–5 kg of traction, the procedure is performed according to the following steps:

Diagnostic Wrist Arthroscopy and TFCC Debridement

Standard diagnostic wrist arthroscopy is performed through 3–4 and 6-R portals, using the dry technique [8] as a routine. Midcarpal inspection (through RMC and UMC portals) is included to rule out associated intercarpal lesions.

After the diagnosis of class 4 TFCC peripheral tear is made, TFCC remnants are debrided with a full-radius or aggressive shaver to expose the fovea ulnaris, using 6-R portal and 4–5 and 6-U portals as accessory portals for instrumentation (Fig. 11.5). The fovea is eventually marked with a radio-frequency probe.

Tendon Graft Harvest and Preparation of the Radial Tunnel

The extra-articular step of the procedure consists of two limited approaches (palmar and dorsal) to the distal radius (Figs. 11.6 and 11.7).

A 2.5-cm palmar longitudinal incision is made from the proximal wrist crease in order to harvest the distal part of the palmaris longus (PL) tendon and to expose the palmar aspect of the distal radius. The PL tendon is divided proximally through a 1-cm transverse incision over the tenomuscular

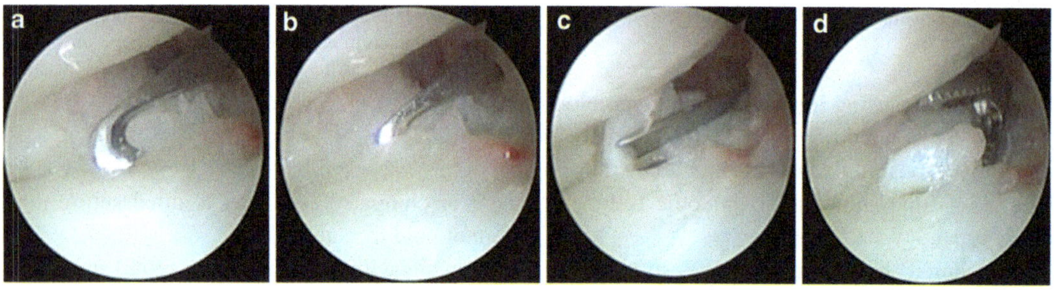

Fig. 11.5 Arthroscopic resection of the central fibrocartilagenous disk of the TFCC with the use of a hook-shaped (**a**, **b**) and frontal (**c**) arthroscopic blade. The disk is removed from the 6-R portal (**d**)

Fig. 11.6 Artistic rendering of the dorsal and palmar aspect of the wrist shows the portals and skin incisions required for arthroscopic reconstruction of the TFCC

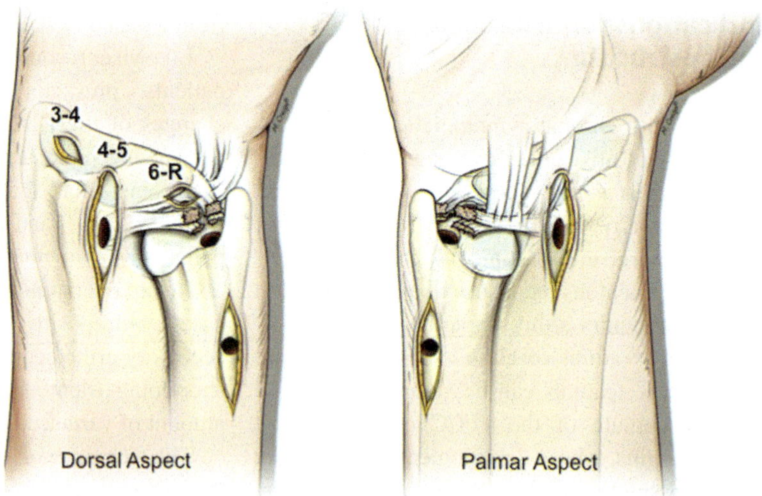

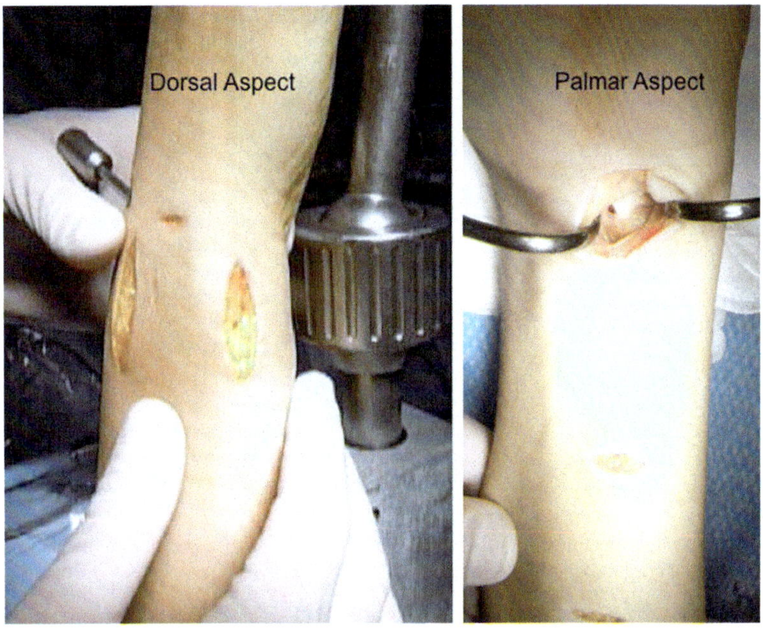

Fig. 11.7 Intraoperative views of the dorsal and palmar aspect of the wrist show the portals and skin incisions required for arthroscopic reconstruction of the TFCC

junction. When PL is absent, the flexor digitorum superficialis tendon of the ring finger or a strip of the FCR may be harvested. In order to expose to the ulnar part of the palmar aspect of the distal radius, the access is deepened in the interval between the ulnar neurovascular bundle and the finger flexor tendons that are retracted ulnarly and radially, respectively. Special care is taken to free and protect the ulnar neurovascular bundle from any adhesions on the palmar aspect of the ulnar carpus to avoid damage during late passage of the tendon graft. The palmar carpal arch is coagulated, and the pronator quadratus is retracted proximally to allow subperiosteal dissection of the ulnar corner of the palmar aspect of the radius.

On the dorsal aspect of the wrist, the skin incision for the 4–5 portal is extended 2–3 cm proximally, the extensor retinaculum is incised over its distal margin, the posterior interosseous nerve is preserved and retracted radially, and the dorsoulnar corner of the distal radius is exposed by subperiosteal dissection. Fluoroscopic control is used to allow for precise positioning of the guidewire and cannulated drilling of the distal radius through the floor of the fourth extensor compartment (Fig. 11.8) and to prevent fracture of the subchondral bone during successive drilling. A 2.4-mm cannulated drill bit is driven over the guidewire through the radius, just a few millimeters proximal to the articular surface of the lunate fossa and radial to the sigmoid notch. The tunnel is progressively enlarged to 3.4–4 mm with standard drill bits according to the size of the graft. A suture shuttle wire (ref. C6004; Concept shuttle relay suture passing system, Linvatec Corp., Largo, FL) or a steel-wire loop is introduced into the tunnel and left for later passage of the tendon graft.

Preparation of the Ulnar Tunnel

The arthroscope is introduced again through the 3–4 portal to visualize the foveal area that was exposed, and eventually marked, previously during TFCC debridement.

In order to prepare the tunnel through the distal ulna, use of an arthroscopic compass is recommended: the ankle arthroscopy compass produced by Dyonics (Ref. 4291; Dyonics, Smith & Nephew Inc., Andover, MA) fits this purpose quite well. The pointing tip of the compass is positioned on the foveal area through the 6-U portal, and the opposite, extra-articular extremity is used to localize the skin incision over the lateral aspect of the distal ulna (Fig. 11.9). The 3-cm skin incision is

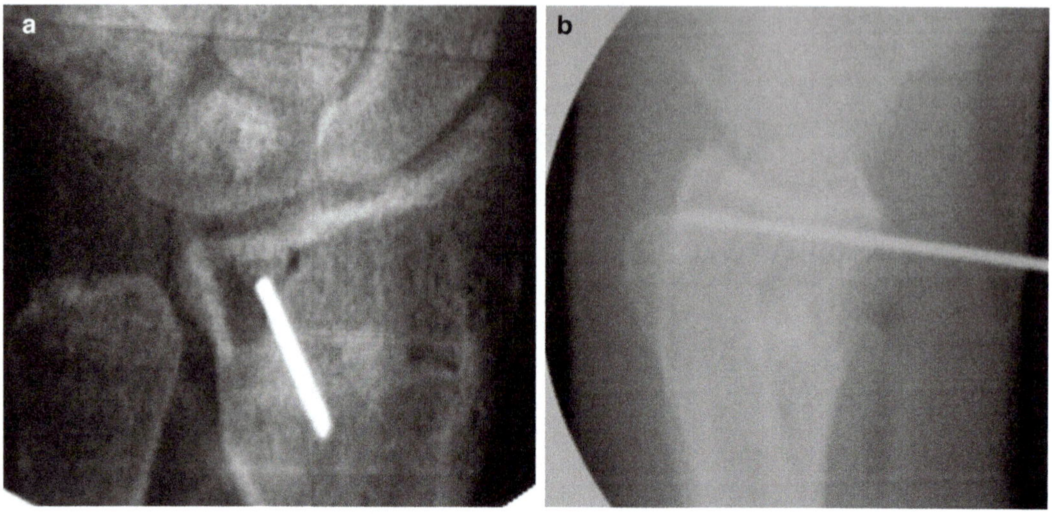

Fig. 11.8 Intraoperative fluoroscopic control showing precise positioning of the guidewire for tunnel preparation on the medial corner of the radius (**a** and **b**: AP and lateral views)

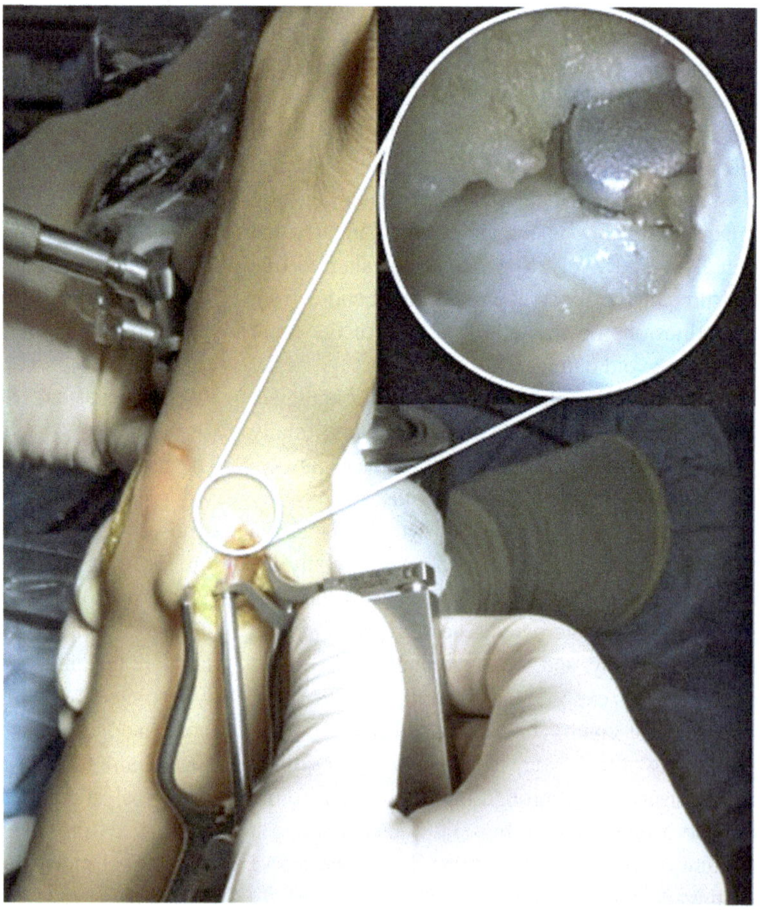

Fig. 11.9 Combined extra-articular and arthroscopic views of the procedure show the compass positioned to aim for the preparation of the ulnar tunnel. The pointing tip is placed over the fovea under arthroscopic control

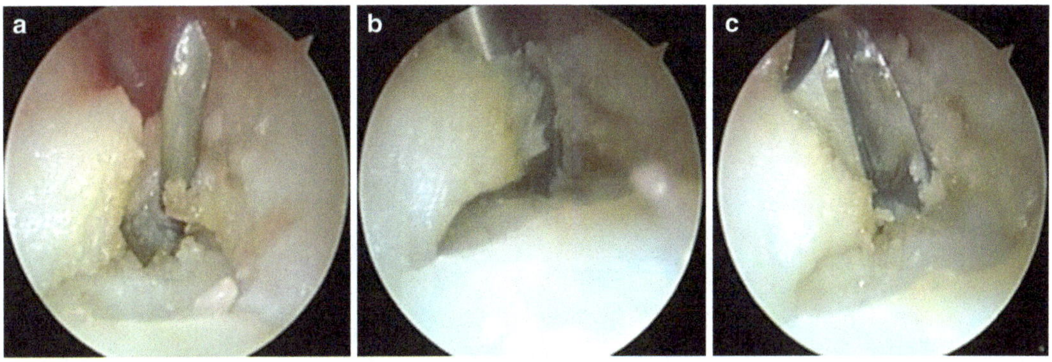

Fig. 11.10 Arthroscopic view of the three basic steps to create the ulnar tunnel. The guidewire drilled through the compass exits at the fovea (**a**) and drives a 3.2-mm cannulated drill bit to create the ulnar tunnel (**b**); this tunnel may be enlarged by a free-hand drill bit to fit the tendon graft with (**c**)

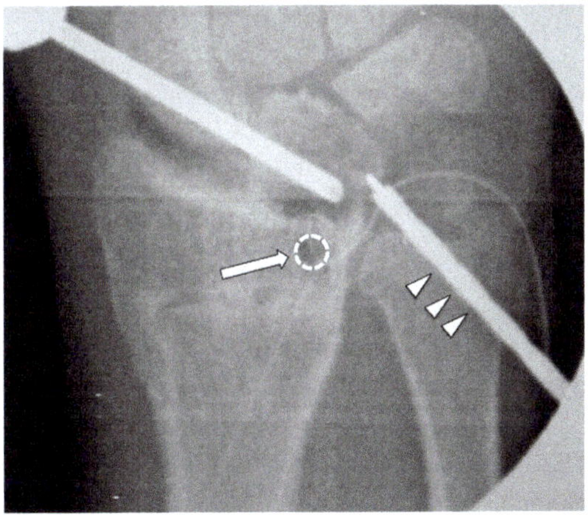

Fig. 11.11 Intraoperative fluoroscopic control confirms proper position of the tunnels on the radius (*arrow*) and ulna (*arrow heads*)

usually located 3–4 cm proximal to the 6-U portal. Care is taken to protect the dorsal sensory branch of the ulnar nerve (DSBUN), and the distal shaft of the ulna is exposed subperiosteally to provide firm rest to the compass tip. Under arthroscopic control, a cannulated drill bit is used from outside-in; then the tunnel may be enlarged to accommodate the tendon graft, usually up to 3.5–4 mm (Fig. 11.10). A fluoroscopic control is recommended to check proper tunnel positions (Fig. 11.11).

Passage of the Palmar End of the Tendon Graft

The scope in the 3–4 portal allows a good view of palmar aspect of the ulnar wrist and an easy location of the interval between the ulnolunate and the ulnotriquetral (UL-UT) ligaments. A blunt trocar is introduced through the 6-R portal to pierce the UL-UT interval just distal to the palmar DRUJ ligament in order to create a passage for an arthroscopic grasper. A grasper is introduced through the 6-R portal and the UL-UT interval to exit through the palmar skin incision (Fig. 11.12) in order to retrieve the shuttle wire holding the palmar end of the tendon graft (PETG) and to pull it inside the ulnocarpal joint.

Once the PETG is inside the joint, the arthroscopic grasper is introduced into the ulnar tunnel for graft retrieval.

At the end of this step, the PETG is entering the ulnocarpal joint through the palmar skin incision and UL-UT interval and exits through the ulnar tunnel and ulnar skin incision (Fig. 11.13).

Passage of the tendon graft in the UL-UT interval, just distal to the TFCC, provides improved stabilization of the ulnar carpus. Due to the improved field of view, arthroscopy allows this passage that would be much more difficult to perform by open technique.

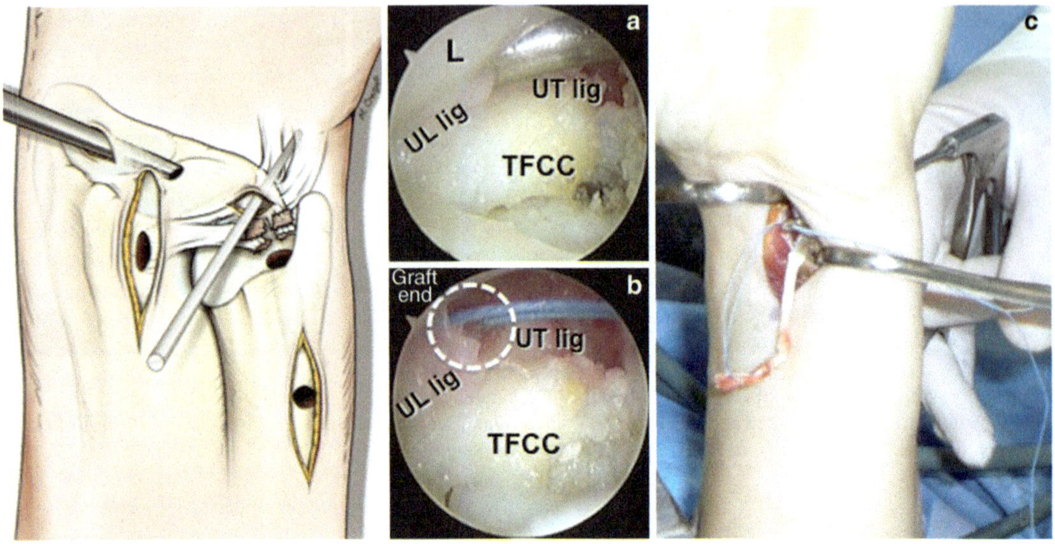

Fig. 11.12 Artistic rendering shows the use of a blunt trocar for the creation of a passage between the UL-UT ligaments. The scope in 3–4 portal visualizes the trocar introduced from 6-R portal, piercing the UL-UT interval. Arthroscopic views of the procedure show the grasper introduced through the UL-UT interval (**a**) and the shuttle suture pulled inside the joint (**b**) through the interval (*circle*). The extra-articular view through the palmar approach shows the grasper catching the shuttle suture carrying the palmar end of the tendon graft (**c**) *L* Lunate

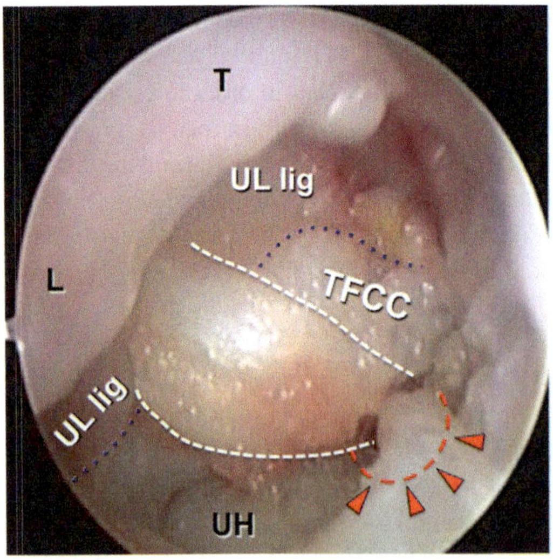

Fig. 11.13 Arthroscopic view of the palmar end of the tendon graft (between the *interrupted lines*) crossing the joint from the UL-UT interval, just distal to the palmar remnants of the TFCC (*dotted line*), to the tunnel (*arrow heads*) on the ulnar head (*UH*) *T* Triquetum, *L* Lunate

Passage of the Dorsal End of the Tendon Graft

The dorsal end of the tendon graft (DETG) is mounted on the shuttle wire and introduced into radial tunnel so that it exits from the floor of the fourth extensor compartment. Then, the shuttle wire is introduced into the joint through the 4–5 portal, passing under the extensor retinaculum (Fig. 11.14). Care should be taken not to harm the posterior interosseous nerve and to avoid entrapment of the extensor tendons that should be retracted. The end of the shuttle wire is easily seen through the scope in 3–4 portal and can be withdrawn through the ulnar tunnel by a grasper introduced from outside-in into the tunnel.

At the end of this step, both ends of the tendon graft are inside the ulnocarpal joint, entering the ulnar tunnel (Fig. 11.15).

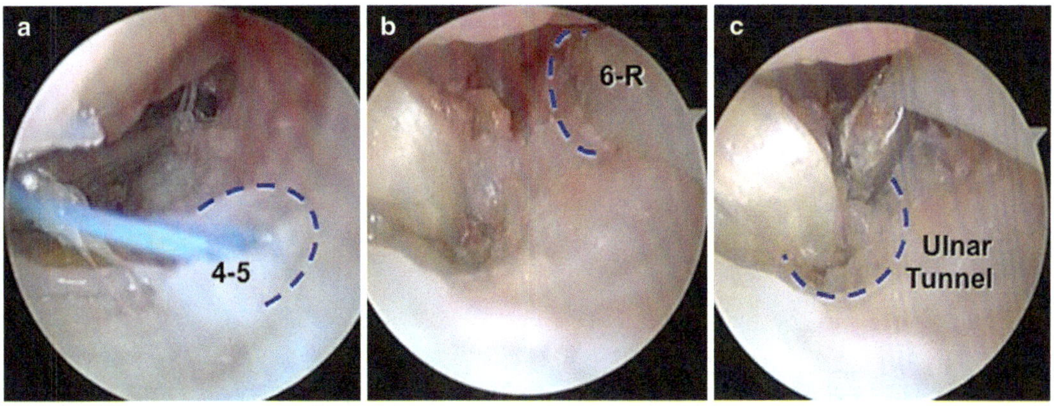

Fig. 11.14 Arthroscopic view of the three basic steps for the passage of the dorsal end of the tendon graft. The shuttle suture is introduced through the 4–5 portal and retrieved through the 6-R portal (**a**). The extremity of the dorsal end of the tendon graft is pulled inside the joint up to the 6-R portal (**b**); then a grasper is introduced through the ulnar tunnel to retrieve the graft and pull it outside the joint (**c**)

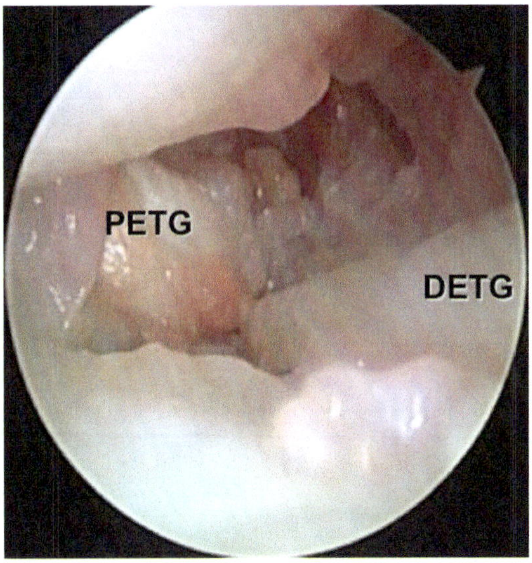

Fig. 11.15 Arthroscopic view at the end of the procedure shows the palmar (*PETG*) and dorsal end of the tendon graft (*DETG*) crossing the joint

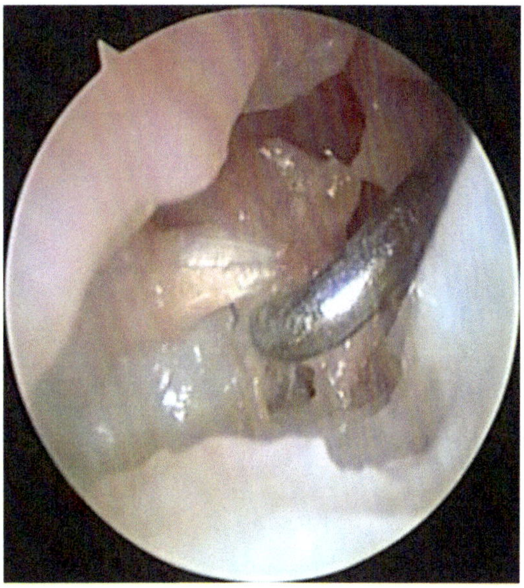

Fig. 11.16 An arthroscopic probe is used to assess preliminary tensioning of the tendon graft

Tensioning and Fixation of the Tendon Graft

When the wrist is held in neutral rotation and the ulnar head is reduced in the sigmoid notch, both ends of the graft exit through the ulnar skin incision (Fig. 11.16). Graft ends are tensioned and temporarily pinned with a hypodermic needle against the edge of the ulnar tunnel. Proper tension should allow full forearm rotation, still preserving physiological DRUJ translation with a "firm" end point. Overtightening the reconstructed ligaments will produce excessive compression of the DRUJ and cause early joint degeneration. Proper tension is also confirmed by arthroscopic examination and probing (Fig. 11.17).

Secure graft fixation is achieved with a 3- or 4-mm interference screw (*Biotenodesis System Screw*® -ref. AR-1530 or 1540, Arthrex Inc., Naples, FL) (Fig. 11.18).

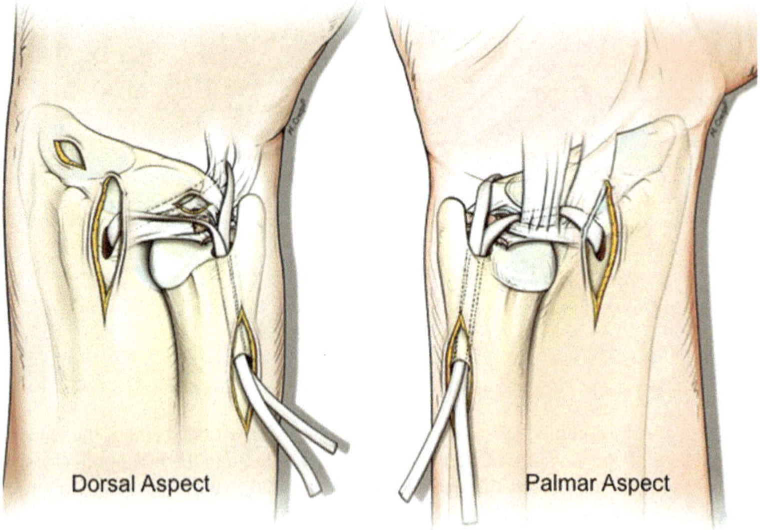

Fig. 11.17 Artistic rendering of the reconstruction at the end of the procedure

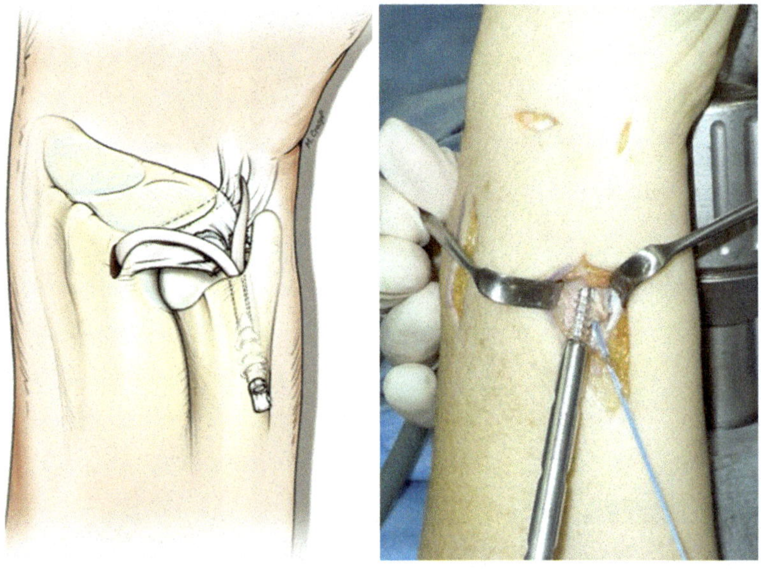

Fig. 11.18 The tendon graft is secured inside the ulnar tunnel with a resorbable interference screw

Postoperative Treatment

The wrist is immobilized in neutral rotation or slight supination in a long-arm cast for 3 weeks, followed by further 4 weeks in a Münster-type splint, during which time the flexion/extension of the elbow is regained. Then, rotation is recovered, but the wrist is protected by a short splint in the intervals between physiotherapy during the following 2 weeks. Progressive resisted wrist and hand strengthening exercises are begun after the eighth week. Complete use is delayed until after 4 months, but heavy loading is avoided for 6 months.

Results and Complications

Authors' experience with this technique started in 2005, and since then 11 patients underwent arthroscopically assisted reconstruction of the TFCC.

Four patients (all males, mean age 28 years) had a minimum follow-up of 1 year (average 22 months, maximum 34 months).

Three patients complained for severe chronic DRUJ instability following distal radius fracture, and one patient had instability due to chondrocalcinosis. The ulnar styloid was ununited in two. In all, arthroscopy revealed a Palmer type 1-B ulnar avulsion of the TFCC which was not reducible in two cases and had too poor TFCC quality and healing potential in the remaining two. One patient had associated lunotriquetral instability (Geissler stage 3).

At follow-up, DRUJ stability was restored in all. The range of motion increased from 85 to 95 % of the contralateral side, and grip strength increased from 65 to 87 %. Pain decreased from 8.7 to 1.7 on a 10-point visual analogue scale. Modified Mayo Wrist Score was excellent in three patients and good in one. All patients were satisfied with the results of the procedure: three resumed manual activities and previous work, and one changed work for unrelated reasons.

Few complications should be encountered during arthroscopic-assisted repair or reconstruction of the TFCC; provided care is taken. The most serious complication is injury to the DSBUN, which depends on the surgeon's experience. Transient neurapraxia of the DSBUN usually recovers spontaneously in 3–4 months. The surgical scar of the ulnar side of wrist may adhere to deeper structures and become painful during the first stages of physiotherapy, especially after prolonged immobilization.

During arthroscopic reconstruction, a nondisplaced fracture in the ulnar tunnel occurred in one case, when the interference screw was inserted.

Conclusions

Advanced arthroscopic classification of TFCC tears helps to decide the appropriate treatment, even for those cases that cannot be treated by direct repair of TFCC remnants.

The primary advantage of the use of an arthroscopic technique is that it is minimally invasive, protects ligaments, and allows for a limited scar adhesion and joint stiffness so that postoperative pain and rehabilitation are usually reduced. However, that is not the only benefit. Above all, it is the improved possibilities for intra-articular visualization. In fact, arthroscopy allows complete joint exploration with magnification of the operating field and therefore provides an improved level of surgical precision. Magnification provided by arthroscopic instrumentation permits more accurate placement of the ulnar tunnel into the fovea and particularly the passage of the graft through the interval between the palmar ulnocarpal ligaments.

This surgical step is rather difficult to perform during open surgery due to the limited space in the ulnar carpus. However, it is very important for a complete restoration of the stabilizing function of the TFCC.

Arthroscopic TFCC foveal reattachment and reconstruction by tendon graft represent an exciting new frontier in arthroscopic wrist procedures.

According to this preliminary experience, arthroscopic-assisted reconstruction retains the potential to overcome the difficulties of open surgery.

It is a complex procedure that demands a specific learning curve. However, once the technique is mastered, the numerous advantages over open surgery, in terms of minimal invasivity and greater accuracy, will give good reason for the specific competence and arthroscopic skills required.

References

1. Adams BD, Berger RA (2002) An anatomic reconstruction of the distal radioulnar ligaments for posttraumatic distal radioulnar joint instability. J Hand Surg Am 27:243–251
2. Atzei A (2009) New trends in arthroscopic management of type 1-B TFCC injuries with DRUJ instability. J Hand Surg Eur 34E:582–591
3. Atzei A, Luchetti R (2005) Clinical approach to the painful wrist. In: Geissler WB (ed) Wrist arthroscopy. Springer/LLC, New York, pp 185–195
4. Atzei A, Luchetti R, Borelli PP, Sgarbossa A, Cugola L (2006) Arthroscopic TFCC reconstruction by tendon graft. Rivista di Chirurgia della Mano 43:370–376

5. Atzei A, Rizzo A, Luchetti R, Fairplay T (2008) Arthroscopic foveal repair of triangular fibrocartilage complex peripheral lesion with distal radioulnar joint instability. Tech Hand Up Extrem Surg 12:226–235
6. Boyes JH (1970) Surgical repair of joints. In: Bunnell S (ed) Bunnell's surgery of the hand. Lippincott, Philadelphia, pp 294–313
7. Breen TF, Jupiter JB (1989) Extensor carpi ulnaris and flexor carpi ulnaris tenodesis of the unstable distal ulna. J Hand Surg Am 14:612–617
8. del Piñal F, Garcia Bernal FJ, Pisani D, Regalado J, Ayala H, Studer A (2007) Dry arthroscopy of the wrist: surgical technique. J Hand Surgery Am 32A:119–123
9. del Piñal F, García-Bernal FJ, Cagigal L, Studer A, Regalado J, Thams C (2010) A technique for arthroscopic all-inside suturing in the wrist. J Hand Surg Eur 35E(6):475–479
10. Eliason EL (1932) An operation for recurrent inferior radioulnar dislocation. Ann Surg 96:27–35
11. Fulcher S, Poehling G (1998) The role of operative arthroscopy for the diagnosis and treatment of lesions about the distal ulna. Hand Clin 14:285–296
12. Hermansdorfer JD, Kleinman WB (1991) Management of chronic peripheral tears of the triangular fibrocartilage complex. J Hand Surg Am 16:340–346
13. Hui FC, Linscheid RL (1982) Ulnotriquetral augmentation tenodesis: a reconstructive procedure for dorsal subluxation of the distal radioulnar joint. J Hand Surg Am 7:230–236
14. Johnson RK, Shrewsbury MM (1976) The pronator quadratus in motions and in stabilization of the radius and ulna at the distal radioulnar joint. J Hand Surg Am 1:205–209
15. King GJ, McMurtry RY, Rubenstem JD, Gertzbein SD (1986) Kmematlcs of the distal radioulnar joint. J Hand Surg Am 11A:798–804
16. Mansat M, Mansat Ch, Martinez Ch (1983) L'articulation radio-cubitale inférieur. Pathologie traumatique. Le poignet. pp 187–195
17. Moritomo H, Murase T, Arimitsu S, Oka K (2008) Change in the length of the ulnocarpal ligaments during radiocarpal motion: possible impact on triangular fibrocartilage complex foveal tears. J Hand Surg Am 33A:1278–1286
18. Moriya T, Aoki M, Iba K et al (2009) Effect of triangular ligament tears on distal radioulnar joint instability and evaluation of three clinical tests: a biomechanical study. J Hand Surg Eur 34:219–223
19. Nakamura T, Makita A (2000) The proximal ligamentous component of the triangular fibrocartilage complex: functional anatomy and three-dimensional changes in length of the radioulnar ligament during pronation-supination. J Hand Surg Br 25B:479–486
20. Nakamura T, Yabe Y, Horiuchi Y (1996) Functional anatomy of the triangular fibrocartilage complex. Hand Surg 21:581–586
21. Nakamura T, Sato K, Okazaki M, Toyama Y, Ikegami H (2011) Repair of foveal detachment of the triangular fibrocartilage complex: open and arthroscopic transosseous techniques. Hand Clin 27:281–290
22. Pederzini L, Luchetti R, Soragni O, Alfarano M, Montagna G, Cerofolini E, Colombini R, Roth J (1992) Evaluation of the triangular fibrocartilage complex tears by arthroscopy, arthrography, and magnetic resonance imaging. Arthroscopy 8:191–197
23. Schuind F, An KN, Berglund L et al (1991) The distal radioulnar ligaments a biomechanical study. J Hand Surg Am 16A:1106–1114
24. Tay SC, Tomita K, Berger RA (2007) The "ulnar fovea sign" for defining ulnar wrist pain: an analysis of sensitivity and specificity. J Hand Surg Am 32:438–444
25. Tsai TM, Stilwell JH (1984) Repair of chronic subluxation of the distal radioulnar joint (ulnar dorsal) using flexor carpi ulnaris tendon. J Hand Surg Br 9:289–294
26. Zanetti M, Bram J, Hodler J (1997) Triangular fibrocartilage and intercarpal ligaments of the wrist: does MR arthrography improve standard MRI? J Magn Reson Imaging 7:590–594

The Carpal Detachment Syndrome

12

Shinji Nishikawa and Satoshi Toh

TFCC injury is recognized as one of the causes of the ulnar-sided pain. The TFCC consists of dorsal and volar radioulnar ligaments, ulnar collateral ligament and disc (TFC) and sheath of ECU [1, 3]. The distal construction of the TFCC was not considered in detail. Therefore, we investigated the TFCC attachment to the carpal bones [4].

Anatomical Study

We conducted anatomical studies on 88 wrists of 51 cadavers (mean ages 74 years: range, 40–99) to further investigate the carpal attachment of the TFCC. Dissections demonstrated a smooth attachment of TFCC to the carpal bones in all cases, and no TFCC was meniscus-shaped or protruding toward the articular surface of the triquetrum. Furthermore, there were no cases of avulsion of the TFCC from the portion of the triquetrum where it is normally attached.

Two types of configurations were seen for the attachment of the TFCC to the carpal bones. In one type, the TFCC was attached to the ulnar edge of the articular surface of the triquetrum (exposed type of triquetrum). In the other, the TFCC was attached to the articular surface of the triquetrum, and thus the whole articular surface of the triquetrum could not be observed (covered type of triquetrum). The exposed type of triquetrum was seen in 82 joints of 45 cadavers (93 %), and the covered type was seen in six joints in six cadavers (7 %) (Fig. 12.1).

The shape of the attachment is unique. If the broad attachment type to the ulnar carpal bones is injured, pain will ensue. We reported this injury as ulnocarpal detachment of TFCC injury (UCD) [4, 5] (Fig. 12.2). In this chapter, we describe the diagnosis and treatment of UCD.

Diagnosis

The symptoms of UCD are the same as TFCC injuries [7]. Sprain of the wrist, falling injury with axially palmar compression and repetitive wrist motion or sport activities were causes of TFCC injury. Ulnar-side tenderness, pain on forearm rotation and pain during the TFCC stress test are recognized as clinical findings. Notably, UCD cases tend to be painful in ulnar deviation stress with forearm supination (see Chap. 3). MRI findings are the most useful information for diagnosis of UCD. In MRI, an injured TFCC shows a flap shape from the carpal bone. Although

S. Nishikawa, M.D. (✉)
Nishikawa Orthopaedic Surgery and Hand Surgery Clinic, Department of Orthopaedic Surgery, Hirosaki University School of Medicine, 2-2-12 Waseda Hirosaki-shi, 036-8087 Aomori, Japan
e-mail: nishikaw@yacht.ocn.ne.jp

S. Toh, M.D.
Department of Orthopaedic Surgery, Hirosaki University School of Medicine, 5 Zaifu-cho Hirosaki-shi, 036-8562 Aomori, Japan
e-mail: toh@cc.hirosaki-u.ac.jp

F. del Piñal et al. (eds.), *Arthroscopic Management of Ulnar Pain*, DOI 10.1007/978-3-642-30544-3_12, © Springer-Verlag Berlin Heidelberg 2012

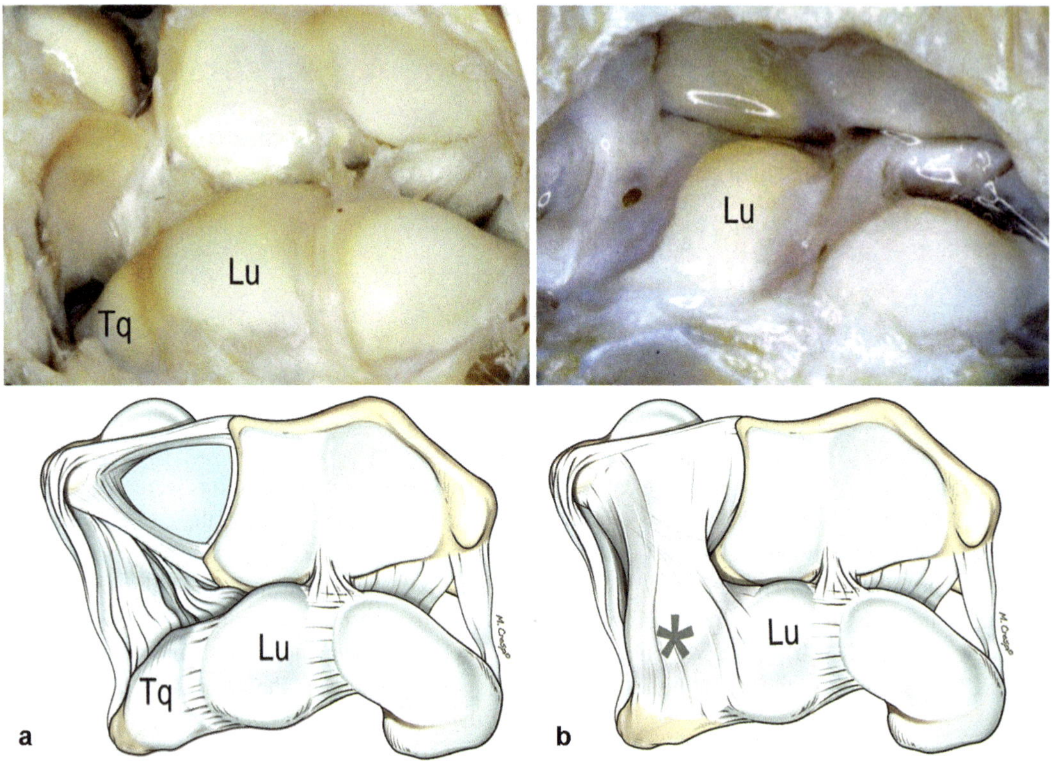

Fig. 12.1 Anatomical study of TFCC attachment to the carpal bones. (**a**) Exposed triquetrum type; (**b**) covered type (*asterisk*)

the finding looks like a TFCC surface tear, the flap of a UCD lesion is recognized more on the ulnar and distal side (Fig. 12.3). Comparing with radial- and ulnar-deviated MRI could show the typical findings of UCD (Fig. 12.4).

We presume that excessive motion stress of the wrist deviation occasions the detachment of the TFCC from the carpal bone, especially in broadly attached type of TFCC (Fig. 12.5).

Treatment

The cases seen within 1 or 2 weeks of onset are treated with short arm casting and anti-inflammatory medications. Steroid injection (triamcinolone acetonide) to the injured lesion is efficacious also but is not effective for cases seen late. These cases are treated with arthroscopic surgery.

Arthroscopic Treatment

We prefer to use a horizontal traction system for wrist joint arthroscopy. Two portals are used: the 3–4 portal for the scope and the 4–5 portal as the working portal. Typically, proliferative synovium which blocks the vision ulnarly needs to be debrided as a preliminary step. Though the shape of a UCD looks the same as a flap tear of the TFC, its stalk is connected to the ulnar edge of the carpal joint surface. The UCD is excised with the shaver. The tissue of the excised UCD is fibrocartilage tissue, same as TFC tissue. The joint cartilage defect is then observed on the ulnar edge of the carpal bone (Figs. 12.6 and 12.7). The TFC disc proper is not injured and has a smooth surface. This is the most important different finding from a surface tear of TFC disc proper (Fig. 12.8). There is no need for rehabilitation after arthroscopic treatment except for a week of rest.

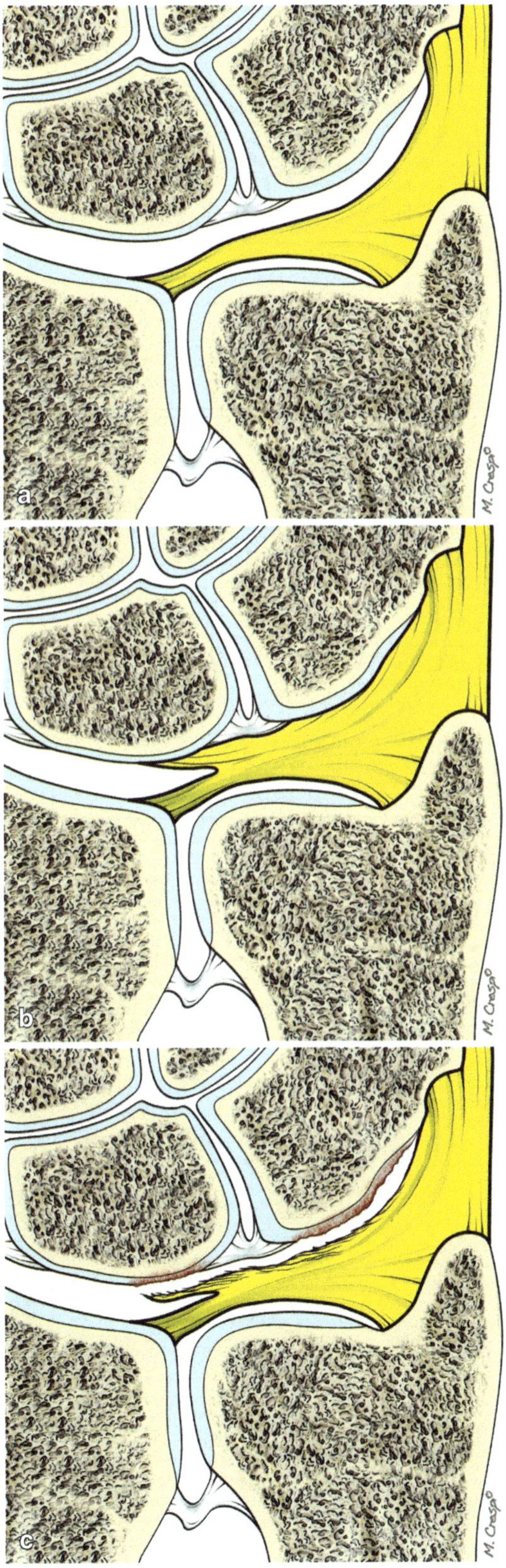

Discussion

There are some variations of TFCC attachment to the carpal bone. Ono et al. [6] described the research of 870 shapes of TFCC with arthrography; there are seven bicompartmentalizations of the radiocarpal joint that congenitally connects widely to the lunotriquetral interosseous ligament and TFCC. Hogikiyan and Louis [2] reported four variations (four types) of anatomical TFCC structures in 18 embryos. Thirty-three per cent of the embryos had wide carpal attachment of the TFCC. These TFCC that were widely attached to the carpal bone were injured and eventually detached from the carpal bone. The triangular impingement ligament tear (TILT) that Watson and Weinzweig [8] reported was impingement of triquetral fibrous tissue that was injured and displaced distally to the ulnar cuff of the wrist. The symptoms and surgical finding of cartilage defect are analogous to UCD. TILT suggested the soft tissue lesion in ulnar side of the wrist. Consequently, UCD was thought to be a TFCC congenitally widely attached to the carpal bone that was injured and avulsed like TILT from the carpal bone.

UCD is a common cause of ulnar pain. It represents 26 % (55/209) of the cases of ulnar pain in our practice. When we perform wrist arthroscopy, we must remember that UCD may exist along with injury of the TFC disc proper.

Fig. 12.2 Diagrams of TFCC attachment to the carpal bones. (**a**) Exposed type of TFCC, (**b**) covered type of TFCC and (**c**) TFCC avulsion from the carpal bones covered type of attachment

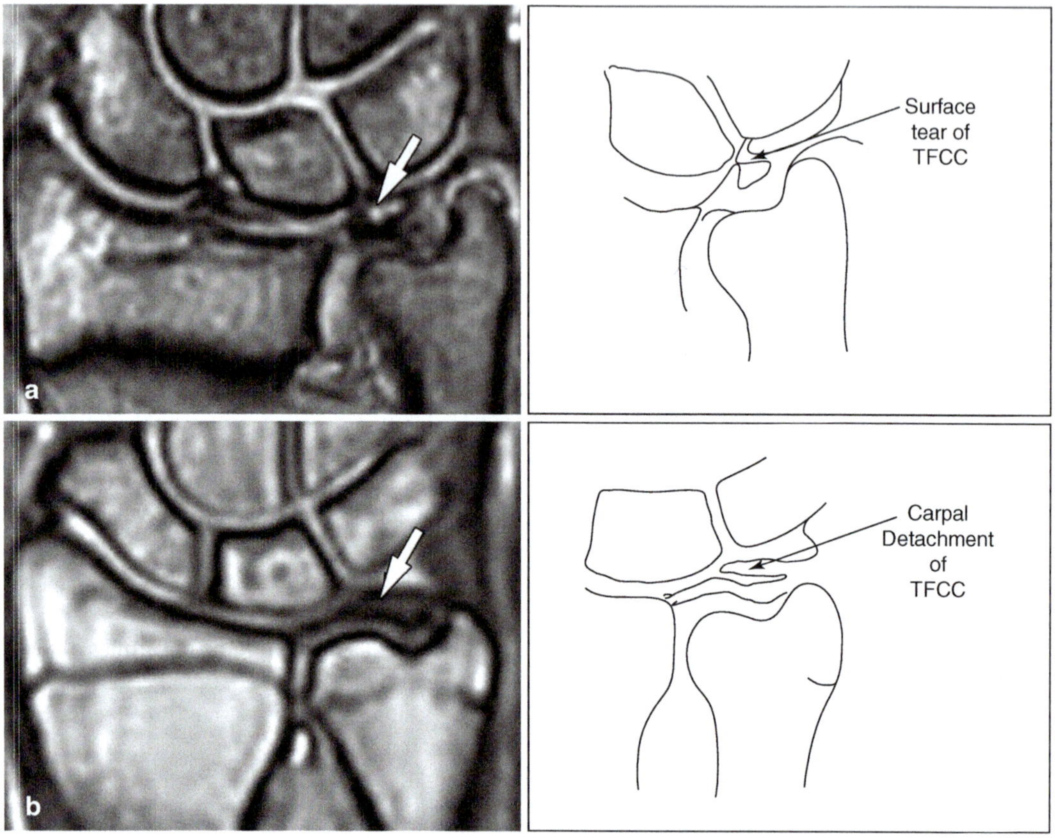

Fig. 12.3 MRI of TFCC injury. (**a**) TFCC surface tear. (**b**) Carpal detachment of TFCC

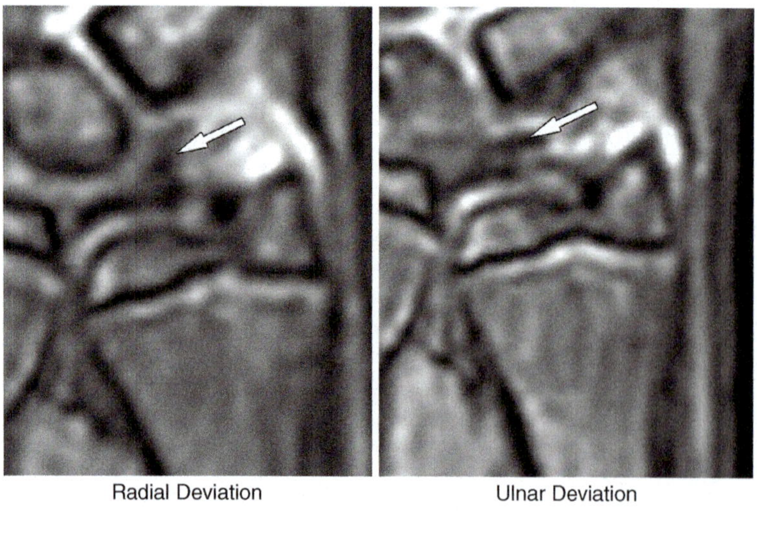

Fig. 12.4 MRI of carpal detachment of TFCC. MRI with full deviation position shows the UCD flap-like motion

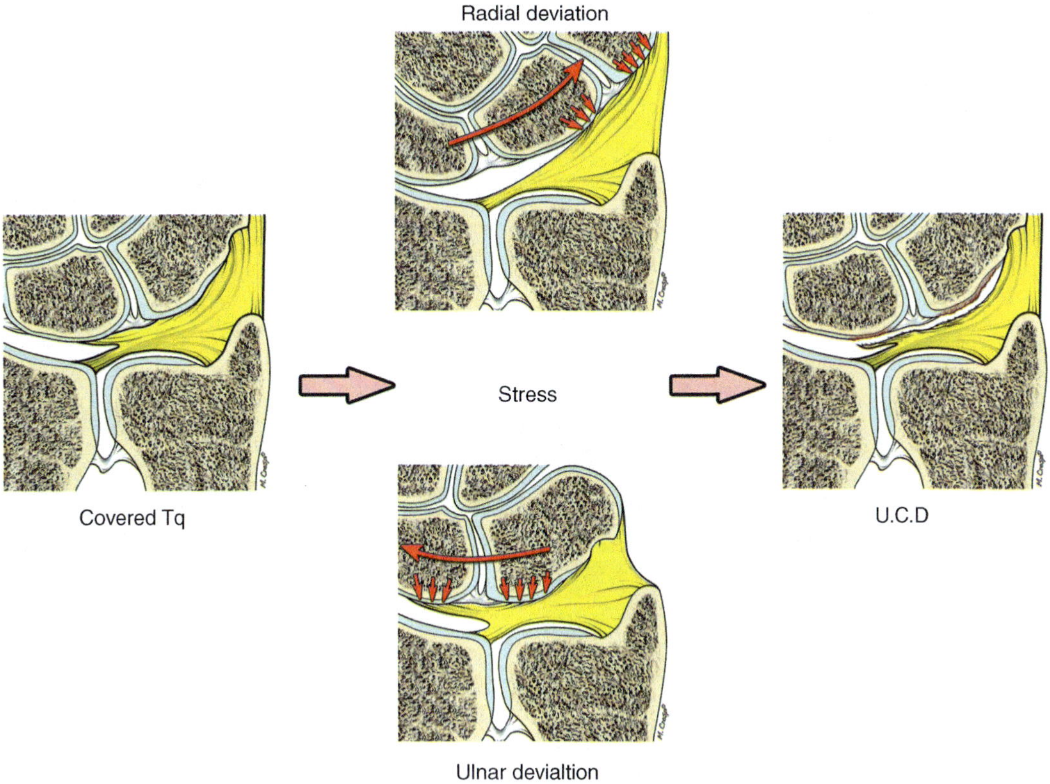

Fig. 12.5 Mechanism of the UCD injury. Radial and ulnar deviation stresses cause TFCC detachment from carpal bones

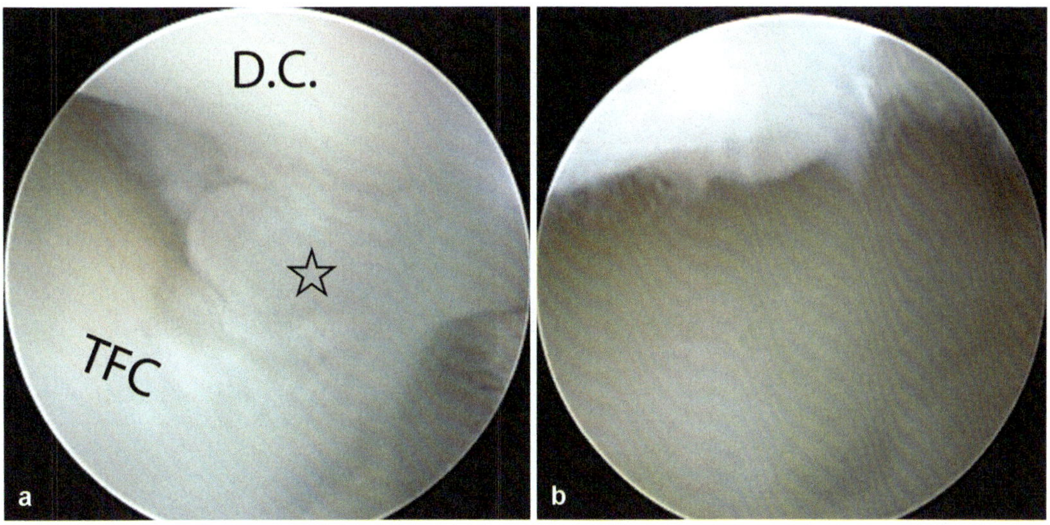

Fig. 12.6 (**a**) Ulno carpal detachment in a 37-year-old female (right wrist). The UCD (*star*) is impinged between dorsal carpal bone (*DC*) and TFC disc (*TFC*). (**b**) After resection of the UCD. Notice that the dorsal capsule surface that was the base of UCD is rough; the TFCC surface is smooth, however

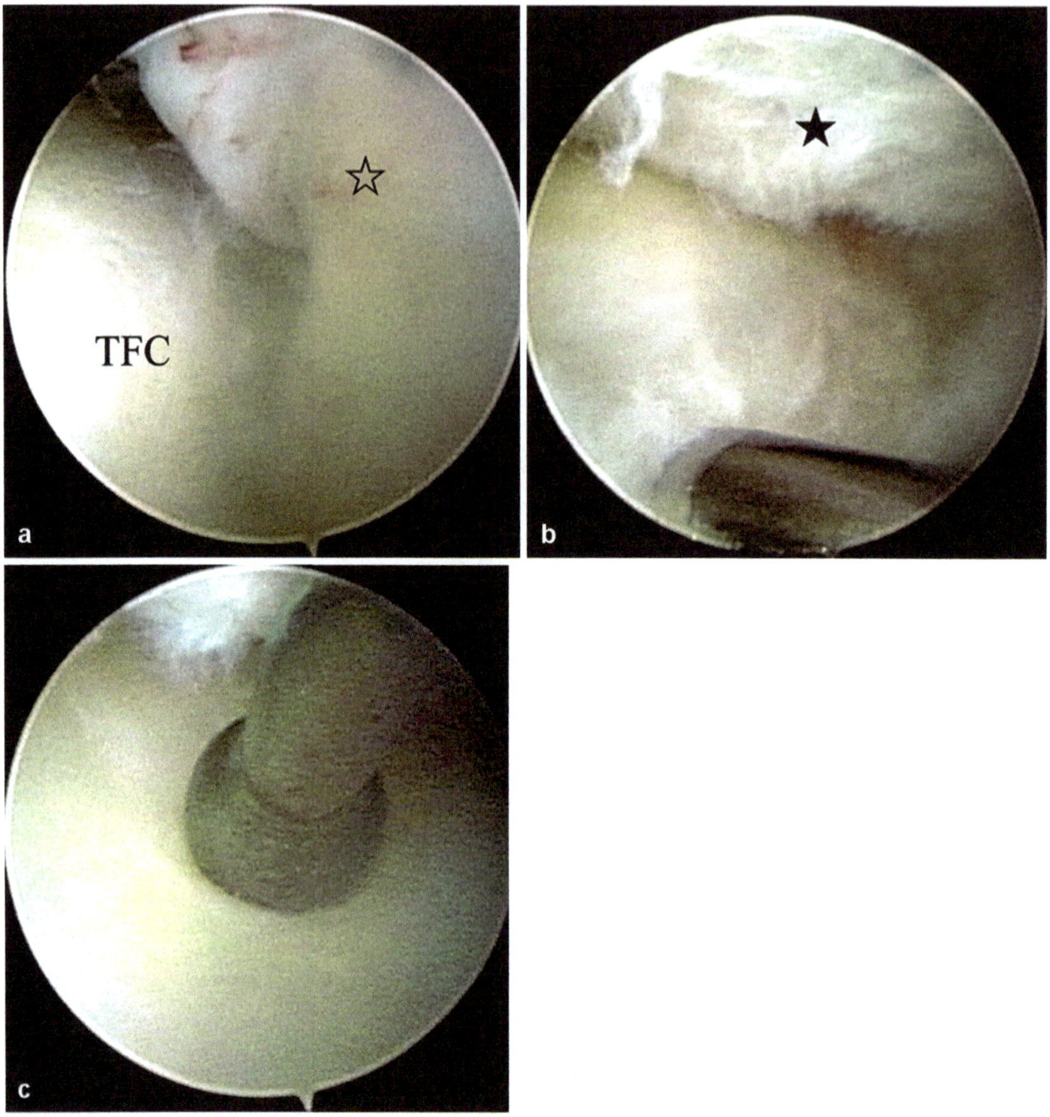

Fig. 12.7 (**a**) A 40-year-old male with a right UCD. UCD (*star*) is observed in the ulnar corner of the wrist joint with hypertrophic synovium. (**b**) Arthroscopic resection of the UCD from ulnar corner of the dorsal capsule. Rough surface of dorsal carpal bone (*black star*) was base of the UCD. (**c**) The TFC surface is shown flat and smooth

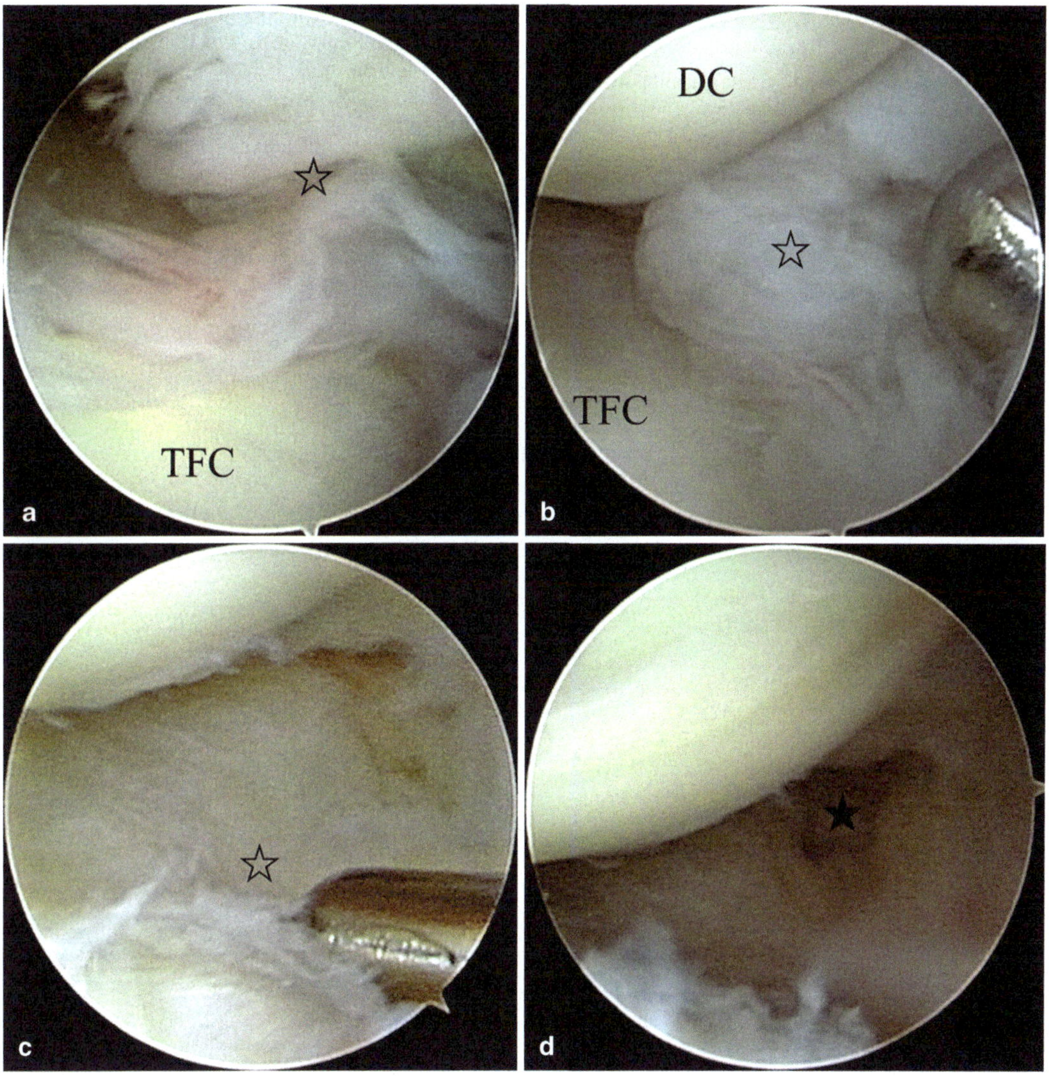

Fig. 12.8 (**a**) TFCC surface tear. A torn TFC and synovitis (*star*) are seen between carpal bone and TFC, apparently a similar picture to an UCD. (**b**) Arthroscopic resection of the impinging tissue (*star*). *DC* dorsal carpal bone. (**c**) After resection of impinged tissue, the TFC surface tear (*star*) was evident with rough surface of TFC and smooth carpal bone surface. (**d**) TFC ulnar corner has normal findings. *Black star* prestyloid recess

References

1. Garcia-Elias M (1998) Soft-tissue anatomy and relationships about the ulna. Hand Clin 14:165–176
2. Hogikyan JV, Louis DS (1992) Embryologic development and variations in the anatomy of the ulnocarpal ligamentous complex. J Hand Surg 17A:719–723
3. Lewis OJ, Hamshere RJ, Bucknill TM (1970) Anatomy of the wrist joint. J Anat 106:539–552
4. Nishikawa S, Toh S (2002) Anatomical study of carpal attachment of triangular fibrocartilage complex. J Bone Joint Surg 84B:1062–1065
5. Nishikawa S, Toh S, Miura H et al (2002) The carpal detachment injury of the triangular fibrocartilage complex. J Hand Surg 27B:86–89
6. Ono H, Gilula LA, Marzke MW et al (1996) Bicompartmentalization of the radiocarpal joint. J Hand Surg 21A:789–793
7. Palmer AK, Werner FW, Eng MM (1981) The triangular fibrocartilage complex of the wrist. Anatomy and function. J Hand Surg 6:153–162
8. Watson HK, Weinzweig J (1999) Triquetral impingement ligament tear (TILT). J Hand Surg 24-B: 321–324

13 Ulnocarpal Abutment: State of the Art and the Role of Arthroscopy

Christophe Mathoulin

Introduction

Ulnocarpal abutment is the inversion of the distal radioulnar index with a positive ulnar variance (long ulna) and is most frequently secondary to distal radius fractures. The relative "shortening of the radius" leads to a conflict between the ulnar head and the proximal lunate (Fig. 13.1). The natural evolution of this condition is usually a central perforation of the TFCC. This lesion eventually leads to arthritis of the medial proximal lunate as well as that of the ulnar head. Persistence of the abutment may further lead to lunotriquetral dissociation (Fig. 13.2a–c).

There are many management options for the distal radioulnar component of distal radius malunions, that cause the most common ulnocarpal abutment, with the radius shortening associated with the dorsal tilt, and the choice depends on clinical evaluation and imaging of this joint. Arthroscopic treatment, when possible, remains the simplest and best solution for these patients.

C. Mathoulin
Institut de la main, Clinique Jouvenet,
6 square Jouvenet, 75016 Paris, France
e-mail: cmathoulin@orange.fr

Indications

Clinical and Paraclinical Assessment

The clinician should differentiate between symptoms related to a pronosupination problem and those arising from proper wrist movements. It is crucial to determine whether the symptoms are caused by the distal radioulnar joint itself or by the ulnocarpal abutment that follows.

The evaluation of functional disability must take into consideration age, dominance, and nature of daily activities whether professional or sports.

Active motion is assessed on flexion-extension and pronation-supination.

Grip strength on both sides is measured using the Jamar.

Posteroanterior and lateral views are taken in neutral position (Fig. 13.3). It is very important to obtain strict PA views in neutral wrist position using radiotransparent plates that sandwich the wrist and forearm. Analysis allows the study of the radioulnar variance usually using the concentric circles of Palmer. The measurements must be comparative as this index is extremely variable. It increases in pronation with a clenched fist and decreases with supination. Dynamic posteroanterior clenched fist views in pronation emphasize the signs of ulnolunate conflict (Fig. 13.4). A CT arthroscanner is useful for showing the state of the cartilage. MRI may also be useful for this purpose (Fig. 13.5).

F. del Piñal et al. (eds.), *Arthroscopic Management of Ulnar Pain*,
DOI 10.1007/978-3-642-30544-3_13, © Springer-Verlag Berlin Heidelberg 2012

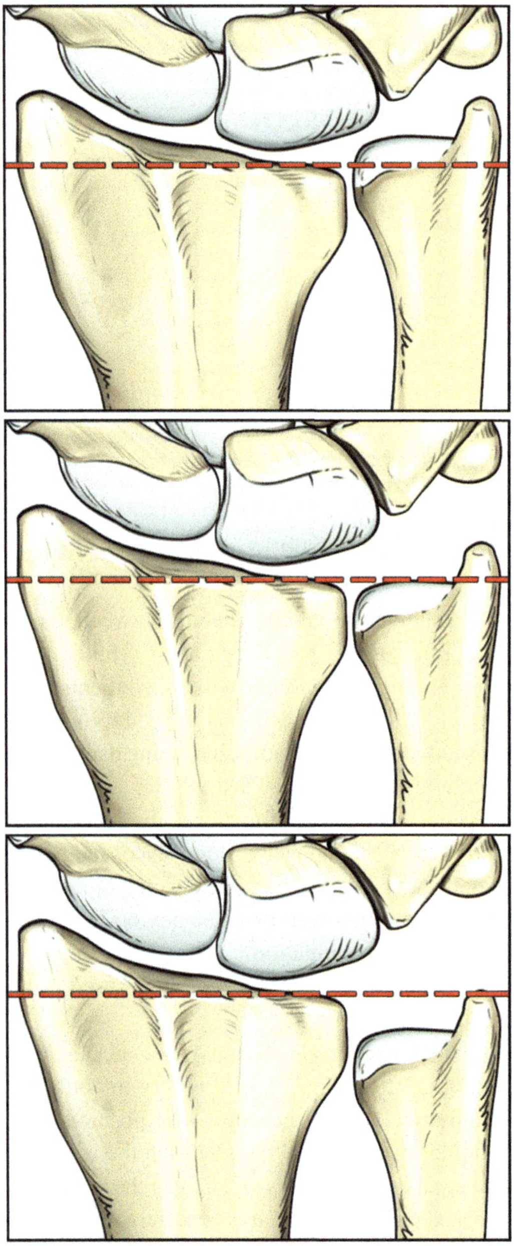

Fig. 13.1 Diagram showing the different relationship between the ulna and radius, measured in neutral position: long ulna, ulna normal, and short ulna

Classical Treatment

1. Ulnar Shortening Osteotomy (USO)
   Described by Milch in 1941, this is the most logical technique. An approach to the inner border of the forearm is required, as the shortening is diaphyseal (Fig. 13.6).

   A dorsoulnar incision is made on the distal one-third of the forearm. The dorsal sensory branch of the ulnar nerve is identified and protected. A 6-hole 3.5-mm DCP plate is positioned at the distal ulna, and the three metaphyseal holes are made. The fragment to be removed is marked using a diathermy blade, and the osteotomy is made using an oscillating saw at low speed under continuous irrigation. The osteotomy may be perpendicular, oblique, or Z shaped. Two parallel saw cuts are made. They are usually from 3 to 8 mm in order to correct the modification of the ulnar variance.

   Fixation and compression are achieved using a plate with 3.5-mm screws. The forearm is immobilized for 21 days postoperatively for pain relief. USO may be associated with radial osteotomy. The most frequent complication of this technique is nonunion.
2. Hemiresection of the Ulnar Head
   Described by Bowers, and modified by Fernandez, this technique involves the hemiresection of the ulnar head through a dorsal approach (Fig. 13.7). A 2-cm flap of the extensor retinaculum is raised over the fourth compartment toward the ulna, taking care not to open the ECU compartment. The EDM is retracted radially. The dorsal capsule of the DRUJ is raised from the sigmoid notch and dissected ulnarly to expose the ulnar head and the TFCC. The ulnar head is resected obliquely from the base of the styloid to the radial side of the neck of the ulna, taking care to preserve the insertion of the TFCC (Fig. 13.8). A musculotendinous flap is harvested using half the ECU, rolled over itself in an anchovy and sutured using absorbable sutures, and inserted into the space left by the resected head (Fig. 13.9). It is fixed to pronator quadratus as well as the dorsal border of the TFCC. The extensor retinaculum and dorsal capsule are closed in one plane using transosseous sutures onto the sigmoid notch (Fig. 13.10).

   Immobilization in a cast for 6 weeks is done, and physiotherapy is commenced afterward.
3. Total Resection of the Ulnar Head (Darrach's Technique)

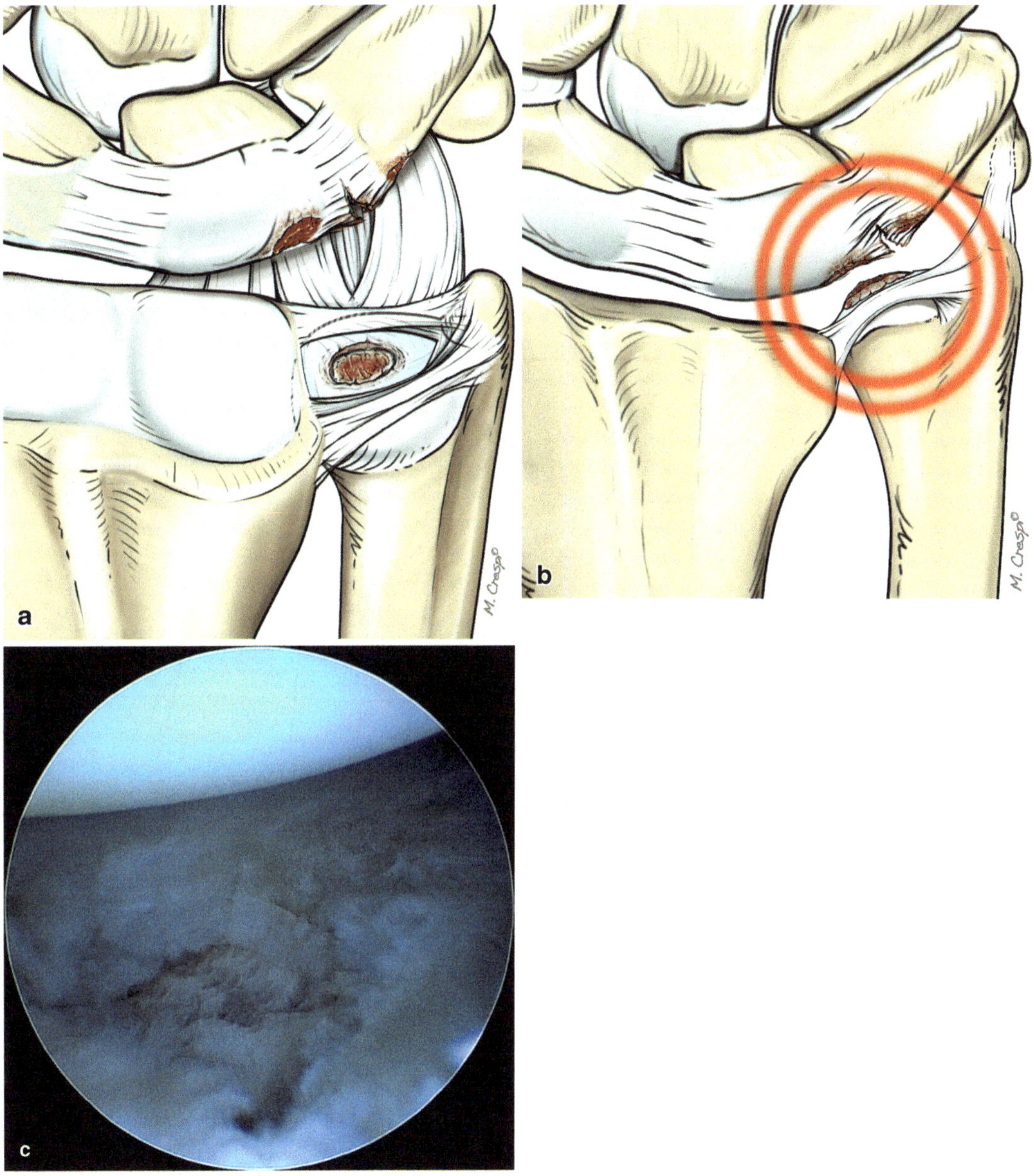

Fig. 13.2 (**a**, **b**) Diagram showing inversion of the distal radioulnar index with abnormal contact between the ulnar head and the internal radiocarpal aspect of the lunate. It is worthy of note that this type of conflict only occurs if the radius has been correctly reduced with a simple axial impaction. Malunions in radial deviation are certainly unsightly, but they protect the ulnar side of the wrist and avoid conflict. (**c**) Operating view showing the central perforation of TFCC with chondral change on ulnar head

This technique was first described by Darrach in 1912 for chronic posttraumatic dislocation of the ulna. The dorsal annular ligament is identified through a dorsal paramedian incision. It is incised on its ulnar border, and a rectangular flap is raised on a radial hinge until the fourth compartment. The capsule is carefully incised axially, identifying both flaps. The ulnar head is approached subperiosteally, preserving the median ligaments. The incision is made as radially as possible, preserving the pronator quadratus insertion. After modeling the ulnar stump to a rounded shape, stabilization

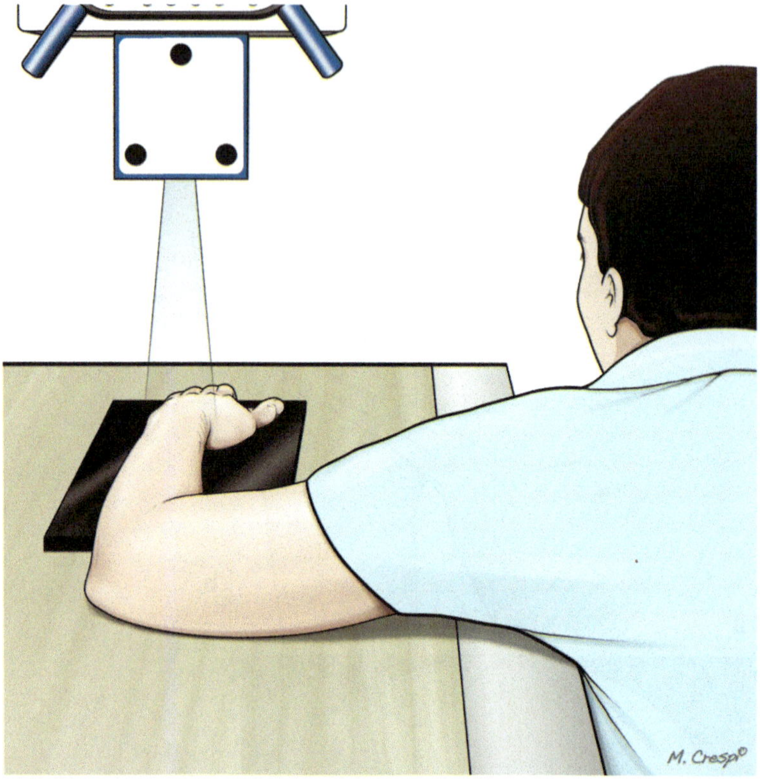

Fig. 13.3 To obtain a neutral pronation position, the arm is at 90° to the body axis with 90° elbow flexion and the hand on the radiology plate

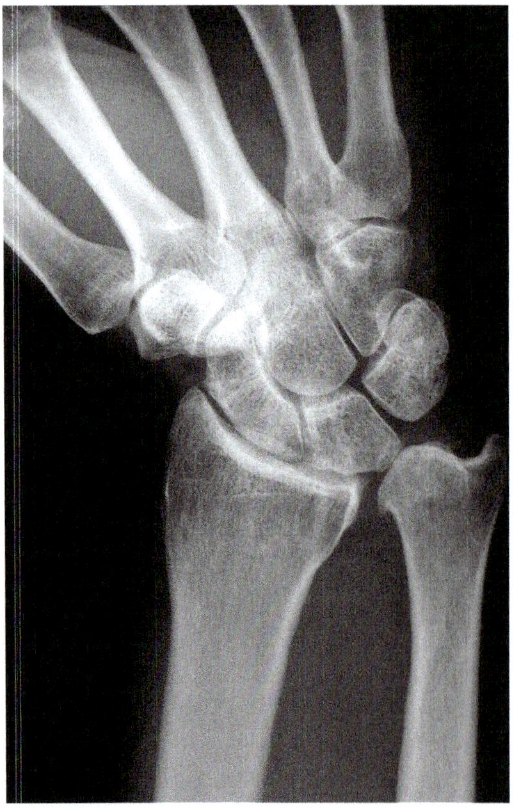

Fig. 13.4 Dynamic view in radial deviation emphasizing the ulnolunate conflict

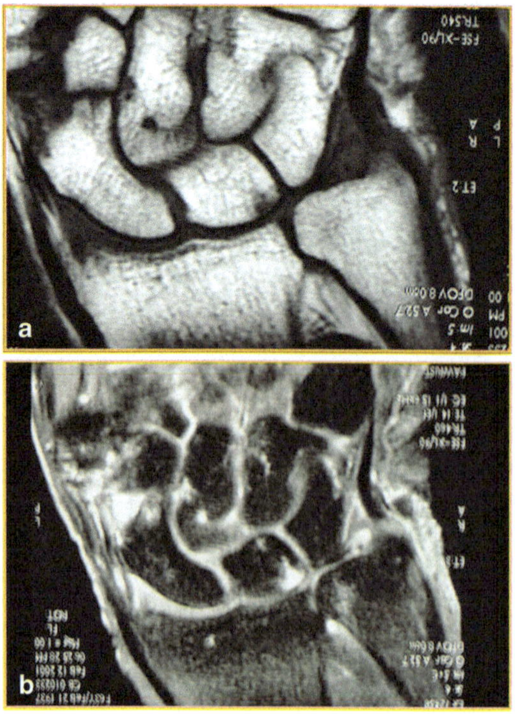

Fig. 13.5 MRI showing the reality of the ulnolunate conflict in two views with cartilage still preserved, but pathological aspect of the subchondral bone especially of the lunate

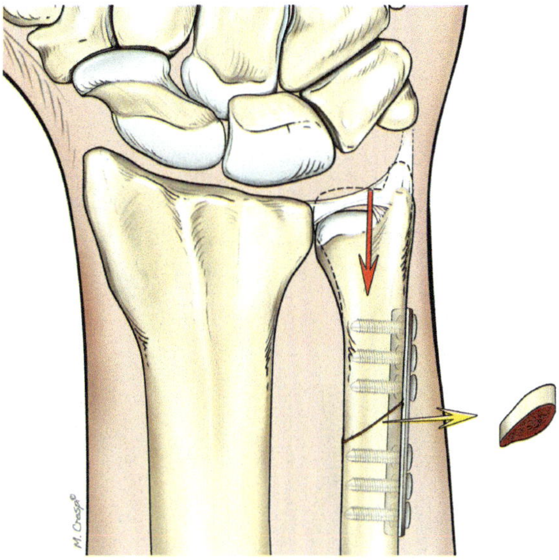

Fig. 13.6 Diagram showing the principle of Milch's ulnar shortening

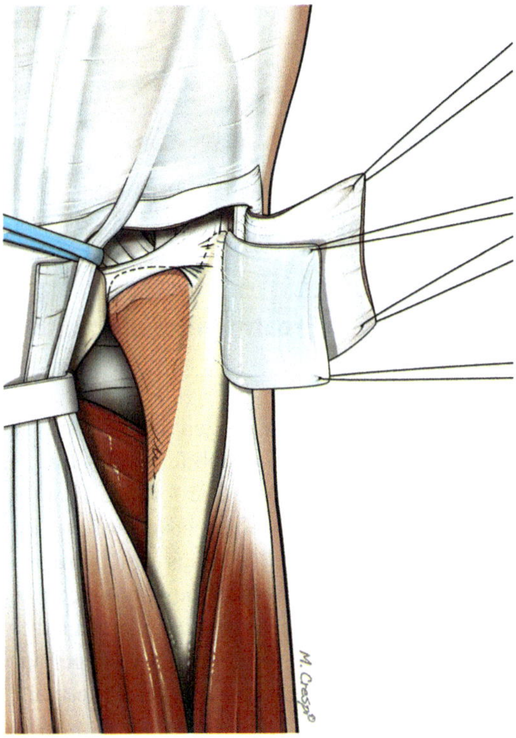

Fig. 13.7 Diagram showing the principle of Fernandez hemiresection

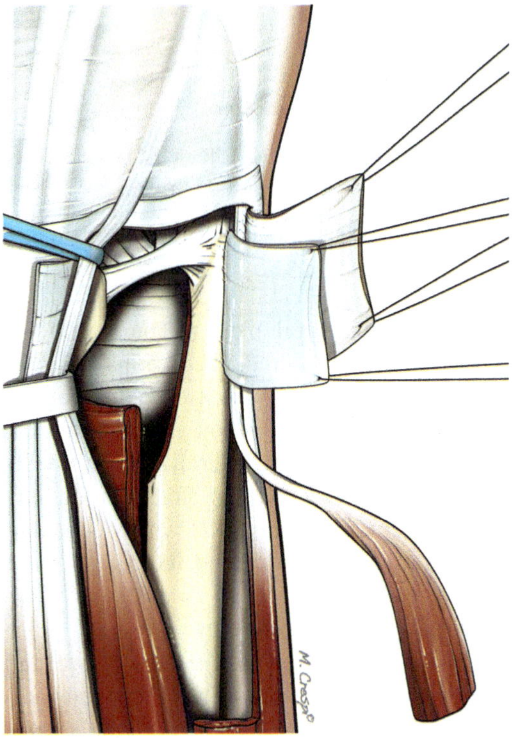

Fig. 13.8 Diagram showing the hemiresection preserving TFCC and harvesting half of ECU

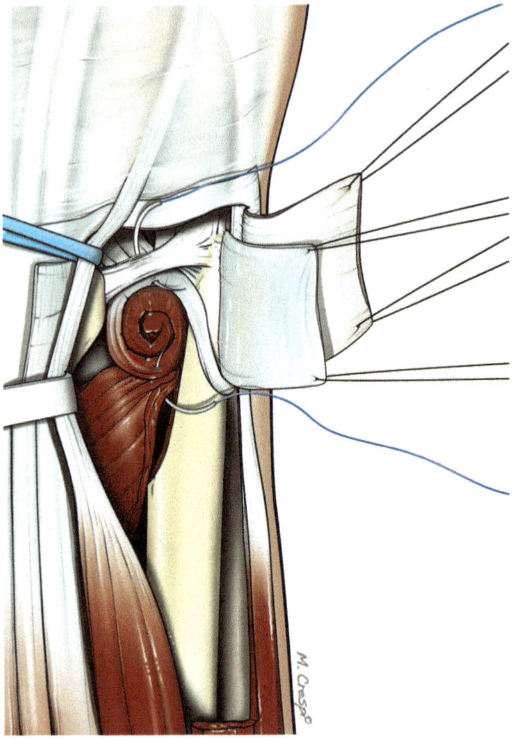

Fig. 13.9 Diagram showing half of ECU rolled over itself and inserted into the space left by the resected head

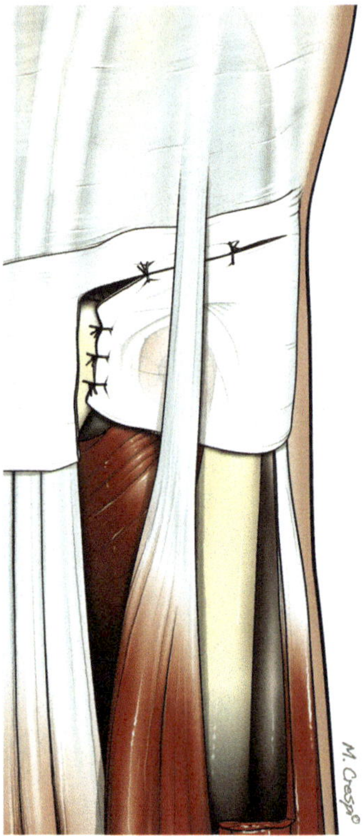

Fig. 13.10 Diagram showing the extensor retinaculum and dorsal capsule closed in one plane using transosseous sutures onto the sigmoid notch

is done at several planes. The capsule is resected and sutured. The retinaculum is reinserted medially onto itself, adjusting the tension and passing below the ECU tendon which is dorsalized, lateralized, and stabilized by a retinacular flap. Stabilization may be easier using hemi-ECU which is passed across the distal ulna and fixed onto itself (Fig. 13.11a, b).

4. Sauvé-Kapandji Technique

   This was described in 1936 by Sauvé and Kapandji.Although described for distal radioulnar dislocations unstable after reduc tion, it can be used for ulnolunate conflict with radioulnar dislocation and is exceptional in pure ulnolunate conflict (Fig. 13.12).
5. Ulnar Head Prosthesis

   Ulnar head prostheses are actually rarely used but could potentially become a therapeutic option.

Arthroscopy in Treatment of Ulnolunate Conflict

Wrist arthroscopy, popularized by Whipple in 1986, has since become a routine examination.

Arthroscopy is the best tool for assessing the gravity of ulnolunate conflict; lesions of the cartilage can be seen directly. This is even more pertinent in early cases where the lesions can be detected only by arthroscopy and are limited to the conflict zone. Arthroscopy at this stage may also show associated lesions in detail especially TFCC lesions which are almost always present. An inversion of the radioulnar index smaller than 5 mm may be treated arthroscopically using Feldon's partial ulnar resection technique. This technique was first done using the same approach as for Bower's partial resection – but we prefer to do it arthroscopically to minimize postoperative pain.

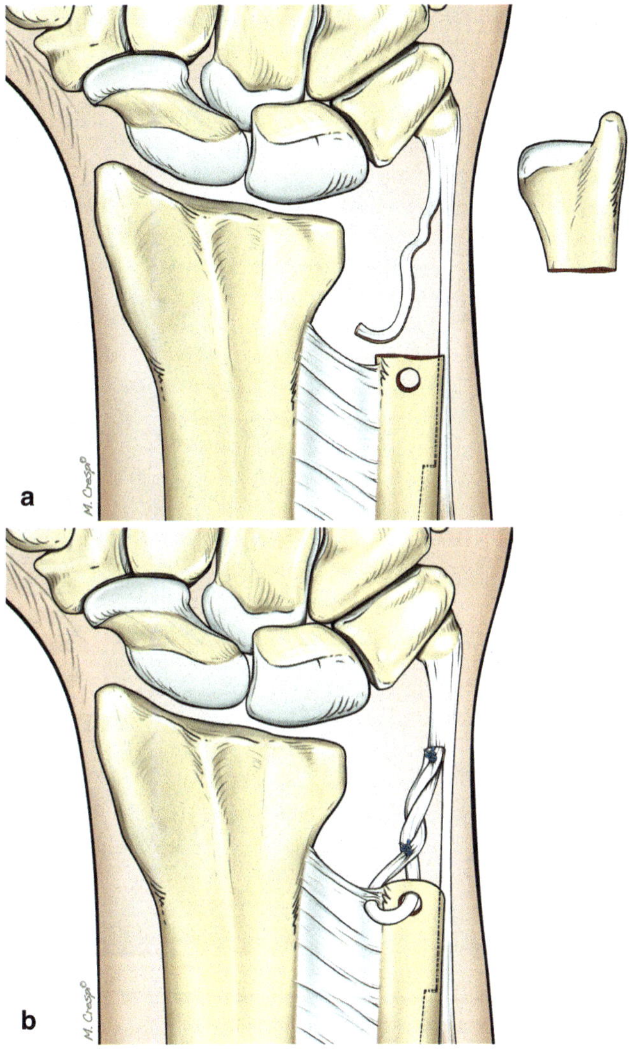

Fig. 13.11 (**a**, **b**) Diagram showing the ulnar head resection and the stabilization using hemi-ECU which is passed across the distal ulna and fixed onto itself

Technique of Partial Resection of the Distal Ulna Under Arthroscopic Control

The patient lies supine with the arm flat and fixed to an arm table. At 90° elbow flexion, the forearm is under axial traction using the arthroscopy tower and Chinese finger traps. It is a day surgery under locoregional anesthesia and arm tourniquet. The scope is introduced through 3–4 portal, allowing exploration of the radiocarpal joint. A 6R portal allows treatment of lesions encountered and the ulnolunate conflict.

I use a 2.4-mm size arthroscope with a 3.0 mm synovitomes and 3.0 mm burr.

Usually, a central perforation of the TFCC is encountered with an ulnar head protruding into the radiocarpal joint. The cartilage on the ulnar head is assessed, and chondropathy is usually found (Fig. 13.13a–c) which is seldom seen on plain films at this stage. This chondropathy is also rarely seen even on arthrogram due to the small size of the lesion which is usually the cause of pain. It is at this stage where partial resection of the distal ulna resolves the ulnolunate conflict and the pain. After introduction of the scope through a 3–4 portal, and a microsuction forceps through

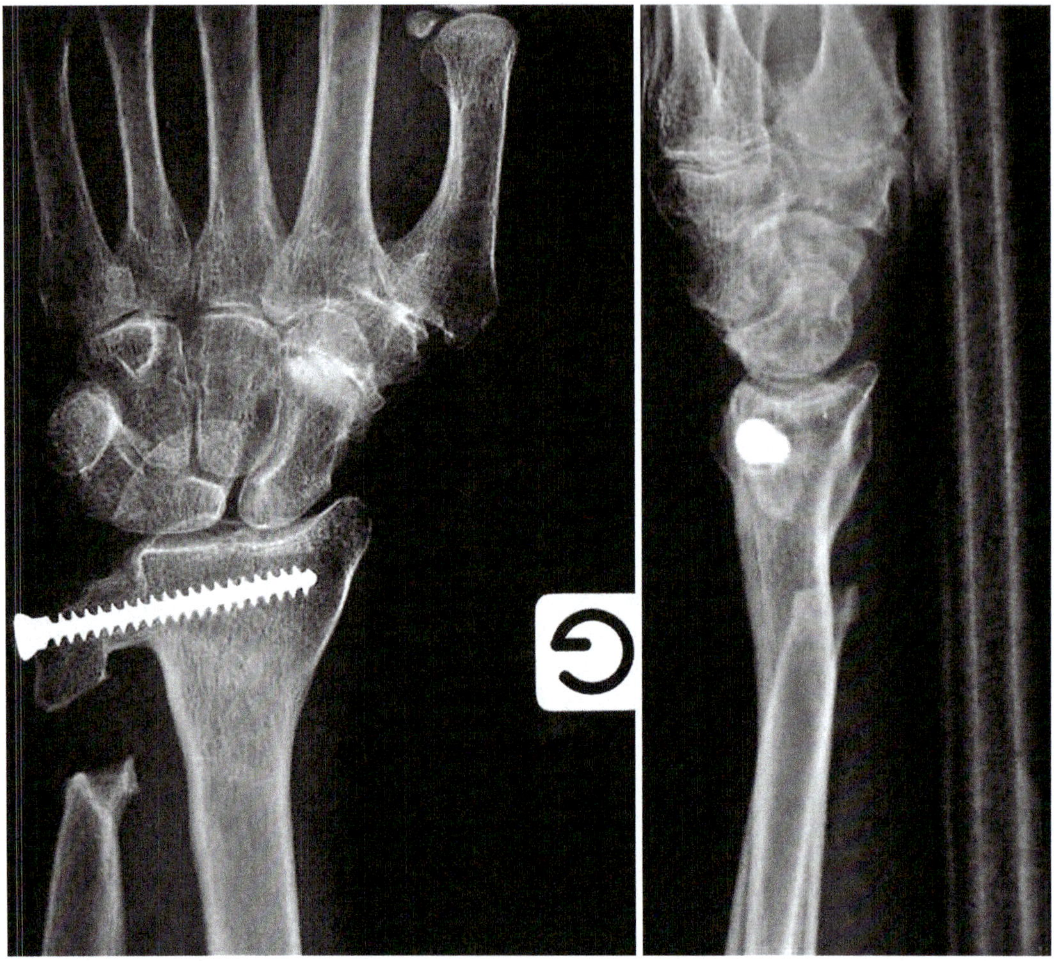

Fig. 13.12 Clinical case showing long-term follow up of Sauvé-Kapandji osteotomy with interposition of a resected ulnar head fragment to preserve carpal breadth

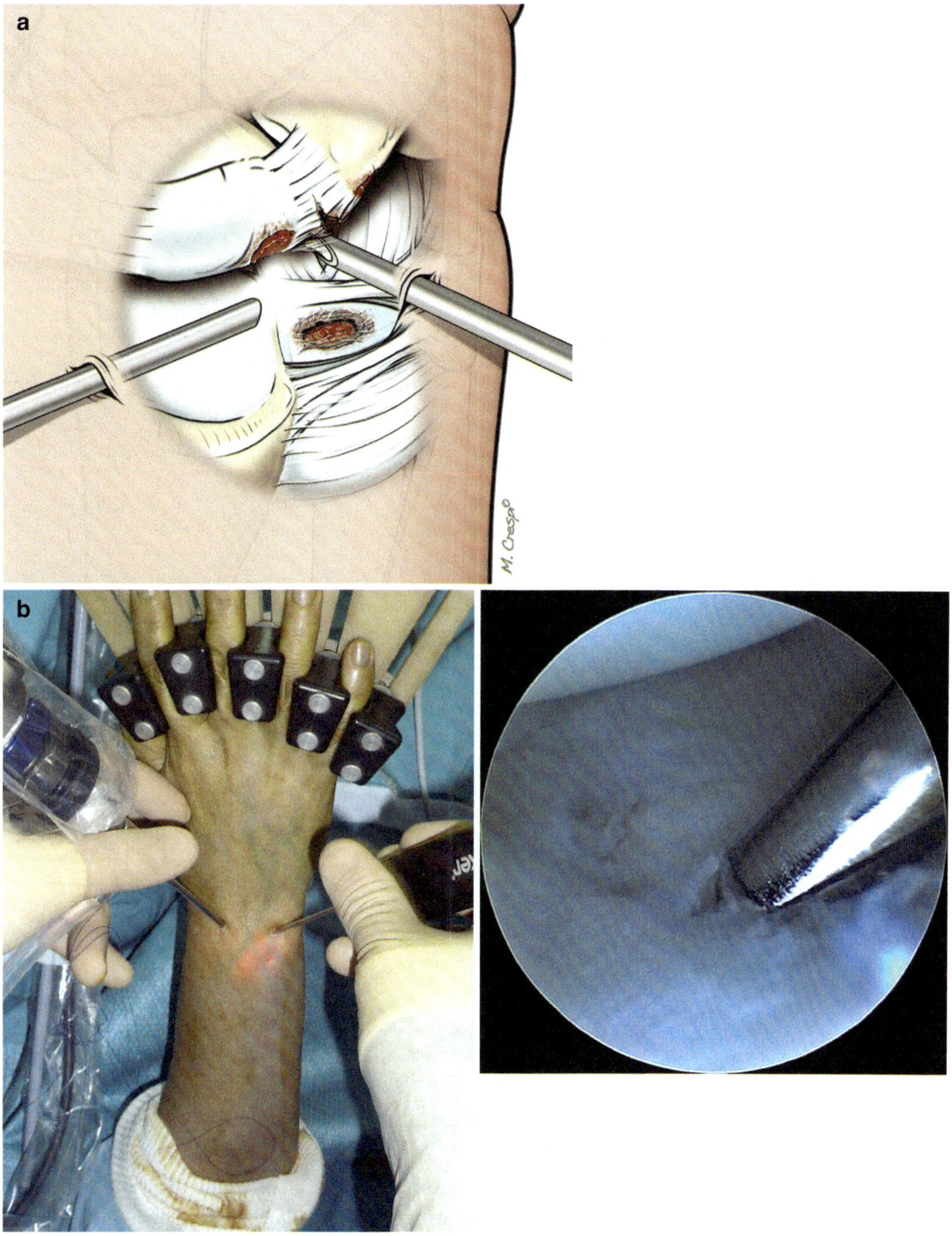

Fig. 13.13 (**a**) Diagram after traction, showing the TFCC central perforation, protrusion of the ulnar head, and cartilage lesions on the lunate. (**b**) Operating view showing the correct position of scope (3–4 radiocarpal portal) and shaver (6R radiocarpal portal). (**c**) Intra-articular operating view showing the central debridement of TFCC with a shaver

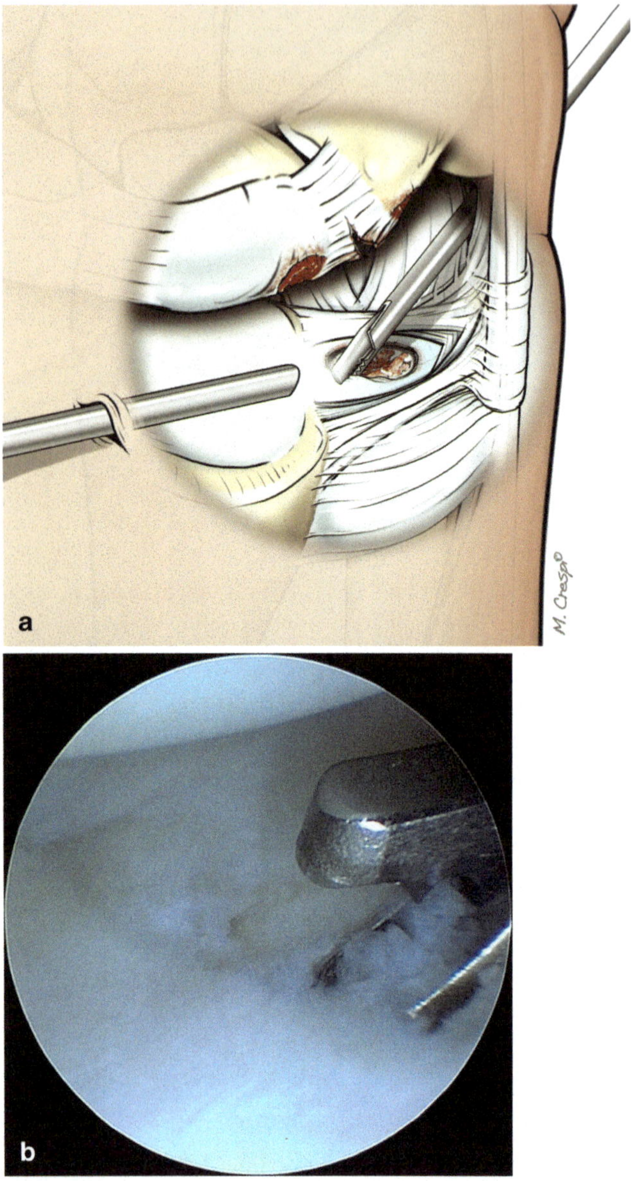

Fig. 13.14 (**a**) Diagram showing arthroscopic setup with central TFCC debridement using basket forceps. (**b**) Intra-articular view showing central debridement of TFCC with a basket forceps

the 6R portal, the central TFCC perforation is first debrided and enlarged (Fig. 13.14a, b). The protruding part of the ulnar head is then resected using a burr under arthroscopic control (Fig. 13.15a, b). If the TFCC is intact, the arthroscope is introduced through the distal radioulnar joint and the burr directly onto the fovea distal and palmar to the ulnar styloid with the wrist in supination to avoid injury to the dorsal sensory branch of the ulnar nerve (see also Chap. 9).

Pronation-supination movements are made to ensure even resection of the anterior and posterior parts of the ulnar head respecting the distal radio ulnar joint (Fig. 13.16a–f).

The ulnar head is not perfectly spherical, and thus, these pronosupinatory movements allow tailored resection of the parts of the head protruding into the TFCC perforation. The resulting osteotomy is usually original, oblique, and helicoidal (Fig. 13.17a, b). This type of osteotomy is

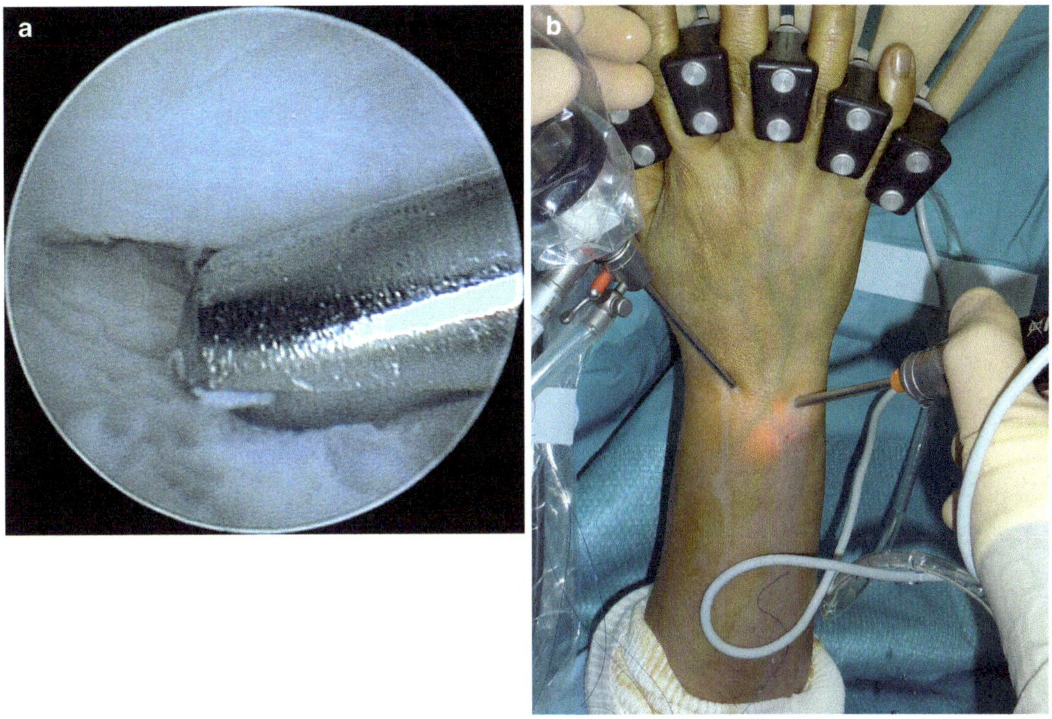

Fig. 13.15 (**a**) Arthroscopic view showing start of ulnar head resection using a burr. (**b**) Operating view showing the correct position of scope (3–4 radiocarpal portal) and burr (6R radiocarpal portal)

not possible through a standard classic open approach using a straight osteotomy blade.

It is crucial to verify the integrity of the DRUJ at the end of the procedure (Fig. 13.18a–c).

Discussion

Ulnolunate conflict is the result of the inversion of the distal radioulnar index, most commonly following a distal radius fracture with impaction in the axis of the distal radius. Ulnolunate conflict causes a central TFCC perforation with cartilage lesions of the distal ulnar head and the lunate. Clinical wrist examination reveals ulnar pain exacerbated in pronation and ulnar deviation of the wrist. This pain may be related to a long congenital ulna (rare lesion), TFCC lesion, lunotriquetral lesion, radioulnar ligament lesion, or chondrocalcinosis of the ulnar head. The variety of possible lesions warrants systematic standard films followed by sophisticated complementary investigations – arthrogram or arthroscopy. Standard bilateral wrist films in supination, pronation, clenched fist, and strict frontal allow an objective measurement of the distal radioulnar index as well as distal radioulnar articular congruency. Complementary arthrogram or arthroscopy accurately shows associated cartilage lesions. The earlier the treatment, the better the results in preventing the inevitable evolution to arthritis.

Between 1998 and 2010, 2,023 wrist arthroscopies including 126 distal ulnar resections (6.23 %) were performed. In three cases with no TFCC lesion, a distal radioulnar approach was used.

In this series, patients included 49 men and 77 women of average age 68 (between 42 and 87 years). All were distal one-fourth radius fractures with axial impaction and inversion of the distal radioulnar index. The ulnar variance was 2.6 mm on average (2–5.5 mm). The mean delay

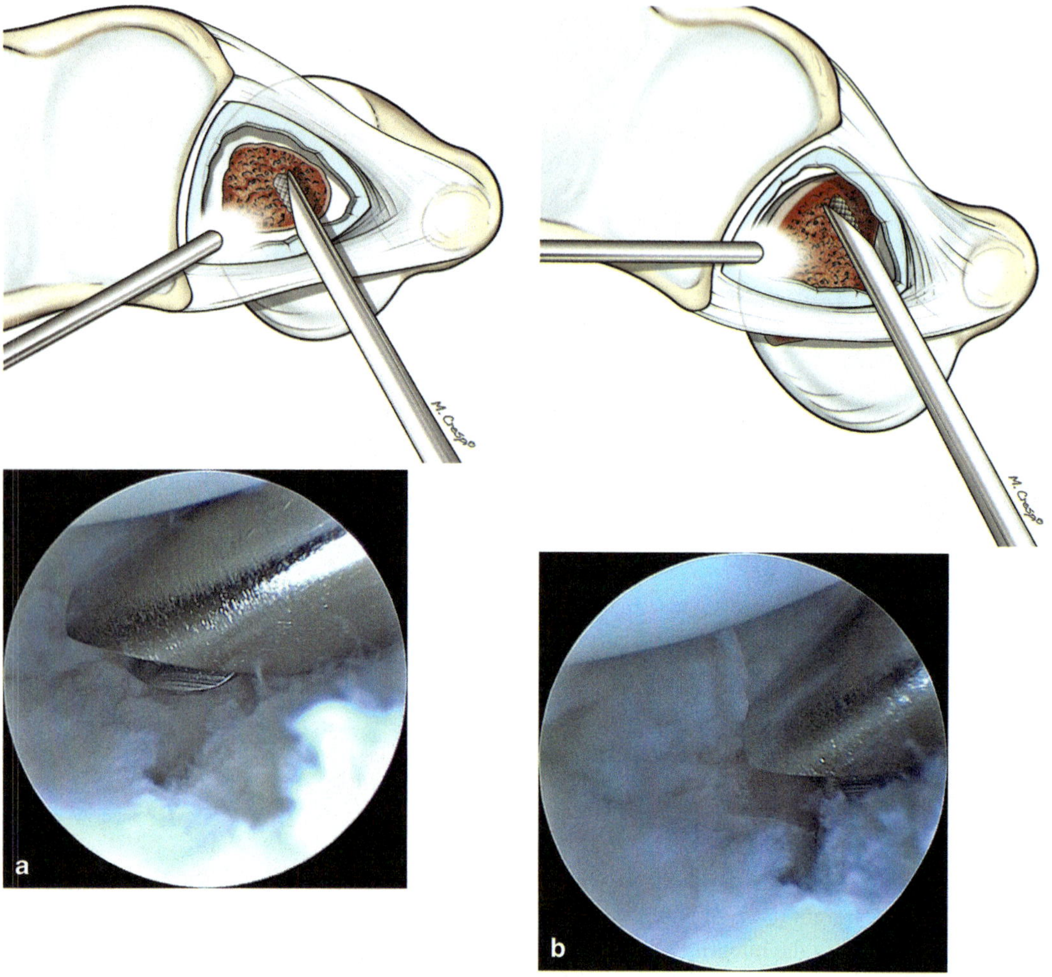

Fig. 13.16 (**a–f**) Diagram and intra-articular view showing arthroscopic resection of ulnar head using a burr with pronation-supination movements to ensure resection of the anterior and posterior parts of the ulnar head

between the fracture and the arthroscopic resection was 9.3 months (2–36 months). Arthroscopic resection was the only procedure performed in all cases. Pain was always present, permanent, and moderate in 80 cases and disabling in 46 cases. Force was diminished by more than half compared to the contralateral side. Mobility was already limited due to the often associated malunion of the distal one-fourth radius fracture. Pronosupination was less than 120° in 93 cases and less than 60° in 33 cases. None of the patients needed postoperative immobilization (Fig. 13.19a, b).

Our average follow-up is 35 months (12–97 months). Recovery of mobility was immediate in all cases with persistence of DRUJ pain in eight cases. In 71 cases, preoperative pain disappeared immediately postoperative. Force increased compared to preoperative values but never reached the value of the healthy contralateral side.

We observed three postoperative hematomas which resolved without treatment, residual limitation of pronosupination in 12 cases and 6 cases of CRPS which were diagnosed early, treated promptly, and recovered completely.

Conclusion

Arthroscopic treatment has proved its efficacy and its safety. It should nevertheless be limited to cases of inversion of small values (inferior

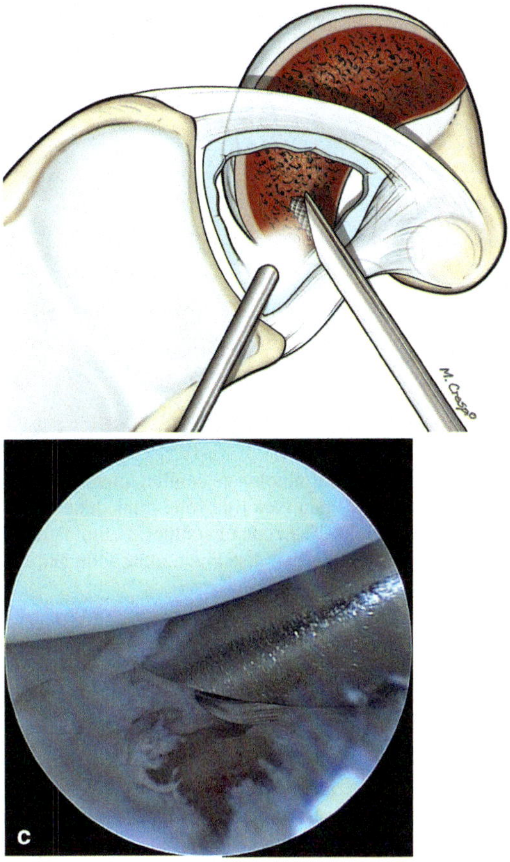

Fig. 13.16 (continued)

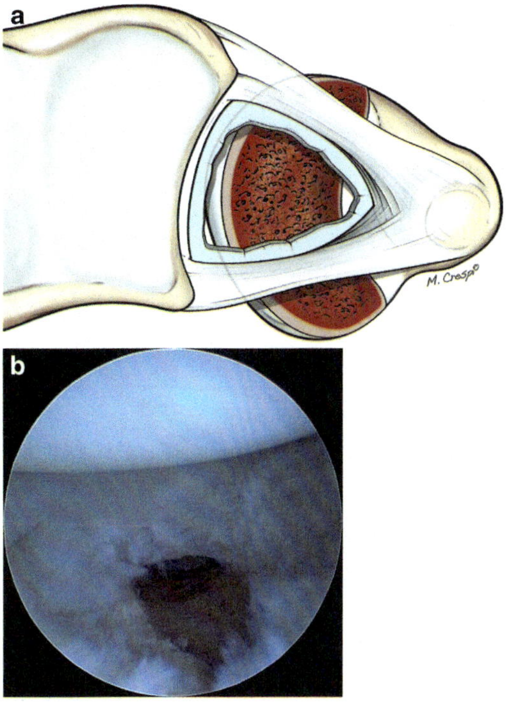

Fig. 13.17 (**a**, **b**) Diagram and intra-articular view showing the final resulting oblique and helicoidal osteotomy

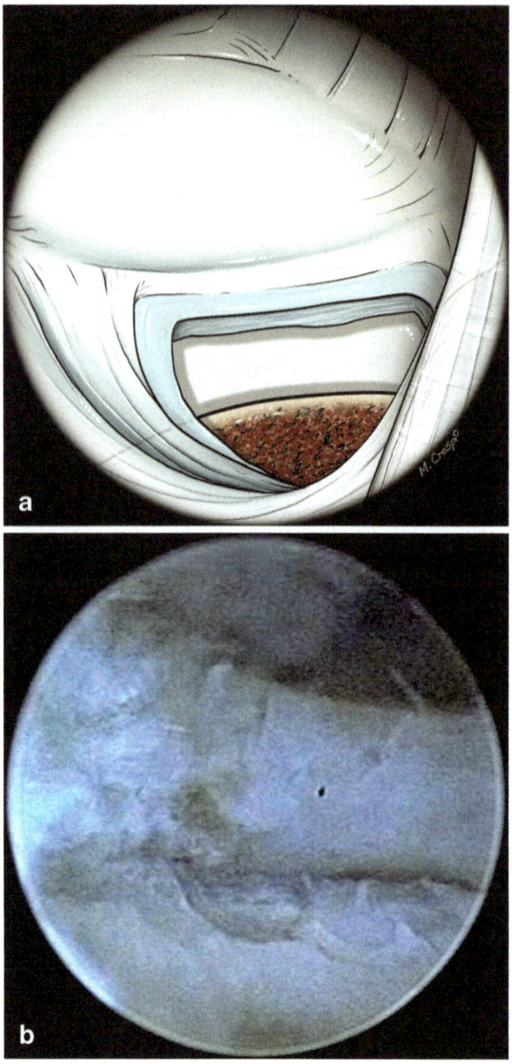

Fig. 13.18 (**a–c**) Diagram and arthroscopic views showing the whole DRUJ intact with arthroscope through 6R

to 5 mm). In greater ulnar variances, we prefer ulnar shortening osteotomy. Other techniques are reserved for cases with altered distal radioulnar joint.

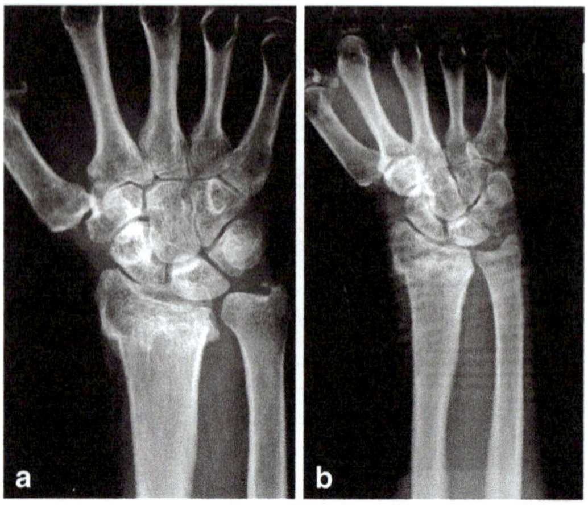

Fig. 13.19 (**a**) Case of ulnolunate conflict after distal radius fracture. (**b**) Plain views showing immediate postoperative results. The zone of conflict is eliminated with preservation of normal distal radioulnar joint and thus normal pronosupination

Bibliography

Bowers WH (1985) Distal radio ulnar joint arthroplasty: the hemi resection-interposition technique. J Hand Surg Am 10-A:169–178

Feldon P, Terrono A, Belsky M (1992) Wafer distal ulna resection for triangular fibrocartilage tears and/or ulna impaction syndrome. J Hand Surg 7A:731–737

Fernandez DL (1988) Radial osteotomy and bowers arthrosplasty for malunited fracture of the distal end of the radius. J Bone Joint Surg Am 26-A:1538–1551

Milch H (1941) Cuff resection of the ulna for malunited colle's fracture. J Bone Joint Surg 23A:311–313

Palmer AK, Glisson RR, Werner FW (1982) Ulnar variance determination. J Hand Surg Am 7:376–379

Sauvé L, Kapandji M (1936) Nouvelles techniques de traitement chirurgical des luxations récidivantes isolées de l'extrémité inférieure du cubitus. J Chir 45:589–594

Arthrosopic Ulnar Styloidectomy for Ulnar Styloid Impaction Syndrome

14

Gregory I. Bain, Mario G.T. Zotti, and Kevin Eng

Ulnar styloid impaction syndrome is characterized by the impaction of the triquetrum against the ulnar styloid causing chondromalacia, synovitis and ulnar-sided wrist pain [15, 16, 18].

Pathology of Ulnar Styloid Impaction Syndrome

In the presence of intact anatomy, the meniscus homologue will be interposed between the tip of the ulnar styloid and the triquetrum [18]. In early stages of the pathology, there is soft tissue erosion before contact of the carpus, specifically the triquetrum, with the exposed tip of the ulnar styloid results in degeneration [16, 18] (Fig. 14.1).

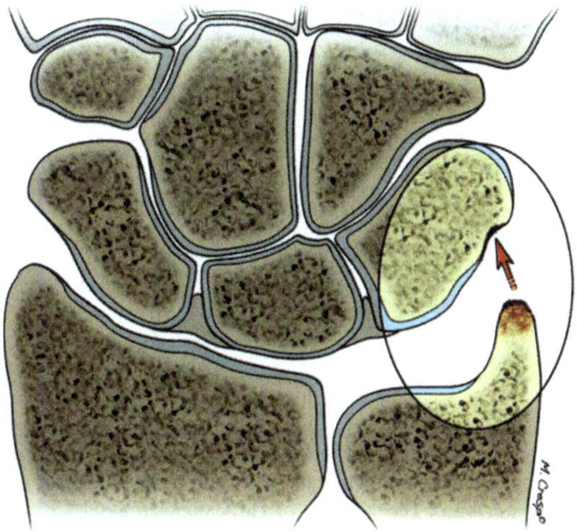

Fig. 14.1 Pathologic sequelae of the ulnar styloid impaction syndrome can include chondromalacia of the triquetrum and subchondral sclerosis of the styloid process. Direction of impaction (*red arrow*) (With permission from Luchetti and Borrelli [11]. Copyright (2010), p. 179, Fig. 13.7)

Aetiology

The ulnar styloid process is a well-differentiated carpal element until it joins to the developing ulnar at around the tenth week of ontogenesis [7] with chondrification usually occurring by around 51 days in utero [12]. The ulnar styloid appears with the adolescent growth spurt, becoming more elongated and adult-like until physeal closure

G.I. Bain (✉)
Department of Orthopaedics Surgery, Discipline of Anatomy and Pathology, University of Adelaide, North Terrace, SA 5000, Australia

Department of Orthopaedics and Trauma, Royal Adelaide Hospital, North Terrace, SA 5000, Australia
e-mail: greg@gregbain.com.au

M.G.T. Zotti
Department of Orthopaedics and Trauma, Royal Adelaide Hospital, North Terrace, SA 5000, Australia
e-mail: mariozotti@gmail.com

K. Eng
Department of Orthopaedics, Modbury Hospital, Smart Road, Modbury, SA 5092, Australia
e-mail: kevinengorthopaedics@gmail.com

F. del Piñal et al. (eds.), *Arthroscopic Management of Ulnar Pain*,
DOI 10.1007/978-3-642-30544-3_14, © Springer-Verlag Berlin Heidelberg 2012

with ossification late in adolescence [13, 14]. Biyani and colleagues [4] in a morphological study of 400 individuals without wrist symptoms found great variation in ulnar styloid processes and defined a standard ulnar styloid process to be 3–6 mm in length with a medial angulation not exceeding 15°.

Giachino [9, 10] classifies the aetiologies being related to:

1. Reduced stylotriquetral distance (bringing the styloid to the triquetrum *or* bringing the triquetrum to the ulnar styloid)
2. Dynamic styloid prominence based on ligamentous laxity, instability or loading activities (such as racquet sports and golf)
3. A combination of the above

Aetiologies classified as bringing the styloid closer to the triquetrum may include a congenitally long ulnar styloid process, styloid overgrowth, for example, from fracture or rheumatoid arthritis-related hypertrophy [5].

Aetiologies bringing the triquetrum to the ulnar styloid include radial shortening related to distal radius fractures, distal radial growth arrest following distal radial physeal injury or Essex-Lopresti lesions, Kienbock's disease and wrist arthrodesis [9].

Clinical Features

The patient with symptomatic ulnar styloid impaction will typically complain of ulnar-sided wrist pain, aggravated by wrist extension and specific positioning, such as having their hands on their hip or in their back pockets [1, 11]. There may be a history of trauma to the distal radius or ulna, surgery to the carpus, generalized ligamentous laxity or other features suggestive of a disturbance to normal wrist mechanics at the lunatotriquetral interval [16].

On examination, there is point tenderness to palpation of the ulnar styloid tip [11], and the patient's pain is classically provoked by Ruby's ulnar styloid provocation test. This is performed with the patient's elbow resting on the examiner's table and the forearm initially in neutral rotation. The dorsiflexed wrist is rotated into full supination (Fig. 14.2). This decreases the distance between the styloid process and triquetrum as the ulnar styloid is positioned dorsally relative to the carpus which is the position of impingement [16]. A positive provocation test is the reproduction of the patient's pain upon performing this manoeuvre.

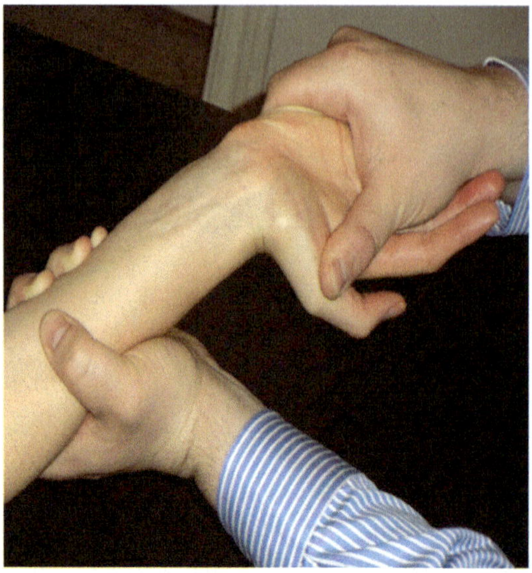

Fig. 14.2 Ulnar styloid provocation test as described by Ruby (1997): Patient's forearm rests on table in neutral rotation with wrist in full extension, brought by examiner into full supination with a positive test ascribed to reproduction of the patient's ulnar-sided wrist pain

This is distinct from ulno-carpal impaction of the ulnar head against the lunate where point tenderness is to the proximal lunate and the ulnar deviation grind test reproduces the pain with the forearm in pronation [9]. Forearm supination in Ruby's test also brings the ulna head into a relatively ulnar negative position, helping to exclude ulno-carpal impaction [16].

The diagnosis is made in patients who have relatively long ulnar styloid process radiographically [6, 17] in combination with a positive ulnar styloid provocation test [16].

Imaging

Patients with this condition tend to have a longer than average ulnar styloid with positive ulnar variance. A long ulnar styloid process can be defined radiographically on standard zero-rotation posteroanterior radiographs as being greater than or equal to 6 mm [17] with their study reporting the mean ulnar styloid length of 4.4 (±1.2 mm).

Two main methods have been described to identify relative ulnar styloid lengths with Garcia-Elias, the first in describing the ulnar styloid process index (USPI) in 1987 with an excessively long styloid having the USPI 0.21 ± 0.07.

Since then, Van der Heijden and colleagues [17] suggested that the ulnar styloid-capitate ratio (SCR) had a stronger correlation with the relative length of the ulnar styloid than did the USPI and also eliminated differences related to gender, with an excessively long styloid defined as having a SCR greater than 0.18 ± 0.05 (Figs. 14.3 and 14.4).

Radiographs may demonstrate degenerative changes including sclerotic and cystic changes in the triquetrum and distal ulna in the early stages before degenerative ulnar-sided progression ensues [18].

Dynamic fluoroscopic assessment and three-dimensional computed tomography can also be used to confirm impingement [1]. The 3D CT scan is performed in the position of provocation, in which case the long ulnar styloid will be seen to impinge on the triquetrum.

In the latter stages of the disease, magnetic resonance imaging may reveal focal subchondral sclerosis and chondromalacia of the styloid tip as well as proximal triquetral chondromalacia [6] (Fig. 14.5).

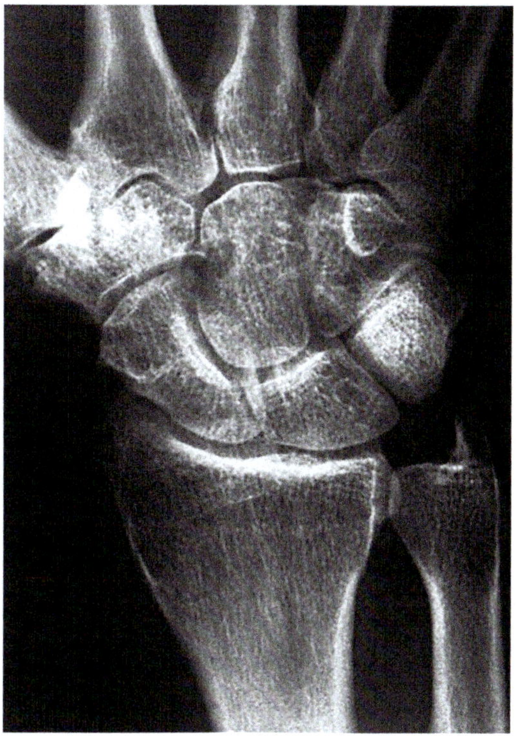

Fig. 14.3 Plain posteroanterior radiograph of a male patient with activity-related ulnar-sided wrist pain and relative prominence of the ulnar styloid (Reprinted from Bain and Bidwell [1]. Copyright (2006), with permission from Elsevier)

The senior author prefers an arthroscopic partial resection of the styloid as it does not compromise the triangular fibrocartilage or ulno-carpal ligaments attached to the base of the styloid, injury to which can lead to ulnar-sided wrist instability [1].

Treatment of Ulnar Styloid Impaction

Non-operative treatment includes wrist splinting, activity modification and analgesia with the addition of injected corticosteroids as necessary [16, 18].

Operative treatment is aimed at correcting the impaction of the ulnar styloid. This can be performed as an open or arthroscopic procedure. If the patient also has ulnar head impaction, then an ulnar shortening procedure may be a viable option and correct the impaction of both the ulnar head and styloid.

Open Ulnar Styloidectomy

Open ulnar styloidectomy can be performed via a dorsal or ulnar approach.

The dorsal approach involves a longitudinal incision on the dorsal-ulnar side of the wrist. The extensor retinaculum between the extensor digiti minimi and extensor carpi ulnaris is incised, with the sheath of the ECU left intact [15]. The DRUJ capsule is then opened with a horseshoe-shaped flap, leaving the radial side of the capsule intact. Following this, the TFCC and ulnar styloid are

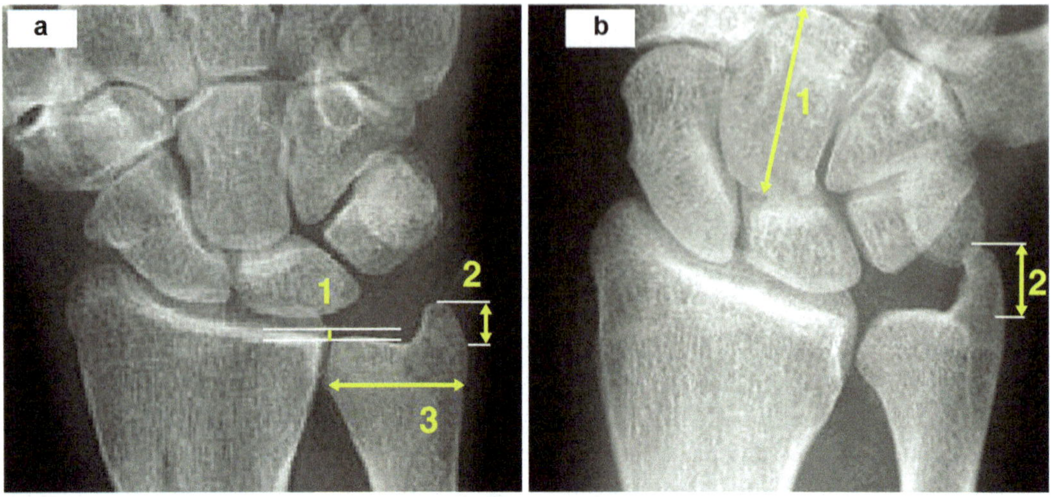

Fig. 14.4 Methods of determining relative ulnar styloid length: (**a**) Ulnar styloid process index (*USPI*) method described by Garcia-Elias [8] – (*1*) ulnar variance, (*2*) ulnar styloid length, and (*3*) ulnar head width; Index = (ulnar styloid length – ulnar variance) divided by ulnar head width. Formula for USPI calculation = ulnar styloid length – ulnar variance (2 – 1)/Ulnar head width (3). (**b**) The ulnar styloid-capitate ratio (*SCR*) method of Van der Heijden and co-authors [17] – (*1*) capitate length, (*2*) ulnar styloid length. Formula for SCR = length of capitate (1)/length of ulnar styloid (2)

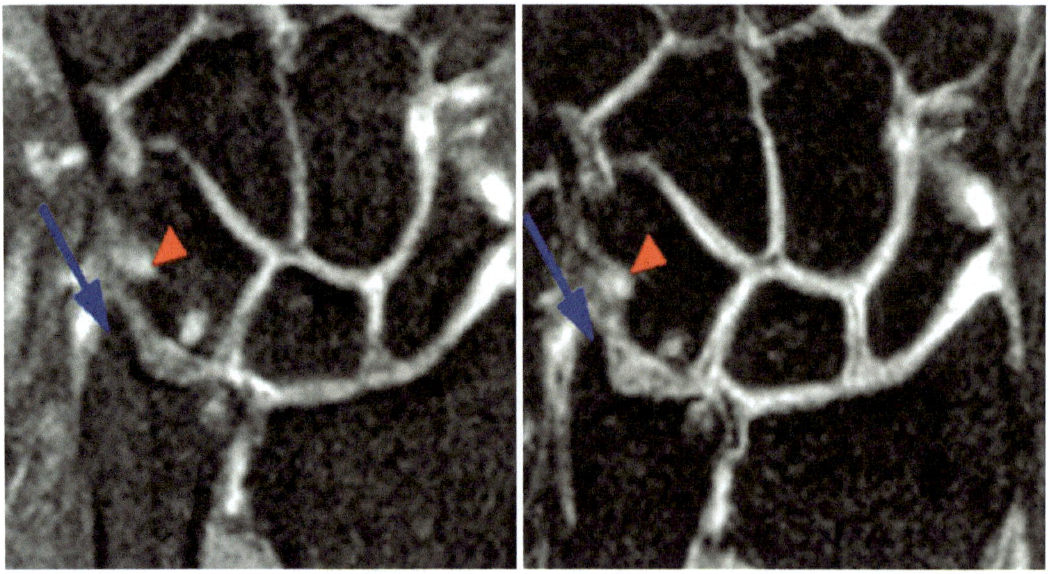

Fig. 14.5 Fat-suppressed proton density and gradient echo coronal images of a patient with ulnar styloid impaction syndrome. An elongated ulnar styloid, lunotriquetral and ulnar styloidchondromalacia, triquetralsubchondral cyst formation and reactive effusion/synovitis are present. There is also a macerated TFC, which is often associated with this condition. Ulnar styloid (*blue arrows*), sunchondral cyst in triquetrum (*red arrowheads*) (Images source with permission http://www.radsource.us/)

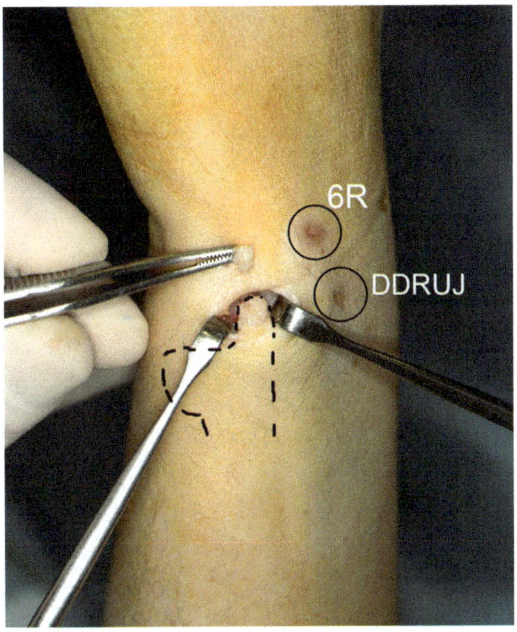

Fig. 14.6 Open ulnar approach to the ulnar styloid. Arm is in full supination; hand pointing to the ceiling. Dorsal branch of the ulnar nerve if protected under a retractor (Image courtesy of Dr. Piñal)

identified with the TFCC (and its attachments) protected. For the resection itself, a small osteotome is used to make a longitudinal cut 2–4 mm in depth along the radial side of the styloid process, and subsequently, a thin oscillating saw is used to remove 2–4 mm from the head of the distal ulnar with the operative goal to create 2 mm of negative ulnar variance. Ligamentous repair and/or TFCC repair (or debridement) can also be performed at this time. Resection to more than 3 mm can potentially destabilize the wrist due to injury to TFCC attachments [15].

The ulnar approach is via a 2 cm ulnar-sided oblique incision with the forearm fully supinated. The ulnar styloid becomes subcutaneous in this position. The dorsal branch of the ulnar nerve is identified and retracted dorsally. The ulnar styloid is approached ulnar to the ECU tendon and subperiosteally identified by sharp dissection and is partially resected [18] (Fig. 14.6).

Typically, the arm and wrist are immobilized for around 4 weeks with recovery being around 3 months with the associated larger incision and soft tissue dissection required [18]. Aside from the potential for prolonged discomfort from retraction of the dorsal branch of the ulnar nerve, poor cosmesis can also result at the site of the incision from scarring. All of these disadvantages are lessened by arthroscopic ulnar styloidectomy.

Arthroscopic Ulnar Styloidectomy

Background

Wrist arthroscopy is a commonly used procedure that has undergone many modifications and improvements since it was first described. The advent of new portals (both dorsal and volar) means that the wrist joint can be viewed from virtually any perspective [2, 3]. Indications for wrist arthroscopy have continued to expand and include diagnostic and reparative procedures and, more recently, reconstructive, soft tissue, and bony procedures [2, 3].

An arthroscopic ulnar styloidectomy has the advantage of being minimally invasive with faster postoperative recovery. It also allows visualization of the TFCC and carpus and an intraarticular assessment of associated pathologies [1]. Previous authors have not recommended arthroscopic ulnar styloidectomy due to the difficulty associated with identifying the styloid and its proximity to the ulnotriquetral and ulnolunate ligaments [16].

In cases where the ulnar styloid is impinging, an eburnated flattened ulnar styloid can be frequently identified. In addition, fluoroscopy can be used to assist in identification of the ulnar styoid.

Author's Technique

The arm is exsanguinated before the tourniquet insufflation, and standard wrist arthroscopy is performed through the 3–4 and 4–5 portals, with an accessory portal, the 6U portal, created with care taken to preserve the dorsal branch of the ulnar nerve.

With the arthroscope positioned in the 3–4 portal, the probe is introduced into the 6R portal. The triangular fibrocartilaginous complex, lunotriquetral ligament complex and pisotriquetral recess are all assessed (Fig. 14.7). By palpation, the burr is placed onto the tip of the ulnar styloid (Fig. 14.8).

Fluoroscopy is then used to confirm correct placement of the burr on the ulnar styloid before resection is carried out (Figs. 14.9 and 14.10). Removal of the desired amount of ulnar styloid can also be confirmed by fluoroscopy with care to preserve and respect the insertion of the TFCC at the base of the ulnar styloid – the goal is to eliminate impingement on intraoperative fluoroscopic assessment. Bain and Bidwell [1] found 3 mm of ulnar styloid resection typically brought the subject into the normal population range of 3–6 mm.

Postoperatively, light dressings are applied and patients advised that they could mobilize the wrist, with formal physiotherapy not required.

Satisfaction is high and complications low in the limited number of arthroscopic ulnar styloidectomies performed in the senior author's practice. Transient ulnar sensory paraesthesia has been noted.

The senior author has also performed arthroscopic resection of symptomatic ulnar styloid non-unions which may produce ulnar-sided wrist pain with loading of the wrist. Again, the

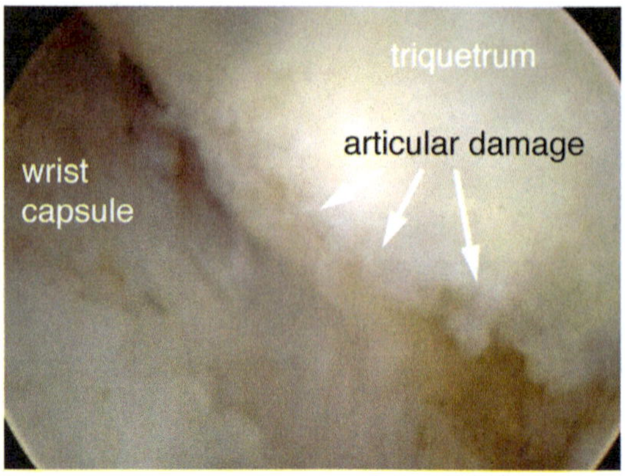

Fig. 14.7 Evidence of articular damage on triquetrum viewed from 3–4 portal

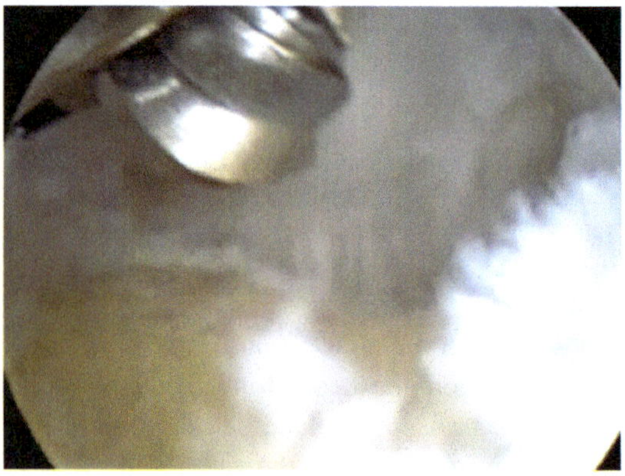

Fig. 14.8 Arthroscopic visualization of the burr on the eburnated ulnar styloid

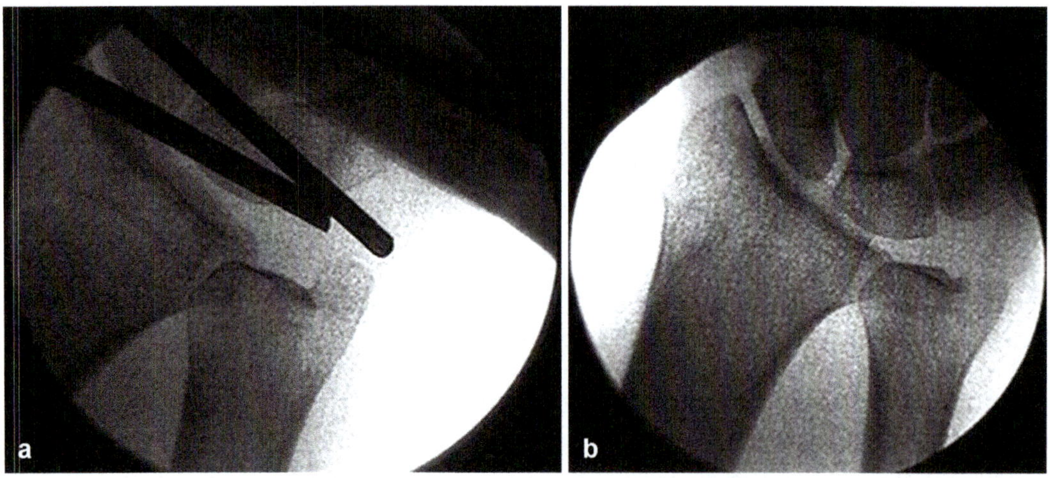

Fig. 14.9 Arthroscopic ulnar styloid resection under fluoroscopic guidance to (**a**) confirm adequate position of the burr relative to the distal ulnar styloid and (**b**) assess effectiveness of resection (Reprinted from Bain and Bidwell [1]. Copyright (2006), with permission from Elsevier)

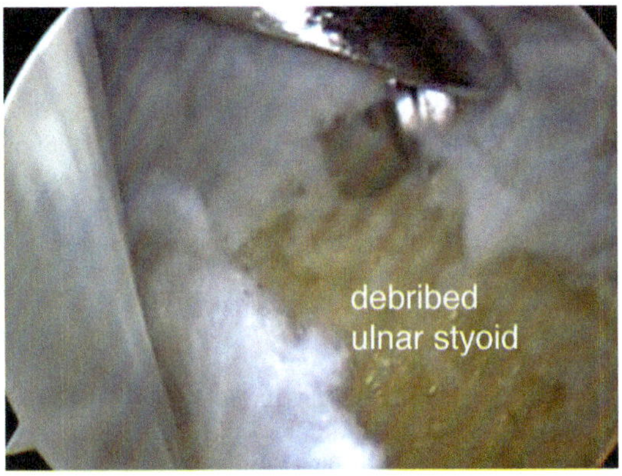

Fig. 14.10 Eburnated bone from distal styloid has been burred to reduce its length and cancellous bone is visible

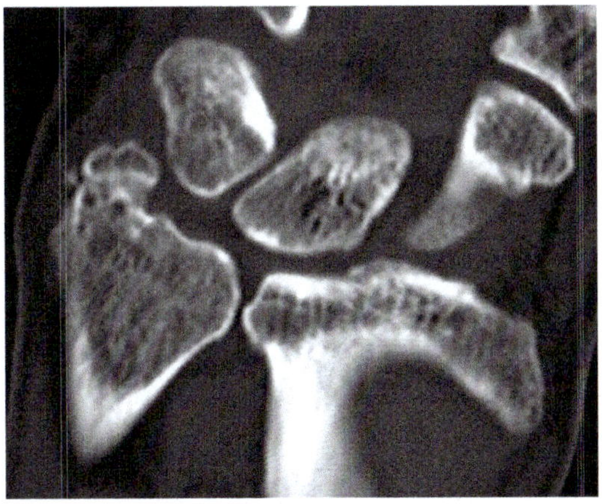

Fig. 14.11 Preoperative CT showing a non-united ulnar styloid fracture

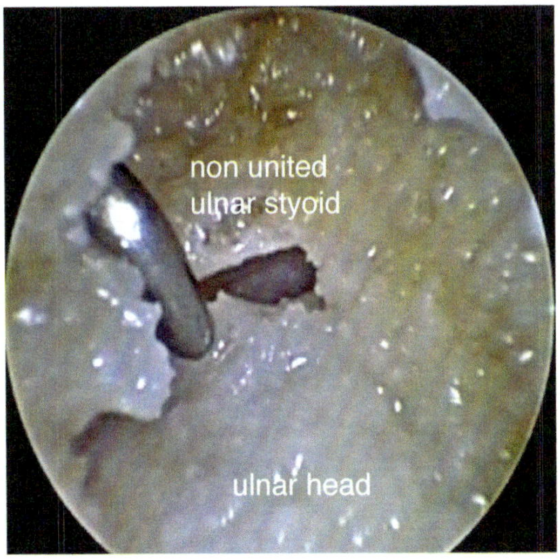

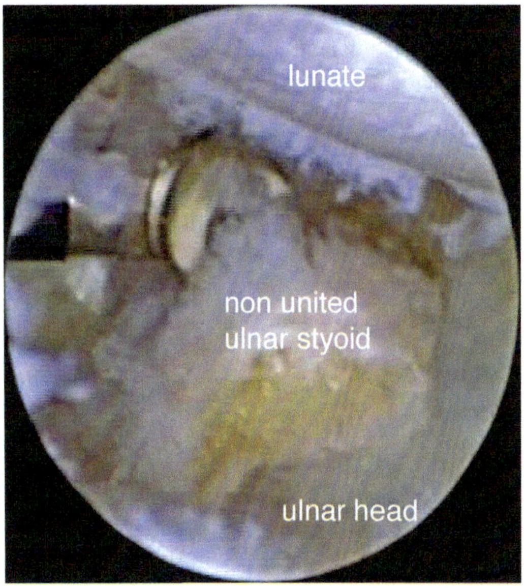

Fig. 14.13 Bipolar cautery used to debride non-united ulnar styloid fragment

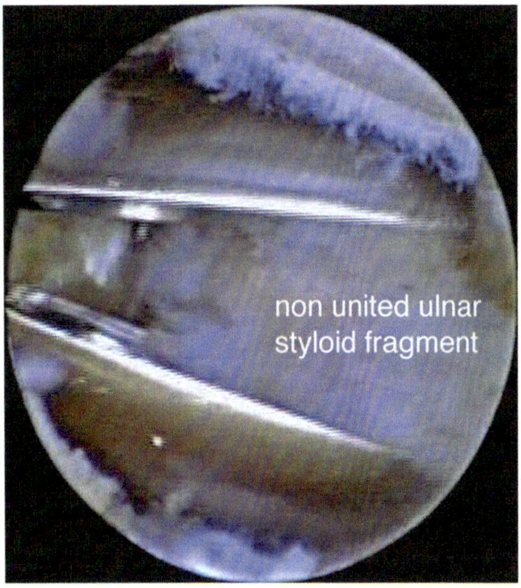

Fig. 14.14 Pituitary rongeur introduced via the 6R portal to remove ulnar styloid fragment

Fig. 14.12 Arthroscopic view of ulnar styloid non-union prior to removal. Probe is lifting the undersurface of the non-united fragment

3–4 portal is used for viewing and the 6R portal used for instrumentation. Palpation of the mobile ulnar styloid with a probe and fluoroscopy helps to identify the fragment (Figs. 14.11 and 14.12). Bipolar diathermy is used to debride the fibrous non-union and soft tissue attachments. The fragment can be removed with a small pituitary rongeur (Figs. 14.13 and 14.14). It is critical to ensure that there is no significant associated DRUJ instability that needs to stabilized.

References

1. Bain GI, Bidwell T (2006) Arthroscopic excision of ulnar styloid in stylocarpal impaction. Arthroscopy 22(6):677.e1–677.e3
2. Bain GI, Munt J, Turner PC (2008) New advances in wrist arthroscopy. Arthroscopy 24(3):355–367
3. Bickel KD (2008) Arthroscopic treatment of ulnar impaction syndrome. J Hand Surg Am 33(8):1420–1423
4. Biyani A, Mehara A, Bhan S (1990) Morphological variations of the ulnar styloid process. J Hand Surg Br 15:352–354
5. Cantor R, Braunstein E (1987) Productive osseous changes about the wrist in rheumatoid arthritis. Skeletal Radiol 16:397–402
6. Cerezal L, del Pinal F, Abascal F (2004) Magnetic resonance imaging findings in ulnar-sided wrist impaction syndromes. Magn Reson Imaging Clin N Am 12(2):281–299
7. Cooney W (2010) The wrist: diagnosis and operative treatment, 2nd edn. Lippincott Williams & Wilkins, Philadelphia, p 26
8. Garcia-Elias M (1987) Dorsal fractures of the triquetrum – avulsion or compression fractures? J Hand Surg Am 12(2):266–268
9. Giachino AA, McIntyre AI, Gui KJ, Conway AF (2007) Ulnar styloid triquetral impaction. Hand Surg 12(2):123–134
10. Giachino A, McIntyre A, Guy K, Conway A (2010) Ulnar styloid triquetral impaction: diagnosis and treatment. In: Slutsky D (ed) Principles and practice of wrist surgery, 1st edn. Elsevier/Saunders, Philadelphia, pp 511–522
11. Luchetti R, Borrelli PP (2010) Treatment of the associated ulnar-sided problems. In: del Piñal F, Mathoulin C, Luchetti R (eds) Arthroscopic management of distal radius fractures, First Editionth edn. Springer, Berlin/Heidelberg, pp 179–183
12. O'Rahilly R, Gardner E (1975) The timing and sequence of events in the development of the limbs in the human embryo. Anat Embryol 148(1):1–23
13. Ogden J, Beall J, Conlogue G, Light T (1981) Radiology of postnatal skeletal development (IV – distal radius and ulna). Skeletal Radiol 6(4): 255–266
14. Scheuer L, Black S (2004) The juvenile skeleton, 1st edn. Academic, London, pp 286–287
15. Tomaino MM, Gainer M, Towers JD (2001) Carpal impaction with the ulnar styloid process: treatment with partial styloid resection. J Hand Surg Br 26:252–255
16. Topper SM, Wood MB, Ruby LK (1997) Ulnar styloid impaction syndrome. J Hand Surg Am 22(4): 699–704
17. Van der Heijden B, Groot S, Schuurman AH (2005) Evaluation of ulnar styloid length. J Hand Surg Am 30(5):954–959
18. Zahiri H, Zahiri C, Ravari F (2010) Ulnar styloid impingement syndrome. Int Orthop 34(8): 1233–1237

15 Hamate Impingement: A Rare Cause of Ulnar Wrist Pain?

Luc De Smet and Ilse Degreef

Introduction

Most causes of ulnar wrist pain are related to the DRUJ and TFCC. However, other structures can be the origin of ulnar pain. Problems in the midcarpal joint, more specifically the interaction between the proximal pole of the hamate and the lunate-triquetrum, are often neglected in the evaluation.

In 1990 and 1993, Viegas et al. described the anatomy of this region in detail. A distinction was made between the type I lunate with one articular facet (with the head of the capitate) and type II with two articular facets (one for the capitate and the other for the hamate) (Fig. 15.1) [10, 12]. According to several authors, type II has been found in 71 % [4], 65.5 % [11], and 55 % [2] of the population.

Cartilage wear on the proximal pole of the hamate is frequent, as it has been observed on several cadaver studies. Nakamura et al. [4] (49 %), Viegas et al. [11] (44 %), and Dautel and Merle [2] (30 %) related this finding with the type II lunates. In fact, arthritis of the hamatolunate joint is probably one of the most frequent localizations of wrist arthritis.

Schuurman et al. [8] did not find a correlation between lunate morphology and ulnar variance in their radiological survey. Furthermore, Pfirrmann et al. [5] in a cadaver/MRI investigation did not find a correlation between the cartilage wear in the hamate and tears of the TFCC. Both surveys are important since in combination, one could suppose that hamatolunate cartilage wear is a specific entity without correlation with the DRUJ/TFCC complex. On the other hand, Burges [1] found an 89 % correlation between hamate arthritis and lunotriquetral ligament tears, confirmed by Harley et al. (91 % association), and introduced the HALT acronym (hamate arthritis lunotriquetral ligament tears).

The clinical features of H-L impaction, however, are not very clear. Ulnar wrist pain with some tenderness distal to the TFCC and increasing pain in extension and ulnar deviation of the wrist are the only clues. At times, dorsal swelling at the level of the UMC due to synovitis can also be seen (Fig. 15.2). Plain radiographs are usually read as normal, but dynamic X-rays may be helpful in some cases (Fig. 15.3). It is not always evident to predict the lunate morphology on plain radiographs. The accuracy was between 64 and 72 % [7]. Often, CT scan is required. MRI is a powerful tool in this pathology. Recently, good correlation between the anatomical findings and high-resolution MRI imaging has been reported [5].

On arthroscopy, the cartilage wear can be seen in several degrees: from discrete fibrillation to obvious cartilage damage, involving both the proximal pole of the hamate as well as the lunate.

L. De Smet, M.D., Ph.D. (✉) • I. Degreef, M.D., Ph.D.
Hand Unit, Department of Orthopaedics,
University Hospitals Leuven,
UZ Pellenberg, Weligerveld 1,
B3212 Lubbeek, Belgium
e-mail: luc.desmet@uzleuven.be

F. del Piñal et al. (eds.), *Arthroscopic Management of Ulnar Pain*,
DOI 10.1007/978-3-642-30544-3_15, © Springer-Verlag Berlin Heidelberg 2012

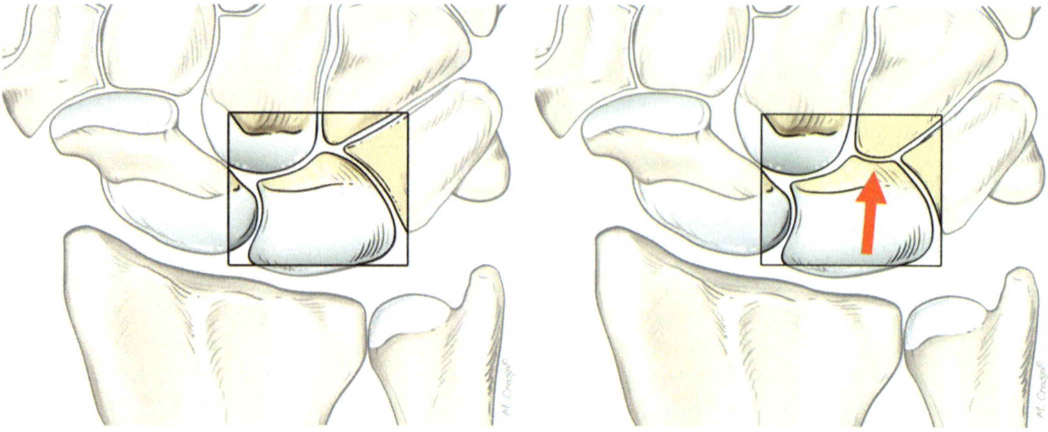

Fig. 15.1 Different shapes of the lunate facet and proximal pole of the hamate. Second facet of the lunate (*arrow*)

Fig. 15.2 Swelling is quite evident in this patient at the level of the UMC portal (*arrow*) (Courtesy Dr. Piñal ©2011)

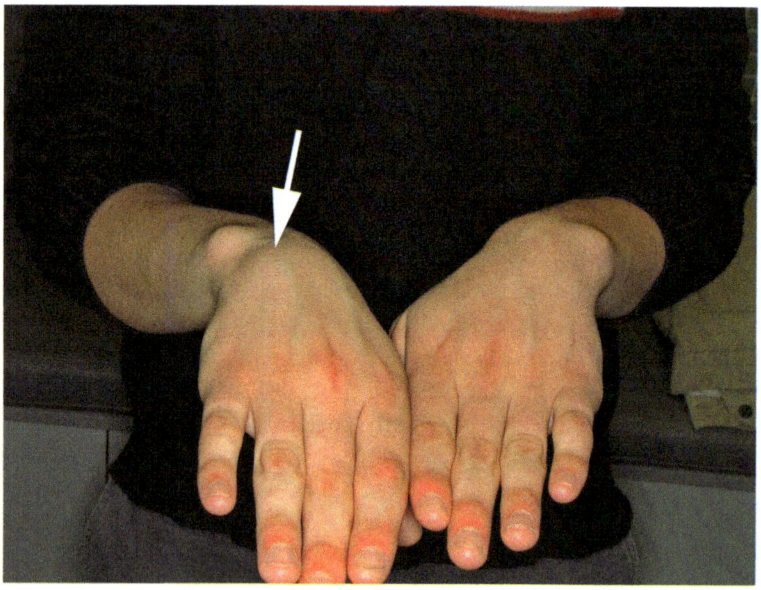

One should take into account, however, that wearing of the proximal pole of the hamate-distal lunate facet is a commonly presented in asymptomatic patients. Correlation of the arthroscopy and the physical examination is paramount (Fig. 15.4).

Most treatment propositions recommend (arthroscopic) resection of the distal pole of the hamate [3, 9, 13]. As far as we know, only two documented patient series were reported: one with five cases, all with good pain relief [9], and the other [3] with 23 patients, of whom 21 were evaluated with 18 excellent or good outcome. Their biomechanical investigations revealed a good decompression with a resection of 2.4 mm of the proximal pole of the hamate.

Surgical Technique

From all arthroscopic procedures, resection of the proximal pole of the hamate is one of the most straightforward procedures. A standard

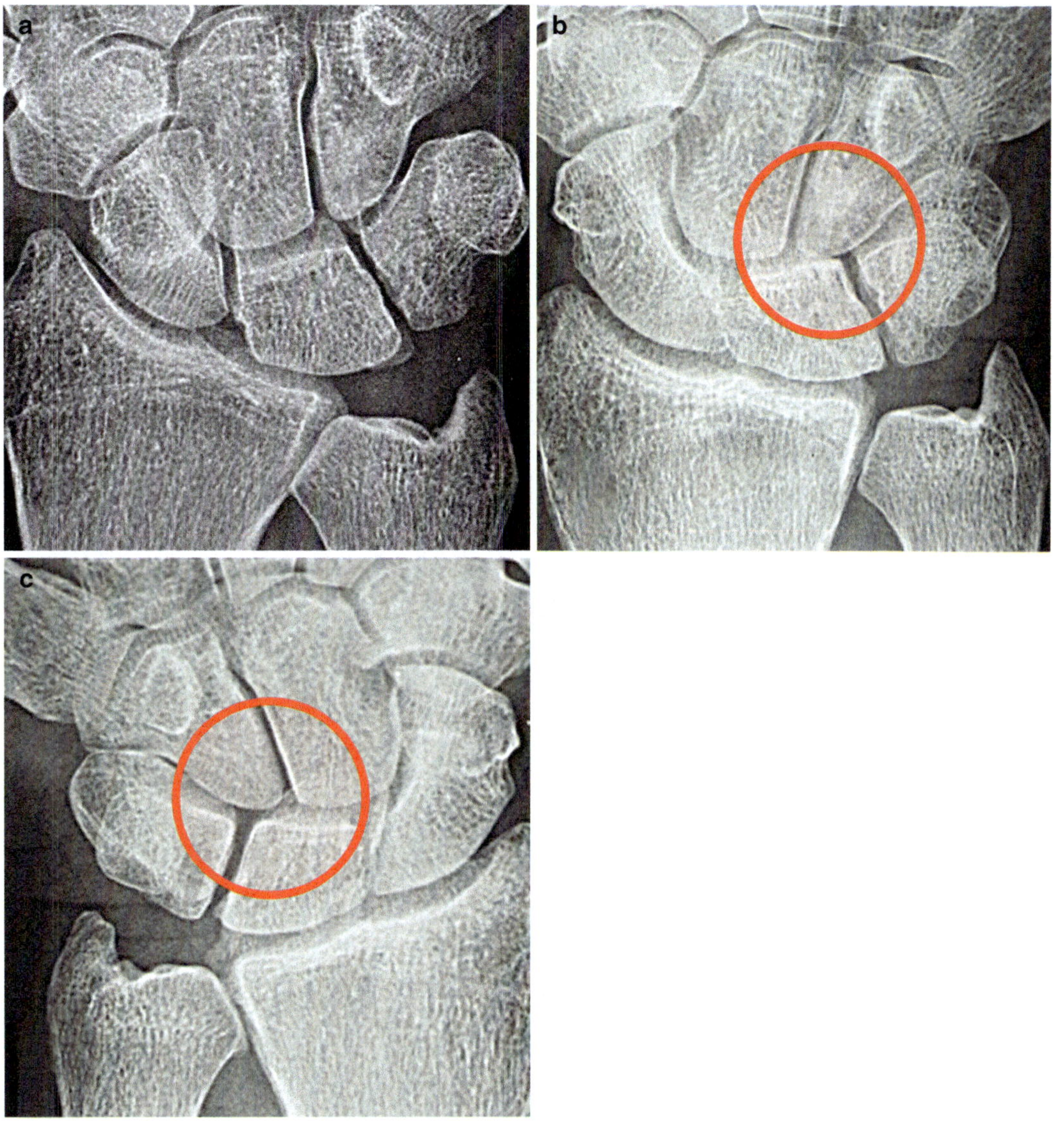

Fig. 15.3 Dynamic radial and ulnar deviation plain PA views may be helpful in some cases. (**a**) In radial deviation, no anomalies are seen, while in ulnar deviation, clear H-L conflict is evident (**b**). Compare the H-L space on the healthy contralateral side in ulnar deviation (**c**). Lunate hamate joint (*circle*) (Courtesy Dr. Piñal ©2011)

setup is used with general (preference) or regional anesthesia and a traction tower. Firstly, the radiocarpal joint and especially the TFCC are inspected with a dry [6] or wet arthroscopy technique. Then, the radial midcarpal (RMC) portal is developed for visualization and the ulnar midcarpal (UMC) portal for instrumentation. Since there is a significant associated lunotriquetral ligament injury, this joint has to be inspected thoroughly. Instability is often not seen as a widening of the joint space but rather as a step-off between lunate and triquetrum (see Chap. 17). Once this has been addressed, the proximal pole of the hamate is inspected and the quality of the cartilage palpated with a hook. Afterward, with a 2.9-mm burr, the proximal 2–3 mm of the proximal pole of the hamate is resected (Fig. 15.5). The hardest task is to remove the anterior part of the proximal pole of the hamate, and hence, other portals may be neces-

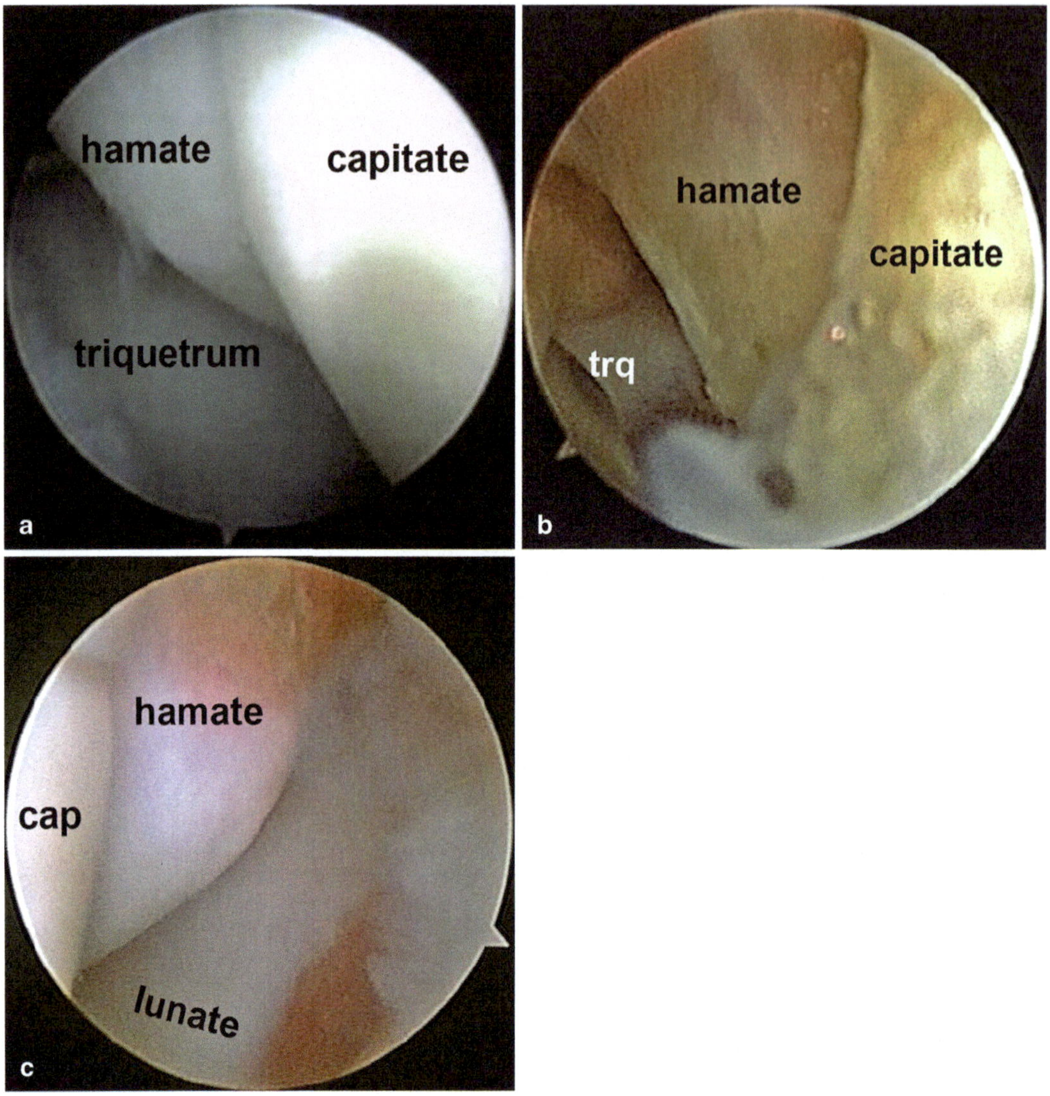

Fig. 15.4 (**a**) Normal aspect of the proximal pole of the hamate viewed from RMC in a right wrist. (**b**) During an arthroscopic ganglionectomy for cosmetic reasons, a totally denuded proximal pole of the hamate was found (arthroscope in RMC left wrist). (**c**) Cartilage wear on the hamate and lunate (scope in RMC right wrist)

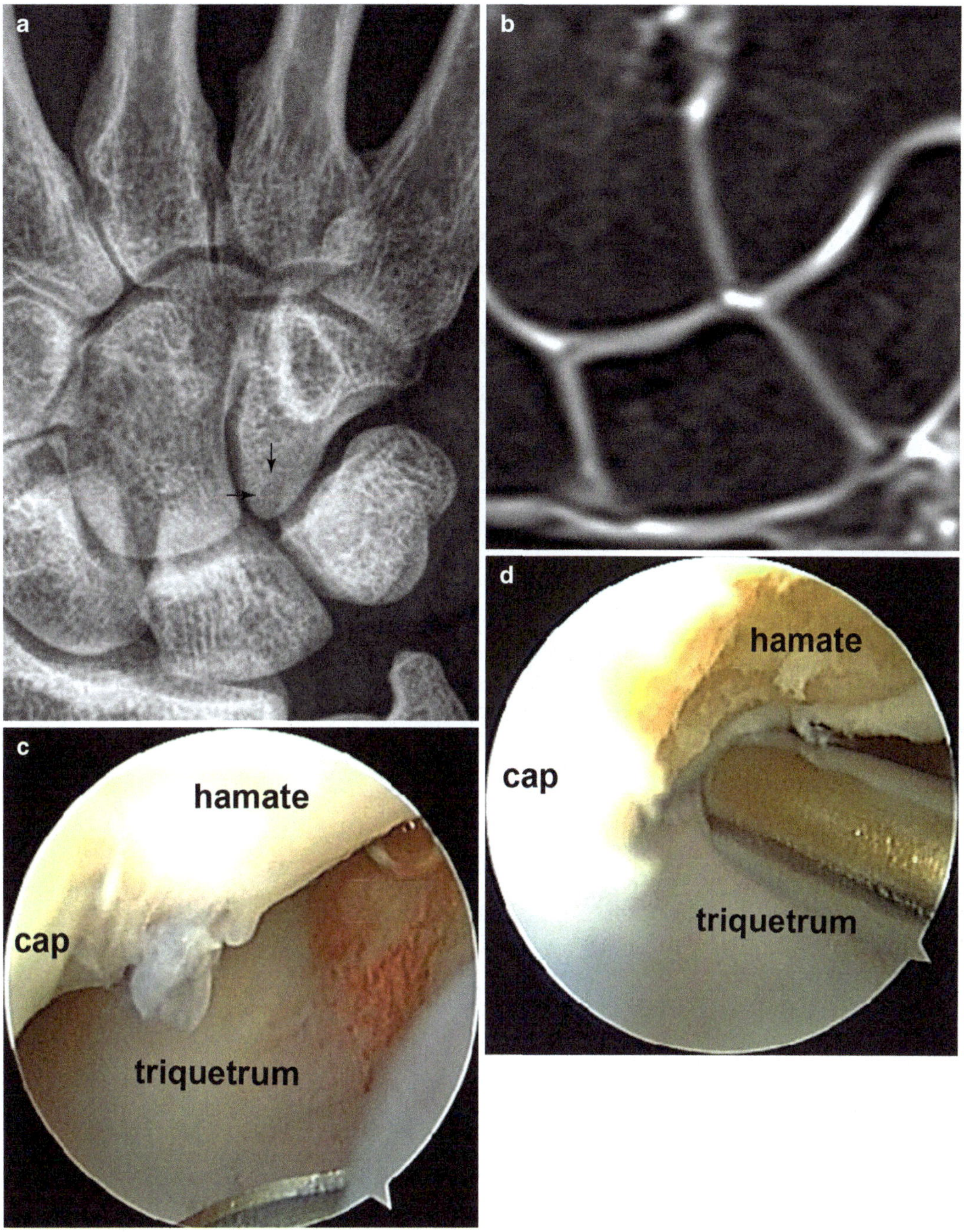

Fig. 15.5 (**a**, **b**) Normal radiographs, type II lunate, and small alterations on the proximal pole of the hamate (*arrows*) on MRI. (**c**) Fibrillation of the proximal pole of the hamate (scope in RMC and instruments in UMC, right wrist). (**d**) Arthroscopic debridement and proximal pole resection gave a favorable outcome in this patient

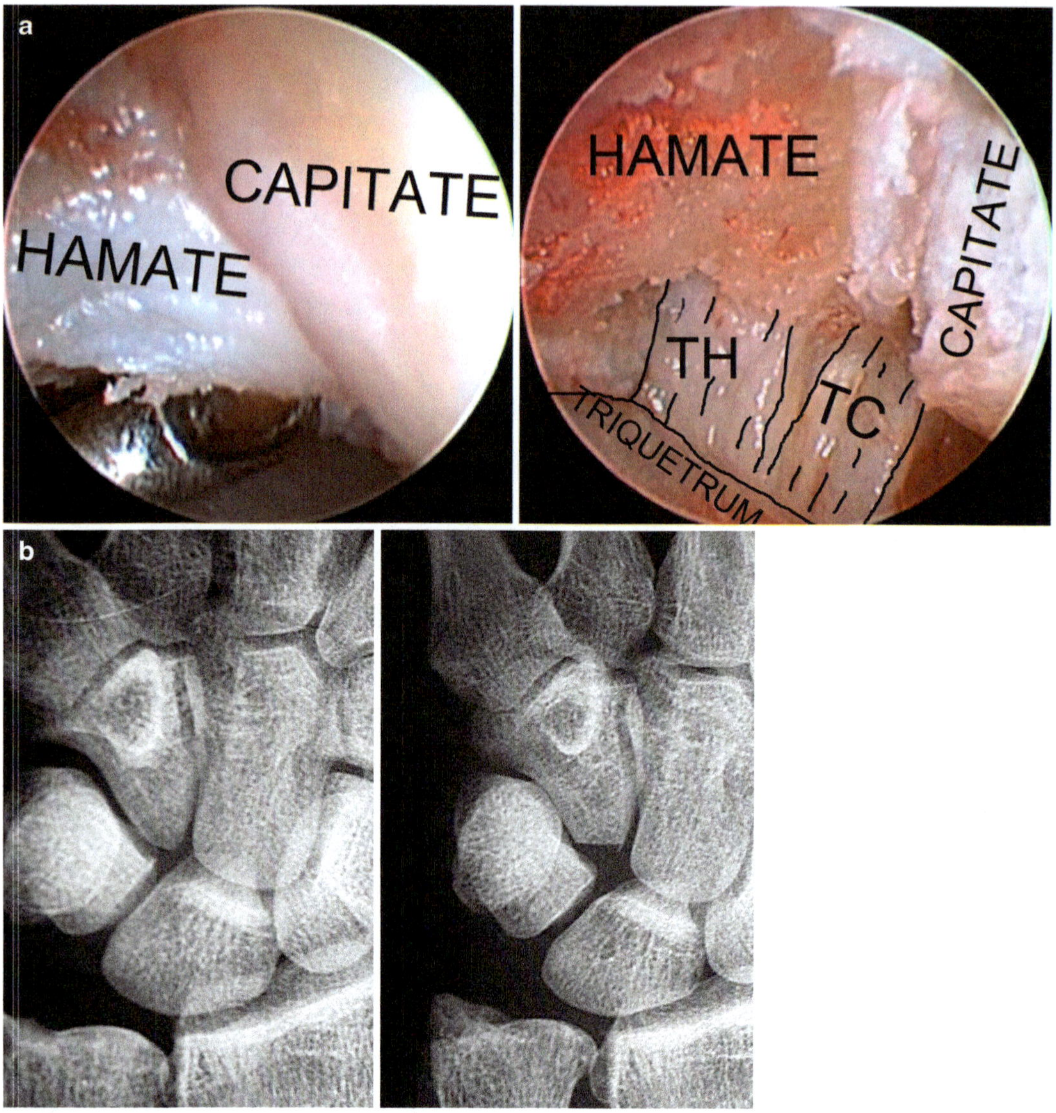

Fig. 15.6 (**a**) A curette may be helpful for clearing the most anterior part of the proximal pole of the hamate (*TH* triquetro-hamate ligament and *TC* triquetro-capitate ligament). (**b**) Resection of the proximal pole of the hamate allows clear visualization of the volar triquetro-hamate and triquetro-capitate ligaments with the scope in UMC. However, only the 2–3 mm of the most proximal aspect of the hamate has to be removed. Overaggressive resection of the hamate is likely to cause carpal instability and static VISI deformity. (**c**, **d**) Preoperative and postoperative plain radiograms of the same patient (Courtesy Dr. Piñal ©2011)

sary in order to obtain a clearer view. Del Piñal (personal communication) often uses the triquetro-hamate (T-H) portal for instrumentation, while the scope is in UMC swapping portals as necessary (Fig. 15.6). A bulky dressing is applied and free mobilization is allowed in the immediate postoperative period. Early disappearance of symptoms and return to activities is the norm. As stated before, the biggest mistake is to focus on "treating" asymptomatic T-H wearing while overlooking the primary pathology of the patient. Thorough inspection of the radiocarpal and midcarpal joints in order to rule out other painful conditions is paramount.

References

1. Burgess RC (1990) Anatomic variations of the midcarpal joint. J Hand Surg Am 15:129–131
2. Dautel G, Merle M (1997) Chondral lesions of the midcarpal joint. Arthroscopy 13:97–102
3. Harly B, Werner F, Boles S, Palmer A (2004) Arthroscopic resection of arthrosis of the proximal hamate: a clinical and biomechanical study. J Hand Surg Am 29:661–667
4. Nakamura K, Patterson R, Moritomo H, Viegas S (2001) Type I versus type II lunates: ligament anatomy and presence of arthrosis. J Hand Surg Am 26:428–436
5. Pfirrmann C, Theumann N, Chung C et al (2002) The hamatolunate facet: characterization and association with cartilage lesions –magnetic resonance arthrography and anatomic correlation in cadaver wrists. Skeletal Radiol 31:451–456
6. del Piñal F, Garcia-Bernal F, Pisani D et al (2007) Dry arthroscopy of the wrist: surgical technique. J Hand Surg Am 32:119–123
7. Sagerman S, Hauck R, Palmer A (1995) Lunate morphology: can it be predicted with routine x-ray film? J Hand Surg Am 20:38–41
8. Schuurman A, Maas M, Dijkstra P, Kauer J (2001) Ulnar variance and the shape of the lunate bone. A radiological investigation. Acta Orthop Belg 67:464–467
9. Thurnston A, Stanley J (2000) Hamato-lunate impingement: an uncommon cause of ulnar-sided wrist pain. Arthroscopy 16:540–544
10. Viegas S (1990) The lunatohamate articulation of the midcarpal joint. Arthroscopy 6:5–10
11. Viegas S, Wagner K, Patterson R, Peterson P (1990) Medial (hamate) facet of the lunate. J Hand Surg Am 15:564–571
12. Viegas S, Patterson R, Hokanson J, Davis J (1993) Wrist anatomy: incidence, distribution, and correlation of anatomic variations, tears, and arthrosis. J Hand Surg Am 18:463–475
13. Yao J, Osterman L (2005) Arthroscopic techniques for wrist arthritis (radial styloidectomy and proximal pole hamate excisions). Hand Clin 21:519–526

Coronal Tears of the TFCC

16

Francisco del Piñal and Toshiyasu Nakamura

Introduction

In a landmark article, Palmer classified traumatic tears of the triangular fibrocartilage into four types [13]. Several articles have appeared in the literature adding new subtypes and locations of traumatic tears [2, 9], underscoring the fact that Palmer's classification was very useful but imperfect. For example, type 1C is very rare, while others, such as 1B, can be subdivided in multiple subtypes that have different prognosis, surgical management, and aftercare [1, and see also Chap. 6]. Although in Palmer's classification degenerative and traumatic tears were clearly separated, overlap can occur. Not uncommonly, one sees patients with asymptomatic degenerative tears who only develop symptoms after a traumatic event. Both the degeneration and the acute tear are clearly seen during arthroscopic inspection (see Fig. 7.6).

In this chapter, we will discuss an entity that we have seen with increasing frequency: a degenerative tear compounded by a traumatic tear. These patients present with ulnar pain and a feeling of instability after a traumatic event (torsion or fall). On clinical examination, they have diffuse ulnar pain, including signs of ulnar head impaction syndrome and moderate instability of the DRUJ. On imaging, they have ulna plus variant and signs of ulnar impaction. And at arthroscopy, a tear in the frontal plane that extends to the fovea is seen. Due to the pattern of the tear, and its responsibility for most of the symptoms, we have termed this entity "coronal tear of the TFCC" (Fig. 16.1).

Pathophysiology

The deep distal radio-ulnar ligaments are found on the proximal aspect of the TFC. They originate in anterior and posterior ulnar corners of the radius and insert into the fovea [10, 11]. In approximately one third of the cases, the ligaments coalesce before inserting in the fovea [12]. This junctional portion reduces the actual functional length of each individual ligament (Fig. 16.2).

If this junctional portion is disrupted, the ligament will be functionally longer, causing a certain degree of instability. This is, in our opinion, the root cause of this syndrome. Because in our cases most patients had an ulna plus variance, it is also quite plausible that as a result of a fall or a hyperpronation injury, the head of the ulna acted as a die-punch, splitting the connection of both distal radio-ulnar ligaments. This is much like a boutonniere deformity, where the head of the

F. del Piñal, M.D., Dr. Med. (✉)
Hand-Wrist and Plastic Surgery,
Private Practice and Mutua Montañesa,
Paseo de Pereda 20-1°,
E-39004 Santander, Spain
e-mail: drpinal@drpinal.com, pacopinal@gmail.com

T. Nakamura
Department of Orthopaedic Surgery,
School of Medicine, Keio University, Tokyo, Japan

F. del Piñal et al. (eds.), *Arthroscopic Management of Ulnar Pain*,
DOI 10.1007/978-3-642-30544-3_16, © Springer-Verlag Berlin Heidelberg 2012

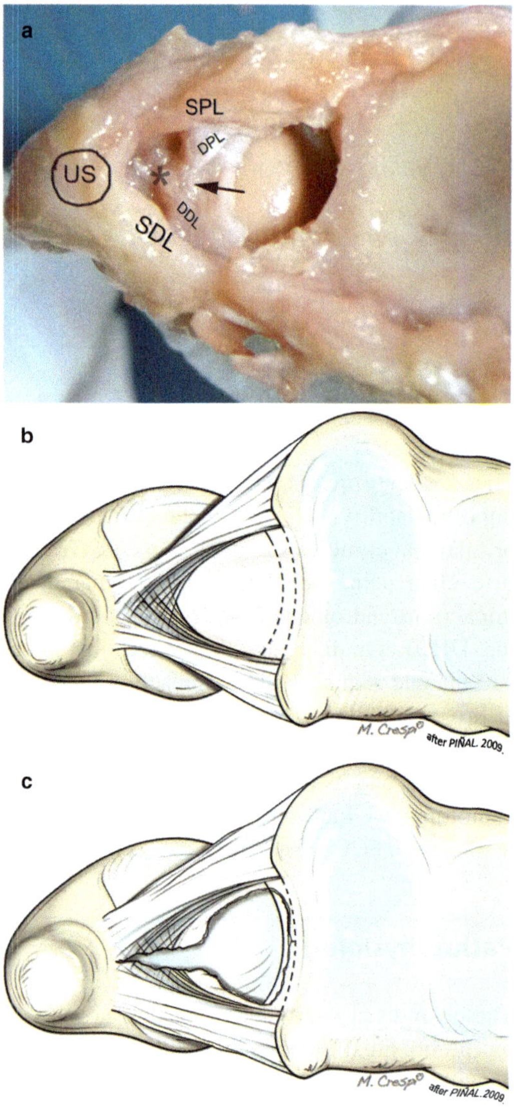

Fig. 16.1 (**a**) Bird's-eye view of the normal anatomy of the conjoined insertion (*arrow*) of the deep palmar and dorsal radio-ulnar ligaments at the base of the fovea (*asterisk*). (*US* ulnar styloid, *SPL* superficial palmar ligament, *SDL* superficial dorsal ligament, *DPL* deep palmar ligament, *DDL* deep dorsal ligament). (**b**) Schematic representation of the same disposition. (**c**) Typical findings of this syndrome: a coronal tear associated to a central (degenerative) perforation (Published with permission of © Dr. Piñal 2012. All Rights Reserved)

proximal phalanx protrudes between both lateral bands (Fig. 16.3).

Biomechanical Study

A cadaver experiment was designed to investigate the deleterious effect of a coronal tear on the stability of the DRUJ and also to investigate the results of ulnar shortening and/or suture repair of the tear. The cadaveric upper extremity was amputated at the midportion of the humerus and mounted in a jig that permitted control of pronation-supination. First, an external fixator was applied to the ulna. Another external fixator was also set to maintain the radiocarpal joint in the neutral position, avoiding any influences on the results by the wrist position other than the pronosupination. The ulna was then cut at its distal fourth. The distal radio-ulnar joint capsule was resected, accessing it by swinging the distal ulna distally. The ulna was then remounted on the external fixator in its native position. The dorsopalmar stiffness of the DRUJ was assessed at neutral position, 60° pronation, and 60° supination (Fig. 16.4). For the second portion of the experiment, the distal ulna was dismounted from the external fixator and swung distally. A coronal tear was created, and the assessment repeated after remounting the distal ulna. For the third portion of the experiment, the effects of ulnar shortening on coronal tears were investigated. Three millimeters of ulna was resected before remounting the ulna and repeating the assessment. Finally, the ulna was once again dismounted from the external fixator and swung distally, and the coronal tear was repaired with two sutures. The ulna was then replaced in the anatomical position and the experiment repeated.

Preliminary data of this experiment revealed that a coronal tear decreased the stiffness of the distal radio-ulnar joint significantly when stress

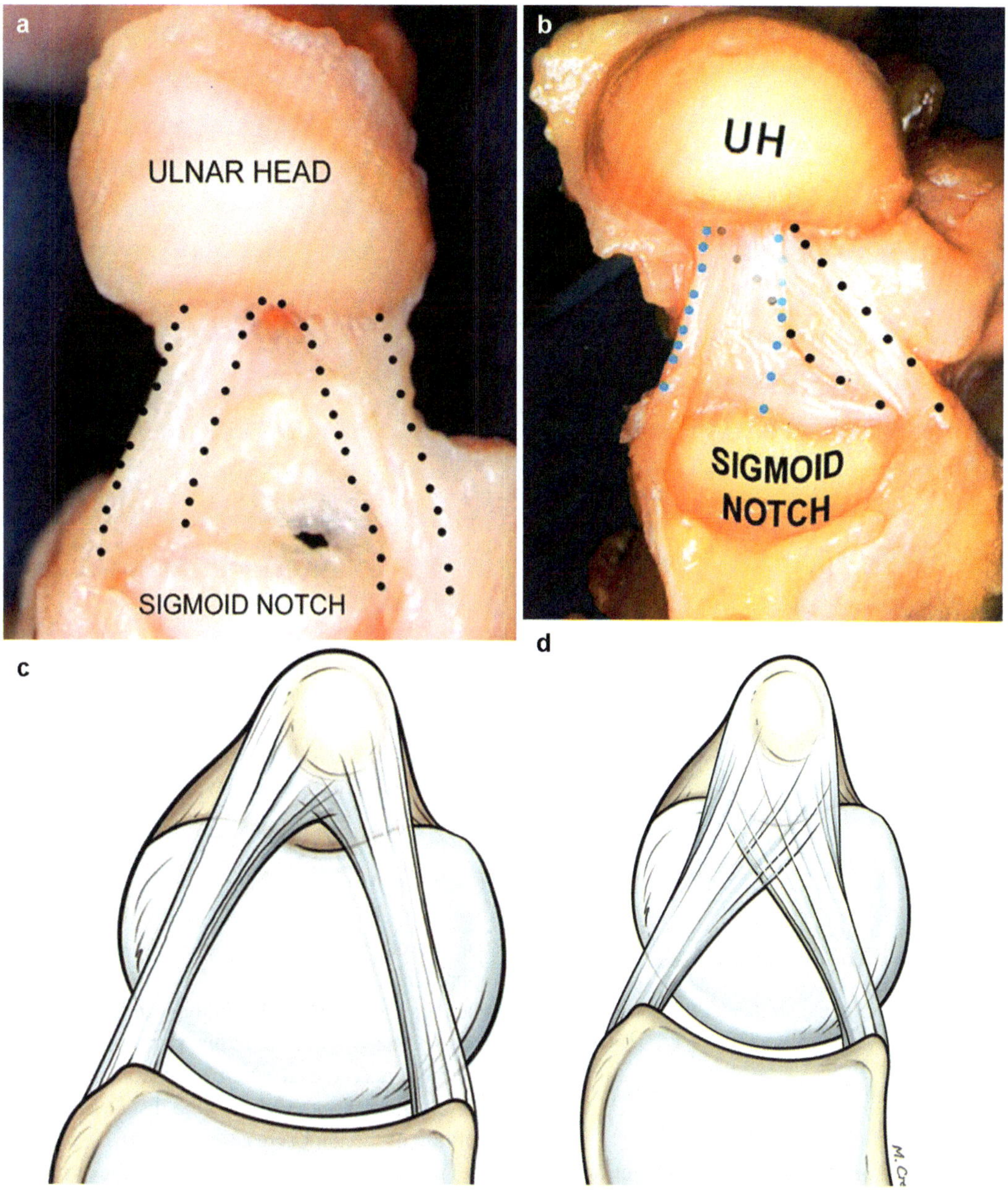

Fig. 16.2 Proximal view of the TFC. The DRUJ has been opened like a book offering an unparalleled view of the proximal anatomy of the TFC and the deep radio-ulnar ligaments. The extreme types are shown. (**a**) Funnel-shaped: both ligaments inserted separately and without crossover in the fovea. (**b**) Fan-shaped: the fibers of the anterior and posterior RUL crossover for half the length of the ligaments. (**c**) Distal view of the deep radio-ulnar ligaments funnel-shaped type. (**d**) Fan-shaped type (coalescing) (Published with permission of © Dr. Piñal 2012. All Rights Reserved)

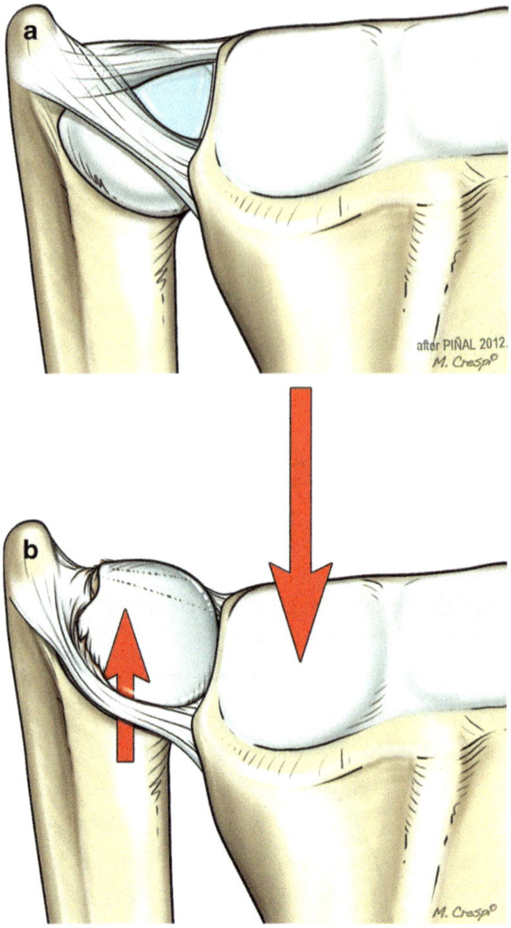

Fig. 16.3 Acute axial protrusion of the ulnar head during axial loading, particularly in pronation, is thought to be the etiology of a boutonniere-like deformity of the ulnar head and rupture of the junction of the distal radio-ulnar ligaments (Published with permission of © Dr. Piñal 2012. All Rights Reserved)

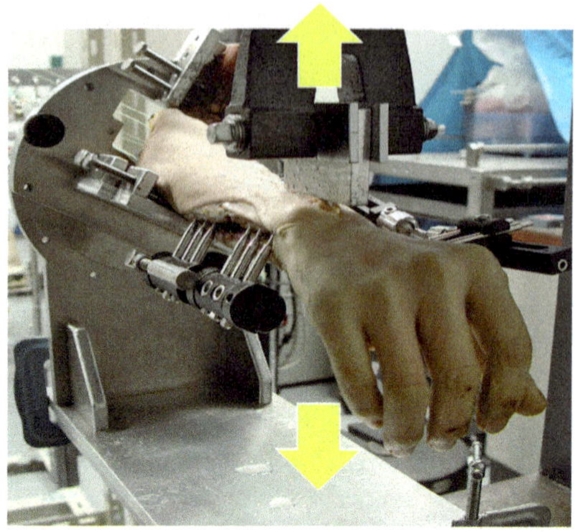

Fig. 16.4 The setup of the experiment. Notice that the proximal ulna and humerus are fixed to the jig to control the position of the forearm. The external fixator on the ulna can be seen (Published with permission of © Dr. Piñal 2012. All Rights Reserved)

was applied in a dorso-palmar direction. This finding was consistent in all positions. Furthermore, both repair of the tear and shortening of the ulnar increased the stiffness, although never to normal values, with the exception of stiffness of the DRUJ in dorsal direction of the radius at pronation, when repairing the TFCC. Ulnar shortening could relatively increase stiffness around 60–85 % when compared to the intact. In supination, DRUJ stiffness in palmar translation of the radius had never influenced by coronal tear. This experiment supports the different approaches we have taken for managing this condition as presented below (Fig. 16.5).

Treatment

One of the authors (TN) opted for a combined approach: an arthroscopic debridement and an open ulnar shortening. The author felt that shortening the ulna would have a dual purpose: the ulnar abutment is corrected, and by increasing distance from the fovea to the edge of the distal radius, the stability of the joint is restored (Fig. 16.6).

The other author (FP) managed the problem arthroscopically by combining repairing the tear with an arthroscopic wafer procedure when needed (Fig. 16.7). The latter technique will be discussed in detail.

The arthroscopy is carried out using the "dry" technique [6], but due to the fact that the portals are not large, it could be carried out equally well under standard (wet) arthroscopy. Typically, a considerable amount of debris is found due to

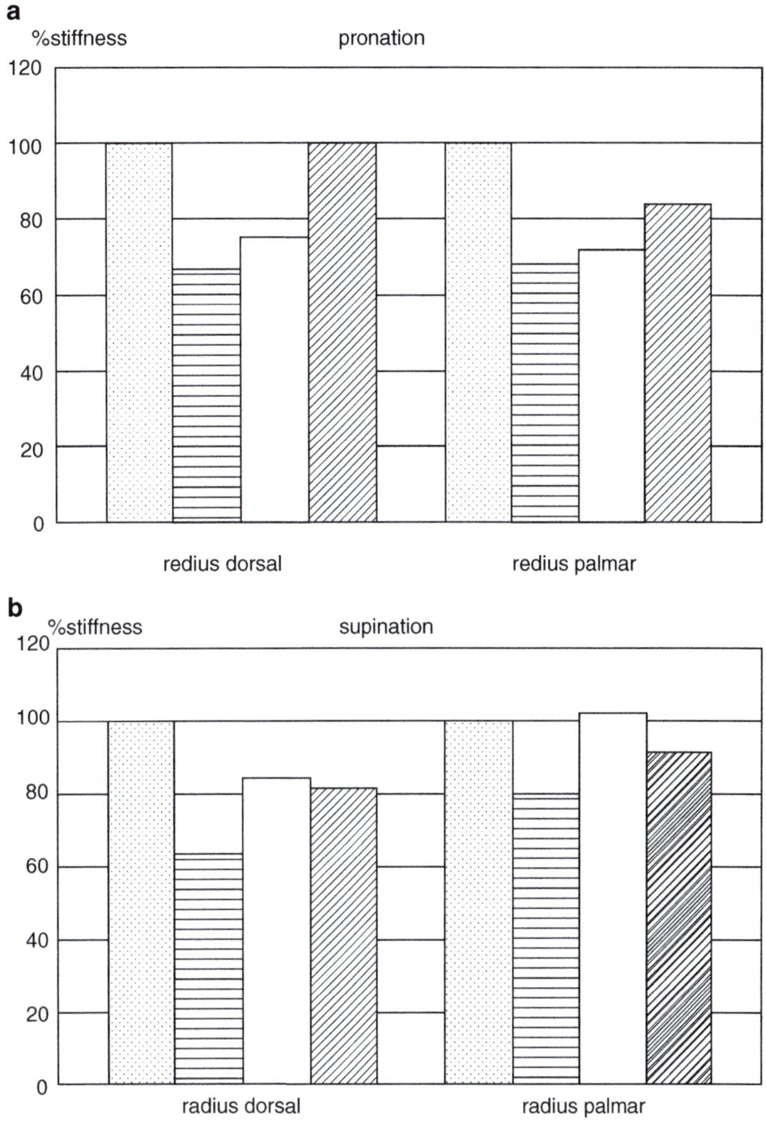

Fig. 16.5 Preliminary result of the restoration of stability by ulnar shortening and repair of the TFC by suturing in an experimental model when the wrist is in pronation and supination. Intact: dotted bar; coronal tear: striped; ulnar shortening: plain; repair: oblique striped ("Published with permission of © Dr. Piñal 2012. All Rights Reserved")

both the long-standing degeneration and the acute synovitis from the recent trauma. As a matter of fact, usually in order to see the tear, it must first be debrided with a 2.9-mm synoviotome inserted through 6R, and the joint needs to be flushed with saline (see below). Rarely, the coronal tear is evident on initial inspection (Fig. 16.8), but probing the tear with the palpator is needed before the diagnosis is made in most cases (Fig. 16.9).

Once the diagnosis is made, we proceed to carry out the arthroscopic wafer procedure only if needed. In our initial experience, we carried out an arthroscopic wafer procedure and sutured both distal radio-ulnar ligaments. In our later experience, despite ulna plus variance and the central perforation, if the cartilage of the lunate and ulna were relatively preserved, we only performed the suture repair of the DRUL. This

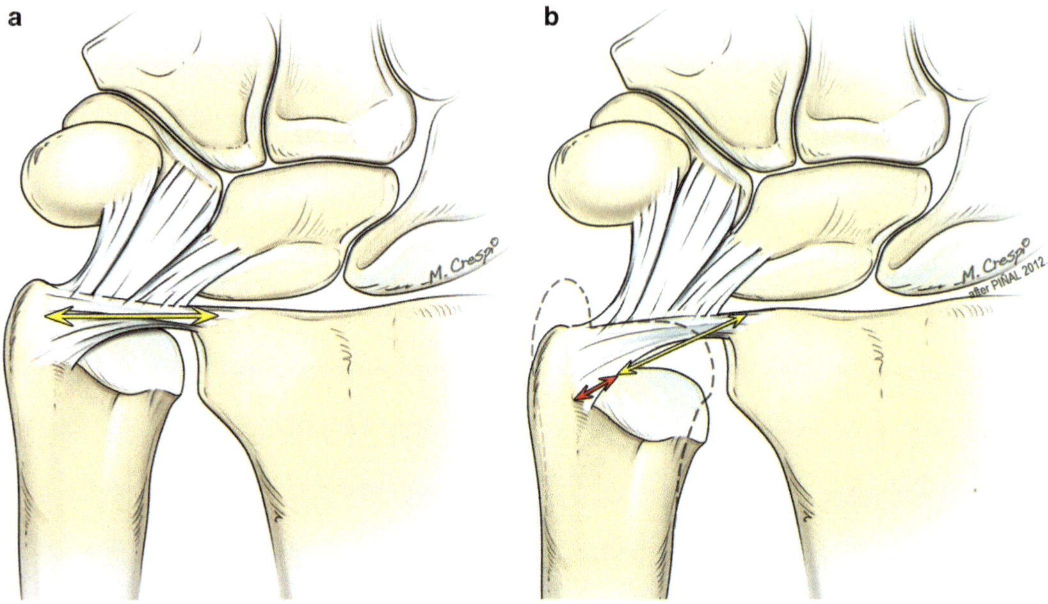

Fig. 16.6 (**a**, **b**) Effect of ulnar shortening on the distal radio-ulnar ligaments (Published with permission of © Dr. Piñal 2012. All Rights Reserved)

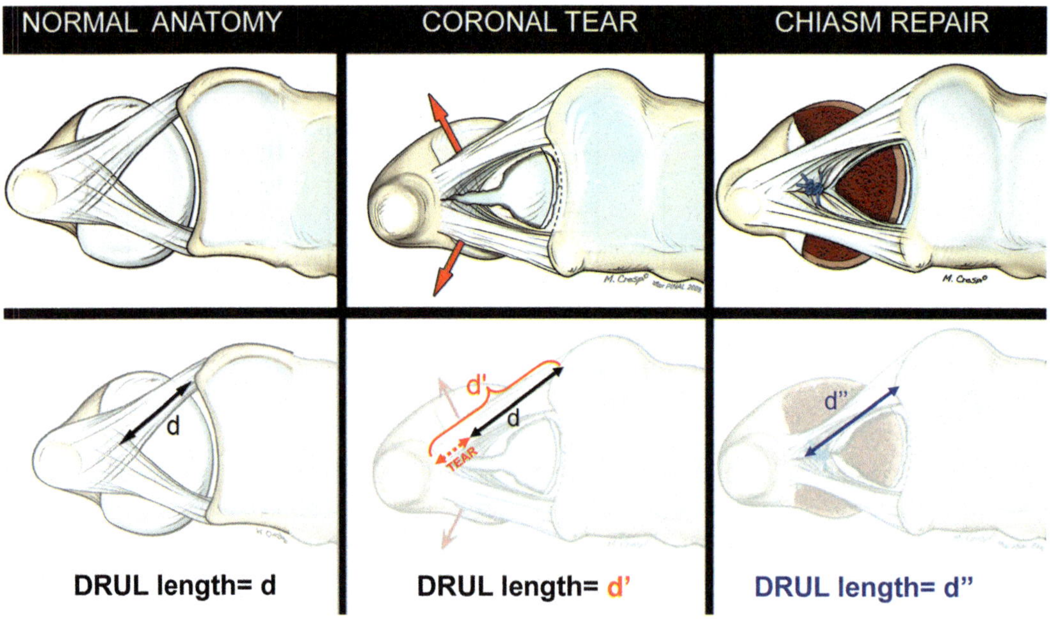

Fig. 16.7 In this bird's-eye view, the effect of distal radio-ulnar lengthening when the junction of the ligaments is disrupted. The restoration of anatomy by arthroscopic DRUL suturing is represented (Published with permission of © Dr. Piñal 2012. All Rights Reserved)

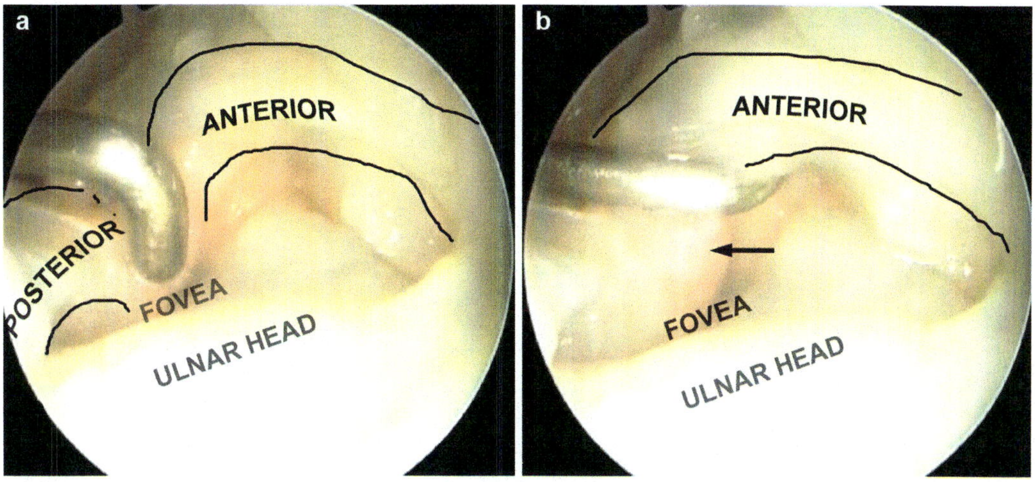

Fig. 16.8 (**a**) In this patient, the splitting of the DRU ligaments extending to the fovea (pointed by the probe) is evident immediately after the debridement. (**b**) Loss of tension on the anterior DRUL is evident as tested by the probe. Notice also slack posterior DRUL. *Arrow* points to synovitis close to the fovea (Published with permission of © Dr. Piñal 2012. All Rights Reserved)

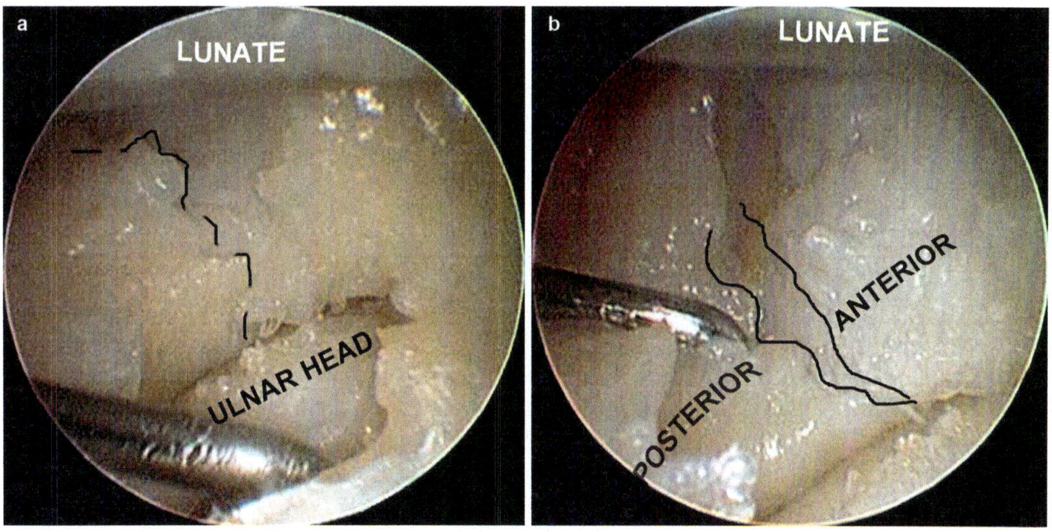

Fig. 16.9 (**a**) A coronal tear (*stripe line*) is barely visible in this apparently simple IIC tear after debridement. (**b**) When probed, splitting of both DRUL goes all the way to the fovea (Published with permission of © Dr. Piñal 2012. All Rights Reserved)

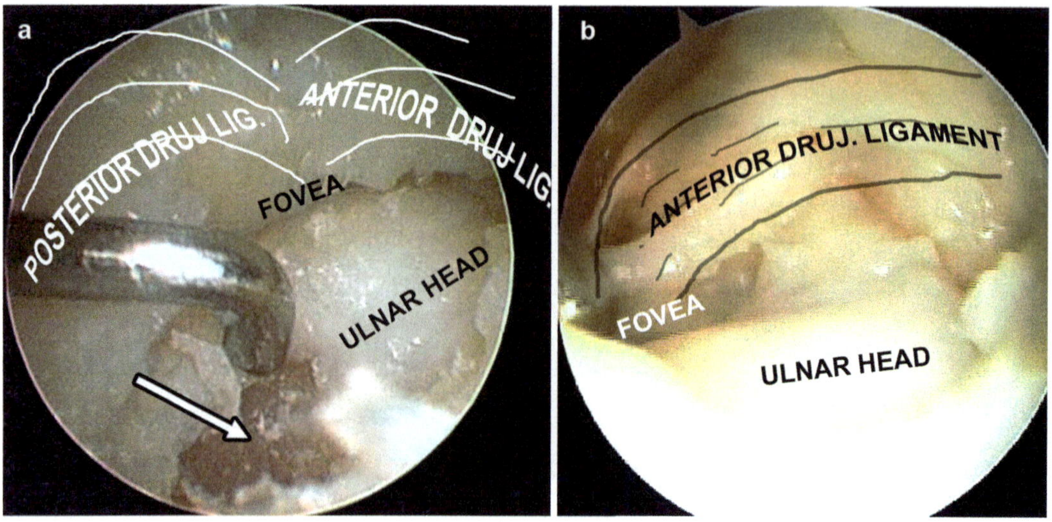

Fig. 16.10 (**a**) Large area devoid of cartilage on the ulnar head (*arrow*) can be seen. (**b**) The cartilage of the ulnar head is intact. Interestingly both patients have a coronal tear that extends to the fovea (In both, the left wrist is involved; the scope is in 3–4 portal and the instruments in 6R) (Published with permission of © Dr. Piñal 2012. All Rights Reserved)

simplifies the technique and is supported by our biomechanical studies (Fig. 16.10).

When loss of cartilage is seen at the ulnar aspect of the lunate and/or the head ulna, the dome of the ulna is burred down to treat the concomitant ulnar impaction. The technique of wafer procedure under dry arthroscopy does not differ significantly from the wet technique, as presented in Chap. 13. However, for a smooth experience while using the dry technique, the following tips need to be underlined [4, 6]:

1. The valve of the sheath of the scope has to be maintained open at all times in order for allowing the air to circulate freely in the joint.
2. The suction of the working instrument (synoviotome or burr) should be used only when needed to clear the contents of the joint. Suction through the shaver stirs up all the debris and makes the vision more difficult as the debris may stick to the tip of the scope.
3. To remove the debris and burred bone, a syringe with 5–10 mL of saline is connected to the side valve of the scope and then aspirated with the arthroscopic shaver. Pressure on the plunger of the syringe is unnecessary, as the negative pressure exerted by the shaver/burr will suck the saline into the joint, thus preventing any extravasation (Fig. 16.11). Once all the fluid has been aspirated, the syringe is removed, and again the suction power of the shaver is enough to dry out the joint sufficiently, thus allowing the surgeon to work. This maneuver should be repeated as needed throughout the procedure. Apart from providing a pristine view of the joint each time the joint is flushed, it has the benefit of cooling down the instrument that may overheat (causing local burns to the skin) when prolonged use of the burr is made. Finally, flushing the joint avoids clogging of the instrument by the dried debris within the burr.
4. In general, I prefer a 2.9-mm pineapple-shaped burr rather than a ball-shaped burr, as the latter tends to produce "holes" instead of an even surface and is easily snagged on the bone.

Once the work of the ulnar head (arthroscopic wafer procedure or debridement) is completed, the diagnosis is evident, even in the cases were some doubt existed during the initial exploration (Fig. 16.12). The suturing now proceeds.

In order to create a raw surface to stimulate healing, the edges of the ligaments are first debrided with the synoviotome all the way to their foveal insertion. Then, a resorbable suture (2/0

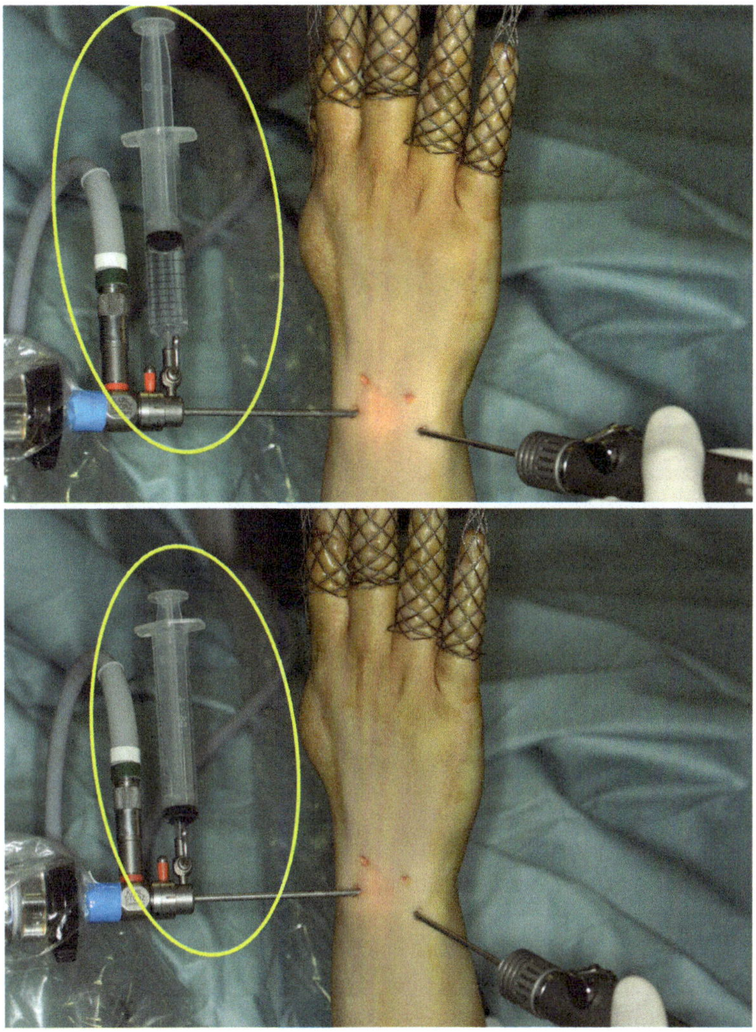

Fig. 16.11 Method used to wash out the joint and clear it of blood. Notice that the negative pressure exerted by the shaver is sufficient to aspirate the saline without extravasation of fluid (From del Piñal [3])

PDS) is placed with an all-inside technique. This technique follows exactly the same principles as previously described for TFC and volar scapholunate ligaments [7, 8] and is adapted for this anatomical problem (see also Appendix A).

With the scope in 3–4 portal, a Tuohy needle is inserted into the joint proximal to the TFC, aiming at the junction of the anterior ligament and the capsule (Fig. 16.13). Because this may require several attempts before the position is satisfactory, an intramuscular needle, which has a smaller bore than the Tuohy, may be used to minimize local insult. Next, the Tuohy needle is inserted following the same path.

The Tuohy needle is now loaded with a (colored) 2/0 PDS suture; the end of which is retrieved with a grasper via the 6R portal and out of the joint (Fig. 16.13a, b).

The needle is then withdrawn slightly under arthroscopic control. Once the tip of the needle has passed the dorsal radio-ulnar ligament, but before it exits the dorsal capsule, it is directed distally and advanced to penetrate the dorsal radio-ulnar ligament. The thread is now pushed in through the Tuohy needle, so as to have a loop inside the joint (Fig. 16.13c). Grabbing this loop with the grasper and pulling it out of the joint via the 6R will allow both ends of the thread to be outside the joint, while the hitch will be on the

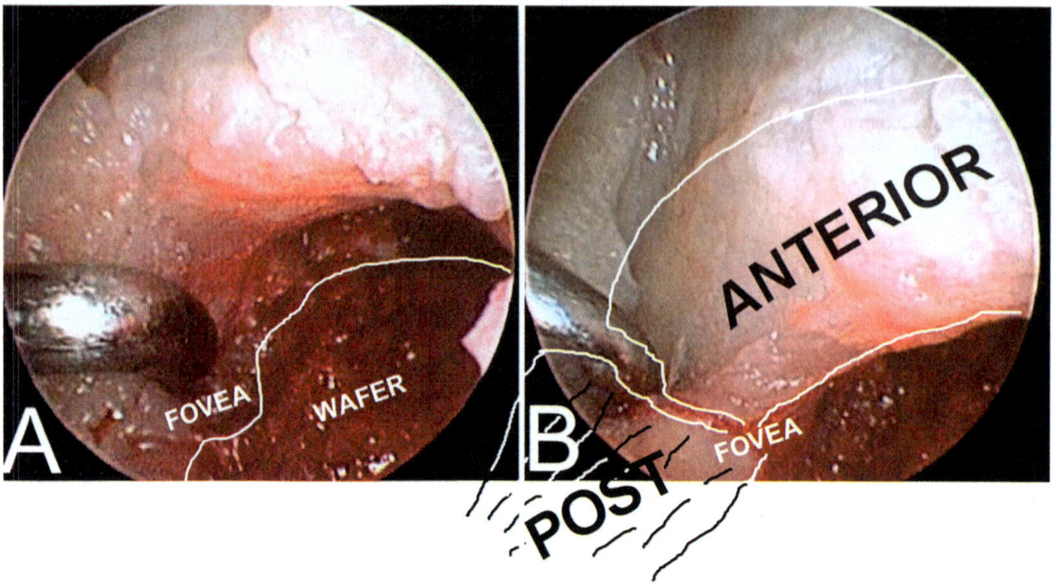

Fig. 16.12 Notice in this sequence how clearly, after the debridement and wafer procedure, the ligaments (anterior and posterior) are shown to be split all the way to the fovea (same patient as Fig. 16.9) (Published with permission of © Dr. Piñal 2012. All Rights Reserved)

proximal aspect (foveal side) on both sides of the distal radio-ulnar ligaments (Fig. 16.13d). By performing a gliding knot, the throw will go all the way to the distal aspect (carpal side) of the TFC (Fig. 16.13e). A knot pusher is now used to tighten the knot bringing together both distal radio-ulnar ligaments and thus reconstructing the chiasm (Figs. 16.13f and 16.14).

Before making the gliding knot, it is crucial that both ends of the suture are withdrawn from the joint through the same path in 6R portal. If *any* tissue is interposed, the gliding knot will be blocked as it passes volarly. A suture hook can be used to make sure that both suture ends follow a single tunnel (see Appendix A for further details).

Postoperatively, the patients were kept in a sugar tong splint for 4 weeks, allowing flexion-extension of the elbow, but blocking pronation-supination. Then they were allowed to start progressive ROM and unlimited activities after 4 months.

All our patients reported a significant improvement at a mean of 1.5-year follow-up with complete resolution of symptoms [5].

Discussion

In a busy biased practice as ours, coronal tears are an infrequent (only eight cases) but definite cause of subtle instability and ulnar pain. Our biomechanical studies confirm the existence of this entity and the efficacy of addressing it by suture repair or by ulna shortening. Because both methods of treatment have provided similar biomechanical results in our experimental model, arthroscopic repair may be recommended. The technique as described is quite straightforward, but is not for a novice: in addition to a well-executed wafer procedure, one has to add the time needed for arthroscopic suturing. The latter has a tricky step, which is piercing of the volar radio-ulnar ligament without damaging any volar structure, i.e., piercing the volar ligament but staying dorsal to the volar capsule. It follows that the needle has to exit more dorsal than the junction of the volar radio-ulnar ligament and the volar capsule. Because the space available to the surgeon to maneuver the needle is quite tight (proximally impeded by the head of the ulna and distally by the dorsal radio-ulnar ligament), it is

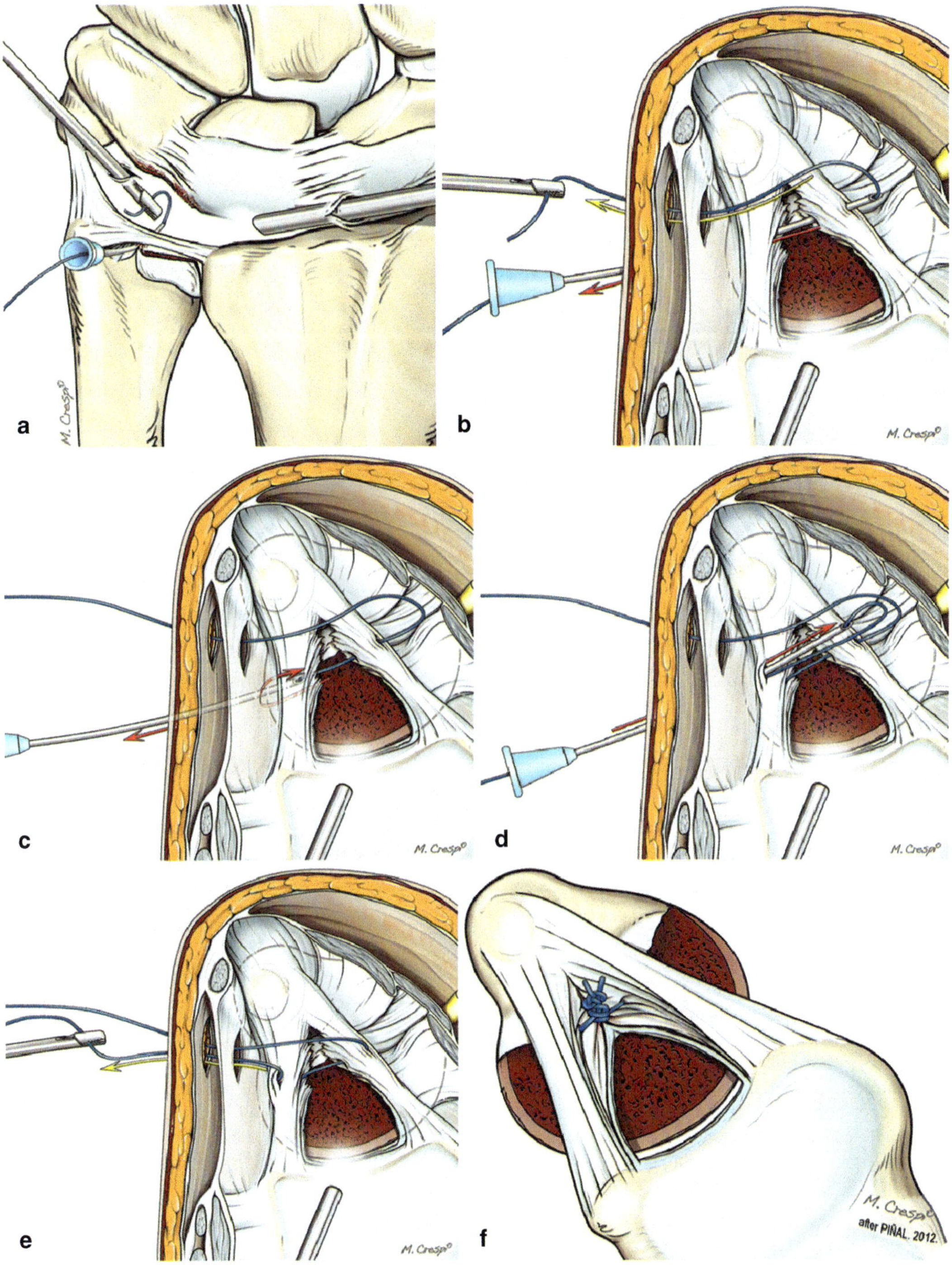

Fig. 16.13 See text for technical details (Published with permission of © Dr. Piñal 2012. All Rights Reserved)

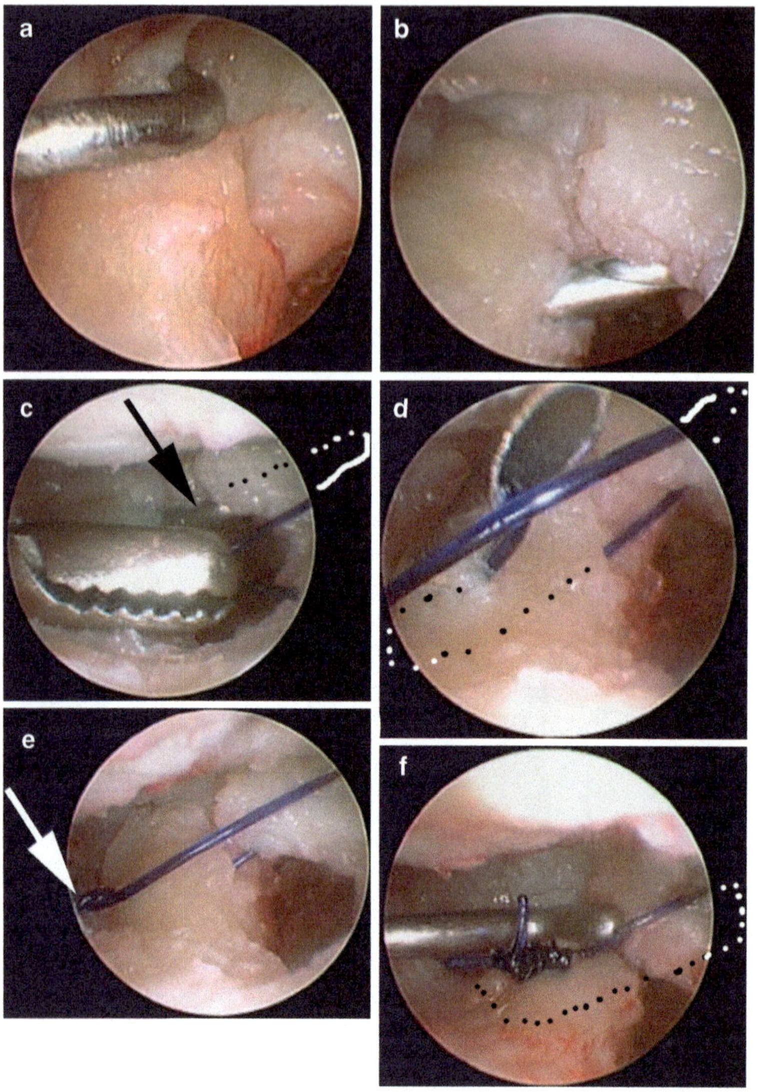

Fig. 16.14 Suture placement in a coronal tear of the TFC at the fovea. (**a**) The tear is being explored. The probe is in 6R in a left wrist. (**b**) A loaded Tuohy needle is passing from the posterior part through the frontal tear to perforate the anterior portion. (**c**) The suture is advanced through the needle and a grasper is now pulling the end of the suture (*arrow*) to be pulled out through 6R portal (in this case). (**d**) The loaded needle is now perforating the posterior part of the tear. The suture end will be pulled out of the joint with a grasper, as in (**c**). (**e**) Both suture ends are now being knotted outside and the gliding knot is now being pushed (*white arrow*). (**f**) Final result [7], with permission from the British Society for Surgery of the Hand. 2010)

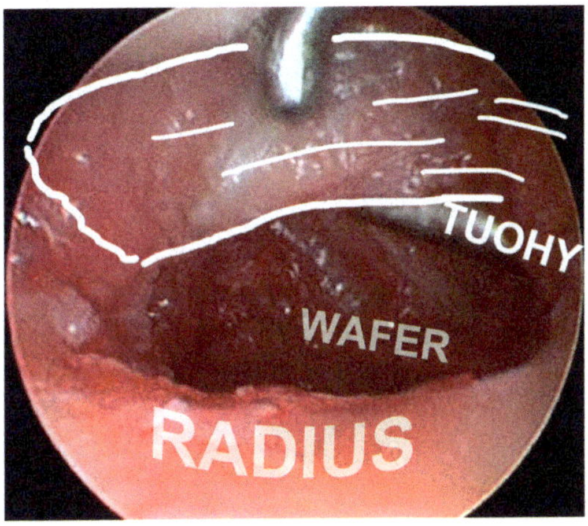

Fig. 16.15 The probe is hooking the volar DRU ligament, while the Tuohy needle is piercing it but not penetrating the volar capsule (Published with permission of © Dr. Piñal 2012. All Rights Reserved)

really difficult to penetrate the volar RUL only. We have sometimes gently bent the Tuohy needle distally in order to facilitate it, and it is also helpful to use a probe in 6R to act as a counterpressure inside the joint (Fig. 16.15). However, when the ulnar head is not resected, the space may be so tight that in one instance, we had to resort to another technique to allow the suture be placed inside the joint (see Appendix A).

The limitation of this study derives from the fact that this is a retrospective study from two different surgeons with different treatment algorithms. The clinical and intraoperative findings however are very similar in both groups, and the biomechanical study supports the pathomechanics of the condition accounts for how both surgical treatments resulted in resolution of symptoms. Although the results were similar, the arthroscopic approach will be employed in the future as the anatomic relationships at the sigmoid notch will remain unaltered if an ulnar resection is avoided. To ascertain if one treatment option described here is superior to the other, a prospective randomized trial is ideal. Unfortunately, due to the rarity of the condition, this is very difficult to perform.

In summary, one should consider this entity in the patient that refers instability of the wrist after a traumatic event in the setting of a degenerative tear.

References

1. Atzei A (2009) New trends in arthroscopic management of type 1-B TFCC injuries with DRUJ instability. J Hand Surg Eur 34:582–591
2. Cooney WP, Linscheid RL, Dobyns JH (1994) Triangular fibrocartilage tears. J Hand Surg Am 19(1): 143–154. PubMed PMID: 8169359
3. del Piñal F (2010) Treatment of explosion-type distal radius fractures. In: del Piñal F, Mathoulin C, Luchetti C (eds) Arthroscopic management of distal radius fractures. Springer, Berlin
4. del Piñal F (2011) Dry arthroscopy and its applications. Hand Clin 27:335–345
5. del Piñal, Nakamura T (2010) Coronal tears of the TFCC. In: Presented at the 26th International Wrist Investigator's workshop, Boston, 2010
6. del Piñal F, García-Bernal FJ, Pisani D, Regalado J, Ayala H, Studer A (2007) Dry arthroscopy of the wrist: surgical technique. J Hand Surg Am 32:119–123
7. del Piñal F, García-Bernal FJ, Cagigal L, Studer A, Regalado J, Thams C (2010) A technique for arthroscopic all-inside suturing in the wrist. J Hand Surg Eur 35:475–479
8. del Piñal F, Studer A, Thams C, Glasberg A (2011) An all-inside technique for arthroscopic suturing of the volar scapholunate ligament. J Hand Surg Am 36: 2044–2046
9. Estrella EP, Hung LK, Ho PC, Tse WL (2007) Arthroscopic repair of triangular fibrocartilage complex tears. Arthroscopy 23:729–737
10. Ishii S, Palmer AK, Werner FW, Short WH, Fortino MD (1998) An anatomic study of the ligamentous structure of the triangular fibrocartilage complex. J Hand Surg Am 23:977–985
11. Nakamura T, Yabe Y, Horiuchi Y (1996) Functional anatomy of the triangular fibrocartilage complex. J Hand Surg Br 21:581–586
12. Nakamura T, Makita A (2000) The proximal ligamentous component of the triangular fibrocartilage complex. J Hand Surg 25(5):479–486
13. Palmer AK (1989) Triangular fibrocartilage complex lesions: a classification. J Hand Surg Am 14:594–606

17 LT Tears and Arthroscopic Repair

Jan-Ragnar Haugstvedt

Background

Tears of the ligament between the lunate and the triquetrum (LT lig) are said to occur approximately 15–20 % as common as injuries of the scapholunate (SL) ligament [33]. It has been reported that isolated LT lig injuries can result from a direct blow to a fall on an outstretched hand; however, these injuries are often described as part of more extensive injuries of the wrist involving other ligaments as well as bones [15, 25, 30]. A true incidence of an isolated LT lig injury is thus difficult to assess.

Anatomy and Biomechanics

The wrist ligaments are typically found within the joint capsule composed of parallel collagen fascicles, small caliber nerves, and blood vessels lined by synoviocytes [4]. The LT lig has an interosseous ligament covering the dorsal, proximal, and palmar aspect of the LT joint, leaving the distal aspect of the joint open to communicate with the midcarpal joint. The ligaments are divided into dorsal, proximal, and palmar regions (Fig. 17.1). Contrary to the SL lig, where the dorsal region is the thickest and strongest, the palmar region of the LT lig is the thickest and strongest region of this interosseous ligament and is together with the thinner dorsal region found to be a true ligament [21]. The proximal region is composed of fibrocartilage without collagen orientation, blood vessels, or nerves. A meniscal projection distally into the joint cleft is described [4].

In a normal wrist, the scaphoid will, on the radial side of the carpus, impart a flexion moment to the proximal carpal row. On the ulnar side, the triquetrum imparts an extension moment. The lunate is well balanced by its ligamentous attachments to the scaphoid and the triquetrum. In flexion-extension of a normal hand, the proximal

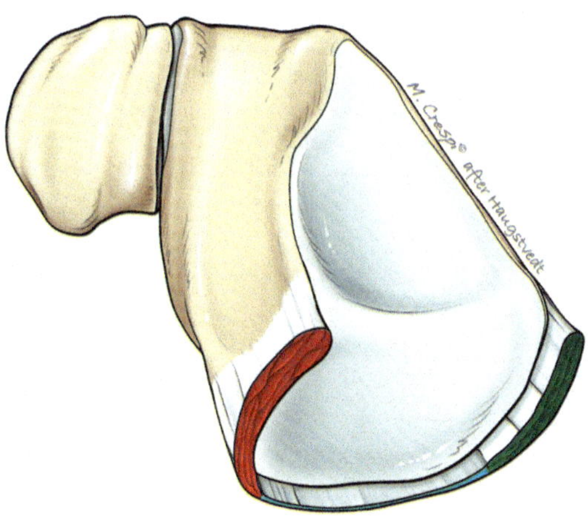

Fig. 17.1 Illustration of the triquetrum and the lunotriquetral joint including the LT ligament covering the dorsal, proximal, and palmar aspect of the LT joint. The palmar region of the LT lig is the thickest and strongest region of this interosseous ligament and is together with the thinner dorsal region a true ligament

J.-R. Haugstvedt, M.D., Ph.D.
Department of Orthopedics, Østfold Hospital Trust, Moss, Norway
e-mail: jrhaugstvedt@gmail.com

F. del Piñal et al. (eds.), *Arthroscopic Management of Ulnar Pain*,
DOI 10.1007/978-3-642-30544-3_17, © Springer-Verlag Berlin Heidelberg 2012

row bones act synergistically and will move with the hand. In radial-ulnar deviation the proximal row moves synergistically from a flexed position in radial deviation to an extended position in ulnar deviation.

Pathomechanics

When a rupture of the SL lig occurs, the scaphoid will tend to flex, while the lunate, still attached to the triquetrum, will extend together with the triquetrum. This will cause a dorsal intercalated segmental instability (DISI) pattern (Fig. 17.2).

Investigations on cadaveric specimens have shown that sectioning of the proximal and dorsal parts of the LT lig had little effect on carpal kinematics. For a volar intercalated segment instability pattern (VISI) to occur, sectioning of both the proximal and the palmar components had to be performed, while a greater VISI occurred after additional sectioning of the dorsal radiocarpal (dorsal radio-triquetral) and intercarpal ligaments, implying a considerable compressive force [11, 20, 22, 32, 34]. In these situations, the lunate will tend to go into a flexed position with the scaphoid (Fig. 17.3).

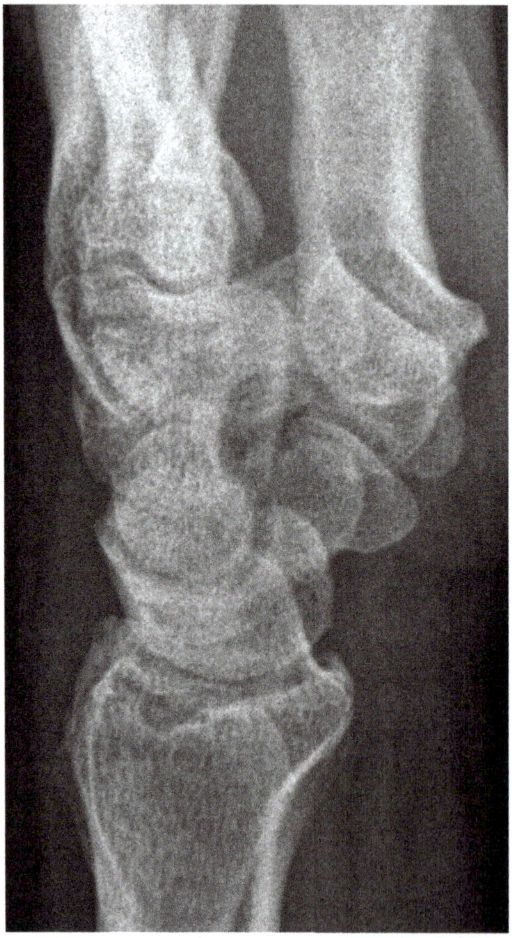

Fig. 17.2 A side view of the carpus showing a dorsal intercalated segmental instability (*DISI*) as could be seen following a rupture of the SL lig

Mechanism of Injury

The exact mechanism of an injury leading to an LT lig injury is yet to be proven. In the radial side of the wrist, a progressive injury pattern has been described when a force is applied to the thenar area with the wrist in a dorsiflexed and ulnarly deviated position. This has been shown

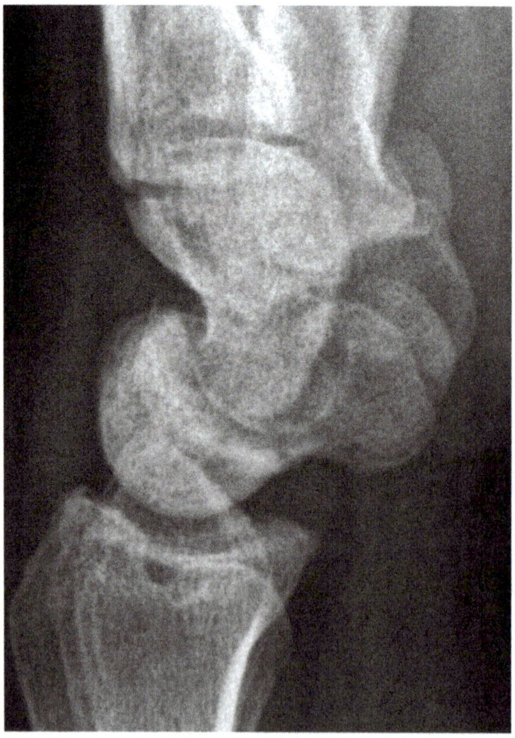

Fig. 17.3 A side view of the carpus showing a volar intercalated segmental instability (*VISI*) as could be seen following ruptures of the LT lig and the dorsal radiocarpal and intercarpal ligaments

to give a progressive injury pattern in a radial to ulnar direction. The injury will pass through ligaments and/or bones, and dependent on the force and direction of the impact a perilunar dislocation may occur [16]. An isolated LT lig injury may be the result of a reverse perilunate injury where the wrist is forcefully twisted into extension, radial deviation, and pronation, thus displacing the triquetrum dorsally relative to the lunate [34]. From the cadaver study, Viegas et al. have defined three stages of ulnar-sided perilunate instability pattern. In stage I, a tear of the interosseous LT lig showed increased motion between the lunate and the triquetrum. In stage II, after having sectioned the palmar LT lig, an increased laxity between the lunate and triquetrum was noted; however, a VISI deformity could be produced only while maintaining a translational force to the dorsum of a neutral or flexed wrist. If there was an additional disruption of the extrinsic ligaments, a VISI deformity was present (stage III). Due to the secondary joint stabilizers of the LT joint, a true static instability, or VISI, is very rare, and most of the LT lig injuries are found to be dynamic.

In most reports, a history of trauma is presented along with the ulnar-sided wrist pain [6, 12, 24, 26]. Other causes may be the result of TFCC tears, positive ulnar variance, degenerative LT lesions, inflammatory arthritis, midcarpal instability, or fractures [23].

Diagnosis

An injury, especially a fall on a dorsiflexed wrist with an impact on the ulnar side of a pronated hand, should give suspicion of a possible LT lig injury in a patient with ulnar-sided wrist pain. Symptoms are often intermittent and are prominent in special positions of the wrist such as ulnar deviation or pronation. Examination should include the entire arm, especially focusing on the ulnar side of the wrist (Fig. 17.4a, b). Comparison

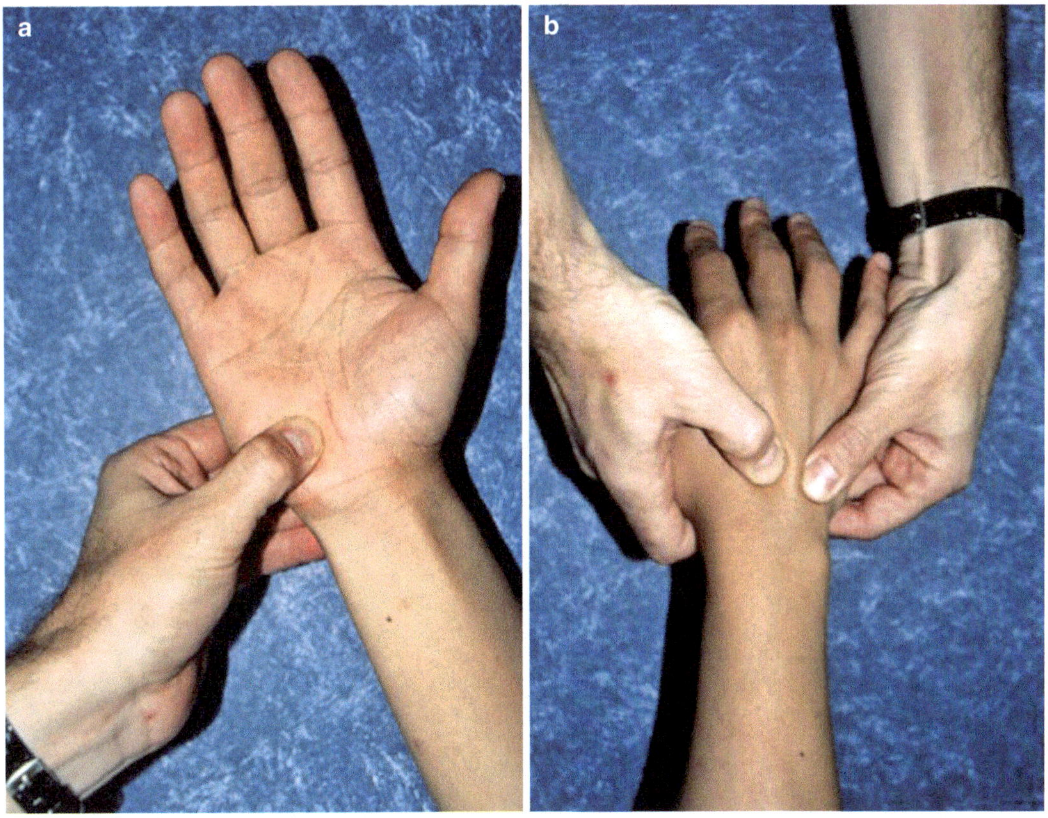

Fig. 17.4 (**a**, **b**) Clinical examination should focus on the ulnar side of the wrist and the LT interval

to the other hand/wrist is essential. (For further details, see Chap. 3).

Provocative Tests

Several tests have been described to diagnose pathology of the LT ligament (see also Chap. 3). Reagan and his coworkers [20] described what has been called the ballottement test. Stabilizing the lunate between the thumb and index finger of one hand, while the pisotriquetral unit is displaced in a dorsal-palmar direction using the thumb and index finger of the other hand carries out the test. As the two hands are moved in opposite directions, stress is created across the LT joint. A positive test elicits pain, crepitus, and laxity during manipulation of the joint (Fig. 17.5).

The shear test [13] is another provocative test for dynamic LT instability. The examiner's fingers are placed dorsal to the lunate, while the thumb is placed on the volar side to load the pisotriquetral joint in a dorsal direction. This load will create a shearing vector across the LT joint that may result in crepitation or clicking reproducing pain in the patient (Fig. 17.6).

In still another test [1], lateral pressure is applied to the so-called ulnar snuffbox, located between the extensor carpi ulnaris and the flexor carpi ulnaris tendons, distal to the ulnar head over the medial aspect of the triquetrum. Reproduction of the patient's pain while radially deviating the wrist when applying the pressure is considered a positive test suggesting LT lig injury or an ulnar styloid triquetrum impingement.

Whipple presented a somewhat similar test at an IWIW meeting (personal communication). The examiner grips the patient's involved wrist with one hand, placing his thumb on the triquetrum and his fingers on the radial border of the distal radius and squeezes (Whipple proximal row squeeze (PRS) test). Reproduction of the

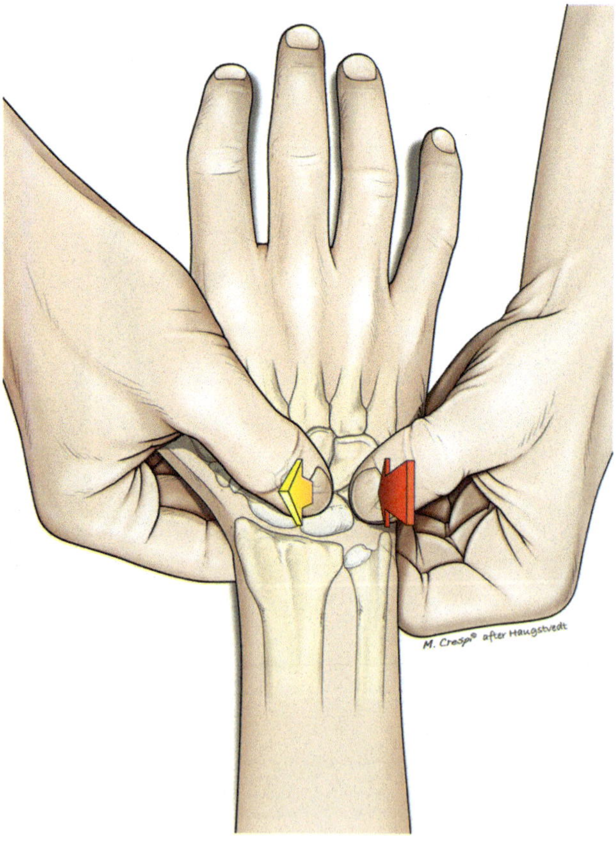

Fig. 17.5 Ballottement test. The lunate should be stabilized between the thumb and the index finger of one hand, while the pisotriquetral unit is displaced in a dorsal-palmar direction using the thumb and index finger of the other hand. As stress is created across the LT joint, a positive test elicits pain, crepitus, and laxity during manipulation of the joint

patient's pain on the dorsal, ulnar aspect of the wrist means the triquetrum slides distally on the ulnar slope of the lunate due to disruption of the LT lig. There is no other structure that is stressed with this test, so the pain reproduction isolates the LT lig injury/instability (Fig. 17.7a, b).

While performing these different tests, it should once again be emphasized the importance of making comparisons to the non-injured contralateral side. For other causes of ulnar-sided wrist pain, see Chap. 3.

Imaging

Radiographs

Radiographs obtained with the forearm in neutral rotation position should include standard posterior-anterior (PA), lateral, and oblique images. Stress views including radial and ulnar deviation, and clenched-fist views, are often helpful to demonstrate instability. The images should at least be examined for ulnar positive variance, type of lunate, and widening of the LT interval. The standard views often appear normal in patients with dynamic LT instability caused by a partial tear of the LT lig. When there is a complete tear of the intrinsic and the extrinsic ligaments supporting the lunate and the triquetrum (see section "Pathomechanics"), a static carpal collapse will occur resulting in disruption of the so-called Gilula's arcs [10] (Fig. 17.8a–d). This is visualized as a step-off between the lunate and the triquetrum on a PA view, rarely though, there is a widening of the gap between the two bones (like the one seen in an SL dissociation). The VISI (see section "Pathomechanics") is more easily recognized in a side view.

Arthrography

Arthrography can be useful in identifying LT lig tears, demonstrating leakage of dye at the LT inter-

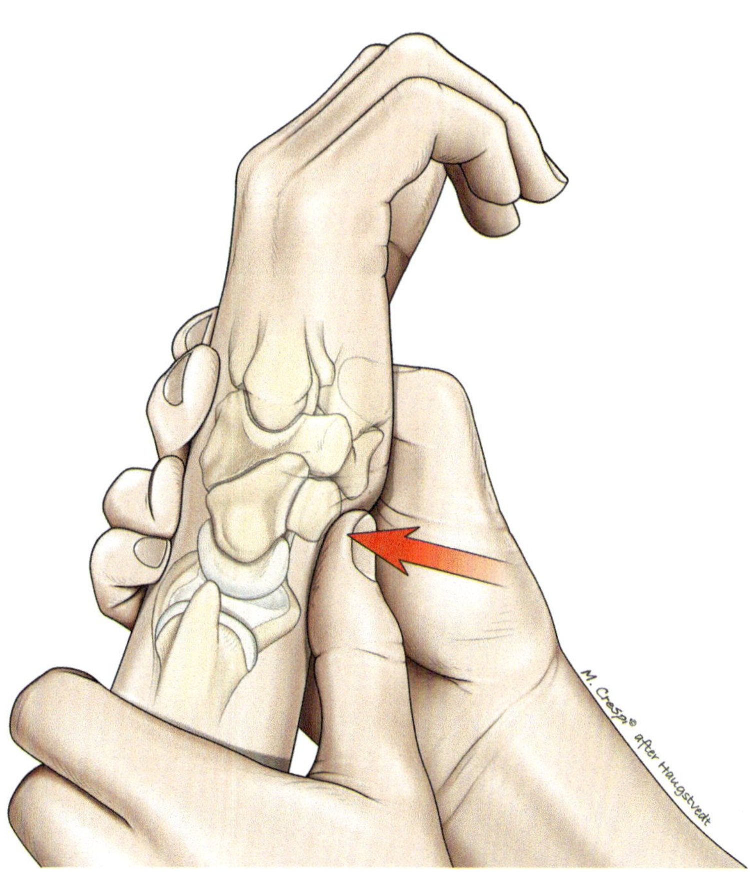

Fig. 17.6 Shear test. The examiner's fingers are placed dorsal to the lunate, while the thumb is placed on the volar side to load the pisotriquetral joint in a dorsal direction. This load will create a shearing vector across the LT joint that may result in crepitation or clicking reproducing pain in the patient

Fig. 17.7 (**a**, **b**) Proximal row squeeze test. The examiner grips the patient's wrist with one hand, placing his thumb on the triquetrum and his fingers on the radial border of the distal radius and squeezes (**a**). If the LT lig is ruptured, the triquetrum will slide distally and radially along the articular slope of the lunate reproducing pain from the LT instability (**b**)

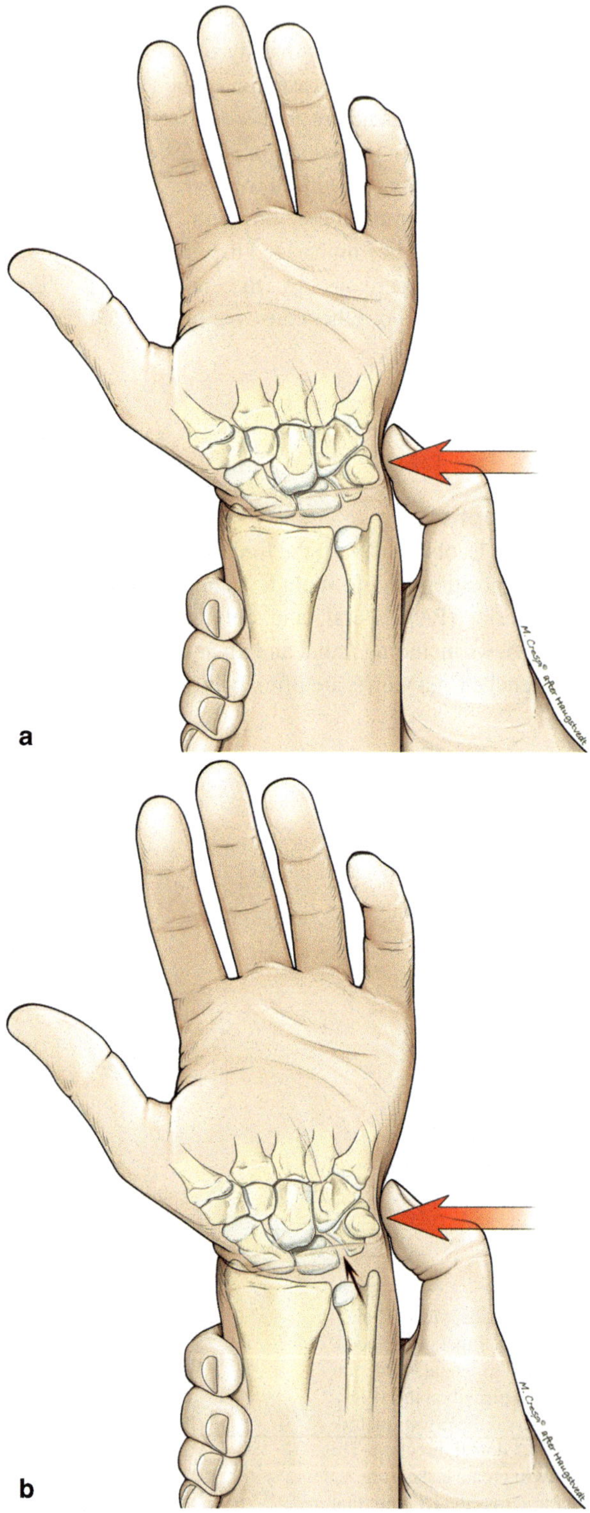

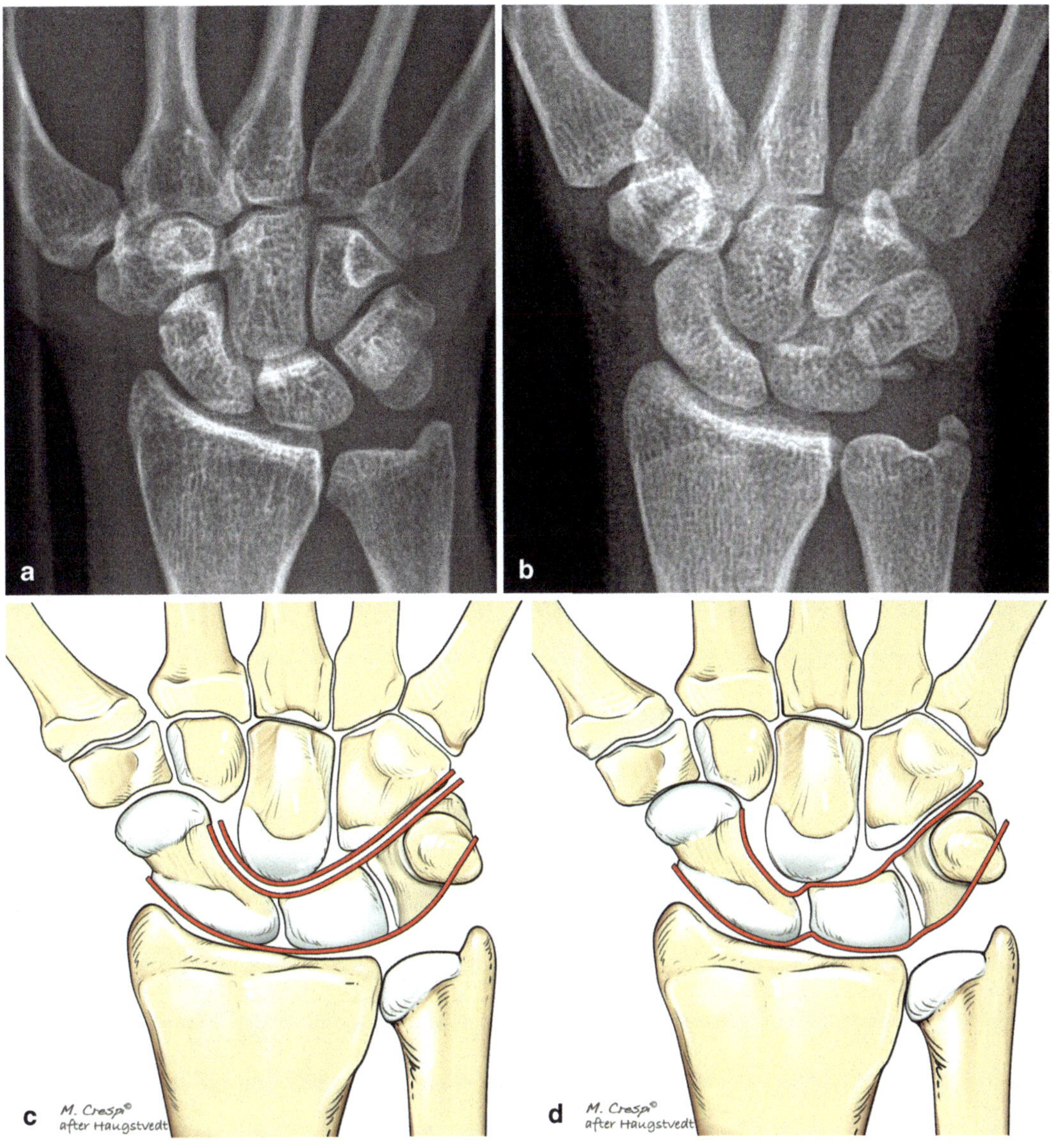

Fig. 17.8 (**a–d**) When there is a normal alignment of the proximal row bones, no disruption of the so-called Gilula's lines is seen (**a**, **c**). Disruption of Gilula's lines gives an indication of an injury of intercarpal ligament(s) of the proximal row (**b**, **d**)

space. The injection could be into the radiocarpal or the midcarpal joint. In cases with perforations of the LT membrane due to age-related changes, or wear and tear from an ulnar impaction syndrome, a positive arthrography does not imply a traumatic LT lig tear. The sensitivity and specificity of arthrograpy is variable, and positive findings should be interpreted with caution [6, 17, 36]. Good quality images could reveal the diagnosis (Fig. 17.9a).

Magnetic Resonance Imaging

It has been said that the utility of magnetic resonance imaging (MRI) in LT lig diagnostic imaging has not proven reliable to date [27, 38, 39]. However, as the method has been refined, the quality of MRI studies is improving and the images thus obtained will be of good help in diagnosing LT lig tears in the future (Fig. 17.9b).

Video Fluoroscopy

The use of video fluoroscopy is possible to demonstrate the sudden movement of the triquetrum into extension as the wrist moves from a radial into a maximal ulnar deviated position. A video fluoroscope could also be used when performing injection studies of the wrist in order to confirm the leakage of dye into the LT interval.

Other Imaging Techniques

CT imaging of the wrist will not add new information to the imaging techniques already mentioned. Bone scanning is also a technique of lower specificity, and compared to other available techniques, this examination should today not be high on the list [10].

Arthroscopy

Using arthrotomy as the diagnostic tool, Cooney [6] showed that arthroscopy had no false-positive

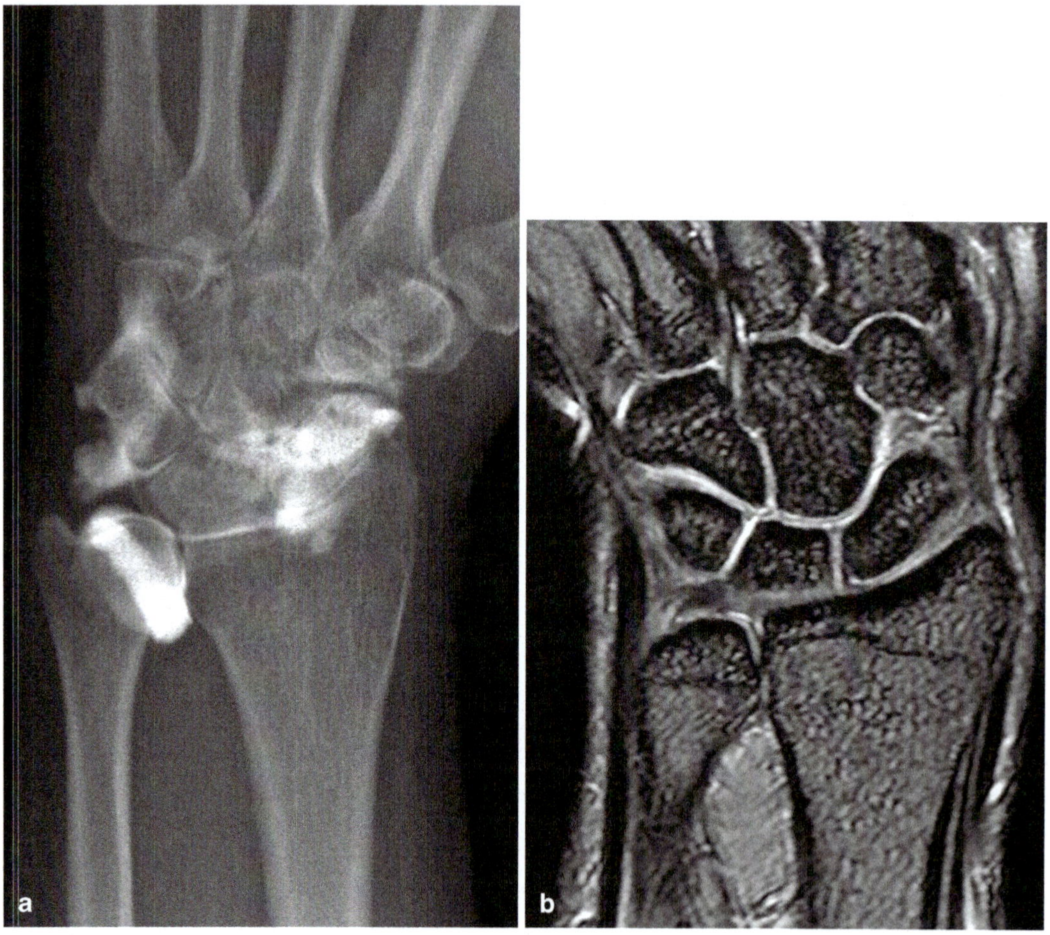

Fig. 17.9 (**a**, **b**) Arthrography and MRI from the same patient showing changes in the LT lig on the midcarpal surface (Courtesy: Toshiyasu Nakamura)

or false-negative intercarpal ligament tears, being the most precise diagnostic tool in indicating the location, size, and extent of ligament injuries of the wrist. Wrist arthroscopy should be considered the gold standard for examining the wrist and LT lig injuries.

Using the well-known setup for wrist arthroscopy, the LT lig can be difficult to view from the 3–4 portal in the radiocarpal joint, however, is best visualized with the scope in the 4–5 or the 6-R portal. When viewing volarly, the ulnolunate (UL) and ulnotriquetral (UT) ligaments could be traced distally to identify the interval between these ligaments as the LT joint and the LT lig [3]. Using a probe, the integrity of the different parts of the LT ligament should be examined. In a normal wrist, the smooth surface of the proximal interosseous LT ligament could be difficult to identify; however, bulging or frayed edges in the interval between the bones indicate an injury. It is, however, through a midcarpal arthroscopy the LT interval can be thoroughly evaluated. The scope should be in the radial midcarpal (MCR) portal, while the probe is in the ulnar MC (MCU) portal. From both the wrist and the midcarpal joints, the dorsal, membranous, and palmar portions of the ligament should be tested to verify the extent of the lesion(s). It should be mentioned that Viegas and coworkers have described a separate facet of the lunate [35]. The shape of this lunate can sometimes interfere a good view from the MCR, making a switch to the ulnar portal necessary (Fig. 17.10a, b).

If a wet arthroscopy is performed, placing a needle in the midcarpal joint will yield fluid if there is a disruption, or a rupture of the intercarpal ligaments ("a poor man's arthrogram") [19]. While the SL interval is normally tight and congruent without any step-off when viewed from the midcarpal space (MCS), a small step-off of 1 mm is occasionally found when viewing the LT interval. There is likewise normally slight motion between the lunate and the triquetrum viewed from the MCS, while no such motion is normally found between the scaphoid and the lunate. Using a probe to assess the LT interval will enable a more precise description of the injury/instability (Fig. 17.11a, b). An arthroscopic classification of carpal interosseous ligament tears has been presented [9], from Grade I describing an attenuation and/or hemorrhage of the ligament with no incongruence of carpal alignment, to Grade IV where incongruence and/or step-off of the carpal alignment are observed in both the radiocarpal and midcarpal space. In Grade IV, a small-joint arthroscope may be passed through the gap between the bones. After having verified the extent of the LT lig tear, the arthroscopic examination should also reveal any injuries to other ligaments, as well as to the TFCC, the

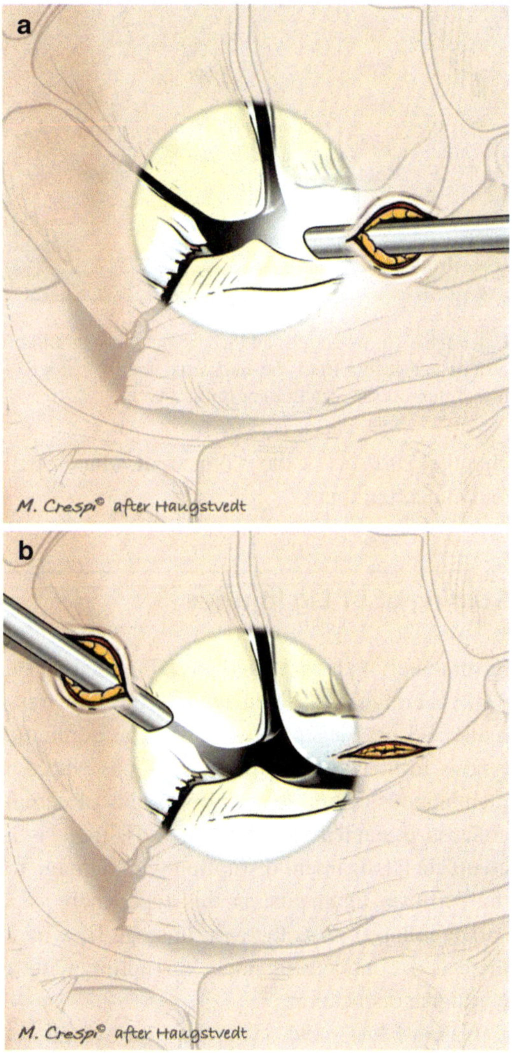

Fig. 17.10 (**a**, **b**) When a lunate type II is found, a good view of the LT interval from the MCR portal may not be possible necessitating the use of the MCU portal for the scope for a better view

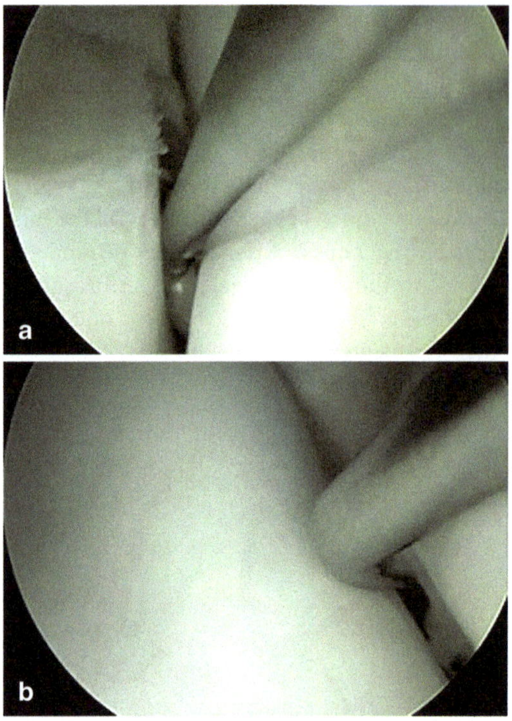

Fig. 17.11 (**a**, **b**) The SL and LT lig intervals should be probed and tested from the midcarpal joint in order to reveal step-off (as seen in **a**) or instability

chondral surfaces of the radiocarpal, ulnocarpal, and midcarpal joints.

Staging of LT Lig Injuries

Several authors have staged the LT lig tears [19, 34]. Osterman and Seidman describe one traumatic and one degenerative type. The traumatic type is further divided into three types where a membranous central tear without signs of carpal collapse is named type I. In type II, there is a complete LT ligament disruption with damage to the extrinsic ligaments; in this type, there is a carpal collapse, as is the case in stage III where there is a complete ligament disruption with a perilunate dislocation.

Garcia-Elias and Geissler presented a modification of Osterman and Seidman's classification [8]. They recognized six different types of LT lig injuries: acute dynamic, chronic dynamic, static, acute perilunate instability, chronic perilunate instability, and degenerative ulnocarpal abutment.

Treatment

Treatment of LT lig injuries could be challenging, and there is, to the author's knowledge, no prospective randomized study evaluating the different treatment options for this entity of injuries. The following recommendations are thus based on retrospective studies, case reports, and author's own experience. The treatment should be according to the injury, acute or chronic, and the state of instability, dynamic or static, taking into consideration concomitant injuries and/or degenerative changes.

Some treatment modalities described in the section of acute injuries have also been used for treatment of more chronic cases. A true acute injury should be considered as one treated within 6 (−12) weeks. However, some of the results referred to in the following describe the same treatment used from 3 days to 84 months after injury [2, 14]. When the treatment is performed, the edges of the healing sites should be debrided, and the bones should be able to be reduced to normal alignment without difficulties.

Acute Injuries

Conservative Treatment

There are reports on conservative treatments of LT lig injuries without a static VISI. These injuries have been treated with immobilization using a well-molded cast or a splint giving support underneath the pisiform and over the dorsum of the distal radius [5, 8, 20, 28]. The arm should be immobilized in an above-the-elbow cast (to prevent rotation of the forearm with proximal-distal movement of the ulna) for 4 weeks followed by a forearm splint for another 4 weeks. It has been reported ligament healing in more than 80 % of the cases with immobilization in a cast [5], while complete symptom resolution may take months.

Others [8] discuss the failures of conservative treatment with cases progressing from a dynamic carpal instability to a static VISI type due to lack of ligament healing and subsequent attenuation of the secondary constraints. The problem, as previously discussed, is to confirm the correct diagnosis of an LT lig tear. As the use of wrist arthroscopy is becoming more popular, and is now widely performed for exploration and diagnosis of wrist injuries, the treatment of the acute injuries has changed as well.

Debridement

The technique for diagnosing an LT lig tear is previously described in this Chapter. The scope is placed in the 3–4 portal or the MCR portal, while the probe is in the 6-R or MCU portal. When evaluating the LT interval, there is normally, as previously mentioned, a slight motion that takes some experience to judge as "normal" or "pathologic." When instability is found, potential frayed edges should be debrided from the radiocarpal as well as from the midcarpal joint. The arthroscope should be in a radial (3–4 or MCR) portal, while the shaver is handled and debridement performed in an ulnar (4–5 or MCU) portal, although the portals may be switched for better views.

Debridement of the torn ligament ends has been thought of inciting a scar and a healing reaction that could provide stability to the carpus (Fig. 17.12). Weiss and coworkers [37] report good results of arthroscopic debridement alone in patients with intercarpal ligament tears. After debridement, all patients had immobilization of the forearm in a splint for 14 days followed by hand therapy. After an average of 27 months to follow-up, seven out of nine patients with a complete LT lig tear were found to have almost complete resolution of symptoms. Of the six patients found to have partial LT lig tears, all six reported complete resolution of symptoms, or only occasional symptoms with heavy-use activities.

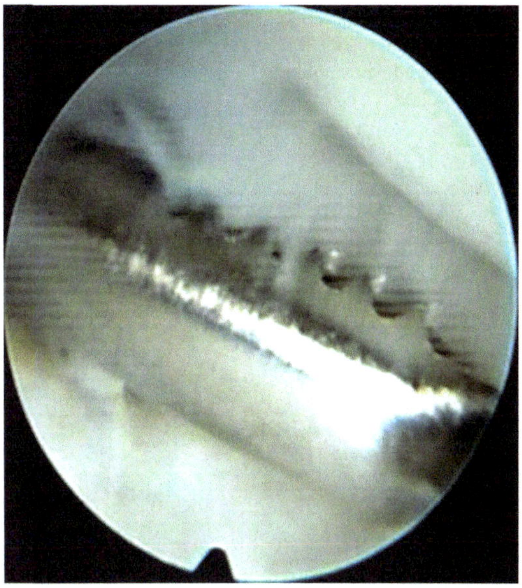

Fig. 17.12 The frayed edges of the injured LT lig are debrided

Pin Fixation of LT Interval

Debridement followed by pin fixation of the LT interval using several K-wires is widely used, a technique that has been described by several authors [12, 19]. With the scope in the MCR portal, examination of the tear should be performed (Fig. 17.13) followed by reduction of the LT interval. To facilitate this, K-wires could be inserted in the lunate and triquetrum to be used as joysticks (Fig. 17.14a, b). When reduction has been achieved, multiple pins are advanced through the triquetrum into the lunate. A fluoroscope is needed for the introduction of the K-wires. If the arm is in a traction tower, the beam of the fluoroscope has to be horizontal. The alternative is to take the hand out of the traction and put it on the table to insert the K-wires into the triquetrum. A small incision should be made on the ulnar border of the carpus, or a soft-tissue protector or a 14- to 16- gauge needle should be used to avoid injury of the dorsal sensory branch of the ulnar nerve. When inserting the K-wires over the LT interval, the hand should be in the traction tower, and the arthroscope should be used to verify reduction and closing of the gap. The radial articular edge of the triquetrum should be aligned with the ulnar articular edge of the lunate. Multiple 1.25 mm K-wires are used; the positions of which are controlled in the

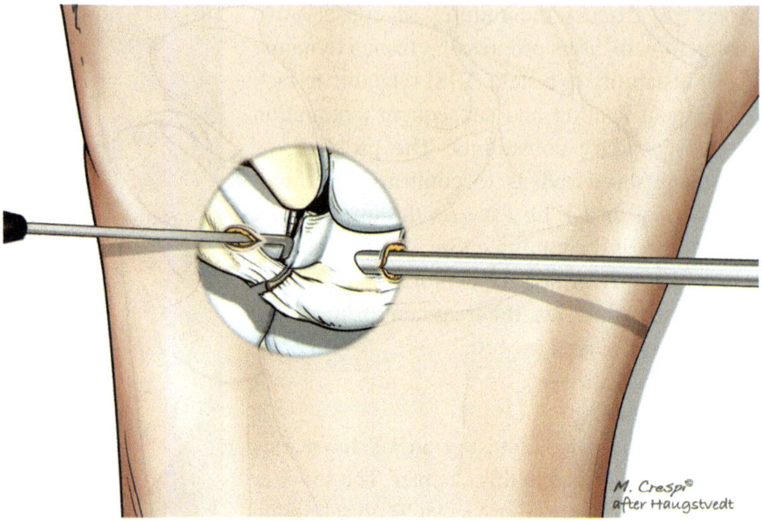

Fig. 17.13 With the scope in the MCR portal, the LT lig interval should be examined using a probe

fluoroscope in the PA and lateral planes. Marrow fat droplets may be seen "boiling" up from the LT interval in the MCS as the K-wires are drilled across the LT interval. The goal of this treatment is to stabilize the joint while the ligament heals and to create a fibrodesis over the joint (Fig. 17.15a, b). The author recommends immobilization as previously mentioned; the K-wires are removed when the cast is removed after 8 weeks (Fig. 17.16a–c).

Osterman and Seidman [19] have reported the results of this treatment in 20 patients with LT lig tears without a VISI. After a follow-up averaging 32 months, 16 patients had good to excellent relief of pain and preoperative symptoms. Loss of wrist extension was 17 %, wrist flexion 25 %, and grip strength 30 % as compared with the contralateral uninjured hand. In 18 out of 20 patients, the grip strength improved.

As an injury of the LT lig is often a part of a more extensive injury, the result of the LT lig repair is difficult to evaluate as other factors may influence on the result. Ritter et al. [23] report on 11 patients in which arthroscopic debridement of a partial or complete LT lig injury was performed. In cases of LT instability, K-wires were used to stabilize the LT joint. In patients with concomitant injuries, central or peripheral TFCC tears were repaired, arthrosis was debrided, and, in two cases with a distal radius fracture, arthroscopically assisted reduction and fixation were carried out. At final follow-up, eight patients had significant improvement in their symptoms, while three had only moderate improvement, two of the last mentioned had TFCC tears with persistent DRUJ instability. In another paper, arthroscopic treatment of simultaneous complete tears of the scapholunate and lunotriquetral ligaments is reported [2]. In a retrospective study, they reviewed 13 patients with gross arthroscopic carpal instability treated with debridement of the torn ligaments followed by stabilization of the SL and LT intervals with K-wires. The arms were immobilized for 8 weeks. At the final follow-up (20–84 months), ten patients had no pain, one had mild pain, and two had moderate pain. The ROM was good with an average grip strength of 67 % compared to the non-injured side. The average DASH score was 10.7.

In the last study, the authors present one patient who was treated acutely with arthroscopic

Fig. 17.14 (**a, b**) To reduce and stabilize the LT interval, the arthroscope should be in the midcarpal joint, and the fluoroscope should be placed with the beam in a horizontal direction. K-wires are placed in the lunate and the triquetrum to be used as joysticks to facilitate the reduction. When reduction is achieved, as verified by the arthroscope and the fluoroscope, K-wires are inserted through the triquetrum into the lunate

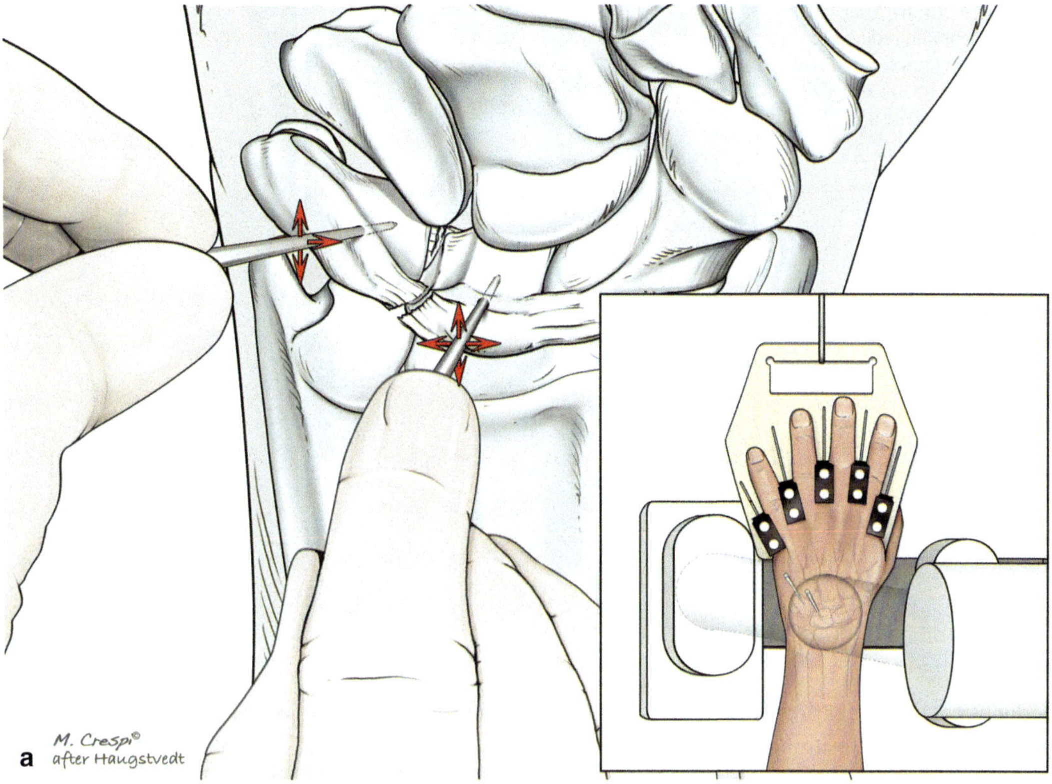

a M. Crespi© after Haugstvedt

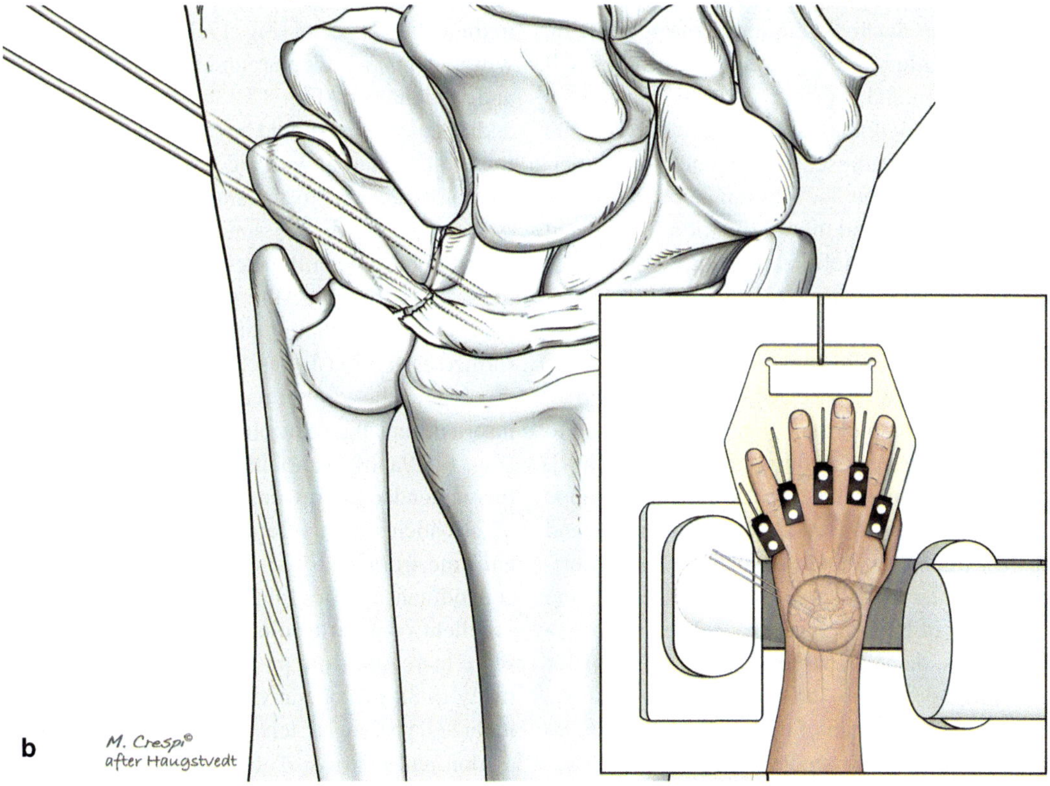

b M. Crespi© after Haugstvedt

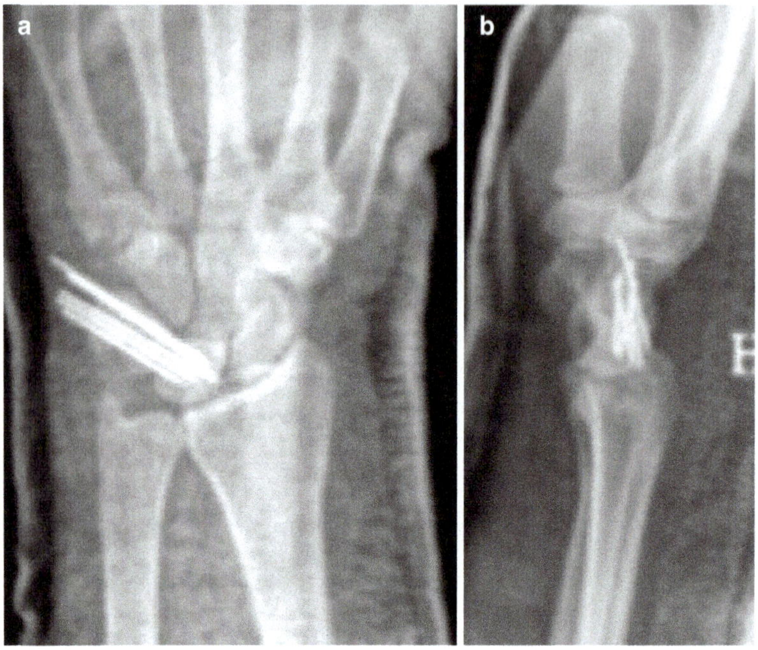

Fig. 17.15 (**a**, **b**) After debridement and reduction, the LT interval is secured with multiple K-wires to stabilize the joint and create a fibrodesis

reduction and pin fixation of both SL and LT lig injuries [2]. Arthroscopic reduction and pinning could be combined with ligament repairs using bone anchors. In an acute perilunate instability injury, however, most colleagues will still recommend open reduction through a palmar and a dorsal approach, repair of the ligaments (the radioscaphocapitate, the lunotriquetral, and the scapholunate ligaments), K-wire fixation, and immobilization [8]. Closed reduction and immobilization only should not be the treatment of choice.

Plication of LT Lig Tears

Suture plication of the UC lig is performed to shorten the length of the ligaments, thus trying to prevent excessive lunotriquetral motion [14]. With the arm in the traction tower, and the scope in the 3–4 portal, the interval between the UL and the UT ligaments should be identified and debrided. A volar portal is then established on the ulnar side in the soft spot adjacent to the prestyloid recess, the volar 6U portal (Fig. 17.17). After having made a skin incision and identified the dorsal sensory branch of the ulnar nerve, a spinal or epidural (Tuohy) needle is used to pass along the immediate volar side of the UT and UL lig to enter the radiocarpal joint at the radial side of the UL lig. From inside the joint, a suture passed through the needle is retrieved and brought back to the volar 6U portal (Fig. 17.18a, b). The suture will now make a loop around the UT and UL lig and is tightened (Fig. 17.18c, d). The need for additional sutures should be evaluated by inspecting the LT interval with the scope in the MCJ as tension is applied to the sutures, one at a time. Additional one or two suture loops are placed, each suture some millimeters distal to the former; the goal is to reduce the gap over the LT joint (Fig. 17.18e, f). Pinning of the LT interval is performed as previously described together with this procedure; the joint is reduced, the K-wires are inserted, and then the plication sutures are tied (Fig. 17.19a, b). Immobilization of the forearm is recommended as previously described. In a series of 21 patients with different backgrounds, different time from injury to treatment, and different concomitant injuries, nine out of 21 patients had excellent or good results, while the Mayo wrist score increased from an average of 50 preoperatively to 88 postoperatively [14]. Complications included prolonged tenderness along the ECU tendon and neuritis of the dorsal branch of the ulnar nerve.

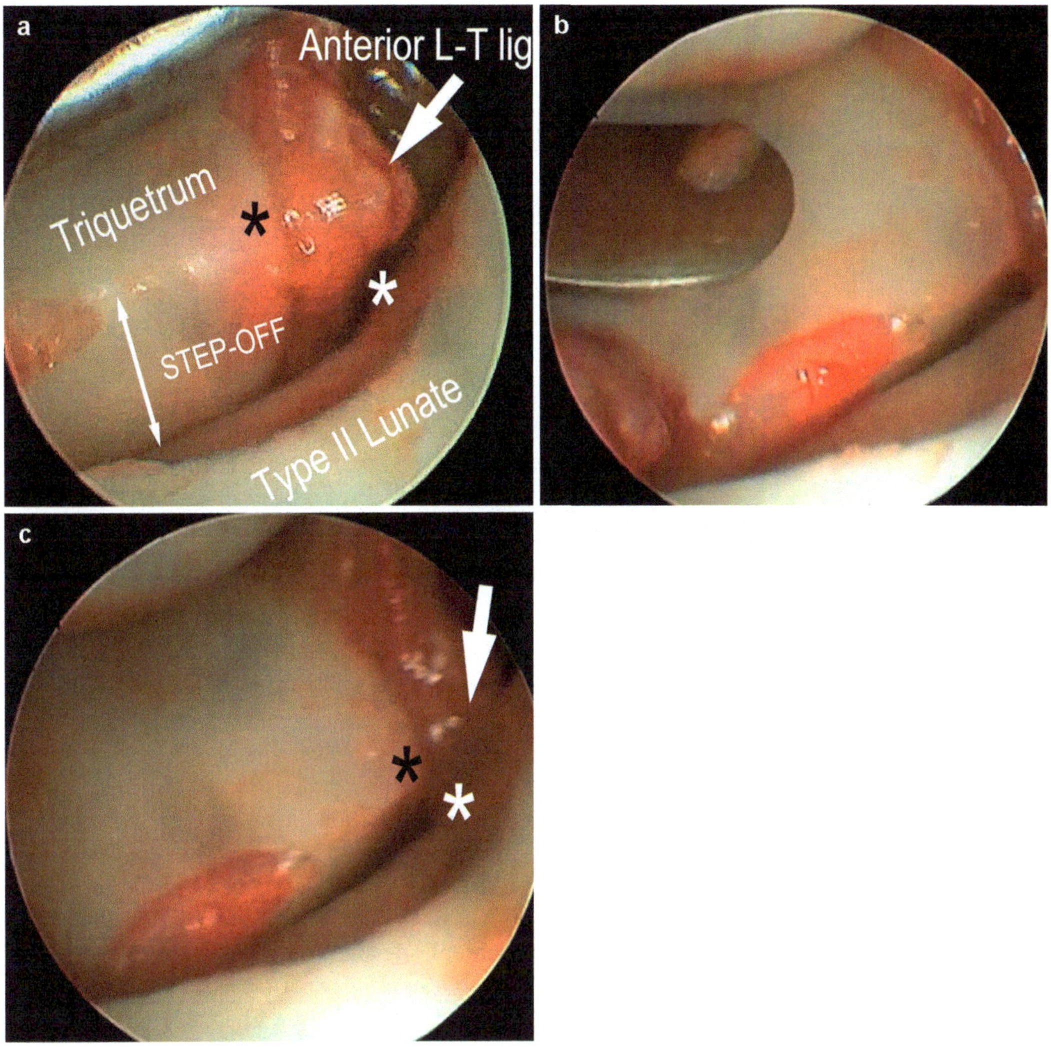

Fig. 17.16 (**a**–**c**) Acute unstable LT dislocation reduced under arthroscopic control. (**a**) *Asterisks* mark the anterior ulnar corner of the lunate and the anterior radial corner of the triquetrum. Most of the LT ligament is still attached to the triquetrum. (**b**) By means of a Freer elevator and external maneuvers, the triquetrum is being reduced to the lunate. (**c**) Preplaced Kirschner wires in the triquetrum have been pushed further into the lunate, thus maintaining the reduction. Notice that the anterior LT ligament is now in contact with the remnants of the LT ligament of the lunate (Case courtesy of Dr. Piñal)

Chronic Tears

Conservative Treatment

Cast immobilization with or without midcarpal corticosteroid injections has been advocated as conservative treatment [5, 25, 28]. The patients may experience temporary relief; however, other options should be used for correction of malalignment and reestablishment of normal proximal row integrity.

Surgery

As already stated, many techniques described in the previous section (acute injuries) are used for chronic tears as well. The results are reported as relatively good; however, the results are difficult to

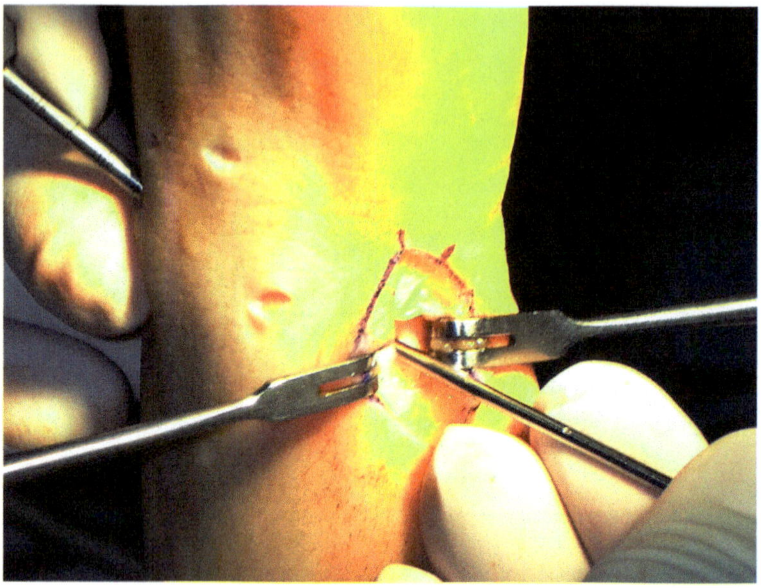

Fig. 17.17 The volar 6U portal has been established

interpret as most of the series are retrospective presenting an inhomogeneous cohort, small groups of patients, or case series [14, 19, 23, 24, 37].

Other treatment options should be considered when debridement and LT pin fixation fail or when a chronic instability is diagnosed with a carpal collapse [31]. These options include ligament reconstruction, capsulodesis, tenodesis, or arthrodesis [18, 26, 29]. Shin and coworkers ([29]; see also Chap. 21) described a reconstruction of the LT lig using a distally based strip of the ECU tendon passed through tunnels in the triquetrum and the lunate to be sutured to itself over the dorsum of the wrist (Fig. 17.20a–g); this method was compared to ligament repair and arthrodesis. They found the probability of remaining free from complications at 5 years to be close to 70 % for the reconstruction, between 10 % and 15 % for the repair, while less than 1 % for arthrodesis. Other authors also report imperfect results for arthrodesis [38], as are our results. The reconstruction has so far been performed as an open procedure; however, as we gain further experience, the arthroscopic-assisted technique might evolve as has been shown for other ligamentoplasties in the wrist [7]. Likewise, the LT arthrodesis is today performed as an arthroscopic-assisted procedure (see Chap. 23).

For chronic LT lig tears on the basis of an ulnar impaction, any treatment of the LT lig complex should be combined with treatment of the ulnar impaction (see Chap. 13).

Fig. 17.18 (**a**–**f**) After having established the volar 6U portal, a spinal needle is passed immediately volar to the UT and UL lig to enter the RC joint on the radial border of the UL lig (**a**). A suture passed through the needle is retrieved and passed back to the volar 6U portal (**b**). While tightening the suture, the gap between the UT and UL ligaments should be inspected (**c**, **d**). Additional suture loops may be placed just distal to the first suture to reduce the gap (**e**, **f**). The arthroscope should be in the MCJ when tightening the sutures to watch the closening of the LT interval

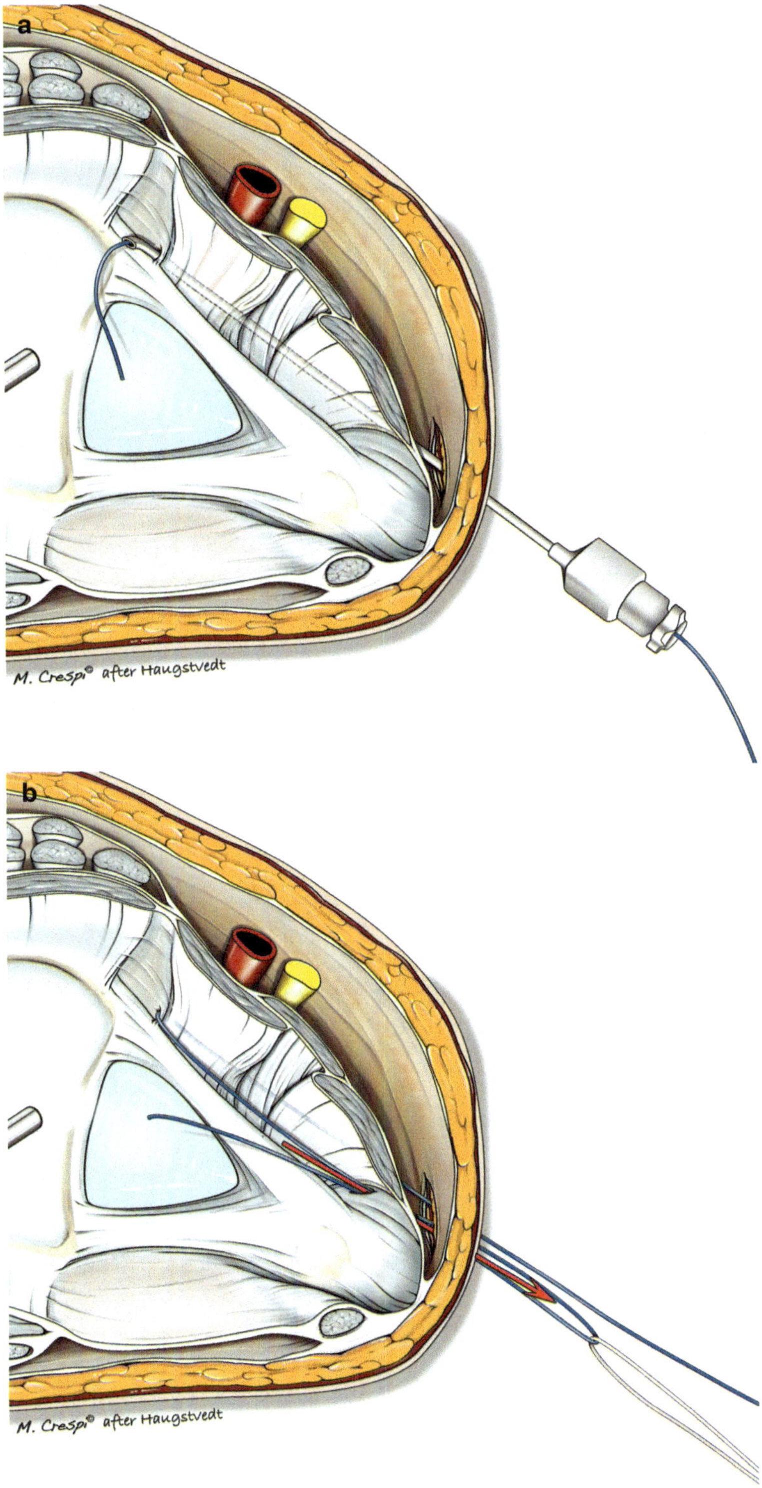
a
M. Crespi© after Haugstvedt
b
M. Crespi© after Haugstvedt

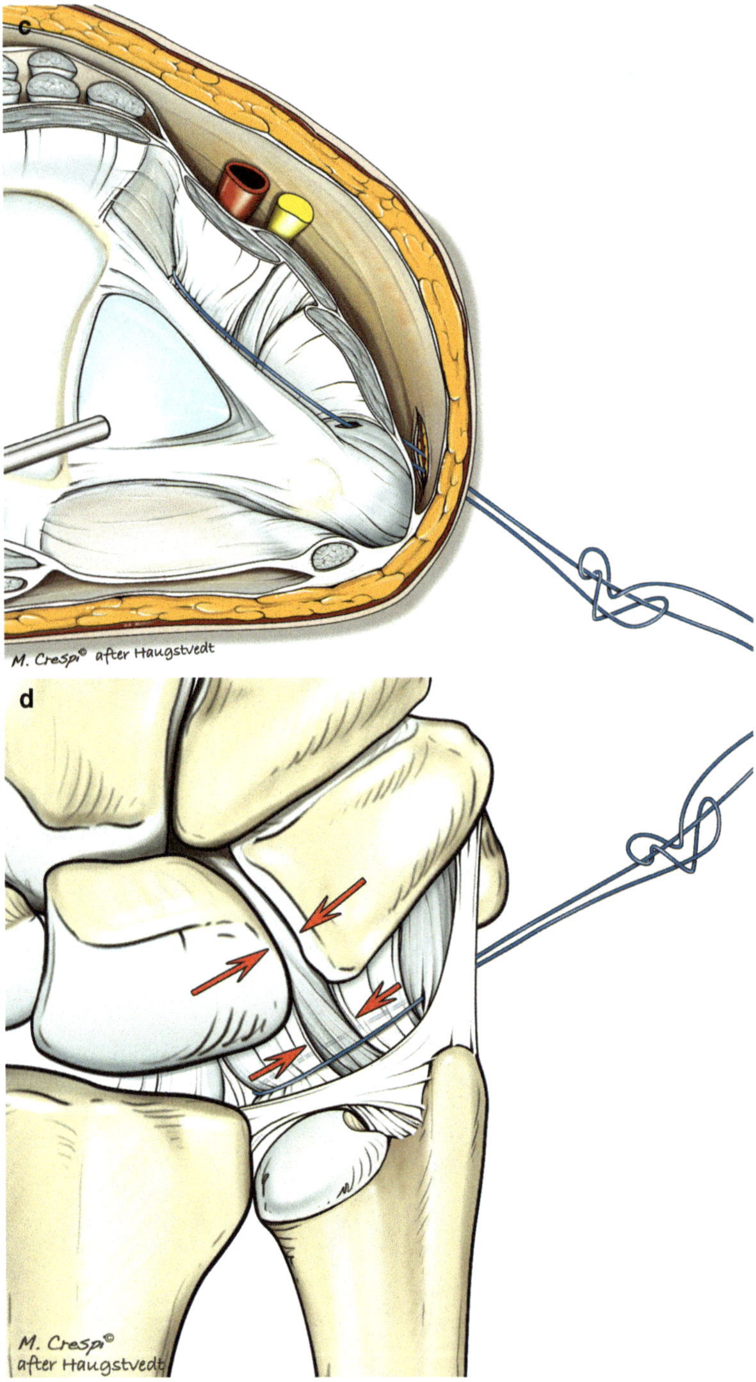

Fig. 17.18 (continued)

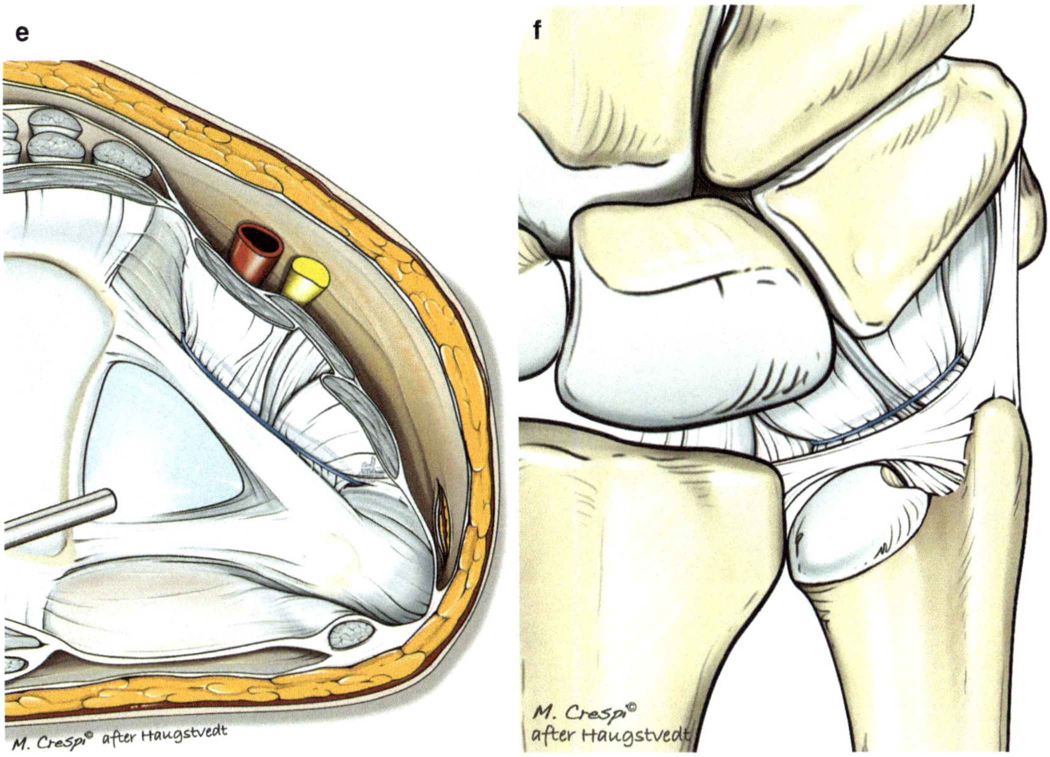

Fig. 17.18 (continued)

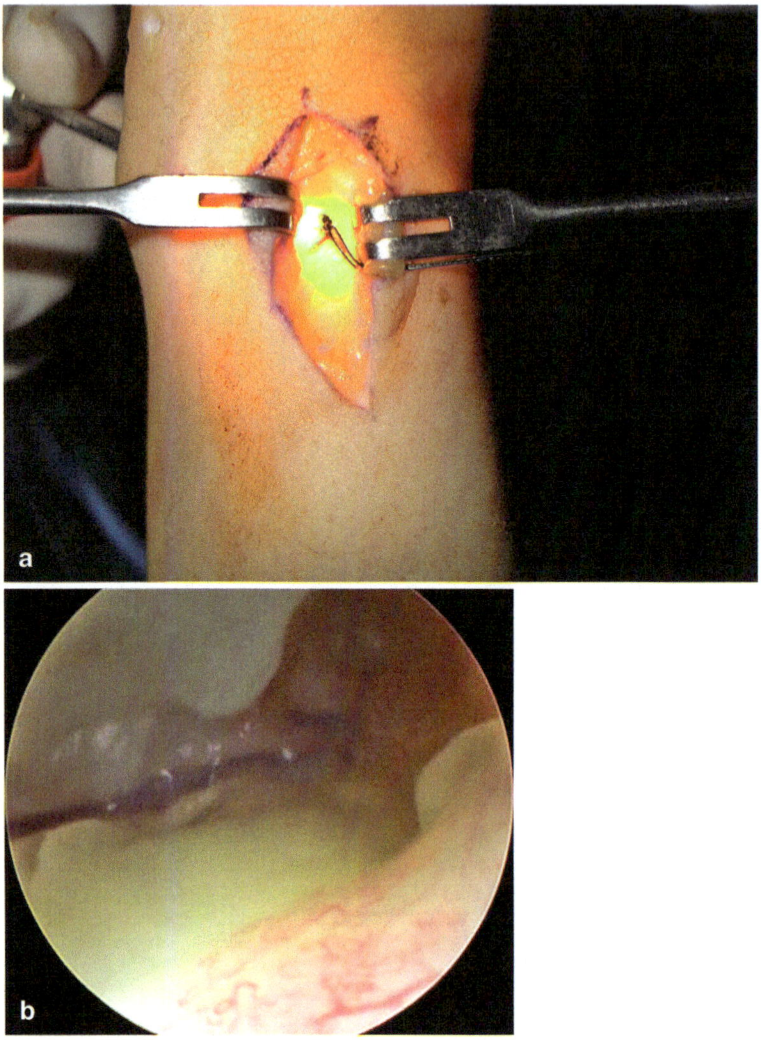

Fig. 17.19 (**a**, **b**) The suture viewed from outside the volar 6U portal (**a**) and through the arthroscope from the RC joint (**b**)

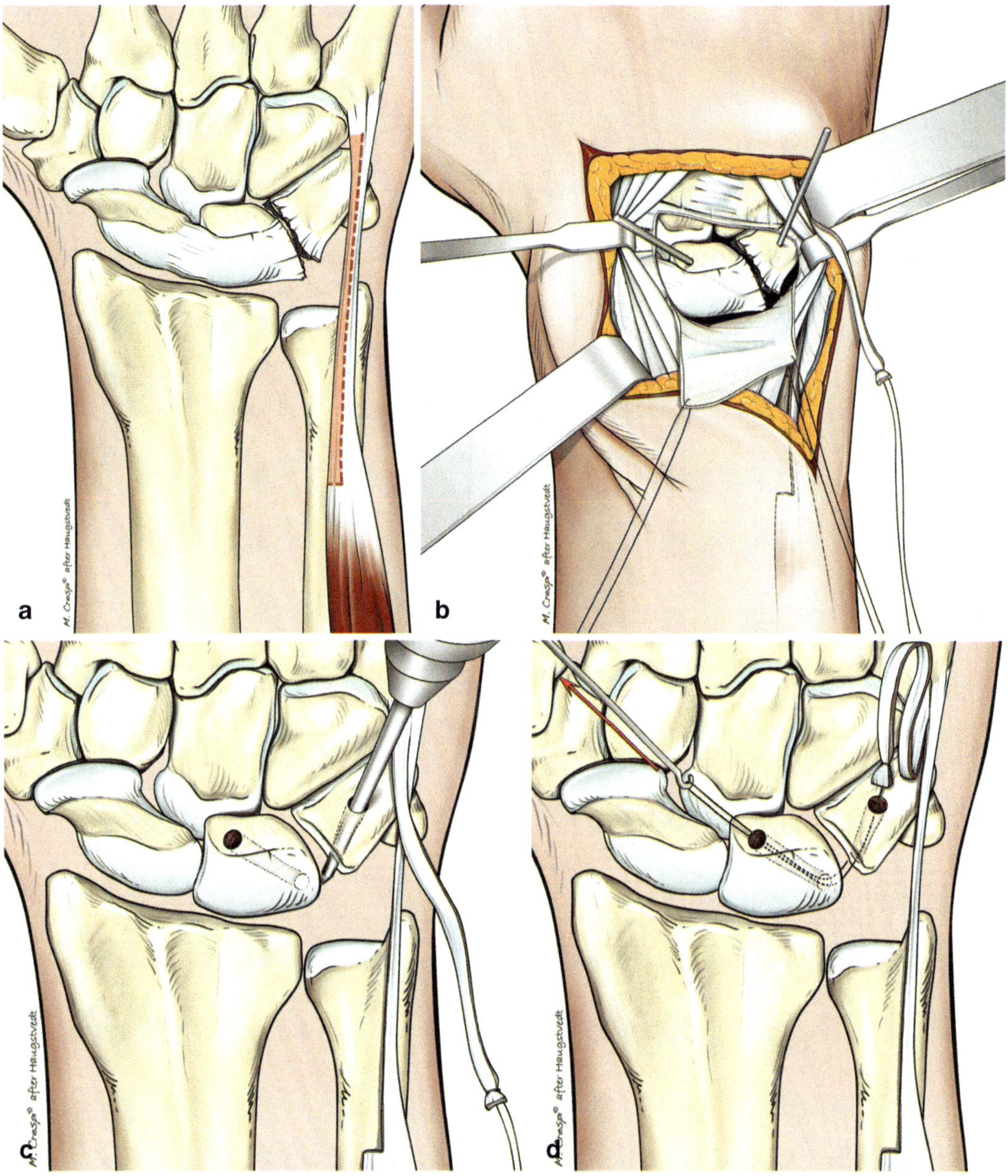

Fig. 17.20 (**a–g**) When a reconstruction of the LT lig is planned for a distally based part of the ECU tendon is prepared (**a**). A capsulotomy is performed and the diagnosis is verified (**b**). A K-wire is drilled into the triquetrum from a dorsal ulnar point in a volar radial direction to come out in the triquetrum close to the volar side of the bone in the LT joint. Another K-wire is drilled into the lunate from a dorsal radial point to come out in the LT joint where the first K-wire (through the triquetrum) exited. After the position of the K-wires is verified, 3-mm drill holes are made (**c**). A suture attached to the tendon is passed through the drill holes (**d**), and the tendon is then pulled through the holes (**e**). The tendon is pulled tight while the gap over the LT interval is closed and reduced and the position is secured by two K-wires. The tendon is then sutured to itself (**f, g**) routed through the triquetrum and the lunate to be secured to itself on the dorsum of the hand

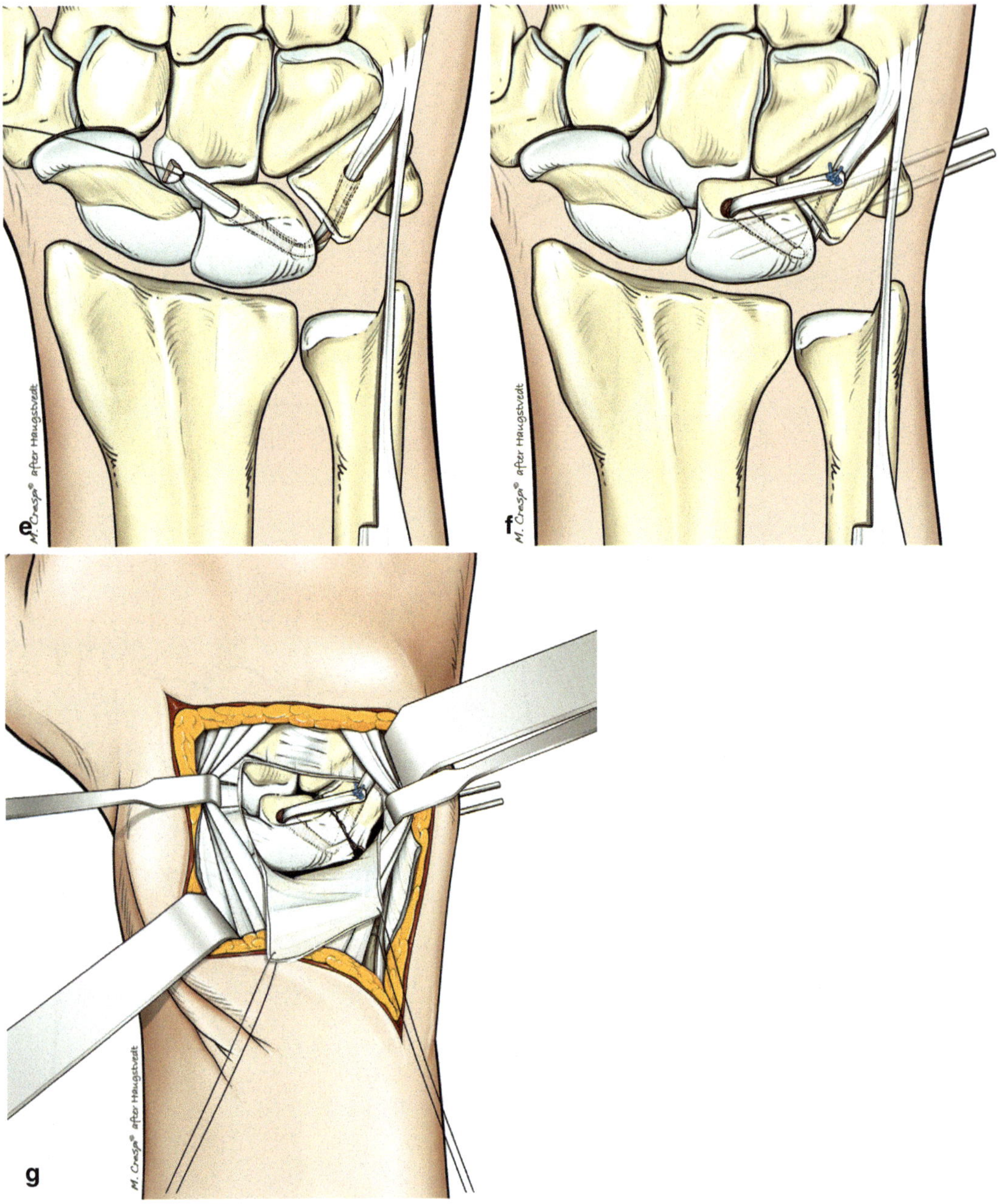

Fig. 17.20 (continued)

References

1. Ambrose L, Posner M (1992) Lunate-triquetral and midcarpal joint instability. Hand Clin 8:653–686
2. Badia A, Khanchandani P (2009) The floating lunate: arthroscopic treatment of simultaneous complete tears of the scapholunate and lunotriquetral ligaments. Hand 4(3):250–255
3. Berger RA (1999) Arthroscopic anatomy of the wrist and the distal radioulnar joint. Hand Clin 15:393–413
4. Berger RA (2001) The anatomy of the ligaments of the wrist and distal radioulnar joints. Clin Orthop Relat Res 383:32–40
5. Cohen MS (1998) Ligamentous injuries of the wrist in the athlete. Clin Sports Med 17:533–552
6. Cooney WP (1993) Evaluation of chronic wrist pain by arthrography, arthroscopy, and arthrotomy. J Hand Surg 18A:815–822
7. Corella F, Cerro MD, Larrainzar-Garijo R, Vázquez T (2011) Arthroscopic ligamentoplasty (bone-tendon-tenodesis). A new surgical technique for scapholunate instability: preliminary cadaver study. J Hand Surg 36E:682–689
8. Garcia-Elias M, Geissler WB (2005) Carpal instability. In: Green DP (ed) Green's operative hand surgery, 5th edn. Elsevier Inc, Philadelphia
9. Geissler WB, Fernandez DL, Lamey DM (1996) Distal radioulnar joint injuries associated with fractures of the distal radius. Clin Orthop Relat Res 327: 135–146
10. Gilula LA, Weeks PM (1978) Post-traumatic ligamentous instabilities of the wrist. Radiology 129:641–651
11. Horii E, Garcia-Elias M, An KN, Bishop AT, Cooney WP III, Linscheid RL, Chao EY (1991) A kinematic study of luno-triquetral dissociations. J Hand Surg 16A:355–362
12. Kirschenbaum D, Coyle MP, Leddy JP (1993) Chronic lunotriquetral instability: diagnosis and treatment. J Hand Surg 18A:1107–1112
13. Kleinmann WB (1985) The luno-triquetral shuck test. Am Soc Surg Hand Corr News:51
14. Levine JW, Savoie FH III, Moskal MJ (2008) Arthroscopic plication of lunotriquetral ligament tears. In: Slutsky DJ, Nagle DJ (eds) Techniques in wrist and hand arthroscopy. Elsevier Inc, Philadelphia
15. Lindau T, Arner M, Hagberg L (1997) Intraarticular lesions in distal fractures of the radius in young adults. A descriptive arthroscopic study in 50 patients. J Hand Surg 22B:638–643
16. Mayfield JK, Johnson RP, Kilcoyne RK (1980) Carpal dislocations: pathomechanics and progressive perilunar instability. J Hand Surg 5A:226–241
17. Metz VM, Mann FA, Gilula LA (1993) Lack of correlation between site of wrist pain and location of noncommunicating defects shown by three-compartment wrist arthrography. AJR Am J Roentgenol 160: 1239–1243
18. Omokawa S, Fujitani R, Inada Y (2009) Dorsal radiocarpal ligament capsulodesis for chronic dynamic lunotriquetral instability. J Hand Surg 34A: 237–243
19. Osterman AL, Seidman GD (1995) The role of arthroscopy in the treatment of lunatotriquetral ligament injuries. Hand Clin 11:41–49
20. Reagan DS, Linscheid RL, Dobyns JH (1984) Lunotriquetral sprains. J Hand Surg 9A:502–514
21. Ritt JPF, Bishop AT, Berger RA, Linscheid RL, Berglund LJ, An KN (1998) Lunotriquetral ligament properties: a comparison of three anatomic subregions. J Hand Surg 23A:425–431
22. Ritt JPF, Linscheid RL, Cooney WP III, Berger RA, An KN (1998) The lunotriquetral joint: kinematic effects of sequential ligament sectioning, ligament repair, and arthrodesis. J Hand Surg 23A:432–445
23. Ritter MR, Chang DS, Ruch DS (1999) The role of arthroscopy in the treatment of lunotriquetral ligament injuries. Hand Clin 15(3):445–454
24. Ruch DS, Poehling GG (1996) Arthroscopic management of partial scapholunate and lunotriquetral injuries of the wrist. J Hand Surg 21A:412–417
25. Sachar K (2008) Ulnar-sided wrist pain: evaluation and treatment of triangular fibrocartilage complex tears, ulnocarpal impaction syndrome, and lunotriquetral ligament tears. J Hand Surg 33A:1669–1679
26. Shahane SA, Trail IA, Takwale VJ, Stilwell JH, Stanley JK (2005) Tenodesis of the extensor carpi ulnaris for chronic, post-traumatic lunotriquetral instability. J Bone Joint Surg Br 87B:1512–1515
27. Schweitzer ME, Brahme SK, Hodler J, Hanker GJ, Lynch TP, Flanningan BD, Godzik CA, Resnik D (1992) Chronic wrist pain: spin-echo and tau inversion recovery MR imaging and conventional arthrography. Radiology 182:205–211
28. Shin AY, Battaglia MH, Bishop AT (2000) Lunotriquetral instability: diagnosis and treatment. J Am Acad Orthop Surg 8:170–179
29. Shin AY, Weinstein LP, Berger RA, Bishop AT (2001) Treatment of isolated injuries of the lunotriquetral ligament. A comparison of arthrodesis, ligament reconstruction and ligament repair. J Bone Joint Surg Br 83B:1023–1028
30. Slutsky DJ (2008) Incidence of dorsal radiocarpal ligament tears in the presence of other intercarpal derangements. Arthroscopy 24(5):526–533
31. Taleisnik J (1987) Pain on the ulnar side of the wrist. Hand Clin 3:51–68
32. Trumble TE, Bour CJ, Smith RJ, Glisson RR (1990) Kinematics of the ulnar carpus related to the volar intercalated segment instability pattern. J Hand Surg 15A:384–392
33. Trumble TE, Bour CJ, Smith RJ, Edwards GS (1988) Intercarpal arthrodesis for static and dynamic palmar intercalated segment instability. J Hand Surg 13A: 396–402

34. Viegas SF, Patterson RM, Peterson PD, Pogue DJ, Jenkins DK, Sweo TD, Hokanson JA (1990) Ulnar-sided perilunate instability: an anatomic and biomechanic study. J Hand Surg 15A:268–278
35. Viegas SF, Wagner K, Patterson R, Peterson P (1990) Medial (hamate) facet of the lunate. J Hand Surg 15A:564–571
36. Weiss APC, Akelman E, Lambiase R (1996) Comparison of the findings of triple-injection cinearthrography of the wrist with those of arthroscopy. J Bone Joint Surg Br 78A:348–356
37. Weiss APC, Sachar K, Glowacki KA (1997) Arthroscopic debridement alone for intercarpal ligament tears. J Hand Surg 22A:344–349
38. Weiss LE, Taras JS, Sweet S, Osterman AL (2000) Lunotriquetral injuries in the athlete. Hand Clin 16(3):433–438
39. Zlatkin MB, Chao PC, Osterman AL, Schnall MD, Dalinka MK, Kressel HY (1989) Chronic wrist pain: evaluation with high resolution MR imaging. Radiology 173:723–729

Arthroscopic Management of Piso-Triquetral Conditions

18

Jon Compson

Introduction

The piso-triquetral (PT) joint is a relatively common site of ulnar-sided wrist pain. The pain arises either from the tendon of flexor carpi ulnaris (FCU), its stabilising ligaments or the joint itself. Though in many cases the symptoms and signs of joint pain are clear-cut, in a few cases, it is difficult to localise the pain especially when wear or instability is early or subtle. The joint is sometimes difficult or impossible to scope, but when it can arthroscopy can be a useful tool in assessing the source of pain (Fig. 18.1).

Arthroscopy of any joint evolves through a series of levels. It probably starts as a desire to see if it can be done and to record the arthroscopic anatomy. Then comes diagnosis of known general and joint specific pathology. Further to this and an important use of any small joint arthroscopy is the assessment of the degree of wear or soft tissue injury which is important when proceeding either to further arthroscopic or open surgery. This is especially important in areas where the non-invasive imaging techniques are poor. The last stage is the development of therapeutic techniques.

With the piso-triquetral joint, we are probably at the assessment level rather than therapeutic since the anatomy, especially the proximity of the ulnar nerve makes intervention risky. The advantage of being able to assess the joint arthroscopically is that the joint can be a very important component of ulnar-sided wrist pain, either the primary problem or secondary to changes in ulnar-sided mechanics. Unfortunately, x-rays, MRI, CT and radionuclear scans can be misleading. An important reason to get the diagnosis right is that one cannot see the joint surface of the pisiform during pisiformectomy through standard approaches until the bone is completely removed. Though pisiformectomy is now a fairly common and validated procedure [14], there are still a significant number of patients, particularly where there is little wear that have poor

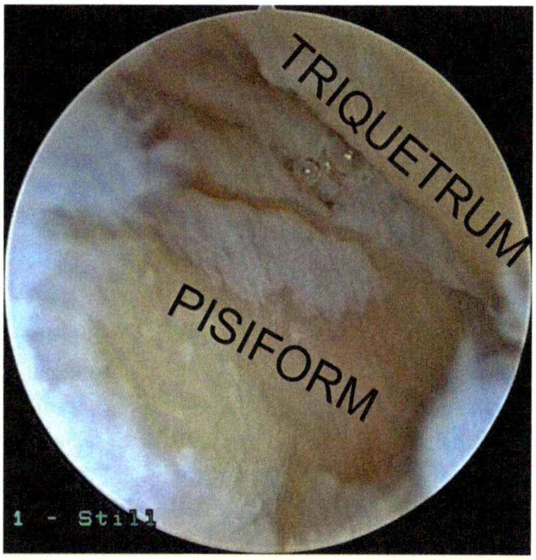

Fig. 18.1 Osteoarthritis of the piso-triquetral joint, well seen from 6R portal. Triquetrum is *top right* and pisiform below and to the *left*

J. Compson
Upper Limb Unit, Kings College Hospital,
Denmark Hill, London SE5 9RS, UK
e-mail: jonathan.compson@nhs.net

F. del Piñal et al. (eds.), *Arthroscopic Management of Ulnar Pain*,
DOI 10.1007/978-3-642-30544-3_18, © Springer-Verlag Berlin Heidelberg 2012

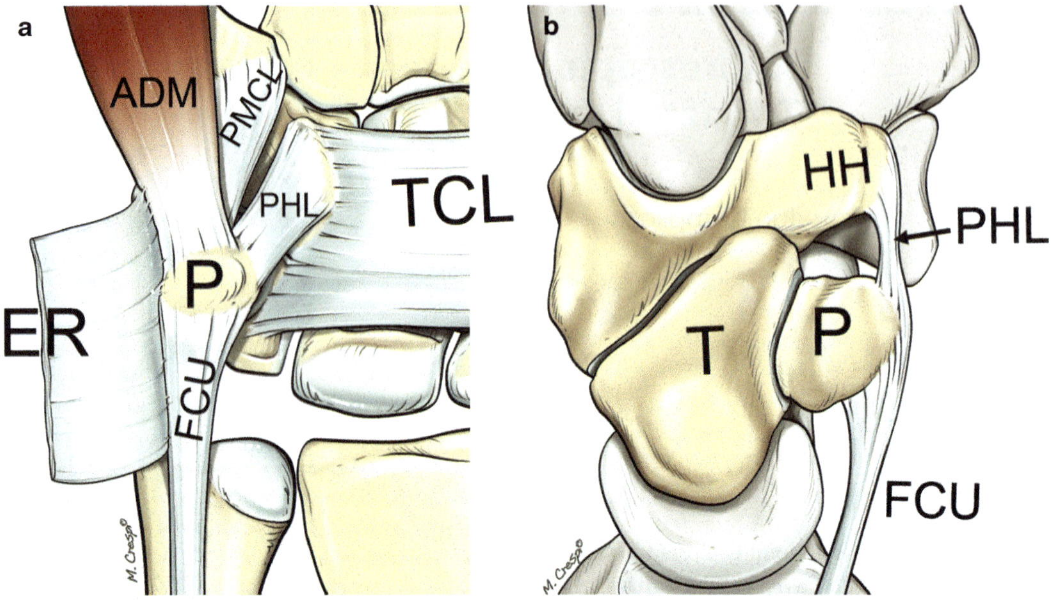

Fig. 18.2 The superficial volar stabiliser of the pisiform. Volar view (**a**) and sagittal view (**b**). Pisiform (*P*), flexor carpi ulnaris (*FCU*), transverse carpal ligament (*TCL*), extensor retinaculum (*ER*), piso-hamate ligament (*PHL*), piso-metacarpal ligament (*PMCL*), abductor digiti minimi (*ADM*), hook of hamate (*HH*)

results [31]. It is better to be sure of the pathology before surgery rather than when too late! Arthroscopy of the piso-triquetral joint is very useful both in confirming and excluding piso-triquetral pathology, especially when the clinical findings and imaging are not specific. The problem is that one cannot see the joint easily in some patients, but if it can it should be a routine part of any wrist arthroscopy.

Anatomy of the Piso-Triquetral Joint

The pisiform though said to be a carpal bone and part of the proximal carpal row is in many aspects unique. It is considered by most people to be a sesamoid bone lying in the tendon of flexor carpi ulnaris (FCU) and acts separately to the intercalated proximal row. In many ways, it acts similar to the patella in the knee in that it increases the lever arm and therefore the strength of the FCU by holding the tendon away from its centre of rotation and to some degree stabilising it. It articulates with the volar surface of the triquetrum by a separate oval joint surface. Though one could consider the FCU inserts into the pisiform, in many ways, the tendon extends distal to the bone as the piso-hamate and piso-metacarpal ligaments.

The stability of the piso-triquetral joint relies on its soft tissue attachment since the joint itself is almost flat with only a slight concavity of the pisiform and convexity of the triquetrum. The volar stabilisers (Fig. 18.2a, b) are the transverse carpal ligament, the extensor retinaculum, the piso-hamate and the piso-metacarpal ligaments helped by the flexor carpi ulnaris tendon and the abductor digiti minimi muscle, which act as a single continuous structure [24]. There is variability. Yamaguchi et al. [33] found three types of distal tendon/ligament attachments to the hook of hamate and the base of the metacarpal.

Around the joint itself, the capsule is weak; however, on the ulnar side the extensor retinaculum overlies the capsule making this, the subcutaneous side, more stable. The radial side is relatively weak so any maltracking, subluxation or dislocation will be towards the ulnar side (Fig. 18.3).

When considering arthroscopic visualisation of the joint and potential portals, one needs to know the anatomy of the structures around the joint and in particular the ulnar nerve and its cutaneous branches. The main ulnar nerve lies intimately to the radial side of the joint [22] between it and the artery (Fig. 18.3). On the ulnar side of the joint, there is the capsule and extensor retinaculum. Between this and the skin are cutaneous branches of the ulnar nerve. The main dorsal branches lie proximal and dorsal to the joint, though there may be some branches supplying the ulnar side of the hand overlying the joint itself. Distal and ulnar lie branches of the proper digital nerve to the little finger and its branches. The most likely direct portal to the piso-triquetral joint, from the ulnar side, lies in the watershed between these nerves so it is theoretically safe from producing nerve damage (Fig. 18.4). Saying that, despite the many extensive studies on the cutaneous nerve supply he hand [5, 17, 23, 30], more anatomical studies are needed to verify this and also look for high-risk variations which are quite common in the cutaneous nerves of the hand.

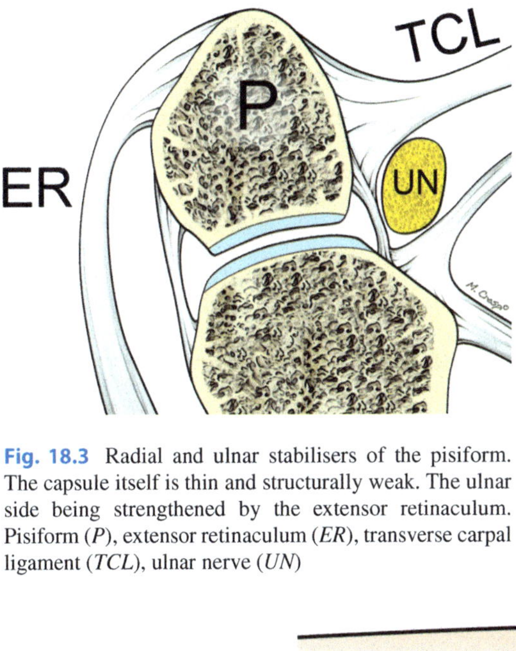

Fig. 18.3 Radial and ulnar stabilisers of the pisiform. The capsule itself is thin and structurally weak. The ulnar side being strengthened by the extensor retinaculum. Pisiform (*P*), extensor retinaculum (*ER*), transverse carpal ligament (*TCL*), ulnar nerve (*UN*)

There is in most wrist joints a natural connection between the main radio-carpal joint and the piso-triquetral which Berger [6] describes as passing through the substance of the ulno-triquetral ligament. The number of people with this connection has been evaluated by anatomists and radiologists. It was originally thought that less than a third of wrists have this connection [15, 20]. However, Keopp [13] found it present in 76 % of anatomical specimens, and in a large study Viegas and colleagues [32] found it present in 88 % of unembalmed specimens. Arthrography has confirmed a similar frequency [21]. We felt that the best way to see the piso-triquetral joint arthroscopically was from the radio-carpal joint [3]. However, we were not sure how large the hole was or if we would need to open a passage. We therefore recorded the type of connection and their frequency in a series of cases. We found that there are four types of connection (see Table 18.1) (Fig. 18.5a–f). We found in most cases the hole was big enough not to require dilatation or constructing.

Biomechanics/Kinematics

The pisiform moves both proximal and distal and transversely across the surface of the triquetrum. In vivo studies [18] show contact is maximum on wrist extension and ulnar deviation which corresponds to the areas of articular surface wear (radial and distal). It is thought that the main

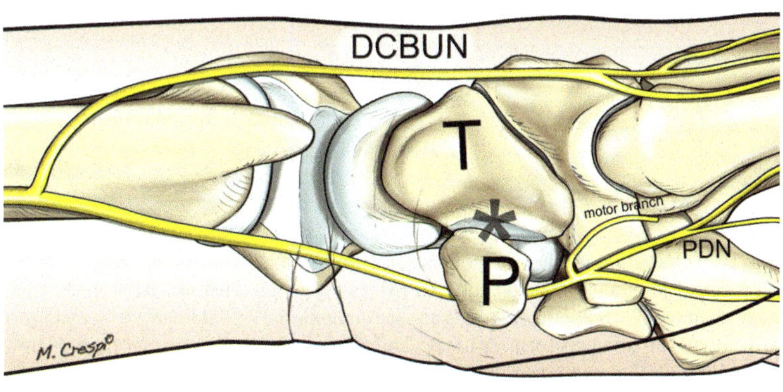

Fig. 18.4 Ulnar-sided cutaneous nerves and their relationship to the piso-triquetral joint *. A potential safe portal to view the joint. Dorsal cutaneous branch of the ulnar nerve (*DCBUN*), proper digital nerve to the little finger (*PDN*), triquetrum (*T*); pisiform (*P*)

Table 18.1 Types of communication between the radio-carpal and piso-triquetral joints [3]

Type 1: Thick synovial membrane preventing joint visualisation	23 %
Type 2: Thin synovial covering allowing for visualisation of pisiform and joint space	15 %
Type 3: Small fenestration in synovial covering	7 %
Type 4: Large fenestration in membrane or no covering	55 %

cause of wear is due to disruption of the normal stabilising ligaments.

Pathology of the Piso-Triquetral Joint

The piso-triquetral joint can suffer all the conditions affecting sesamoid bones. In many ways, it also behaves and suffers like the patella in the knee. Osteoarthritis is the commonest

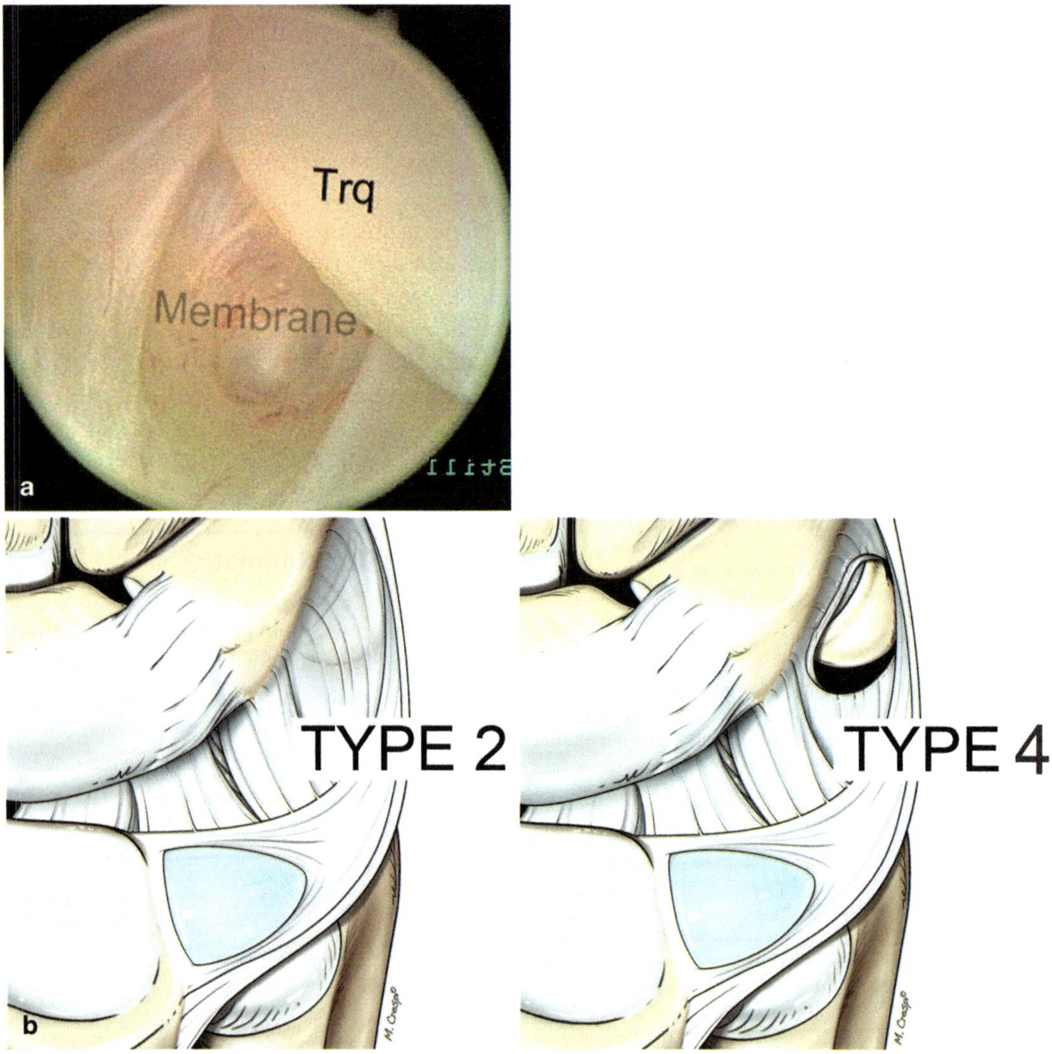

Fig. 18.5 Variation in the communication between the radio-carpal joint and the piso-triquetral [3]. (**a**) Type 1: thick membrane. Sometimes one can see membrane move when palpating pisiform. (**b**) Type 2 allows visualisation through the membrane, whereas type 4 is a large hole. (**c**) Type 2. Thin membrane showing PT joint behind. (**d**) Type 3: small hole allows fluid and air to pass but unable to see pisiform. (**e**) Type 4: large hole. PT joint easily seen from radio-carpal joint and (**f**) after passage of the scope

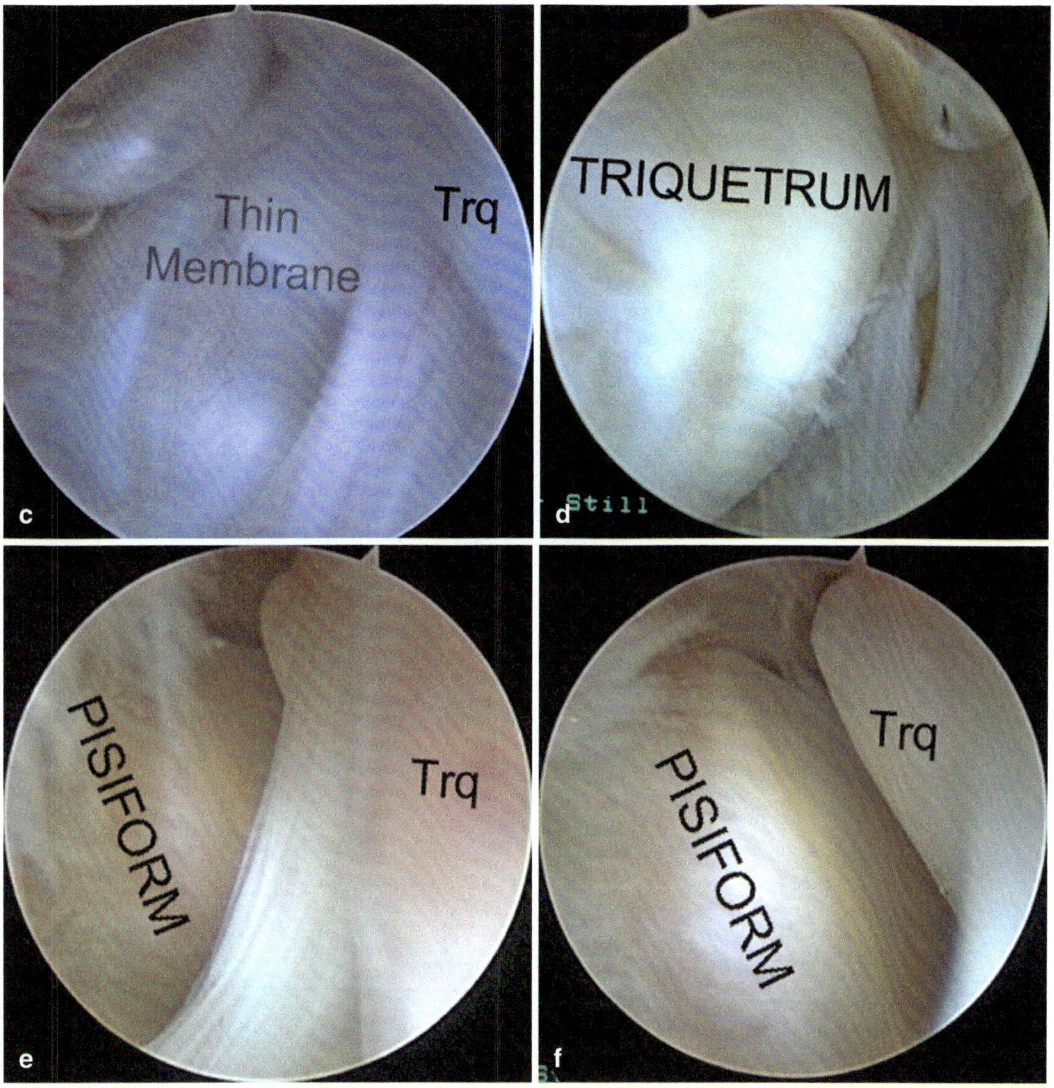

Fig. 18.5 (continued)

affliction, either isolated or associated with arthritis in other parts of the wrist [11], or more commonly, especially in symptomatic patients, secondary to trauma. The wear patterns found in cadaver specimens have been described and divided into five types [33] (see Table 18.2 and Fig. 18.6).

Table 18.2 Types of patterns of degenerative changes in the piso-triquetral joint [33]

Type 1: Central
Type 2: Peripheral
Type 3: Fan-shaped
Type 4: Mix
Type 5: Total

However, it must be remembered that wear is common and is the normal finding in the cadavers used in anatomical studies. Many of which were probably asymptomatic. Pevny et al. [22] found at least mild wear on both the pisiform and triquetrum present in all 29 cadavers they studied. Similarly, Rayan et al. [24] found it in 10 out of 12 specimens. Yamaguchi et al. [33]

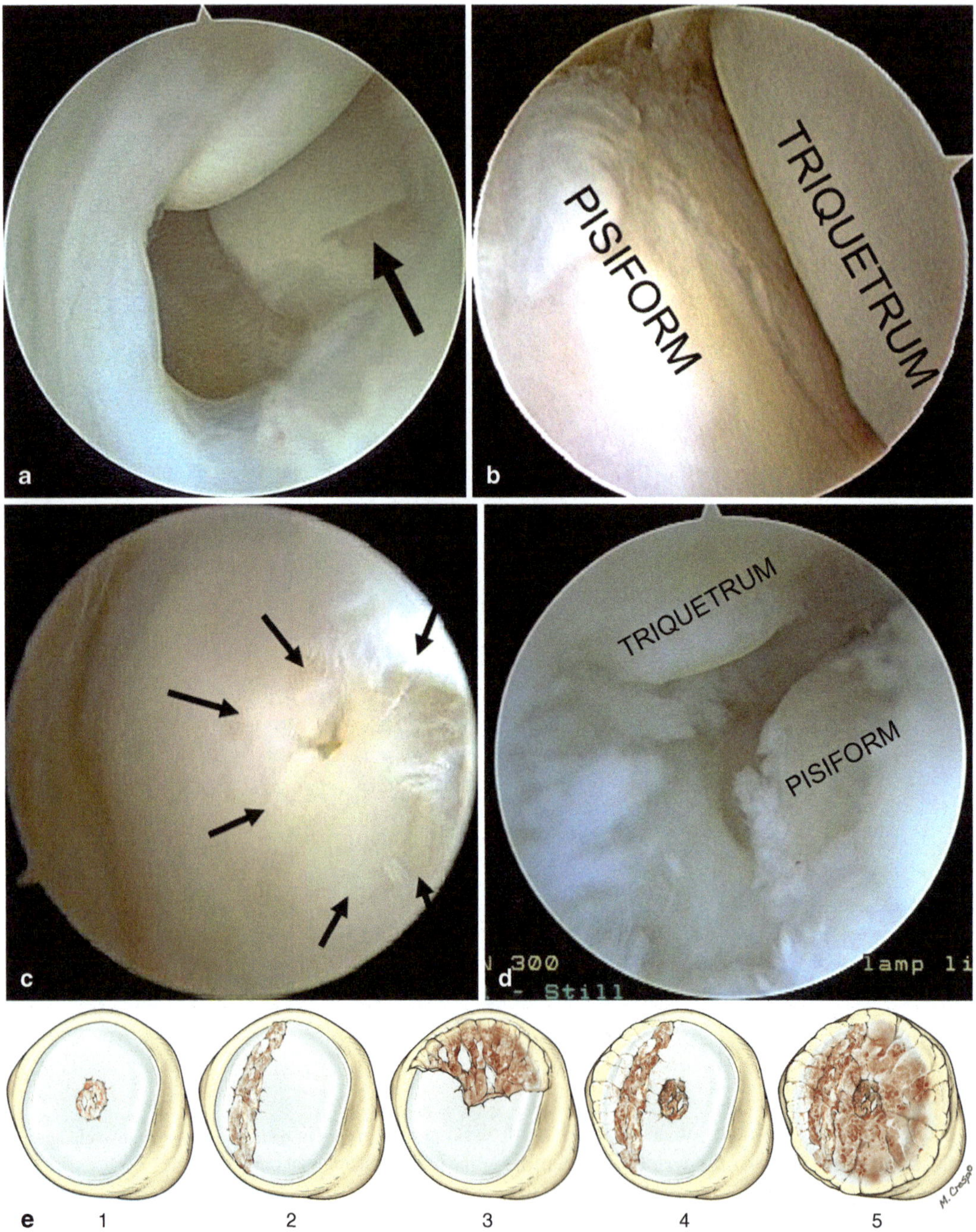

Fig. 18.6 Wear in the piso-triquetral joint as seen arthroscopically. (**a**) Bare areas on side of pisiform (*arrow*). Probably normal. (**b**) Chondromalacia, (**c**) fissuring and chondral ulceration (*limited by arrows*), (**d**) full-thickness wear and (**e**) wear patterns (after Yamaguchi et al. [33])

also showed about 80 % of their cadavers had wear but also that there was a steady increase in both sexes from middle age onwards and often there was wear in both hands. Therefore, it appears chondromalacia and osteoarthritis are normal age-related conditions, and most will be asymptomatic. We must take this into account when attributing ulnar-sided pain to piso-triquetral joint arthritis.

The pisiform is very vulnerable to trauma either from repetitive loads, for instance, from bicycle handlebars or crutches, or the direct trauma when falling on the ulnar side of the outstretch hand, the latter resulting in fractures of the triquetrum, pisiform or crush injuries to the chondral surface. Post-traumatic osteoarthritis can occur after displaced pisiform fractures, triquetral mal-unions [2] or the chondral injuries [27]. It can also result from injuries to the stabilising ligaments with consequent maltracking, subluxation, dislocation and secondary wear. Instability and maltracking are thought by several authors to be the main causes of chronic pain and secondary arthritis.

Loose bodies are uncommon and have only rarely been reported in the literature [9, 19, 26]. They can either arise in isolation in the piso-triquetral joint, be associated with isolated osteoarthritis of the piso-triquetral joint [26], move there from the radio-carpal joint or be part of a more generalised osteoarthritis. Occasional cases of synovial chondromatosis have been reported.

Instability, recurrent dislocation and fixed dislocation have all been reported [8, 10, 16] mostly post-traumatic, though anatomically maltracking is also common. Pain has been reported in the piso-triquetral joint following wrist arthrodesis, arthroplasty and carpal tunnel decompression.

Clinical Examination of the Piso-Triquetral Joint

As with the rest of the carpus, diagnosis is dependent on careful systematic clinical examination [28]. One cannot rely on either imaging or arthroscopy. What one has to rely on is knowledge of the three-dimensional and surface anatomy of the carpus and an ability to visualise this. The points of tenderness are very important in an area with so many structures which can produce pain (see Table 18.3).

Table 18.3 Differential diagnosis of volar ulnar-sided wrist pain

1. Piso-triquetral arthritis. Normally osteoarthritis, either primary or post-traumatic
2. Piso-triquetral instability
3. Piso-triquetral loose bodies
4. Flexor carpi ulnaris tendonitis
5. Detachment tears of TFC from the fovea and the distal limb
6. Ulno-triquetral ligament tears
7. Volar TFC ganglions
8. DRUJ instability and arthritis
9. Non-union of hook of hamate fracture

Examination of the piso-triquetral joint (Fig. 18.7) should start by asking the patient to point, with one finger, to the site of maximal pain. This can be surprisingly accurate! Then to ask if the pain and/or tenderness is worse on any particular movement. If it is, I again ask the patient to point to the site of pain as it is being demonstrated. This can pinpoint pathology in the FCU, the hook of hamate and injuries to the foveal attachment of the TFC. To provoke the pain, sometimes the patient has to press down on the desktop or push the wrists together in a praying position. The pisiform is then easily palpated on the volar side of the wrist at the ulnar end of the distal volar wrist crease. Palpating the ulnar joint line and stressing the PT joint in a radial direction can help localise the pain as can a grind test. Direct pressure on the bone in varying degrees of extension can also be useful.

However, because of the closeness of many of the potentially painful structures, all these must be palpated or tested.

1. Palpate hook of hamate.
2. Palpate FCU and stress testing of the tendon in extension and radial deviation against resistance. This will also provoke the piso-triquetral joint.
3. Palpate each side of the FCU for ganglions.
4. Look for an ulnar foveal sign [29]. Pressure in this area, the soft spot between FCU, the ulnar styloid and the pisiform can indicate pathology in the TFC insertion in the fovea or the ulno-triquetral ligament.

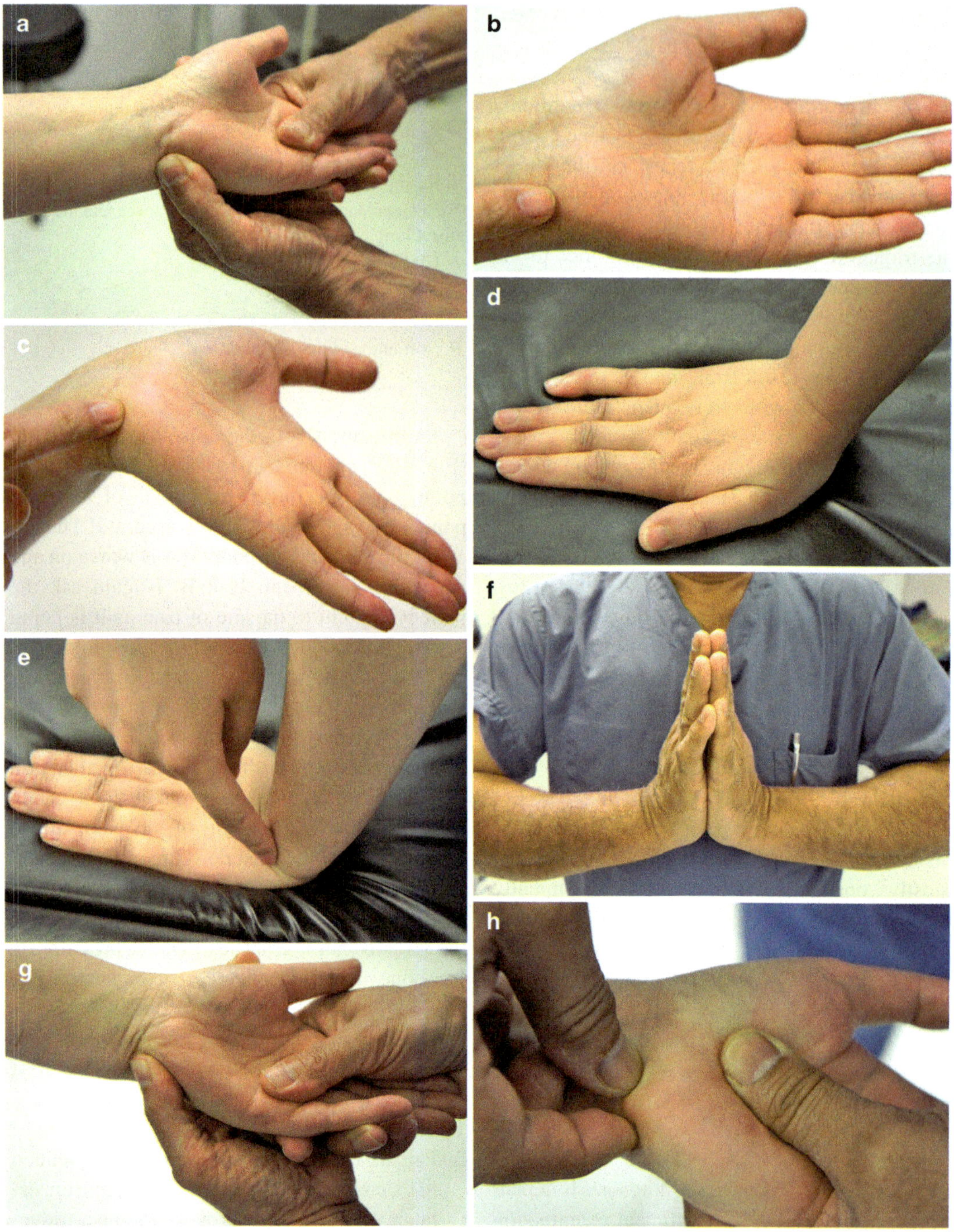

Fig. 18.7 Examination of the piso-triquetral joint. (**a**) The pisiform is easily palpated at the ulnar end of the distal wrist crease. (**b**) It is worth asking the patient to point to the site of maximum pain using one finger! (**c**) Also, to point to pain on maximum range of movement. (**d–f**) Demonstrating what movements produces the pain. (**g**) Stressing the piso-triquetral joint from the ulnar side. (**h**) Grind testing the piso-triquetral joint in varying positions. (**i**) Palpating the hook of hamate (**j**) and flexor carpi ulnaris (**k**). (**l**) Foveal sign, testing attachment of TFC and ulno-triquetral ligaments. (**m**) Testing for ulnar abutment and (**n**) ballottement of luno-triquetral joint

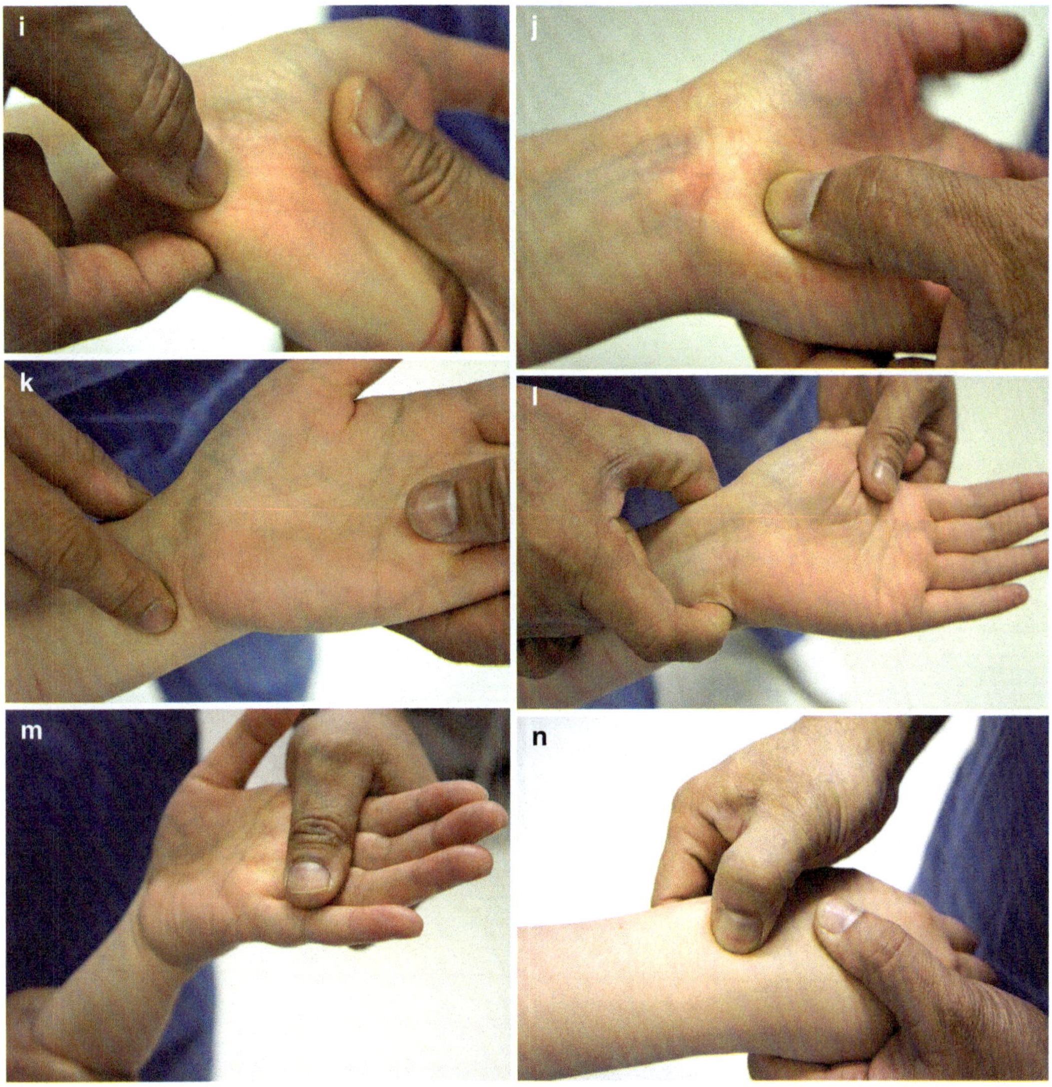

Fig. 18.7 (continued)

5. Make sure there is no pain on ulnar abutment, i.e. passive ulnar deviation.
6. Test the luno-triquetral joint. Remembering ballottement requires holding the pisiform tight to the triquetrum so the pain may be coming from the PT joint itself.
7. Test DRUJ and TFC.

Unfortunately, not all patients are accurate or consistent! I am also not convinced; local anaesthetic injections can actually be that accurate in differentiating the source of pain when there are so many structures in a very confined area.

Imaging of Piso-Triquetral Joint

Imaging of the piso-triquetral joint should be used to confirm the clinical diagnosis made by examination and to help in the exclusion of differential diagnoses. Because standard radiographs of the wrist do not show the piso-triquetral joint well due to overlap of other carpal bone, special views are needed which include the ball catchers and carpal tunnel views (Fig. 18.8a–d). This normally shows the joint line clearly and most pathology including fractures, moderate

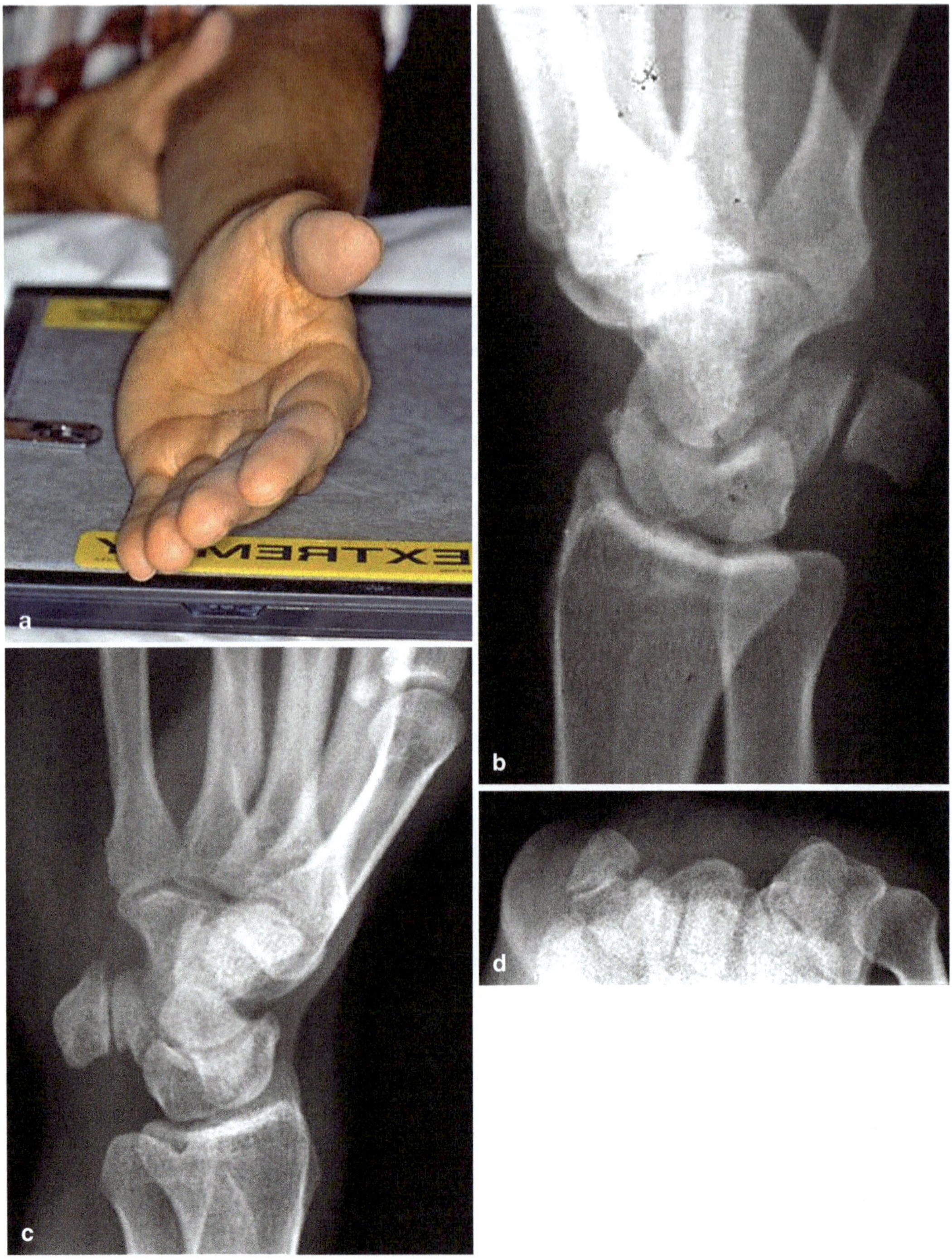

Fig. 18.8 Radiology of the piso-triquetral joint. (**a**) Ball catchers, semisupinated or 45-degree AP (antero-posterior) oblique. (**b**) Normal view of PT joint. (**c**) Osteoarthritic PT joint. (**d**) Carpal tunnel view showing marked wear

and severe wear, calcification of the FCU and loose bodies. However, the main problem is in chondromalacia and early stages of wear when x-ray changes are minimal or non-existent. Tracking of the pisiform or instability obviously cannot be seen on plain x-rays.

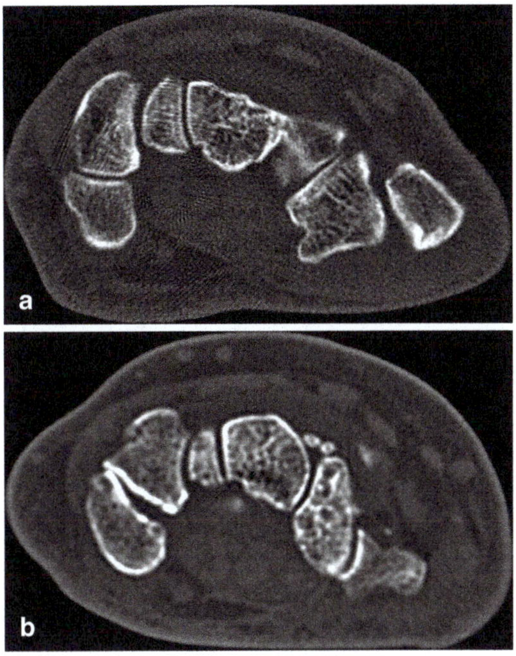

Fig. 18.9 Computerised tomography shows axial view well. Both normal (**a**) and worn (**b**) also shows any subluxation or dislocation (normally ulnarwards)

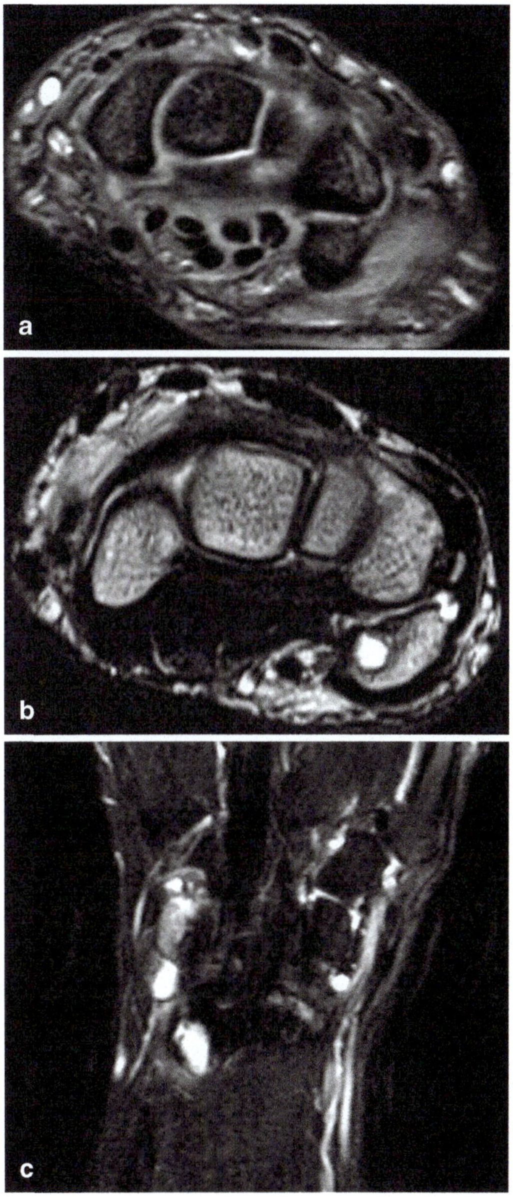

Fig. 18.10 MRI scanning. (**a**) Normal view. (**b**) Severe osteoarthritis. (**c**) Fluid in piso-triquetral joint may not actual arise there

Computerised tomography (CT), because of its ability to show a transverse plane, is good at showing subluxation and dislocation. It also shows unevenness in the width of the joint suggesting partial loss of articular surface and increased sclerosis and cyst formation suggestive of advanced wear. This does not show well on radiographs, and CT is often better than an MRI for this (Fig. 18.9a–b). I tend to use CT as my imaging of choice if the x-ray does not give me the answer. It can show maltracking if cuts are taken in different wrist positions.

Magnetic resonance imaging can be misleading. For instance, fluid in the piso-triquetral joint need not come from the joint itself but from the radio-carpal joint, the piso-triquetral acting as a sump to the main joint collecting the effusion (Fig. 18.10a–c). Also the quality of MRI scans is highly variable, and subtle changes in the articular surface require very good films with no movement artefacts. It can show subchondral cysts better than x-rays and bone oedema indicative of localised loading of the bone or trauma. Its main use for myself is to exclude soft tissue abnormalities like FCU tendonitis and TFC tears.

We used to use SPECT nuclear isotope bone scanning which in the delayed phase can show up both wear and increased loading. SPECT or registration is needed since single-plane scans can be misleading due to overlap of the anatomy.

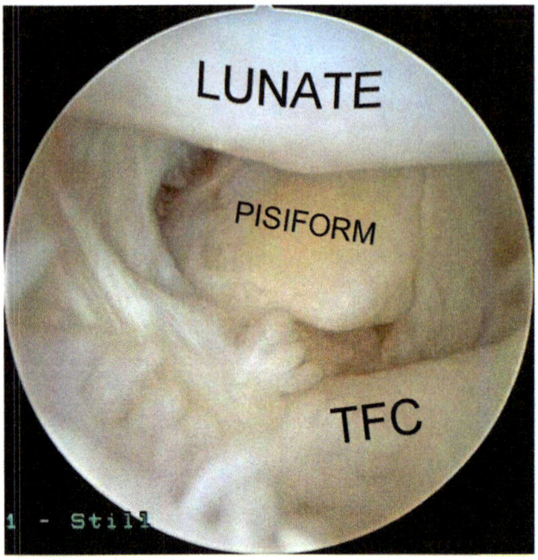

Fig. 18.11 Good view from 3/4 portal. A rare sight!

I tend to use this modality in the cases where there is clinical pain on stressing the PT joint, equivocal x-rays and CT scans, and a complete membrane has prevented me from seeing the joint surfaces arthroscopically. I am not convinced about its anatomic accuracy in many cases so now rarely use it.

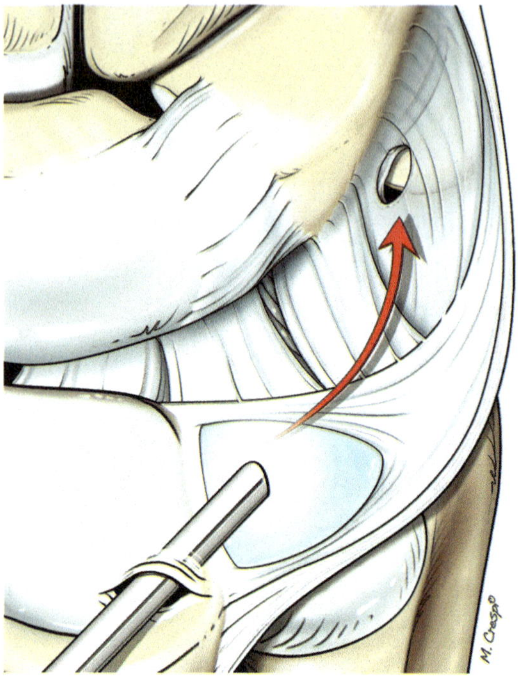

Fig. 18.12 Arthroscopic visualisation of the PT joint from the radio-carpal joint. Looking through the 6R or 4/5 portal, one starts at the TFC/radius junction. Then sweep the scope ulnarwards past the luno-triquetral joint and further into the recess above the distal reflection of the TFC. And then even further! Persistence pays off in difficult cases!

Visualisation Through Standard Portals

As yet, the only way we believe to visualise the piso-triquetral joint is through the standard ulnar-sided radio-carpal portals. Unfortunately, a clear view of the joint is only possible in half of cases. Very occasionally, one can see the pisiform from the 3/4 portal, but this is extremely rare (Fig. 18.11). We tend to use the 4/5 portal more frequently than the 6R to avoid potential damage to the dorsal branch of the ulnar nerve. The visualisation is normally easy but requires persistence since the communication is always more ulnar than one believes. We make this part of our standard arthroscopic examination of the wrist and is particularly important when there is ulnar-sided pain.

The technique (Fig. 18.12) is to start by looking at the lunate then sweeping the scope ulnarwards past the luno-triquetral joint which, if normal, appears like a step. The lower border of the triquetrum is followed, as far as possible, ulnarwards. In the recess, there is either an opening, normally large but occasionally small, or a membrane of variable thickness. The fluid pressure should be increased to either open the passage or to clear synovium away from the membrane. We use handheld syringes for fluid insufflation in our wrist arthroscopies which makes pressure control easier. Often the pisiform can be seen through a thin membrane by manipulating the bone. Relaxing the pressure often produces an air bubble which helps to see a small connecting hole as it moves in or out.

The main tip is to keep going since a thick membrane is rare, and the commonest reason not to see the joint is technique and lack of persistence. Also, it is often better to back off with the scope since it can be difficult to see if one is too close. Moving the scope is best done by rotating into the corner. To see it best in the right hand, a

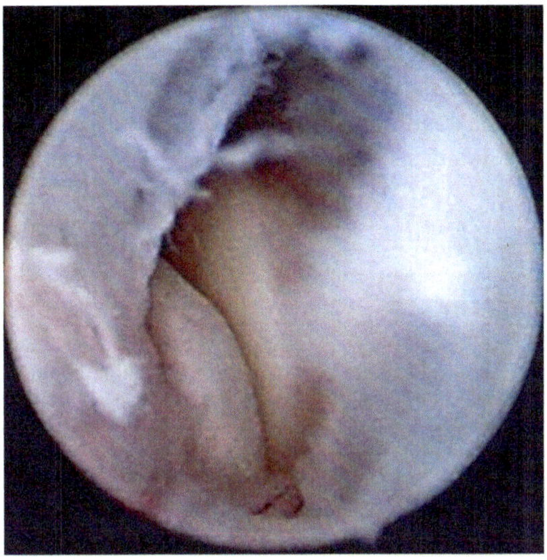

Fig. 18.13 The view of the PT joint following dilatation and arthroscopic excision of the membrane

clockwise rotation as one sweeps the scope ulnarwards is better than a pure ulnarwards swing.

If the hole in the membrane is small, then one can dilate it. I do so by moving the scope right up to the hole. Keeping the sheath in position, I remove the camera and replace it with the pointed obturator and use it to dilate. Since I tend to use the 4–5 portal on, I can use the 6R portal to bring in instruments to do the same under direct vision. The main problem, however, is that once the second instrument is in the joint, it obscures the piso-triquetral joint until it is removed and it is difficult to triangulate (Fig. 18.13).

Therapeutic Uses of the Arthroscope

In the past, open removal with or without pisiform excision for associated osteoarthritis was the normal treatment for symptomatic piso-triquetral loose bodies [9, 19, 26]. However, nowadays, arthroscopic rather than open removal of loose bodies is the method of choice in most joints. In the piso-triquetral joint, it is probably best performed by moving the loose body into the main radio-carpal joint where it can be removed easily. This obviously can only be done easily in joints with a large connection (type 4). If there is a small hole or complete membrane, one can access the joint by dilatation or creation of a passage through the membrane [12].

Future Development

Many of the future developments will be conversion of techniques used in other joints. Compared with them, the piso-triquetral joint has limited pathology, so the range of potential therapeutic manoeuvres is also limited. However, to advance, because of the difficulty in access, either instrumentation which can be used through a single portal needs to be developed, or more likely a second more direct but safe portal has to be used. This portal is most likely to be from the ulnar side. However, though the joint is close to the skin, further anatomical studies need to be undertaken to assess the position of the ulnar nerve cutaneous branches and their variability (Fig. 18.4). This may either produce areas in which portals can be safely made or show us that limited open visualisation and protection of the nerve is needed.

A potential goal is to perform pisiformectomy arthroscopically. However, the pisiform is much larger than one presumes from the surface anatomy. To arthroscopically remove the whole bone would be a major and time-consuming undertaking. Also in osteoarthritic joints, the most likely ones to be removed, the osteophytes which arise around the joint and base of the bone on the radial side are very close to the ulnar nerve (Fig. 18.14). One appreciates this most clearly when doing an open pisiformectomy. Even in relatively normal-shaped bones, the nerve is only a thin sheet of tissue away. Arthroscopic removal though a 'tour de force' may actually be too risky to be undertaken as a standard operation.

Saying that, piso-triquetral arthrodesis has been reported as a successful alternative to pisiformectomy in high-demand athletes with painful pisiform instability [1, 25] since it probably results in less weakening of wrist strength. In other joints, for instance, the ankle, arthroscopic-assisted arthrodesis is a standard technique. For the piso-triquetral joint, removal of the articular surface

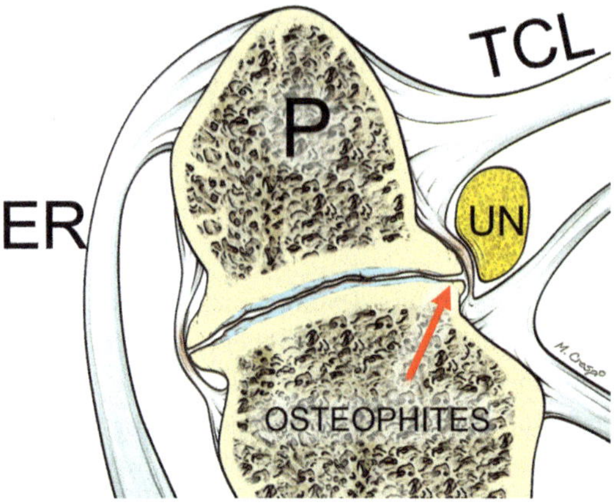

Fig. 18.14 The closeness of the ulnar nerve to the radial osteophytes in severe osteoarthritis. Too close for comfort? Pisiform (*P*), extensor retinaculum (*ER*), transverse carpal ligament (*TCL*), ulnar nerve (*UN*)

arthroscopically and screw fixation under radiographic control are certainly a potential advance. It also has the advantage of reducing scar tenderness which may be particularly good for sportspeople, like moutain bikers, who not only are susceptible to piso-triquetral pathology but also will continue to load the ulnar side of the palm.

A further area of development may be partial excision with interposition of materials as is already being performed in the carpometacarpal joint of the thumb and other small joints [4, 7]. This being either synthetic spacers, for instance, pyrocarbon, or biological materials like tendons.

Conclusion

1. Pain from the piso-triquetral joint or the flexor carpi ulnaris tendon is a common cause of ulnar-sided wrist pain.
2. Past middle age articular surface wear is normal and probably not painful.
3. The main symptomatic pathology is post-traumatic osteoarthritis, instability and maltracking.
4. The joint can be easily seen and assessed arthroscopically in two thirds of patient from the radio-carpal joint.
5. The main use of arthroscopy is to confirm wear and assess the degree of articular surface wear.
6. Therapeutic manoeuvres remain limited, though removal of loose bodies is straightforward. Partial pisiformectomy with interpositional arthroplasty and arthroscopic-assisted arthrodesis is a possibility.

References

1. Abrams R, Tontz W (2006) Pisotriquetral arthrodesis as an alternative to excision for pisotriquetral instability in high demand patients: a case report in a gymnast. J Hand Surg Am 31A:611–614
2. Aiki H, Wada T, Yamashita T (2006) Pisotriquetral arthrosis after triquetral malunion: a case report. J Hand Surg Am 31A(7):1157–1159
3. Arya AP, Kulshreshtha R, Kakarala GK, Singh R, Compson JP (2007) Visualisation of the pisotriquetral joint through standard portals for arthroscopy of the wrist: a clinical and anatomical study. J Bone Joint Surg Br 89B:202–205
4. Badia A (2007) Arthroscopy of the trapeziometacarpal and metacarpophalangeal joints. J Hand Surg Am 32A:707–724
5. Bas H, Kleinert JM (1999) Anatomic variations in sensory innervations of the hand and digits. J Hand Surg 24A:1171–1184
6. Berger RA (1999) Arthroscopic anatomy of the wrist and distal radioulnar joint. Hand Clin 15:393–413
7. Cobb T, Sterbank P, Lemke J (2011) Arthroscopic resection arthroplasty for treatment of combined carpometacarpal and scaphotrapeziotrapezoid (pantrapezial) arthritis. J Hand Surg Am 36A:413–419
8. Corten EML, Van den Broecke DG, Kon M, Schurrman AH (2004) Pisotriquetral instability causing an unusual flexor tendon rupture. J Hand Surg Am 29A:236–239
9. Hall TD (1981) Loose body in the pisotriquetral joint (report of two cases). J Bone Joint Surg 63A:498–500
10. Ishizuki M, Nakagawa T, Itoh S (1991) Positional dislocation of the pisiform. J Hand Surg Am 16A:533–535
11. Jenkins SA (1951) Osteoarthritis of the pisiform-triquetral joint. J Bone Joint Surg 33B:532–534
12. Katolik LI (2008) Arthroscopic resection of pisotriquetral joint loose body: a case report. J Hand Surg Am 33A:206–209
13. Keopp BN (1945) A note on the piso-triquetral joint. Anat Rec 92:91–92
14. Le Nen D, Saraux A, Yaacoub C, Hu W, Le Goff P, Lefevre C (1997) Osteoarthritis of the pisiform-triquetral compartment. A review of eight cases of an under recognized entity. Rev Rhum Engl Ed 64(6):396–401
15. Lewis OJ, Hamshere RJ, Bucknill TM (1970) The anatomy of the wrist joint. J Anat 106:539–552
16. Minami M, Yamazaki J, Ishii S (1984) Isolated dislocation of the pisiform: a case report and review of the literature. J Hand Surg 9A:125–127

17. Mok D, Nikolis A, Harris PG (2006) The cutaneous innervations of the dorsal hand: detailed anatomy with clinical implications. J Hand Surg Am 31A:564–574
18. Moojen TM, Snel JG, Ritt MJPF, Venema HW, Den Heeten GJ, Bos KE (2001) Pisiform kinematics in vivo. J Hand Surg Am 26A:901–907
19. Needoff M, Frostick SP (1994) Pisotriquetral loose body (an unusual cause of wrist pain). J Hand Surg 19B:215–216
20. Palmer AK, Werner FW (1981) The triangular fibrocartilage complex of the wrist: anatomy and function. J Hand Surg Am 6:153–162
21. Pessis E, Drape J-L, Bach F, Feydy A, Guerini H, Chevrot A (2006) Direct arthrography of the pisotriquetral joint. AJR Am J Roentgenol 186:800–804
22. Pevny T, Rayan GM, Egle D (1995) Ligamentous and tendinous support of the pisiform, anatomic and biomechanical study. J Hand Surg Am 20A:299–301
23. Puna R, Poon P (2010) The anatomy of the dorsal cutaneous branch of the ulnar nerve. J Hand Surg 35E:583–585
24. Rayan GM, Jameson BH, Chung KW (2005) The pisotriquetral joint: anatomic, biomechanical, and radiographic analysis. J Hand Surg Am 30A:596–602
25. Singer G, Eberl R, Hoellwarth ME (2011) Pisotriquetral arthrodesis for pisotriquetral instability: case report. J Hand Surg Am 36A:299–303
26. Steinmann SP, Linscheid RL (1997) Pisotriquetral loose bodies. J Hand Surg Am 22A:918–921
27. Suzuki T, Nakatsuchi Y, Tateiwa Y, Tsukada A, Yotsumoto N (2002) Osteochondral fracture of the triquetrum: a case report. J Hand Surg 27A:98–100
28. Taleisnik J (1988) Clinical and technological evaluation of ulnar sided wrist pain. J Hand Surg 13A: 801–802
29. Tay SC, Tomita K, Berger RA (2007) The "ulnar foveal sign" for defining ulnar wrist pain: an analysis of sensitivity and specificity. J Hand Surg 32A: 438–444
30. Tindall A, Patel M, Frost A, Shetty A, Compson J (2006) The anatomy of the dorsal cutaneous branch of the ulnar nerve–a safe zone for positioning of the 6R portal in wrist arthroscopy. J Hand Surg Br 31: 203–205
31. Trail IA, Linscheid RL (1992) Pisiformectomy in young patients. J Hand Surg Br 17B:346–348
32. Viegas SF, Patterson RM, Hokanson JA, Davis J (1993) Wrist anatomy: incidence, distribution, and correlation of anatomic variations, tears and arthrosis. J Hand Surg Am 18A:463–475
33. Yamaguchi S, Viegas SF, Patterson RM (1998) Anatomic study of the pisotriquetral joint: ligament anatomy and cartilaginous change. J Hand Surg Am 23A:600–606

Wrist Arthroscopy and Its Role in Kienböck's Disease

19

George S. Gluck, Gary G. Poehling, Terry L. Whipple, and Gregory I. Bain

Introduction

The purpose of this chapter is to discuss wrist arthroscopy and its value in the staging and treatment of osteonecrosis of the lunate, or Kienböck's disease. A brief review of the condition will also be included to help support wrist arthroscopy as a useful tool in the management of this difficult problem. Additional tips for use of arthroscopy in Kienböck's disease, for both diagnostic and treatment purposes, are also discussed here. Please note that the content of this chapter largely reflects what is available in published literature, but also includes the opinions of the authors.

In order to understand how wrist arthroscopy can be beneficial in Kienböck's disease, it is important to understand the etiology, natural history, and current management concepts. The true etiology remains uncertain, but it is thought to be related to both joint mechanics and vascularity [29]. Significant controversy remains in the treatment of this condition. Negative ulnar variance has been identified as a commonly accepted association in the literature, but even this is subject to debate [5, 7, 8, 21]. The source of this uncertainty largely stems from the fact that the incidence is low, and that patients may be asymptomatic or have vague symptoms [21]. This makes it a difficult problem to study and an important condition to include in the differential diagnosis of ulnar-sided wrist pain.

As with many other conditions, it is likely to be multifactorial. Two prominent concepts that have emerged are vascular compromise and repetitive trauma [17]. While the dominant or primary cause has yet to be determined, the end result is necrosis and collapse. The initial insult may also differ among patients [12]. Ideally, the natural history of any pathology should serve as a basis upon which treatment is measured. Large natural history studies are lacking, but smaller studies are available which provide an acceptable foundation upon which the outcomes of various treatments can be analyzed [4, 14, 24]. Indeed, the disease progresses through a predictable

G.S. Gluck, M.D. (✉) • G.G. Poehling, M.D.
Department of Orthopaedic Surgery, Medical Center BLVD, Winston-Salem, NC 27157, USA
e-mail: gluckortho@gmail.com

T.L. Whipple, M.D.
Chief of Orthopaedics, American Self, PLC, Richmond, VA, USA

Associate Professor of Orthopaedic Surgery, Virginia Commonwealth University, Richmond, VA, USA

Director, Orthopaedic Research of Virginia, Richmond, VA, USA
e-mail: whipple@americanself.com

G.I. Bain, M.B.B.S., FRACS, FA(Ortho)A, Ph.D.
Department of Orthopaedics Surgery, Discipline of Anatomy and Pathology, University of Adelaide, North Terrace, SA, Australia

Department of Orthopaedic Surgery, Royal Adelaide Hospital, North Terrace, SA 5000, Australia
e-mail: greg@gregbain.com.au

F. del Piñal et al. (eds.), *Arthroscopic Management of Ulnar Pain*,
DOI 10.1007/978-3-642-30544-3_19, © Springer-Verlag Berlin Heidelberg 2012

Table 19.1 Radiographic staging of Kienböck's disease [11, 12]

Stage	Radiographic findings
I	Normal (MRI shows decreased signal intensity on T1 image)
II	Increased radiodensity with possible mild decrease in lunate height on radial side
IIIA	Lunate bone collapse, no scaphoid rotation
IIIB	Lunate bone collapse, fixed scaphoid flexion
IV	Degenerative changes around the lunate

series of radiographic changes and is associated with decreased grip strength and wrist motion [12]. Currently, many studies in the literature evaluating treatment outcomes utilize this radiographic progression for staging in a system developed by Stahl and Lichtman [16, 25] (Table 19.1).

Multiple treatment options can be found in the literature with varying levels of complexity. Most of these options are based on the two dominant theories in the pathology of the disease. Therefore, the surgical options mainly include some form of revascularization, some form of unloading, or some type of salvage procedure. These are also dependent on the stage of disease, using the established radiographic classification. Prior to lunate collapse, and even after collapse, there is a large body of published patient outcomes literature and biomechanical data that supports surgical intervention aimed at unloading the lunate, with or without revascularization [1, 6 ,10, 11, 13, 18, 19, 27, 28, 30].

For more advanced stages where collapse has occurred, no one treatment aimed at lunate salvage has proven more effective than the rest [10]. Symptom reduction with possible slowing or stopping of disease progression has been noted, but few comparative studies exist. One study by Salmon et al. [24] compared the nonoperative treatment of 18 patients with radial shortening osteotomy in 15 patients. Patients were all Lichtman stages 2 and 3 by radiographic criteria. Follow-up averaged 3.6 years. They found small improvements in grip strength and pain in the surgical group. They also found that, while progression seemed to be slower in the surgical group, both cohorts still had disease progression. While the authors recommended shortening osteotomy, they did note that one surgical patient developed chronic regional pain syndrome and that there were multiple patients who underwent diagnostic arthroscopy that identified chondral damage and arthritis not seen on plain radiographs. No statistical analysis was discussed in the study.

Age of the patient also needs to be considered when it relates to healing potential and durability of treatment. Kho et al. [13] looked at their radial shortening osteotomies with a minimum 10-year follow-up. There was no control group, and they were able to demonstrate small improvements with surgery. They also noted that younger patients tended to do better, although this trend did not reach statistical significance. When considering this, and the available literature, physiologically younger patients may be more appropriately treated with attempts at lunate preservation prior to salvage procedures. Preventing progression is certainly worthwhile. The most potential for truly altering the natural history of the disease likely exists prior to articular compromise and collapse.

The treatment methods for various stages are criticized on the basis that they lack appropriate controls, which is not surprising when considering the relatively low prevalence of the disease. In this instance, the natural history of the condition is the next best comparison. Unfortunately, it has been difficult to show consistent improvement over the natural history with regard to either radiographic progression or patient symptoms in long-term follow-up [10]. It may be that we do not understand the true etiology of the disease, but one must also consider the ability of the current staging system to determine the ideal treatment. Perhaps the algorithms for treatment need to include more information in order to improve on the reproducibility of desired outcomes. Plain radiographs are excellent for evaluating alignment and osseous structures. Magnetic resonance imaging can also play a role in providing valuable information regarding vascularity and necrosis [26], but it is not reliable for evaluat-

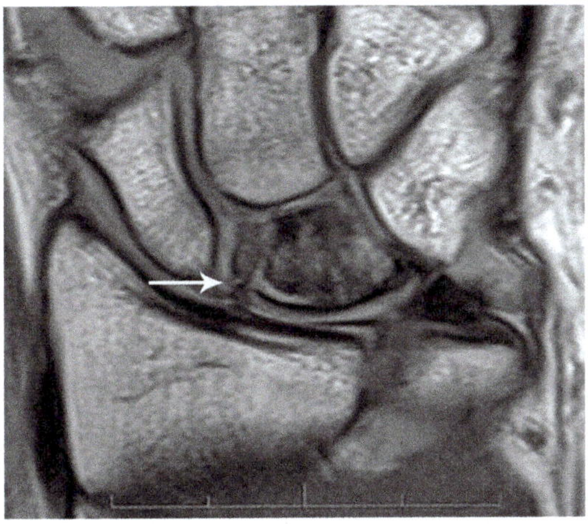

Fig. 19.1 Magnetic resonance imaging scan showing the lunate with some fragmentation and a subchondral fracture extending distally (*arrow*). The articular cartilage has some irregularity. At this stage, the resolution of the articular cartilage is not sufficient to recommend treatment. Arthroscopy is essential to evaluate the integrity of the articular surface in this case (Used with permission – [3])

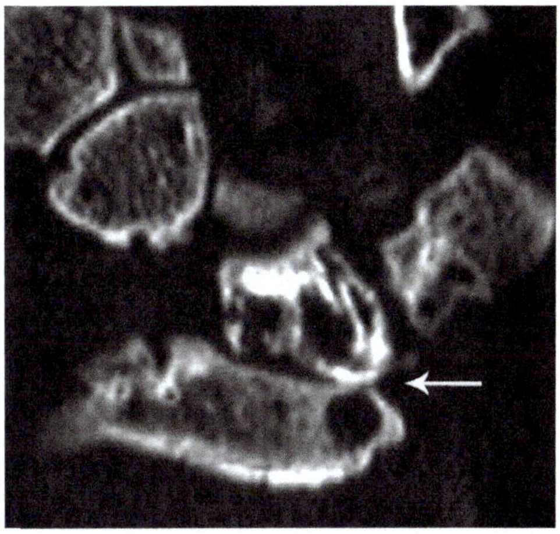

Fig. 19.2 Computed tomographic scan of the wrist with sclerosis and fragmentation of the lunate. There must be full-thickness loss of the articular cartilage of the lunate and lunate facet, as bone-on-bone degenerative arthritis is present (*arrow*). Arthroscopy will be of value to assess the midcarpal joint (Used with permission – [3])

ing articular cartilage [9]. It can clearly delineate necrosis and fracture, as seen in Fig. 19.1, but the integrity of the articular cartilage is better assessed through arthroscopy before the decision is made on whether or not the patient has enough functional joint surfaces to support a proximal row carpectomy in this example. Perhaps attempts at lunate preservation would be reasonable in a young patient if, at the time of arthroscopy, the lunate articular surfaces were intact despite fracture and underlying necrosis. This information cannot be reliably obtained from MRI in the absence of complete joint collapse on plain radiographs or CT scan, as seen in Fig. 19.2.

Arthroscopy of the wrist allows both evaluation and palpation of articular surfaces. This information can play a valuable role in staging and clinical decision making in Kienböck's disease. High-quality MRI provides a great deal of information about the integrity of the radiocarpal and midcarpal articulations, but arthroscopy remains the gold standard upon which all noninvasive diagnostic modalities are based [9]. In an attempt to guide surgical decision making and to potentially improve surgical outcomes, Bain and Begg have developed an arthroscopic staging system based on the number of nonfunctional articular surfaces, seen in Fig. 19.3. The grade simply represents the number of nonfunctional articular surfaces [2].

In grade 0, all articular surfaces are functional. An arthroscopic synovectomy is performed. An extra-articular unloading procedure may be indicated. If there is negative ulnar variance, a radial shortening osteotomy is performed. For neutral or positive ulnar variance, a capitate shortening procedure can be performed. A revascularization procedure could also be indicated in this group. The authors have also managed patients with arthroscopic-assisted drilling of the lunate.

In grade 1, a nonfunctional proximal lunate articular surface is identified as the only articular abnormality. A healthy midcarpal joint and lunate facet of the distal radius are seen on arthroscopy. Proximal row carpectomy or radioscapholunate fusion may be indicated.

In grade 2, there are two nonfunctional articular surfaces. This grade is subdivided based on the location of articular compromise. *Grade 2a* involves the proximal articular

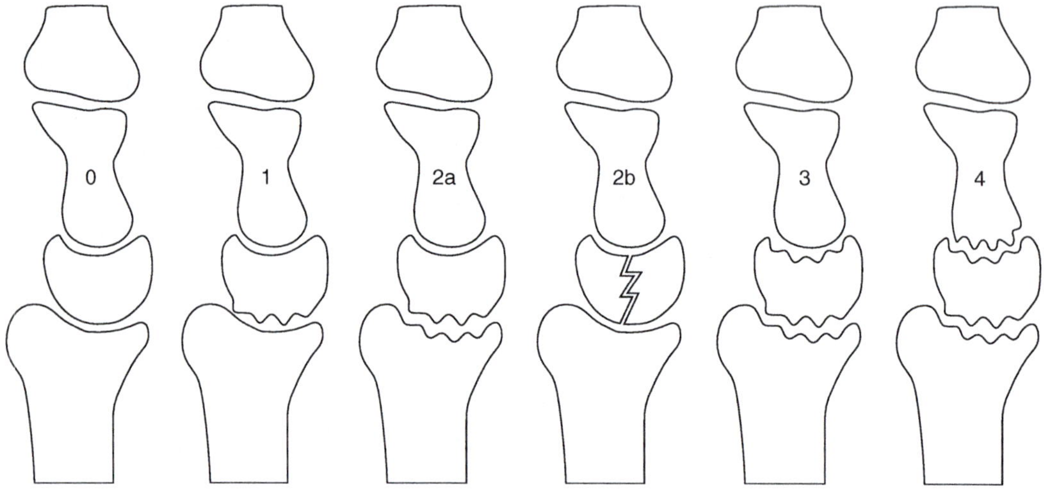

Fig. 19.3 Bain and Begg arthroscopic classification of Kienböck's disease. The grade is determined by the number of nonfunctional articular surfaces. The grading system assists the surgeon to determine the best surgical option, based on the pathoanatomic findings (Used with permission – [2])

surface of the lunate and the lunate facet of the distal radius. A radioscapholunate fusion will remove both nonfunctional articular surfaces and enable the wrist to articulate through the normal midcarpal joint. *Grade 2b* involves the proximal and distal articular surfaces of the lunate. This typically occurs when there is a coronal fracture in the lunate extending between the radiocarpal and midcarpal joints. The lunate fossa of the radius and the head of the capitate are normal. This is best managed with a proximal row carpectomy. Lunate replacement is another alternative. These patients often do not do well with more complex procedures such as internal fixation or vascularized bone grafting.

In grade 3, there are three articular surfaces that are nonfunctional. Most likely, it will be the capitate articular surface which remains functional. This situation could be managed with a hemiarthroplasty. Alternatively, in a salvage procedure such as scaphocapitate fusion with capitate head resection, a total wrist fusion or total wrist arthroplasty may be performed, depending on patient age and activity level.

In grade 4, all four articular surfaces are nonfunctional. A total wrist fusion or arthroplasty is indicated. Arthroscopic debridement may be considered for grades 3 and 4 as a less-invasive, temporizing measure for symptomatic relief. Debridement may also be performed in association with extra-articular procedures, such as radial shortening, to remove debris in the setting of mechanical symptoms.

This grading system utilizes direct visual assessment of the articulations of the lunate and a probe to assess the degree of softening of the articular surfaces. Correlating this arthroscopic assessment with the traditional investigations can help the clinician make better informed management decisions. A study on arthroscopic assessment of Kienböck's disease found that synovitis was present in all cases; the degree of synovitis correlated with the degree of articular damage, the severity of articular changes was often underestimated by plain radiographs, and that arthroscopic findings commonly changed the recommendation for treatment. Eighty-two percent of cases had at least one nonfunctional articulation, whereas 61 % had at least two nonfunctional articulations [2]. The authors identified cases in which the chondral envelope was intact, although softening and collapse of the subchondral bone plate were noted. This was considered an important subgroup where attempts at revascularization and unloading of the lunate should be considered, especially in the younger individual where there is more potential to heal and stabilize. The spectrum of arthroscopic findings appeared to fit into a continuum, which were placed into the proposed arthroscopic classification with a proposed treatment algorithm [2].

The advantage to this method is that functional joint surfaces determine treatment. The normal arthroscopic appearance of articular cartilage is defined as having a white, smooth, glistening appearance. Minor fibrillation is still classified as a normal articular surface. The subchondral bone should be firm to palpation without significant softening. Articular surfaces that display extensive fibrillation, fissuring, localized or extensive loss, a floating articular surface, or fracture are considered nonfunctional (Fig. 19.4). The aim of surgical treatment is to maintain functional motion with normal articulations. The articular-based classification directs treatment based on sound surgical principles. If all articular surfaces are intact, then a procedure that does not violate the articular surfaces is indicated, such as synovectomy, vascularized bone grafting, drilling, or joint leveling. With nonfunctioning articular surfaces, an articular reconstructive procedure is required to leave the carpus mobile with only functional articular surfaces remaining, such as proximal row carpectomy, radioscapholunate fusion, lunate replacement, or hemiarthroplasty. More extensive joint involvement requires a salvage procedure.

It has puzzled one of the authors (GIB) for some years that the recommended principles of management of Kienböck's disease are different from that of the scapholunate advanced collapse wrist. A more unified principle respecting articular damage is discussed in this chapter. The importance of the articular changes is better appreciated when they are seen as part of the overall pathologic process. The classification and concepts presented in this study [2] are pathoanatomic, and not just anatomic. The approach that is presented respects the articular cartilage in patients with Kienböck's disease. It places the pathoanatomic aspects of the articular cartilage at the forefront of the decision-making process.

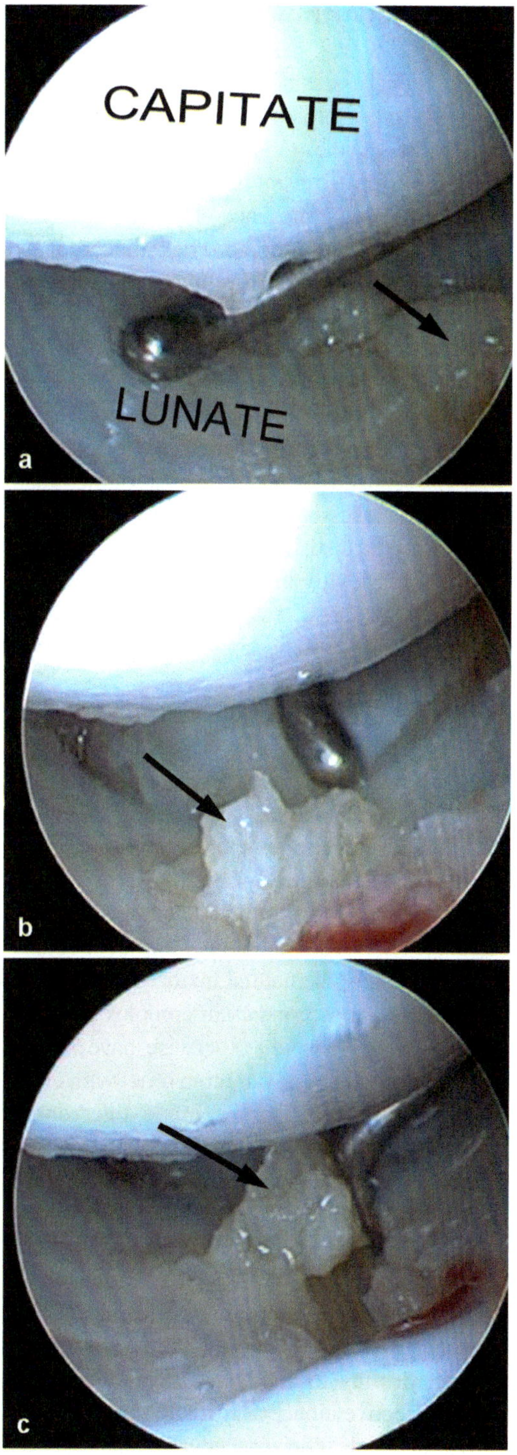

Fig. 19.4 (**a**, **b**) In the midcarpal space, the lunate cartilage seems normal – only a loose body could be seen on first inspection (*arrow*). (**c**) When probing, a clear coronal fracture (*arrow*) can be seen at the junction of the dorsal and middle lunate thirds (scope in UMC and probe in RMC) (Courtesy of Dr. Piñal)

Technique: Arthroscopic Assessment

Arthroscopic assessment is carried out using standard wrist arthroscopic techniques. A general assessment of the radiocarpal and midcarpal joints is performed using the 3–4, 6R, and midcarpal portals. The presence or absence of synovitis or loose bodies is noted. The radiocarpal and capitolunate surfaces of the lunate are assessed, as are the corresponding articular facets on the distal radius and the head of the capitate. The surfaces are palpated with a probe, and the presence of softening, "floating" (unsupported) articular surfaces or gross degenerative changes are noted (Fig. 19.5). Any associated fractures of the lunate can also be assessed. Debridement of the joints can be performed in all patients, including removal of synovitis and loose bodies, in addition to other procedures. If no further surgical intervention is planned, debridement alone can acutely help with symptoms.

In the early stages of Kienböck's disease, the goals of treatment should be to either halt progression or reverse osseous changes prior to compromise of subchondral support and subsequent articular degeneration. Arthroscopy, as a diagnostic tool, should ideally help the surgeon identify which patients fall into a truly reversible category. This would potentially allow for consistent alteration of the natural history and also prevent unnecessary secondary or complex surgeries in a patient who would otherwise have similar long-term outcomes or symptom relief with either no intervention or a more simple intervention with more rapid recovery.

Arthroscopy can be a valuable treatment tool in early Kienböck's disease. It offers a less morbid option through guided drilling of the lunate as a form of revascularization. This has been shown to be effective in the hip in some studies [23] in early stages of osteonecrosis. It is not known whether drilling to encourage revascularization can be effective alone, or if it should be used as an adjunct with other procedures, such as joint leveling or unloading procedures. A case report was published of Kienböck's diagnosed prior to evidence of necrosis on MRI or sclerosis on plain radiographs that was managed with drilling alone after failure of nonoperative treatment. This led

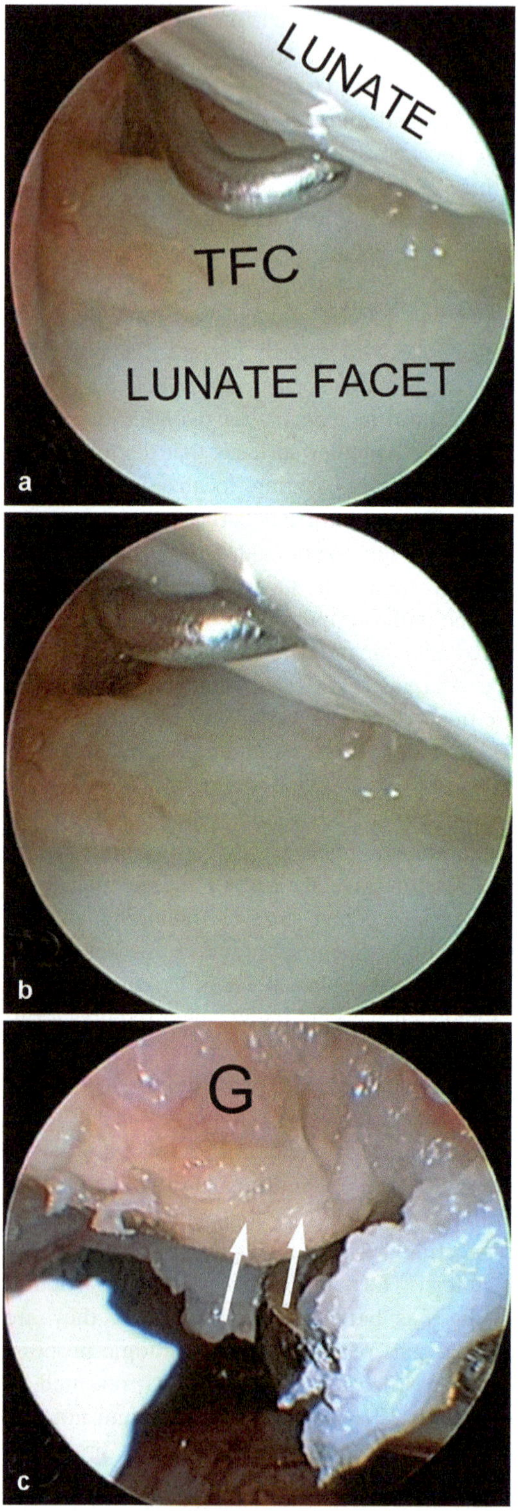

Fig. 19.5 (**a**, **b**) "Bag of worms" sign, pathognomonic of Kienböck's. (**c**) After removing the cartilage shell of the lunate, necrotic bone (*arrows*) and granulating tissue (*G*) can be seen (scope in 3–4 and probe in 6R) (Courtesy of Dr. Piñal)

to complete reversal of symptoms and imaging abnormalities after a 6-year follow-up period. Of note, a second patient in this case report had already progressed to sclerosis on plain radiographs but chose drilling as a less-invasive option. Although the patient improved clinically during the follow-up period, radiographs showed progression and collapse in accordance with the natural history of the disease [3]. Further supporting this approach, a recent study was published including 20 patients treated by lunate drilling alone [20]. This study included mainly Lichtman stage 1 and 2 patients. There were four patients that were subcategorized as Lichtman stage 3a or 3b. In this study, the lunate was decompressed using an open technique. Average 5-year follow-up showed improvement using objective, standardized outcome measures with no radiographic progression. Two of the four patients identified as stage 3 required additional surgery consisting of radial shortening osteotomy. The authors showed significant, lasting improvement in all stage 1 and 2 patients. The ideal patient for this procedure is one with positive or neutral ulnar variance who desires a less-invasive alternative to capitate shortening or vascularized bone grafting. Radiographic changes should be absent, and all articular surfaces should be functional at the time of arthroscopy. Should revascularization not be evident on MRI at the 3–6-month postoperative mark, unloading and vascularized bone grafting still remain as treatment options.

Technique: Arthroscopic-Assisted Drilling of the Lunate

Standard wrist arthroscopy is carried out with a 3–4 and a 6R portal. A brachial tourniquet and standard traction tower are used to aid in visualization. Any synovitis is removed with a motorized resector. Assessment of the lunate, adjacent articular surfaces, and interosseous ligaments are made with a 2.7-mm, 30-degree arthroscope in the 6R portal and a probe through the 3–4 portal. The midcarpal joint is also evaluated through the midcarpal radial and ulnar portals in a standard fashion. Once the integrity of the articular surfaces has been confirmed, an arthroscopic grade 0, attention is turned to drilling the lunate. The dorsal aspect of the lunate is drilled with a 2.5-mm drill through an arthroscopic cannula using the 3–4 portal. Alternatively, a drill sleeve may be used to protect the extensor tendons. The position of the drill can be confirmed with fluoroscopy (Fig. 19.6). Two or more passes of the drill are made at the discretion of the surgeon. Both the angle of the drill and the position of the wrist may be adjusted to ensure the drilling on the areas of necrosis to encourage vascular ingrowth. Surgical planning can be made based on preoperative MRI to identify areas of necrosis. Entry holes will also serve to decompress intraosseous pressure. Any debris is then removed from the joint. Postoperatively, patients are advised to wear a removable wrist splint for comfort, and they are prescribed therapy to focus on wrist range of motion and forearm muscle strengthening.

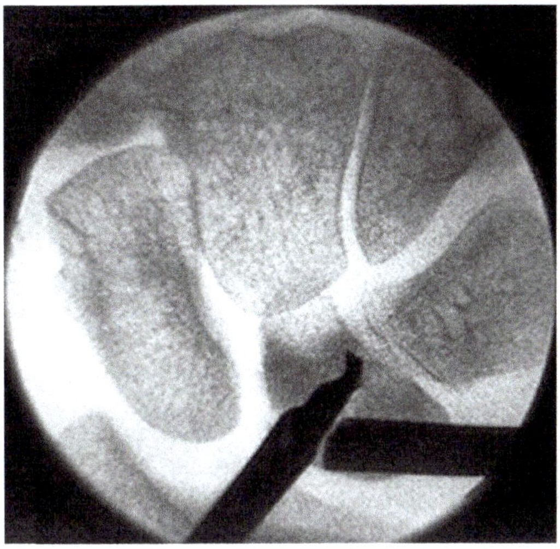

Fig. 19.6 Arthroscopic-directed drilling of the lunate in a patient with arthroscopic grade 0 Kienbock's disease

Arthroscopic debridement has also been shown to be a valuable treatment option in those patients where the lunate has already progressed to collapse or fracture. Menth-Chiari et al. looked at a small cohort of patients with Lichtman stages 3A and 3B Kienböck's disease [22]. Patients were managed with arthroscopic debridement alone. The authors achieved consistent, significant improvements in pain, motion, and grip strength

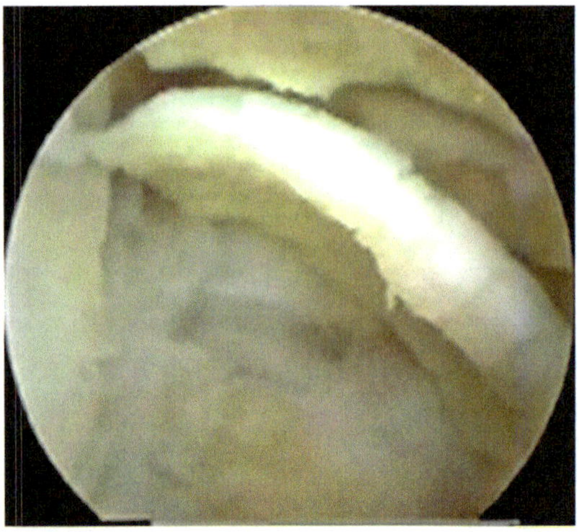

Fig. 19.7 Large, free-floating, osteochondral lunate fragment

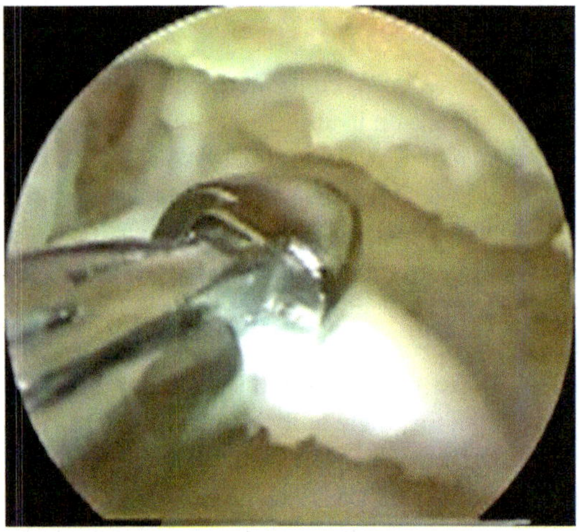

Fig. 19.8 Removal of loose, osetochondral fragments of the lunate

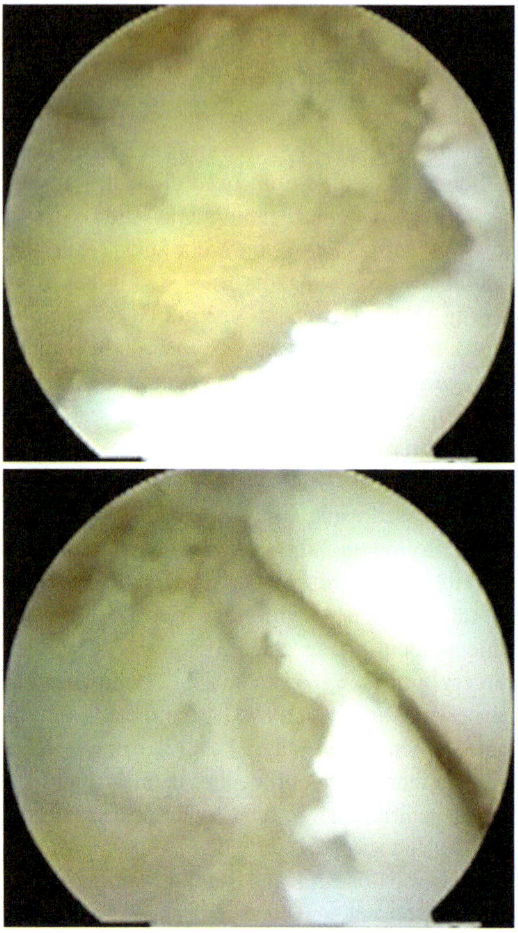

Figs. 19.9 and 19.10 Defect in the necrotic lunate after debridement of loose bodies

with minimal morbidity. In addition, all patients returned to their prior level of activity or occupation within 4 weeks of surgery. After an average follow-up of 19 months, about half had progression of lunate sclerosis. Clinical results were maintained, and none of the patients had further carpal collapse or symptomatic instability during the study period (Figs. 19.7, 19.8, 19.9 and 19.10).

As arthroscopic techniques and technology have evolved, so too have the capabilities of the wrist arthroscopist to perform previously open procedures in a minimally invasive fashion. Intercarpal fusion and proximal row carpectomy are two examples of procedures that can be done arthroscopically and still be done efficiently in experienced hands. Arthroscopic proximal row carpectomy is not only technically possible, but it can also allow for faster recovery and earlier range of motion [31]. Limited intercarpal fusion, such as scaphocapitate fusion, can serve to prevent collapse of the distal carpal row and stabilize scaphoid rotation in the setting of Kienböck's disease. Resection of the proximal pole of the capitate can also serve to unload the lunate. A prospective, randomized study was performed to compare open versus arthroscopic scaphocapitate fusion in Kienböck's disease [15]. The open group also had a revascularization procedure for the lunate. The arthroscopic group included resection of the proximal pole of the capitate. The lunate was preserved in both groups. All patients had radiographic stage III disease. There were 16 patients in the study. Average follow-up was about 3 years. Objective clinical and radiographic grading criteria were used in postoperative analysis. The arthroscopic group without revascularization experienced shorter surgical times with a faster recovery of 6 weeks versus 15 weeks before returning to regular daily activities. Overall modified Mayo Wrist Scores were slightly better in the arthroscopic group versus the open group, but did not reach statistical significance secondary to the small number of patients. Revascularization did not appear to have any effect on clinical or radiographic outcome at 3 years. There were no nonunions.

Technique for Arthroscopic Scaphocapitate Fusion

Arthroscopy of the wrist is performed in a standardized technique. The hand is held in traction of 4–7 kg across the wrist joint. The surface landmarks are drawn, and the joint is distended with 5–10 mL of normal saline solution through the 3–4 portal with an 18-gauge needle. The 4–5, 5–6, 6R, and midcarpal portals are prepared for instrumentation and arthroscopy. A 2.4-mm, 30° arthroscope is preferred, but a 2.7-mm arthroscope may be used. The radiocarpal and midcarpal joints are thoroughly examined, with special emphasis on the cartilage of the lunate surfaces. Both radiocarpal and midcarpal surfaces of the lunate are also examined. The radioscaphoid space, scapholunate ligament, lunotriquetral interval, and ulnar side of the wrist are visualized and documented. Probing is always used to evaluate the stability of the scapholunate and lunotriquetral intervals and the triangular fibrocartilage complex. Provisional shaving and removal of loose bodies are then performed. At the midcarpal space, capitate pole, scapholunate, lunotriquetral, and scaphocapitate intervals are identified. The capitate pole is excised using an oscillating shaver. Alternatively, a 2- or 3-mm round or barrel burr may be used. This shaving is continued until the midcarpal surface of the lunate is free of the capitate pole, as shown in Fig. 19.11. The arthroscope is directed toward the scaphocapitate joint through the ulnar midcarpal portal. The cartilage at the adjacent surfaces of the capitate and scaphoid is removed using shavers through the radial midcarpal portal, exposing the subchondral bone. With the arthroscope in the interval between the radial styloid and the scaphoid, a guide wire for the surgeon's preferred cannulated screw system is inserted in the scaphoid through the anatomic snuffbox, in a radial to ulnar, palmar to dorsal, and proximal to distal directions. The arthroscope is then introduced to the midcarpal space to visualize the previously prepared scaphocapitate joint. The guide wire is further inserted into the capitate under arthroscopic visualization. The wrist is dorsiflexed and ulnarly deviated as much as the instrumentation allows to extend the scaphoid prior to crossing the arthrodesis site. With the arthroscope in the scaphocapitate joint and the guide wire in place, an appropriate sized screw is placed after length measurement and overdrilling. It is recommend to drill across the arthrodesis site but not to the end of the guide wire to avoid displacing the wire. Exact placement of the screw can be checked with the arthroscope and intraoperative fluoroscopy if desired. The arthroscope is then slightly withdrawn, and the screw is tightened to observe compression between the scaphoid and the capitate (Fig. 19.12). A second screw may be used for added fixation. The lunate is left in situ. Loose synovial tissue is consistently found at the radioscaphoid interval, and a full-radius resector is used for arthroscopic synovial debridement. The scapholunate interosseal ligament is often elongated and loose, but not ruptured. Laser thermal modification (Omnipulse Holmium-Yag Laser; Trimedyne, San Francisco, CA) can be used to shrink the scapholunate ligament. Postoperatively, the wrist is immobilized in a short arm splint in a position of 15° of dorsiflexion and 10° of ulnar deviation for 4 weeks. A follow-up radiograph

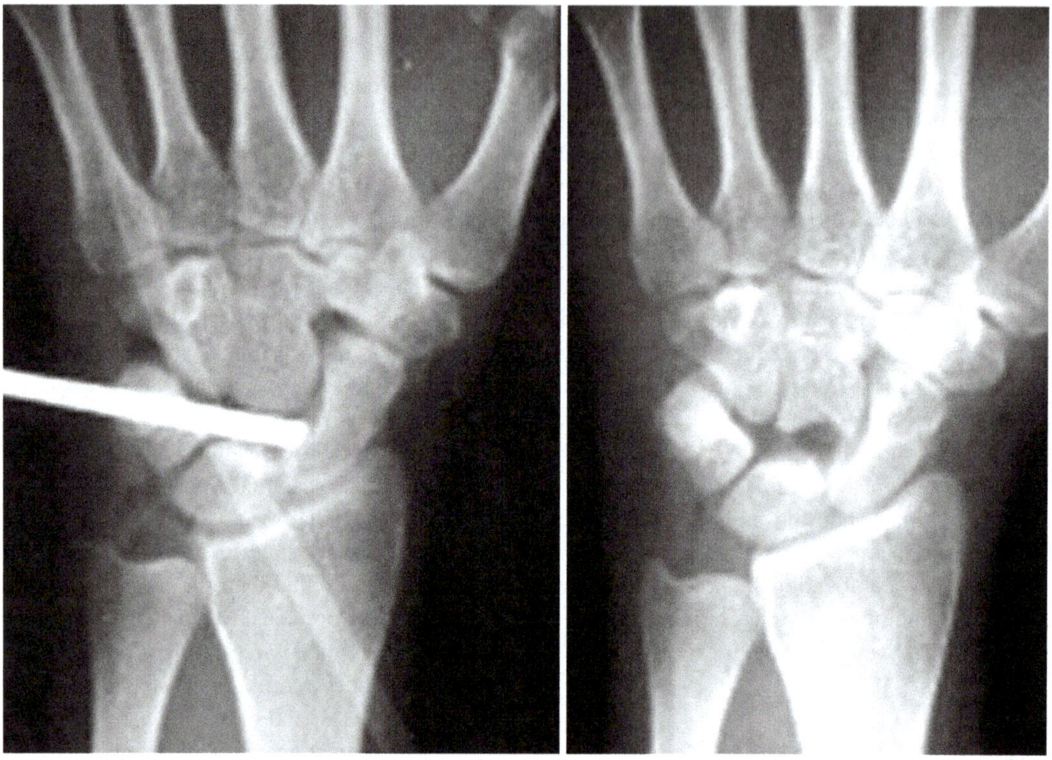

Fig. 19.11 Radiograph of the arthroscope in the midcarpal joint and after arthroscopic resection of the head of the capitate

is obtained to establish a new baseline. After removal of the splint, the patients are allowed to passively mobilize the wrist three times a day to regain motion [15].

The majority of the literature regarding Kienböck's disease does not include wrist arthroscopy for either diagnosis or for treatment. Hopefully, this chapter has demonstrated how wrist arthroscopy can serve as a valuable tool in the management of this challenging disease. It provides direct evidence of articular surface involvement and allows the surgeon to design a logical solution to maintain as much function as possible. Consensus has not yet been achieved on which interventions at the various stages of the disease will achieve results that are consistently better than the natural history. Moving forward, it is the authors' hope that arthroscopy will be incorporated into future studies in order to both gain additional diagnostic information and to potentially provide less-invasive treatment options for patients.

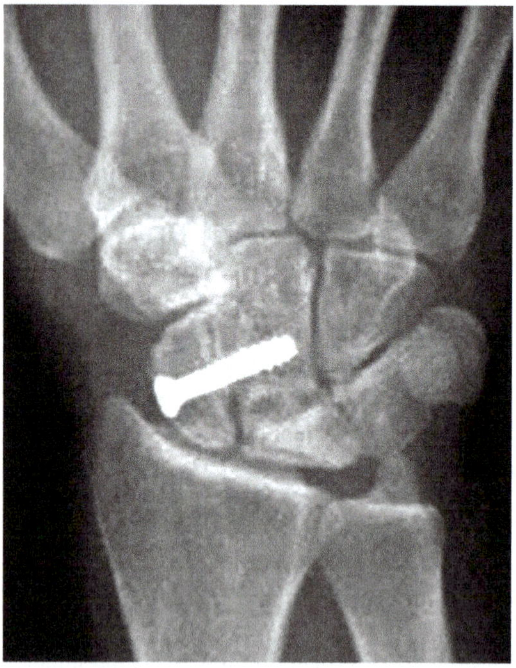

Fig. 19.12 Radiograph showing final fixation for the arthroscopically assisted scaphocapitate arthrodesis

References

1. Afshar A (2010) Lunate revascularization after capitate shortening osteotomy in Kienbock's disease. J Hand Surg 35(Dec):1943–1946
2. Bain GI, Begg M (2006) Arthroscopic assessment and classification of Kienbock's disease. Tech Hand Up Extrem Surg 10(1):8–13
3. Bain GI, Durrant A (2011) An articular-based approach to Kienbock avascular necrosis of the lunate. Tech Hand Up Extrem Surg 15(1):41–47
4. Beckenbaugh RD, Shives TC, Dobyns JH, Linscheid RL (1980) Kienböck's disease: the natural history of Kienböck's disease and considerations of lunate fractures. Clin Orthop 149:98–106
5. Bonzar M, Firrell JC, Hainer M, Mah ET, McCabe SJ (1998) Kienbock's disease and negative ulnar variance. J Bone Joint Surg Am 30A:1154–1157
6. Calfee RP, Van Steyn MO, Gyuricza C, Adams A, Weiland AJ, Gelberman RH (2010) Joint leveling for advanced Kienbock's disease. J Hand Surg 35A:1947–1954
7. D'Hoore K, DeSmet L, Verellen K, Ural J, Fabry G (1994) Negative ulnar variance is not a risk factor for Kienbock's disease. J Hand Surg 19A:229–231
8. Gelberman RH, Salamon PB, Jurist JM, Posch JL (1975) Ulnar variance in Kienbock's disease. J Bone Joint Surg Am 57A:674–676
9. Haims AH, Moore AE, Schweitzer ME, Morrison WB, Deely D, Culp RW, Forman HP (2004) MRI in the diagnosis of cartilage injury in the wrist. Am J Roentgenol 182:1267–1270
10. Innes L, Strauch RJ (2010) Systematic review of the treatment of Kienbock's disease in its early and late stages. J Hand Surg 35(May):713–717
11. Iwasaki N, Minami A, Ishikawa J, Kato H, Minami M (2005) Radial osteotomies for teenage patients with Kienbock's disease. Clin Orthop Relat Res 439:116–122
12. Keith P, Nuttall D, Trail I (2004) Long-term outcome of nonsurgically managed Kienbock's disease. J Hand Surg 29A(1):63–67
13. Koh S, Nakamura R, Horii E, Nakao E, Inagaki H, Yajima H (2003) Surgical outcome of radial osteotomy for Kienbock's disease – minimum 10 years of follow-up. J Hand Surg 28(6):910–916
14. Kristensen SS, Thomassen E, Christensen F (1986) Kienbock's disease – late results by non-surgical treatment. J Hand Surg 11B(3):422–425
15. Leblebicioglu G, Doral MN, Atay OA, Tetik O, Whipple TL (2003) Open treatment of stage III Kienbock's disease with revascularization compared with arthroscopic treatment without revascularization. Arthroscopy 19(2):117–130
16. Lichtman DM, Alexander AH, Mack GR, Gunther SF (1977) Kienbock's disease: the role of silicone replacement arthroplasty. J Bone Joint Surg Am 59A:899–908
17. Lluch A, Garcia-Elias M (2011) Etiology of Kienbock disease. Tech Hand Up Extrem Surg 15(1):33–37
18. Makabe H, Iwasaki N, Kamishima T, Oizumi N, Tadano S, Minami A (2011) Computed tomography osteoabsorptiometry alterations in stress distribution patterns through wrist after radial shortening osteotomy for Kienbock's disease. J Hand Surg 36:1158–1164
19. Mazur KU, Bishop AT, Berger RA (1997) Vascularized metaphyseal bone grafts from the distal radius in the treatment of Kienböck's disease. Orthop Trans 21:442
20. Mehrpour SR, Kamrani RS, Aghamirsalim MR, Sorbi R, Kaya A (2011) Treatment of Kienbock's disease by lunate core decompression. J Hand Surg 36:1675–1677
21. Memmen U, Sithebe H (2009) The incidence of asymptomatic Kienbock's disease. J Hand Surg Eur Vol 34(3):348–350
22. Menth-Chiari WA, Poehling GG, Wiesler ER, Ruch DS (1999) Arthroscopic debridement for the treatment of Kienbock's disease. Arthroscopy 15(1):12–19
23. Mont MA, Carbone JJ, Fairbank AC (1996) Core decompression versus nonoperative management for osteonecrosis of the hip. Clin Orthop Relat Res 324:169–178
24. Salmon J, Stanley JK, Trail IA (2000) Kienböck's disease: conservative management versus radial shortening. J Bone Joint Surg Br 82B:820–823
25. Stahl F (1947) On lunatomalacia (Kienbock's disease). Acta Chir Scand 5(suppl 126):1–133
26. Trumbe T (1990) Avascular necrosis after scaphoid fracture: a correlation of magnetic resonance imaging and histology. J Hand Surg 15(4):557–564
27. Waitayawinyu T, Chin SH, Luria S, Trumble TE (2008) Capitate shortening osteotomy with vascularized bone grafting for the treatment of Kienbock's disease in the ulnar positive wrist. J Hand Surg 33(8):1267–1273
28. Watanabe T, Takahara M, Tsuchida H, Yamahara S, Kikuchi N, Ogino T (2008) Long-term follow-up of radial shortening osteotomy for Kienbock's disease. J Bone Joint Surg 90(8):1705–1711
29. Watson HK, Guidera PM (1997) Aetiology of Kienbock's disease. J Hand Surg 22:5–7
30. Weiss AP, Weiland AJ, Moore JR, Wilgis EFS (1991) Radial shortening for Kienbock's disease. J Bone Joint Surg 73(3):384–391
31. Weiss ND, Molina RA, Gwin S (2011) Arthroscopic proximal row carpectomy. J Hand Surg 36(4):577–582

Arthroscopic Treatment of Midcarpal Instability

20

David Hargreaves

Introduction

Midcarpal instability (MCI) is a condition in which many wrist surgeons have been rather sceptical of the diagnosis and even more sceptical about its need for treatment. This is primarily because there is no diagnostic test nor investigation, which consistently confirms nor quantifies the condition. Even more disconcerting is the fact that even arthroscopically there are no abnormal clinical findings. In the forward to the Dr. Piñal's sister book, 'Arthroscopic Treatment of Distal radius fracture', Dr. Marc Garcia-Elias stresses that 'seeing is believing'. We all agree that it is much more difficult to believe without seeing. Essentially, MCI is a diagnosis made on clinical history and examination alone. Investigations are required though to exclude other pathological causes for the symptoms, rather than for confirming the diagnosis.

It is essential that the treating clinician understands the difference between the concept of natural existing asymptomatic joint 'laxity' versus the symptomatic pathological state of 'instability'. Nowhere in wrist surgery is this more important than in MCI. The degree of laxity of the wrist joint predisposes one to the condition of MCI but does not directly correlate with the level of symptomatology. The condition is as a consequence of general wrist laxity and the pathology exists in both the radiocarpal and midcarpal joints. The term *midcarpal* instability is therefore somewhat misleading. Wright [12] used the term *instability of the proximal carpal row*, as it more accurately describes the pathology. However and despite this, we continue to use the term *midcarpal instability*.

Kinematics

As there are no tendons or muscles directly attached to the carpus, carpal stability is dependent on the bone architecture, ligamental integrity and proprioception for maintaining normal kinematics. The role of proprioception and muscle control has only recently been investigated and appreciated [10]. This is particularly important when the wrist is under load.

In the normal wrist motion, as the wrist moves from radial deviation to ulnar deviation, the proximal row moves from flexion into a relatively extended position. The integrity and tension of the palmar arcuate ligaments are responsible for the smooth transition of this motion. If the transition of the extending proximal row does not occur synchronously, the triquetrum extends before the lunate and is followed by a sudden extension of the lunate as it catches up with the triquetrum. This is known as the 'catch-up clunk'. Cadaveric studies in which ligaments are sectioned, in order to reproduce the pathological process, have

D. Hargreaves, MBBS, FRCS (Orth)
Department of Orthopaedic Surgery,
University Hospital Southampton,
Tremona Road, Southampton SO16 6YD, UK
e-mail: dgharg@aol.com

F. del Piñal et al. (eds.), *Arthroscopic Management of Ulnar Pain*,
DOI 10.1007/978-3-642-30544-3_20, © Springer-Verlag Berlin Heidelberg 2012

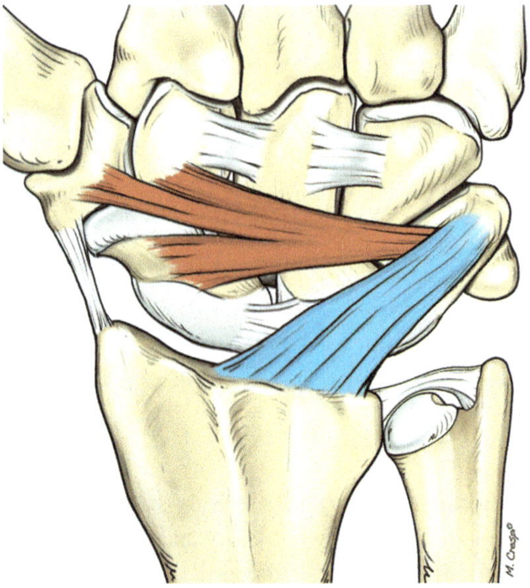

Fig. 20.1 The important dorsal wrist ligaments in palmar MCI are the dorsal radiocarpal (radio-triquetral) ligament (*blue*) and the dorsal intercarpal (scapho-triquetral) ligament (*red*)

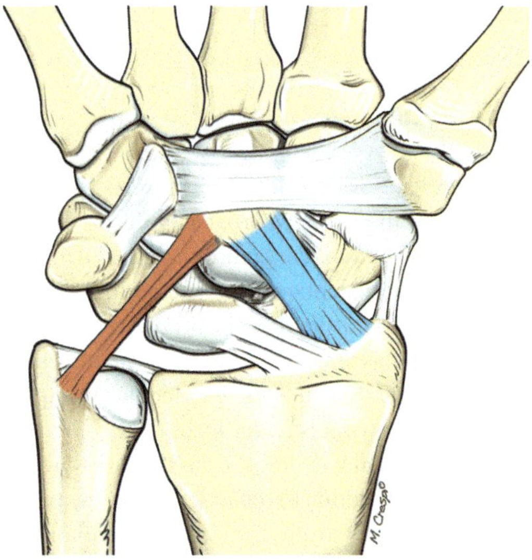

Fig. 20.2 The important volar wrist ligaments in palmar MCI are the radio-scapho-capitate ligament (*blue*) and the ulno-triquetro-capitate ligament (*red*). These make up the palmar arcuate ligament

shown the importance of the dorsal radio-triquetral ligaments (Fig. 20.1) as well as the palmar ulnar arcuate ligaments (Fig. 20.2) [6]. These anatomical studies have helped to show how

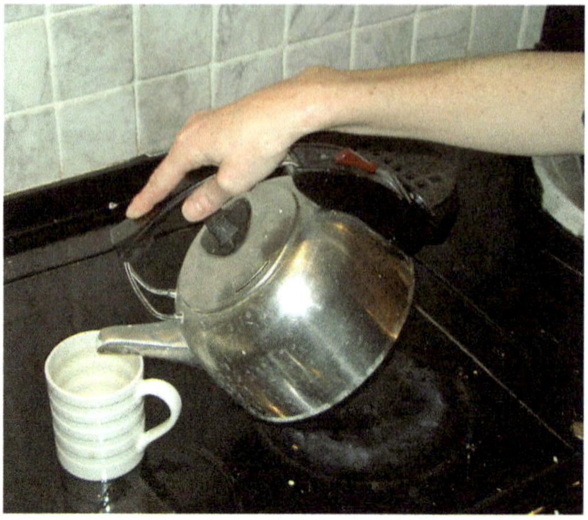

Fig. 20.3 The characteristic position and activity of symptomatic giving way in palmar MCI

treatments need to address both these areas to give consistent results.

I have personally noted that this instability almost only occurs in the pronated wrist. The wrist becomes more stable the further the forearm is supinated. This is most likely to be due to tightening of the ulno-capitate and ulno-lunate ligaments as the wrist supinates.

The nomenclature of the different types of non-dissociative carpal instability (CIND) and midcarpal instability has made this area of wrist surgery difficult to understand. It is best to differentiate MCI into palmar, dorsal or combined. It is likely that the conditions of capitolunate instability pattern (CLIP), chronic capitolunate instability (CCI) and other named conditions are describing one of these three types.

Clinical Findings

The classic symptoms of MCI are a feeling of giving way and clunking when the wrist is under load. This usually occurs during activities which use the pronated forearm, such as pushing open a door or pouring a kettle (Fig. 20.3). This clunking can be asymptomatic or can be associated with pain and ache. It is not uncommon to find that symptoms started

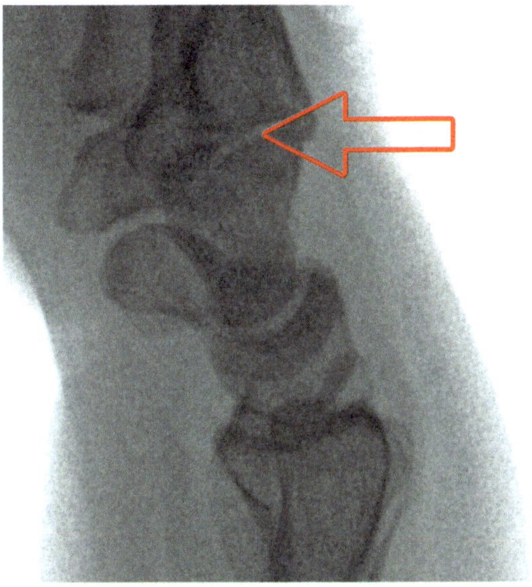

Fig. 20.4 Fluoroscopic imaging of anterior drawer test in palmar MCI. The direction of stress applied (*arrow*)

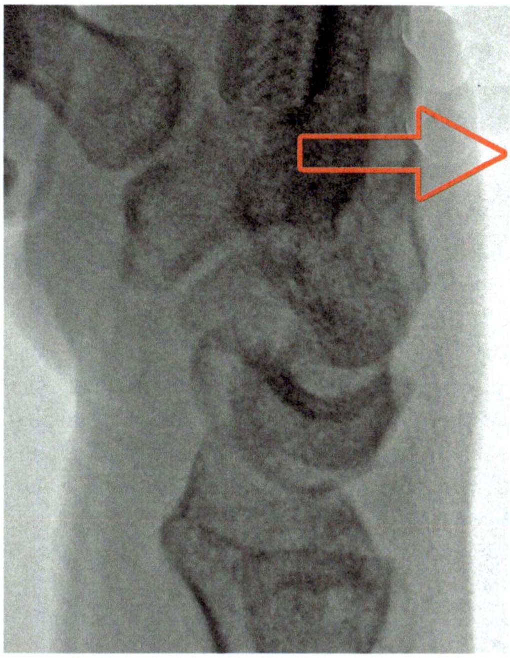

Fig. 20.5 Fluoroscopic imaging of posterior drawer test in dorsal MCI. The direction of stress applied (*arrow*)

shortly after a minor injury or a period of immobilisation. It is likely that this short period of reduced use alters the proprioception, which can thus predispose to symptomatic MCI.

Clinical examination should include the assessment of generalised joint laxity. The Beighton score is useful in quantifying this. Specific assessment of the wrist is crucial in the diagnosis of MCI. There is sometimes some minor joint line tenderness, either at the midcarpal or radiocarpal levels. Some patients have learnt mechanisms to reproduce the clunk that they complain of. These patients usually radially and ulnarly deviate the wrist under stress with a clenched fist. This specific movement can be performed passively, as described by Lichtman [7] in the *midcarpal shift test*. I find the *midcarpal drawer test* to be useful. This involves passively translocating the carpus both anteriorly and posteriorly. It reproduces the same clunk and subluxation feeling that occurs in the symptomatic patient. This test will differentiate between palmar and dorsal MCI (Figs. 20.4 and 20.5). I perform the test initially with the forearm pronated. I then repeat the test in neutral. The subluxation and the instability are usually only present in pronation.

Radiological Findings

Static imaging is unlikely to show any abnormality in MCI, as it is a dynamic instability. It really requires dynamic imaging techniques. Plain X-rays including dynamic instability views should be performed in order to exclude other types of carpal instability (especially scapho-lunate and luno-triquetral instability). Occasionally in the most severe cases of palmar midcarpal instability, a static flexed proximal row is noted (static MCI). In such cases, particular care is required to exclude a luno-triquetral tear. Static MRI scans are routinely performed to exclude other pathology. Usually, in MCI, the MRI scan and X-rays are normal (dynamic MCI). In our series of cases, we have not noticed any abnormality nor high signal in the midcarpal stabilising ligaments (palmar arcuate ligament and dorsal radiocarpal ligament).

The abnormal movements of MCI can be seen and studied in a number of different ways. Video fluoroscopy is probably the most accessible of the useful dynamic imaging modalities. In moving the wrist from radial deviation to ulna deviation, one is able to see the proximal row sag and the failure of smooth extension of the proximal carpus. As the carpus reaches towards maximal ulnar deviation, the lunate snaps into the correct position with a clunk. This 'catch-up clunk' is visible and reproduces the feeling of instability that the patient complains of. Fluoroscopy is also useful for defining the extent of palmar and dorsal translocation that can be achieved with the midcarpal drawer test (as described above). Ultrasound has been used to confirm the 'catch-up clunk', but it is not a very sensitive, nor specific, imaging modality in this situation. Dynamic MRI scans are rather too slow at imaging to pick up the subtle changes that occur. Much faster and more useful dynamic scanning is becoming available with the latest helical CT scans.

Assessment of Severity

A simple method of grading the severity of MCI has been described by Feinstein and Lichtman [1]. This included reproducible self-induced clunking as the most severe group. I have concern over this system as some asymptomatic people are able to perform this manoeuvre. Thus, self-induced clunking is not always a sign of severity of symptoms. Some MCI patients that I have seen have extensive laxity with a strongly positive drawer test but only mild symptoms functionally. I find functional questionnaires (DASH) and visual analogue scores of instability to be most useful marker of severity. We identified that the difficulty in pouring a kettle was consistent with the severity of the instability [8].

Treatment Options

Open procedures such as partial wrist fusion and tenodesis procedures have been the standard techniques used for the last 20 years. There are no large series, nor prospective-controlled studies, as the incidence of patients with MCI requiring surgical intervention is low. Many patients with a short history of symptoms will improve either spontaneously or with a course of physiotherapy.

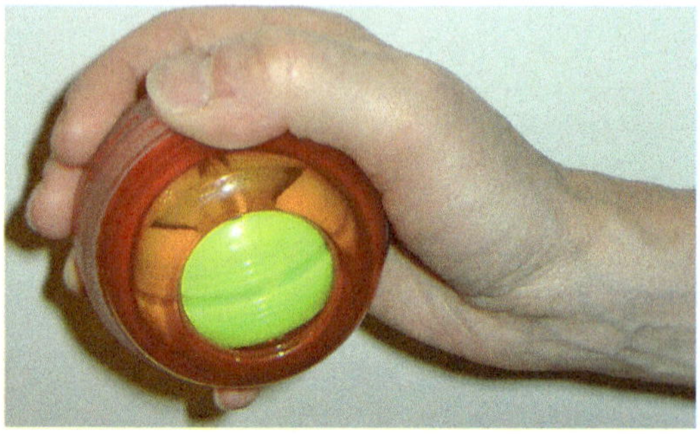

Fig. 20.6 Gyroscopic spinball used for strengthening

Physiotherapy has historically relied upon functional splintage and strengthening. We feel that biofeedback exercises and relearning proprioceptive control is important before progressing to functional strengthening with a gyroscope 'spinball' (Fig. 20.6). We prefer to avoid immobilisation with splints as this may exacerbate the loss of proprioceptive control that we feel is important.

Partial Wrist Fusion

Midcarpal arthrodesis does not guarantee relief of symptoms as some of the instability can also come from the radiocarpal articulation. The majority of patients have been shown to get relief from the clunking [7]. The main disadvantages of fusions are the extreme loss of movement and the development of radio-scaphoid impingement. This can be quite disabling for the typical young female patient. Relatively recently, radio-lunate fusion has been suggested for MCI [4]. This has the advantage of maintaining the functionally important midcarpal dart throwing axis of motion. I preserve wrist fusion procedures only for the most severe cases were radiologically there is a static midcarpal collapse.

Soft Tissue Reconstructions

Open capsular reefing and advancement procedures have had a tendency to fail with a recurrence

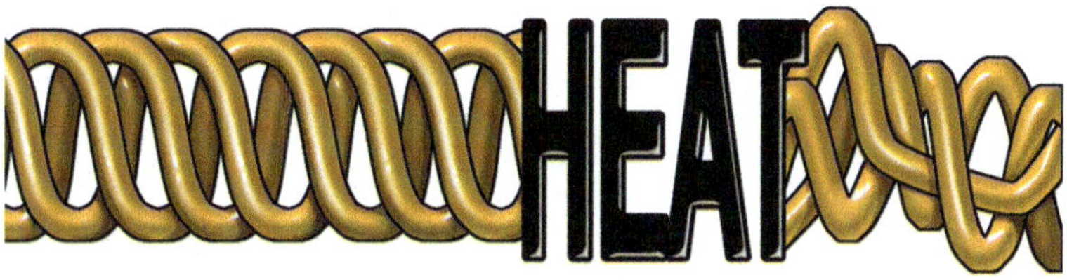

Fig. 20.7 Denaturation and shrinkage of the triple helix collagen fibril when exposed to heat

of symptoms [7]. Elaborated tendon weaves, reconstructing the deficient capsular ligaments of the palmar arcuate ligament, have been used. Such extensive procedures require an extensive approach and have a tendency to improve the stability, but again at the price of mobility. Garcia Elias [3] documented good early results of a tenodesis technique which addresses both the ulnar part of the palmar arcuate ligament and also the dorsal radio-triquetral ligament [2].

Arthroscopic-Assisted Reconstructions

Although some surgeons have previously used arthroscopic assistance whilst performing reefing and tenodesis procedures, results have not been published. Arthroscopy, in these cases, has helped to reduce the trauma of access, but the procedure has essentially been the same as an open tenodesis.

Arthroscopic Thermal Shrinkage

Thermal stabilisation of joints is a concept, which has been used since medieval times. It was used to stabilise the anterior capsule of the shoulder in medieval jousters with recurrent shoulder dislocations. In those days, the thermal injury was applied externally and without anaesthetic! The reinvention of the concept and the clinical application of thermal collagen manipulation was popularised in the shoulder by one of my teachers, Stephen Copeland. Originally, a laser was used, but later simple thermal wands were found to be as effective. Thermal shrinkage for shoulder instability began to fall out of favour as the midterm results showed approximately 40 % recurrence rates [5] despite excellent early results. The surgical technique involved the 'painting' of the capsule with the activated wand. Such continuous use of the wand led to raised fluid temperatures and subsequent chondrolysis in a few cases. The shoulder was not routinely immobilised following such procedures, and thus early stretching out of the collagen may have occurred.

Mechanism

Collagen fibrils are normally found in a triple helix configuration. The fibrils are maintained by covalent bonds between the strands of the fibril. When collagen is exposed to heat, the covalent bonds are lost and a random pattern of the fibril strand occurs (Fig. 20.7). This leads to shortening of the fibril. Animal studies have shown that the collagen is then remodelled as fibroblasts grow back into the injured but contracted matrix [9]. This phase takes approximately 6 weeks. During this time, the collagen is at risk of being stretched back out. Immobilisation of the joint is therefore most important during this period.

Technique

This procedure can be performed under general anaesthetic or regional brachial plexus block. Primarily, an examination of the wrist is performed under fluoroscopic control. I assess the degree of subluxation with a midcarpal drawer test. Dorsal subluxation is also looked for. The hand is then draped and suspended with a sterile arthroscopy tower and disposable Chinese finger traps. A tourniquet is applied to the upper arm. A diagnostic arthroscopy, using standard portals, is then performed of both the radiocarpal and midcarpal joints. Usually in palmar MCI, there are no specific abnormal arthroscopic findings. Inspecting the luno-triquetral ligament and excluding other causes of ulnar sided instability and clunking are important. Having confirmed that there are no other causes of symptoms, it is reasonable to

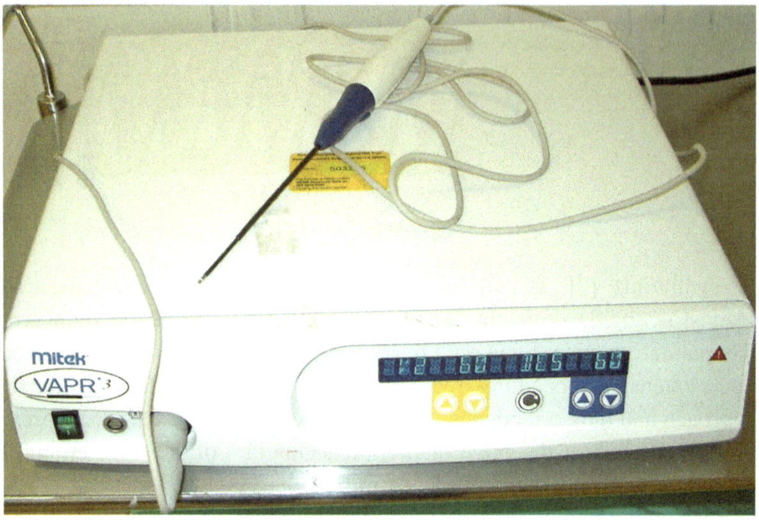

Fig. 20.8 Radiofrequency probe

proceed to the capsular shrinkage. The thermal probe requires the presence of saline, and so caution is required if the primary arthroscopy was performed 'dry'.

I usually start with the midcarpal joint. An outflow portal is inserted into the joint cavity to reduce the risk of overheating of saline. Sotereanos et al. have shown that this can occur, but it is dependent on how much energy is put through the thermal wand and thus ones technique [11].

The aim is to shrink both the palmar arcuate ligaments and also the dorsal capsule.

The arthroscope is inserted through the radial midcarpal portal and the thermal wand through the ulnar midcarpal portal. The type of thermal wand that I use is a 2.3-mm bipolar end-effect probe (Mitek VAPR 3, Depuy, Leeds) (Fig. 20.8). The preset settings create too much energy for safe shrinkage. I therefore reduce the coagulation setting from 90 down to 60. This usually creates temperatures of approximately 70 °C. If the setting is too high, necrosis of the tissues is seen with a visual effect known as 'caramelisation' (Fig. 20.9). This should be avoided to prevent too much thermal penetration and the risk of thermal injury to the adjacent tissues. If such an effect is seen, then the setting should be reduced further. The effect normally seen at the correct setting is a blanching and slight contracture of the tissues (Fig. 20.10). This affects the tissues to a depth of 2 mm from the probe tip. For any effect to occur, the probe must be touching the capsule. The technique for using the wand has been previously described as being used in a continuous manner like a paint brush stroke. This is how it was used in the shoulder. I have concerns that this will create too much heat in the small joint of the wrist. I advise that the effect is used more sparingly. I use the wand statically for a 1-s burst. Then, I move the wand tip to a neighbouring part of the capsule and give a further burst. I prefer to think of the technique as 'spotting' rather than 'brushing'. I do not reapply the wand to an area already treated. If this were to be done, there will

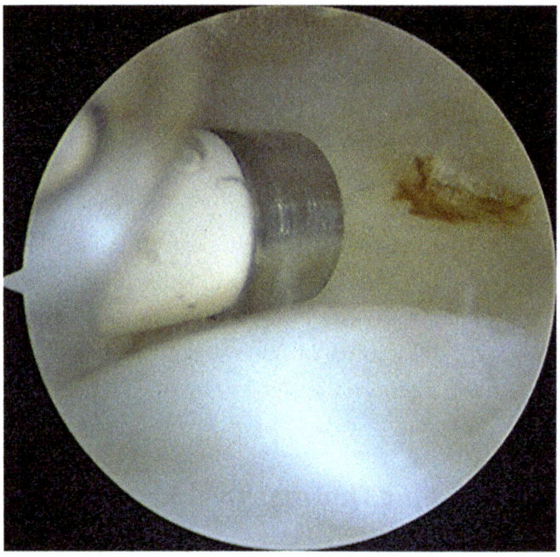

Fig. 20.9 Radiofrequency probe causing thermal injury. Mild 'caramelisation' of capsule noted

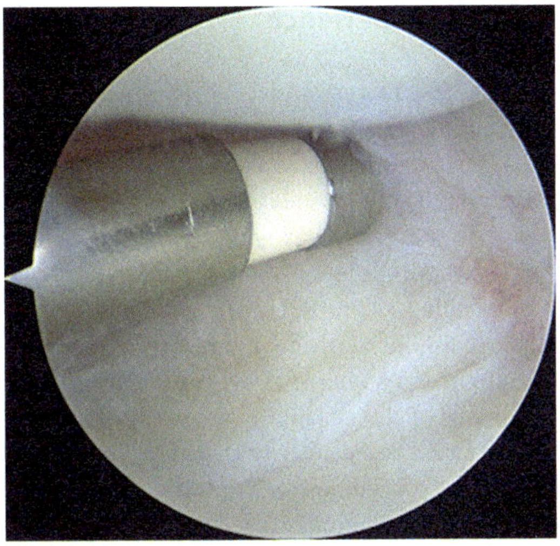

Fig. 20.10 Radiofrequency probe producing thermal shrinkage to volar capsule of radiocarpal joint. Slight blanching is the only visible change, after shrinkage has been performed

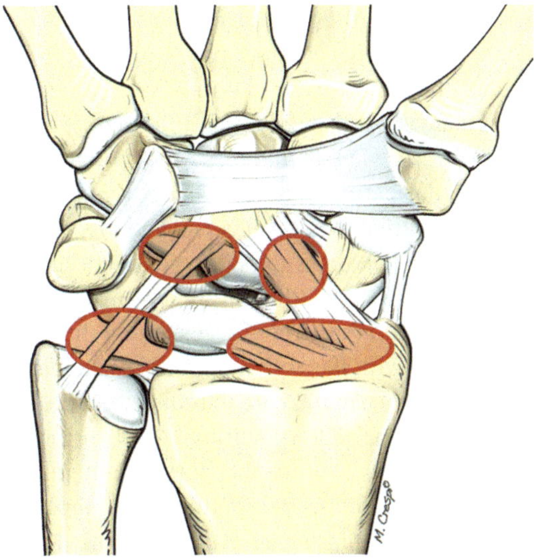

Fig. 20.11 Areas of the palmar ligaments that are treated from the midcarpal and radiocarpal joints are shaded in red

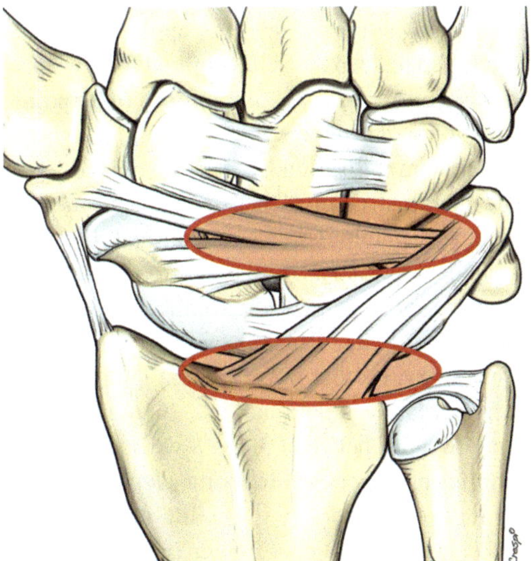

Fig. 20.12 Zones of treatment on the dorsal capsule are shaded in red

not be any further contracture of the collagen, but the risks of injury will increase. Once the collagen fibril has been denatured, no further beneficial change can occur. There is no summative effect. The next stage would be necrosis. Attention to avoid the articular cartilage is important.

The amount of the volar capsule that one can reach with the probe is limited, but the probe is usually able to reach the capsule adjacent to the scapho-lunate articulation and adjacent to the four corner joint. These are the two most important sites as it corresponds to the tissue overlying the palmar arcuate ligament (Fig. 20.11). The ulnar corner of the joint is usually easily reached. The dorsal capsule is then treated from ulnar to radial (Fig. 20.12). Visualisation of this is usually limited and therefore shrinkage here can only be performed blind with pressure of the probe against the capsule. Particular attention to avoid excess burning here must therefore be taken. By performing shrinkage to this area, one is contracting the dorsal intercarpal ligament. Access to the STT joint is limited and I do not treat the capsule in this area, for fear of chondral damage.

Having treated the midcarpal joint, I return and treat the radiocarpal joint. The scope is inserted through the 3–4 portal and the thermal probe through the 6R portal. It is common to swap the portals during the procedure to gain better access to different parts of the joint capsule. Again, I start with the volar capsule, particularly the volar radio-scapho-capitate ligament and working ulnarwards to the long and short radio-lunate ligaments. Access volar to the lunate is often limited and in which case I will move to the capsule anterior to the TFCC (ulno-triquetral ligaments). I will continue to treat the capsule of the ulnar corner and periphery of the TFCC but not the TFCC itself. I do not treat the scapho-lunate ligament nor the lunate-triquetral ligament. My view is that these are too close to the articular cartilage to allow safe treatment. I then finally treat the dorsal capsule across to the radial styloid. Excess dorsal synovial tissue is usually removed by the shrinkage process. If dorsal synovium obstructs access, then this can be removed with the ablation mode of the wand (yellow pedal). Again, care to reduce the setting to 60 (from the factory setting of 90) prior to use is advised. I suture the portals and insert 0.5 % bupivicaine to the joints and wounds. A wrist splint of plaster of Paris is applied for 2 weeks.

Post-operative Rehabilitation

The patient is reviewed at 2 weeks post surgery and a removable wrist splint is applied. Patients are advised to keep the splint applied for 6 weeks. They are informed of the importance of avoiding wrist motion during this time.

Gentle mobilisation is then instigated. The hand therapist is advised to avoid extremes of range and manipulations. Functional use and strengthening is usually all that is required. Most patients have regained approximately 80 % of the preoperative arc of movement by 3 months post surgery. Further improvement in arc occurs with increased functional use. Most patients return to work between 3 and 8 weeks post surgery. It is usually possible for the clerical worker to return to work wearing a splint, but a manual worker would require a longer period of rehabilitation with a phased return to physical activity.

Complications

The main risks are of overheating the local tissues and causing thermal burns to the adjacent neural and tendinous structures. I am aware of perioperative thermal injury to an ulnar nerve, extensor tendon and a case of localised skin burn at a portal site. All these cases occurred with a different type of thermal probe from which I have advised.

Personal Experience

Over the last 11 years, I have performed 26 capsular shrinkage procedures for midcarpal instability. All of these have been for symptomatic palmar midcarpal instability which have failed non-operative treatment with 6 months physiotherapy, concentrating on proprioception and strengthening. Arthroscopically, the appearance of the capsule has been normal. Occasionally, one might see some mild synovitis, but usually just laxity of the capsule is noted. This usually allows access to the anterior capsule with the heat probe. The procedure has been well tolerated by patients with minimal discomfort post-operatively. 85 % of patients have had a good or excellent improvement in instability symptoms from the primary procedure. One patient who had a static flexion deformity of the lunate preoperatively did not benefit and has had continuing pain with no benefit. As one would expect, patients with milder dynamic instability seem to do best.

The range of motion that most patients have at 1 year, is 90 % of the preoperative range. Loss of flexion is most common (Fig. 20.13). No patients have developed stiffness causing a functional deficit. The arc of motion can stretch out with time in some patients. If this were to be the case, then there is a risk that some instability symptoms may start to recur. The majority of cases have continued to do well with minimal symptoms. Approximately 20 % of patients have noticed a slight recurrence in symptoms, but none have recurred to their preoperative level of instability. None of the patients that have initially done well have required further treatment for a recurrence of instability symptoms. It seems that the immobilisation that is afforded to the wrist, which cannot happen in the shoulder, has been beneficial in giving better later results.

Conclusion

Palmar midcarpal instability has become increasingly well recognised and diagnosed in patients with a painful, clunking wrist. Treatments with open surgical techniques have not done consistently well. The loss of movement following partial wrist arthrodesis

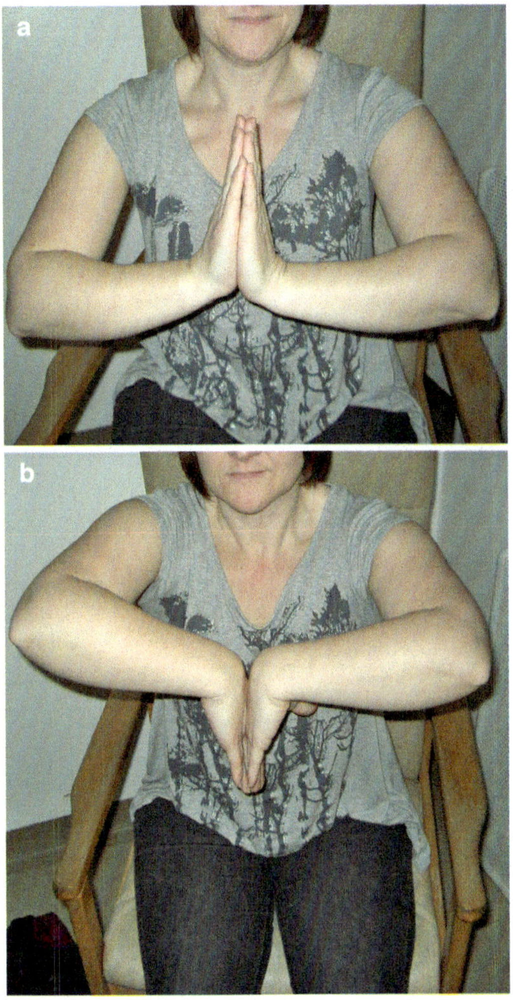

Fig. 20.13 (**a**, **b**) Slight loss of flexion and extension after capsular shrinkage treatment to the right wrist

can be equally disabling. Arthroscopic capsular shrinkage offers a technique, which has given good, reliable functional results, with minimal loss of motion. Care must be taken to avoid thermal injuries to adjacent structures.

References

1. Feinstein WK, Lichtman DM, Noble PC et al (1999) Quantitative assessment of the midcarpal shift test. J Hand Surg Am 24:977–983
2. Garcia-Elias M (2008) The non-dissociative clunking wrist: a personal view. J Hand Surg Eur Vol 33E(6): 698–711
3. Garcia-Elias M (2010) Carpal instability. In: Wolfe K (ed) Green's operative hand surgery, vol 1, 6th edn. Elsevier, Philadelphia, pp 465–522
4. Halikis MN, Colello-Abraham K, Taleisnik J (1997) Radio-lunate fusion: the forgotten partial arthrodesis. Clin Orthop Relat Res 341:30–35
5. Levy O, Wilson M, Williams H et al (2001) Thermal capsular shrinkage for shoulder instability. J Bone Joint Surg Br 5:640–645
6. Lichtman DM, Schneider JR, Swafford AR et al (1981) Ulnar midcarpal instability – clinical and laboratory analysis. J Hand Surg 16A:515–523
7. Lichtman DM, Bruckner JD, Culp RW et al (1993) Palmar midcarpal instability: results of surgical reconstruction. J Hand Surg 18A:307–315
8. Mason WT, Hargreaves DG (2007) Arthroscopic thermal capsulorrhaphy for palmar midcarpal instability. J Hand Surg Eur Vol 32:411–416
9. Nagle D (2005) Lasers and electrothermal devices. In: Geissler W (ed) Wrist arthroscopy. Springer, New York, pp 22–30
10. Salva-Coll G, Garcia-Elias M, Leon-Lopez M et al (2011) Effects of forearm muscles on carpal instability. J Hand Surg Eur Vol 36(7):553–559
11. Sotereanos D, Darlis NA, Kokkalis Z et al (2009) Effects of radiofrequency probe application on irrigation fluid temperature in the wrist joint. J Hand Surg 34(10):1832–1837
12. Wright TW, Dobyns JH, Linscheid RL et al (1994) Carpal instability non-dissociative. J Hand Surg (Br) 19:763–773

21 Capitohamate Axial Carpal Instability of the Wrist

Shian Chao Tay and Alexander Y. Shin

Introduction

Cooney and colleagues coined the term axial-loading dislocation to describe injuries of the carpus where the derangement occurred parallel to the long axis of the forearm [2]. Axial dislocation of the carpus typically occurs after high-energy dorsopalmar compression (crush mechanism), resulting in longitudinal disruption of the carpal arch. The disruption results in the carpus splitting into two axial columns, one remaining normally aligned to the radius and the other becoming unstable and displacing in a radial or ulnar direction. These two patterns are called axial-radial and axial-ulnar fracture-dislocations, respectively [5] (Fig. 21.1).

Such high-energy axial carpal fracture-dislocations are often associated with significant soft tissue injury including disruption of the transverse carpal ligament (Fig. 21.2). In addition, the injury will be obvious from the history and the carpal derangement easily seen on routine wrist radiographs (Fig. 21.3).

In less severe dorsopalmar compressions of the carpal concavity, complete rupture of the transverse intercarpal ligaments between the distal carpal bones may occur without any resulting fractures or dislocations seen on radiographs. If not properly healed, these may result in distal carpal instability and may produce localized pain in the wrist. In such situations, the diagnosis may be suspected from careful clinical examination, together with very subtle findings on computed tomography or magnetic resonance imaging. However, confirmation of diagnosis can typically only be made during wrist arthroscopy.

Much has been written about traumatic carpal instabilities. However, the majority of it has been focused on the proximal carpal row. The distal carpal row has received very little attention, partly because few problems in this area are seen clinically and the distal row is often thought of as a single rigid structure. Of major importance to the stability of the transverse carpal arch of the distal carpal row is the capitohamate joint.

Anatomy and Biomechanics

The capitohamate joint is jointed by three strong transverse carpal ligaments: the dorsal, the palmar, and the deep interosseous ligaments. Garcia-Elias et al. have shown that the palmar capitohamate ligament is of more importance

S.C. Tay, M.D., M.Sc. (✉)
Department of Hand Surgery, Singapore General Hospital, Outram Road, Singapore 169608

Duke-NUS Graduate Medical School, Singapore, Singapore

Mayo Clinic College of Medicine, Rochester, MN, USA
e-mail: tay.shian.chao@sgh.com.sg

A.Y. Shin, M.D.
Department of Orthopedic Surgery, Mayo Clinic, Gonda E14, 200 1st Street SW, Rochester, MN 55905, USA

F. del Piñal et al. (eds.), *Arthroscopic Management of Ulnar Pain*,
DOI 10.1007/978-3-642-30544-3_21, © Springer-Verlag Berlin Heidelberg 2012

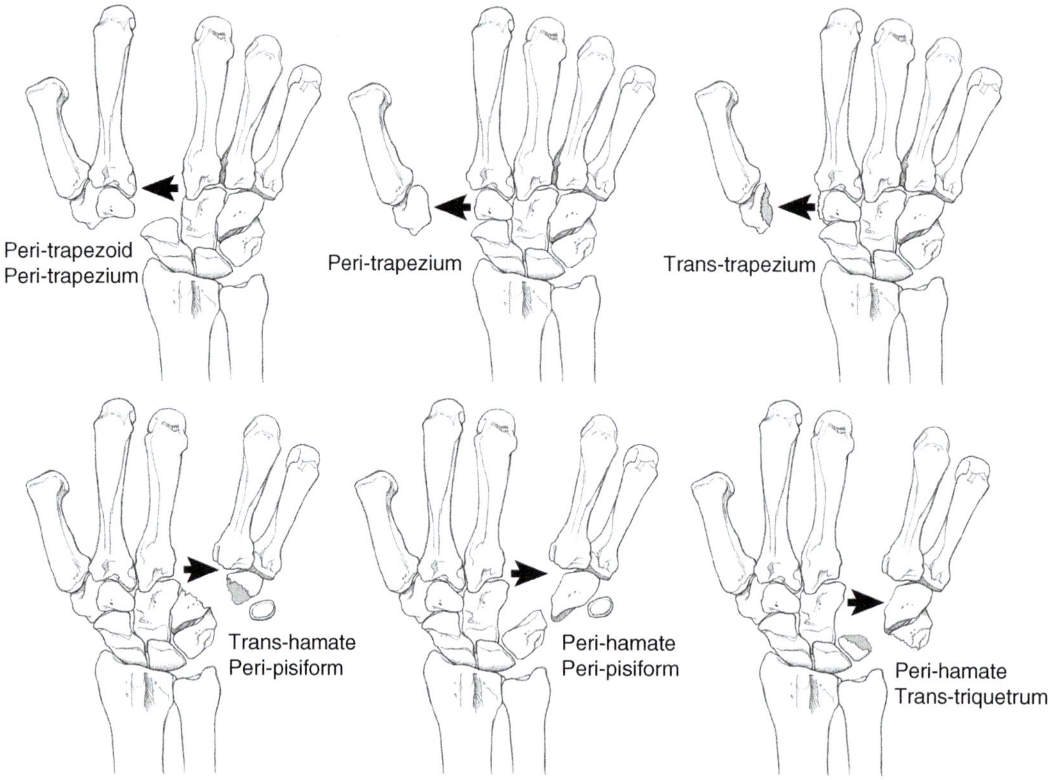

Fig. 21.1 In axial-radial fracture-dislocations, the radial segment is unstable (*top row*). The opposite occurs in axial-ulnar fracture-dislocations, where the ulnar segment is unstable (*bottom row*) (Copyright Mayo Foundation, with permission)

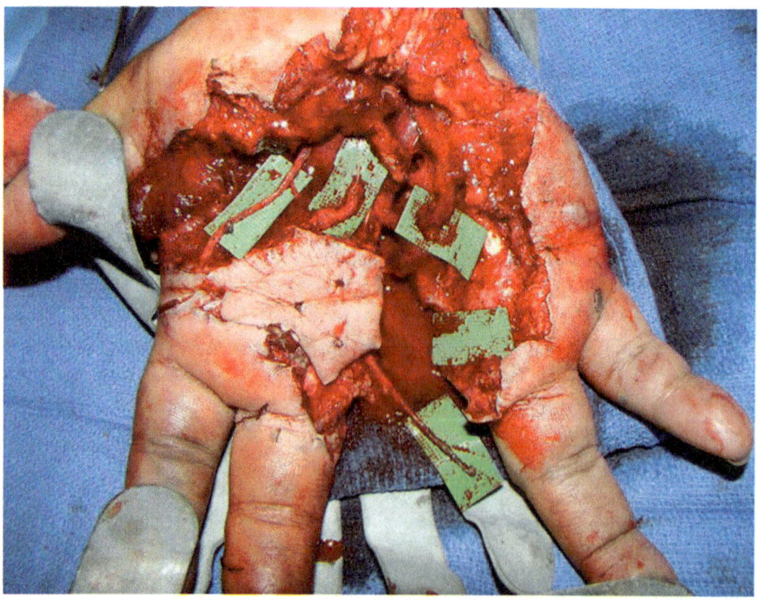

Fig. 21.2 Massive soft tissue injury following a fo`urth of July fireworks blast injury

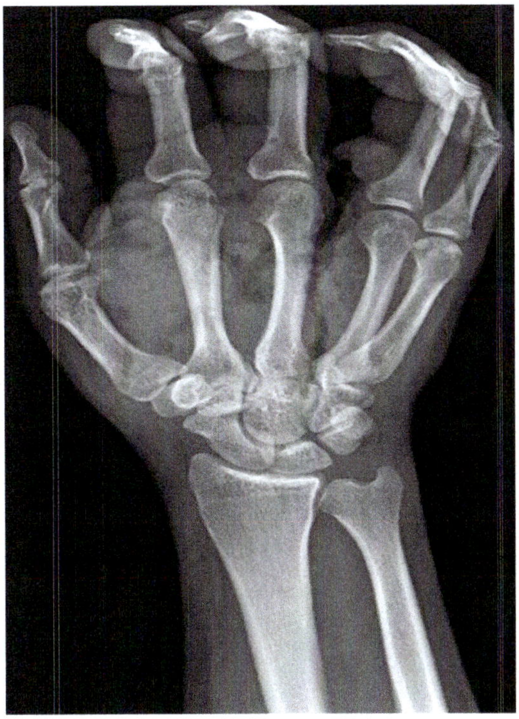

Fig. 21.3 Posteroanterior hand radiograph showing axial-ulnar fracture-dislocation injury

than the transverse carpal ligament in maintaining the stability of the arch [5].

The three ligaments of the capitohamate joint occur only in the distal half of the joint, leaving the proximal half without formal interosseous ligament support (Fig. 21.4) [9]. As such, the capitohamate joint allows more motion proximally than distally. The predominant motion in the capitohamate joint is thus coronal rotation with the pivot point centered at the deep capitohamate ligament [8]. The magnitude of rotation reported to occur at the capitohamate joint ranges from 5° to 12° and occur during extremes of ulnar deviation and finger flexion, or wrist hyperflexion [3]. A cadaveric biomechanical study found that the passive range of motion at the capitohamate joint was as much as 17° [8]. Other passive motions found in the capitohamate joint in the same study were proximal-distal translation (1.2 mm), dorsopalmar translation (1.4 mm), and distraction (0.3 mm).

Despite 4° of passive motion in the capitohamate joint, it is still very limited, and it can be considered to be a single functional unit. The distal carpal row of four carpal bones and the second and third metacarpal rays can be regarded as a central fixed unit in the hand around which the thumb rotates in a large arc on the radial side. On the ulnar side, the mobility of the fourth and fifth carpometacarpal joints is important in gripping, facilitating to a high degree the opposition between the thumb and the ulnar two fingers. Any gripping or pinching motion results in moments at the third carpometacarpal joint and capitohamate joint, where the integrity of the fixed unit is ensured by interlocking bony architecture and strong interosseous ligaments [7, 9].

Clinical

At this point in time, capitohamate axial carpal instability is the only dynamic axial carpal instability reported [10]. It is a rare cause of posttraumatic chronic ulnar-sided wrist pain. Unlike axial dissociations of the distal carpal row which occur following high-energy trauma, capitohamate axial carpal instability requires a large enough force to injure the strong ligaments of the capitohamate joint, but not enough to produce a dislocation. Based on our experience, we have seen the capitohamate instability as a part of an axial carpal dynamic instability pattern. Rarely is capitohamate instability seen in isolation but is most frequently seen with either a scapholunate or lunotriquetral dynamic instability as well, similar to the axial-ulnar or axial-radial patterns described by Garcia-Elias et al. [4, 5]. Since this case report, we have identified this pattern of injury in nearly 20 patients with chronic wrist pain with normal radiographs.

Capitohamate axial carpal instability can occur following moderate injury such as when someone sustains a heavy fall on outstretched hand. The reported mechanism of injury in this case is one of falling on the hypothenar region producing an extension and radial deviation force to the wrist. Other mechanisms of injury include axial loading of the ulnar side, such as from a punching mechanism, or a mild to moderate crushing type of injury.

In the only reported case in the literature, the patient presented after tripping and falling with

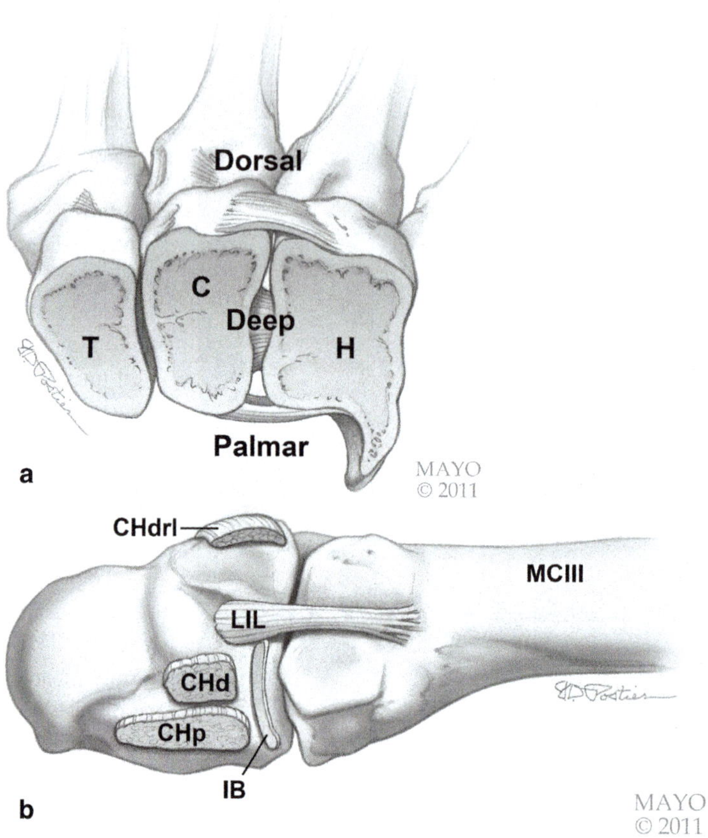

Fig. 21.4 (**a**, **b**) The ligament anatomy of the capitohamate joint consists of three subregions: the dorsal capitohamate ligament (*CHdrl*), the deep capitohamate ligament (*CHd*) (**a**, **b**), and the palmar capitohamate ligament (*CHp*). A longitudinal interosseous ligament (*LIL*), which spans the articular recess of the capitate to the base of the third metacarpal (*MCIII*), can be present. Additionally, an interconnecting band (*IB*) can be found at the distal margin of the CH joint. *T* trapezoid, *C* capitate, *H* hamate (Copyright Mayo Foundation, with permission)

resultant chronic ulnar-sided wrist ache that persisted for 7 months with occasional sharp pain aggravated by lifting and grasping activities. It was found to be particularly associated with little finger flexion. Examination revealed diffuse ulnar-sided wrist tenderness. Mild discomfort was reproduced with wrist ulnar deviation and resisted active finger flexion. Grip strength was also reduced. Diagnostic injections of lidocaine into the midcarpal joint resulted in increased grip strength with near complete resolution of pain.

All imaging modalities had come up with no diagnosis to explain his symptoms. Routine and stress radiographs of the wrist did not show any abnormality. Bone scan only showed increased uptake in the region of the hamate. Magnetic resonance imaging (MRI) was normal. A previous arthrogram revealed a small leak in the triangular fibrocartilage with no other pathologies.

Since this case report, the pattern of injury typically seen include a capitohamate instability in addition to either a scapholunate or lunotriquetral. Between the two, a combined capitohamate and lunotriquetral dynamic instability pattern is more common; based on Garcia-Elias' classification, this would be a dynamic perihamate peritriquetral axial-ulnar instability pattern. An axial load is a typical mechanism of injury such as following a punch with loading on the ulnar side of the wrist.

The radiographs are of an illustrative patient's right hand after punching a wall (Fig. 21.5). Except for mild soft tissue swelling over the dorsum of the wrist, it did not show any fracture or dislocations. Three months later, the patient still complained of ulnar wrist pain. Examination revealed tenderness over the dorso-ulnar carpus, including over the capitohamate joint. There was also pain on capitohamate ballottement. Repeat radiographs were normal with resolution of soft tissue swelling previously seen. A bone scan showed increased uptake in the ulnar carpal bones of the right wrist (Fig. 21.6).

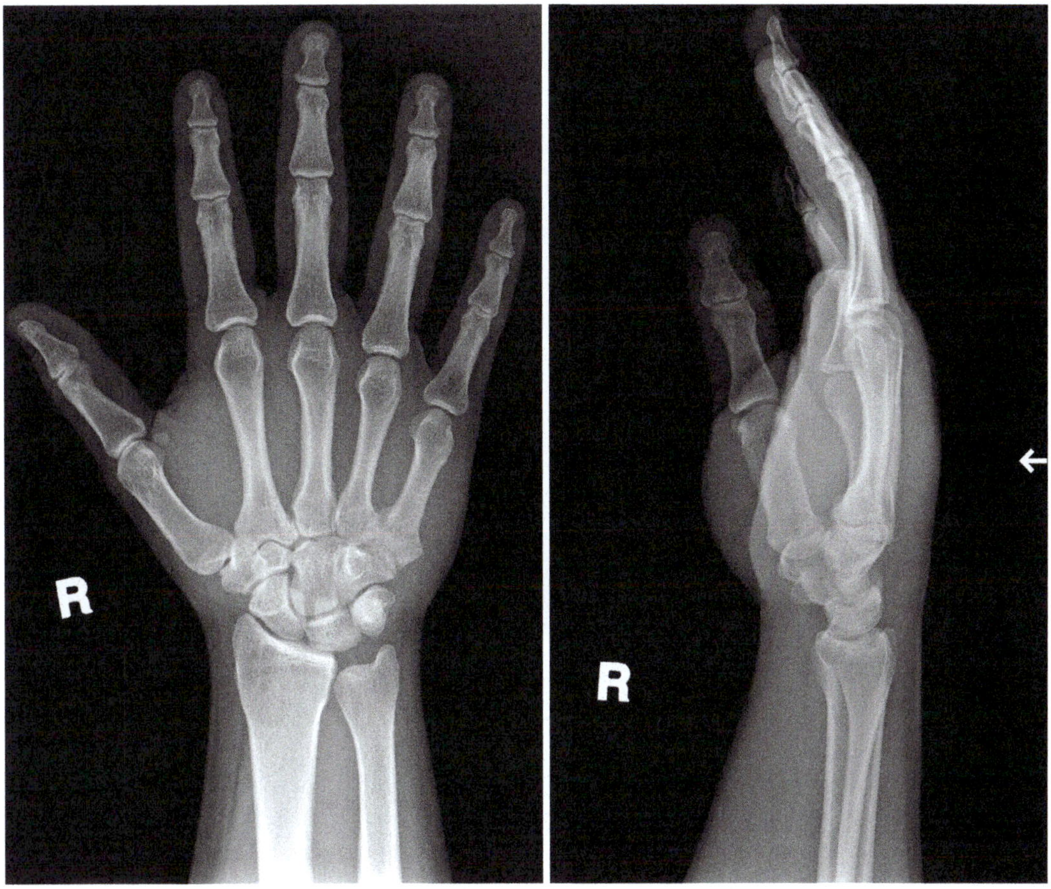

Fig. 21.5 Routine radiographs of a patient with right ulnar wrist pain after punching a wall. There were no fractures or dislocations although soft tissue swelling can be seen over the dorsum of the hand

Indications

Clinical suspicion and exam are likely to yield pain with capitohamate ballottement. Capitohamate ballottement is similar to ballottement of the scapholunate or lunotriquetral joints. The capitate is stabilized with the examiners thumb and index finger, and the hamate is stabilized with the examiners' other thumb and index finger. The capitate and hamate are translated dorsal and palmar with respect to each other. A positive test is one in which there is pain elicited from this maneuver. Occasionally, gross instability can be found in comparison to the contralateral wrist. Radiographic imaging with CT or MRI may demonstrate diastasis or incongruity, but this can be quite subtle. Bone scan can show marked increased uptake but is highly nonspecific. A diagnostic wrist arthroscopy is typically indicated for diagnosis in those individuals with chronic wrist pain in the axial carpal area who has not improved with previous conservative treatment, with no attributable diagnoses found on standard imaging modalities.

Technique

A standard wrist arthroscopy procedure is used with the hand in an arthroscopic tower. No other special instruments are required. Radiocarpal arthroscopy using the standard portals is first performed. Midcarpal arthroscopy using the midcarpal ulnar and midcarpal radial portals is next performed in the routine manner. Following that, the capitohamate joint should be inspected. Any gaps should be noted. The hamate can be balloted

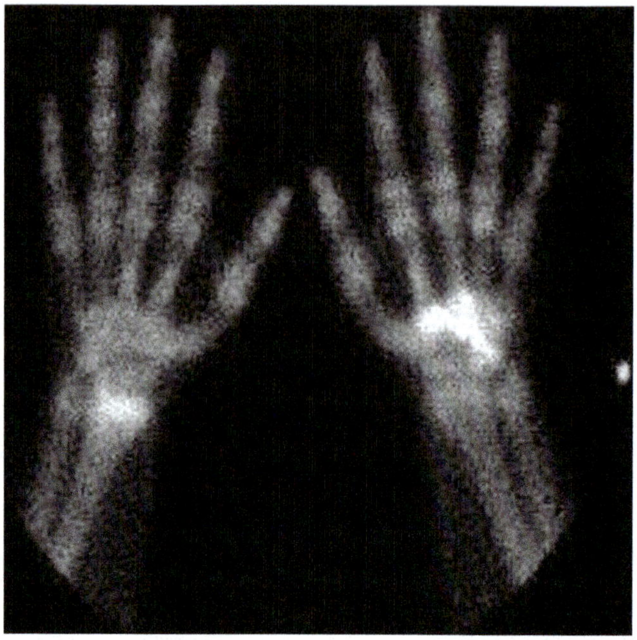

Fig. 21.6 Bone scan show increased uptake in the trapezoid, capitate, hamate, and triquetrum of the right wrist 3 months after the punching injury

and the joint can be inspected at the same time to look for any joint displacement. Alternatively, if available, manually pumping the irrigation may force a gap in the capitohamate joint, if it is unstable, using hydrostatic pressure. Finally, a probe can be inserted into the joint to determine the degree of laxity according to Geissler's classification [6].

This illustrative patient with chronic ulnar wrist pain following a punching injury underwent right wrist arthroscopy which showed Geissler's grade II scapholunate ligament injury, grade III lunotriquetral ligament injury, and grade IV capitohamate ligament injury (Fig. 21.7).

Capitohamate dynamic instability is treated by limited intercarpal fusion. Arthroscopic arthrodesis and placement of a cannulated percutaneous screw could be considered if the capitohamate dynamic instability is found in isolation; however, this is rarely the case. As many of these dynamic instabilities require addressing proximal carpal row instabilities, a formal open surgical procedure is required. A dorsal skin incision is used followed by ligament-sparing dorsal capsulotomy as described by Berger [1, 11]. A posterior interosseous neurectomy is typically performed at the same time. The diagnoses can be reconfirmed at this stage which may include associated instabilities of the lunotriquetral joint (Figs. 21.8 and 21.9). The cartilage between the capitate and hamate is then removed and autologous cancellous bone graft from distal radius or iliac crest inserted. Fixation can be performed using staples, dorsal plate, or intraosseous screws. Concomitant SL or LT instability should be addressed as well and is beyond the scope of this chapter. In our illustrative case, an extensor carpi ulnaris tendon was used to reconstruct the lunotriquetral ligament (Figs. 21.10, 21.11, and 21.12).

Postoperative Outcome

In the case reported in the literature, the capitohamate fusion was healed within 6 weeks confirmed by trispiral tomography. At 3-year follow-up, the patient had complete relief of pain with nearly full motion (wrist extension of 77°, flexion of 60°, ulnar deviation 40°, and radial deviation of 13°). Grip strength increased to an average of 60 kg and radiographs showed complete fusion of the capitohamate joint with no evidence of any dissociative carpal instability.

When associated with concomitant scapholunate or lunotriquetral dynamic instability, the wrist should be immobilized until those

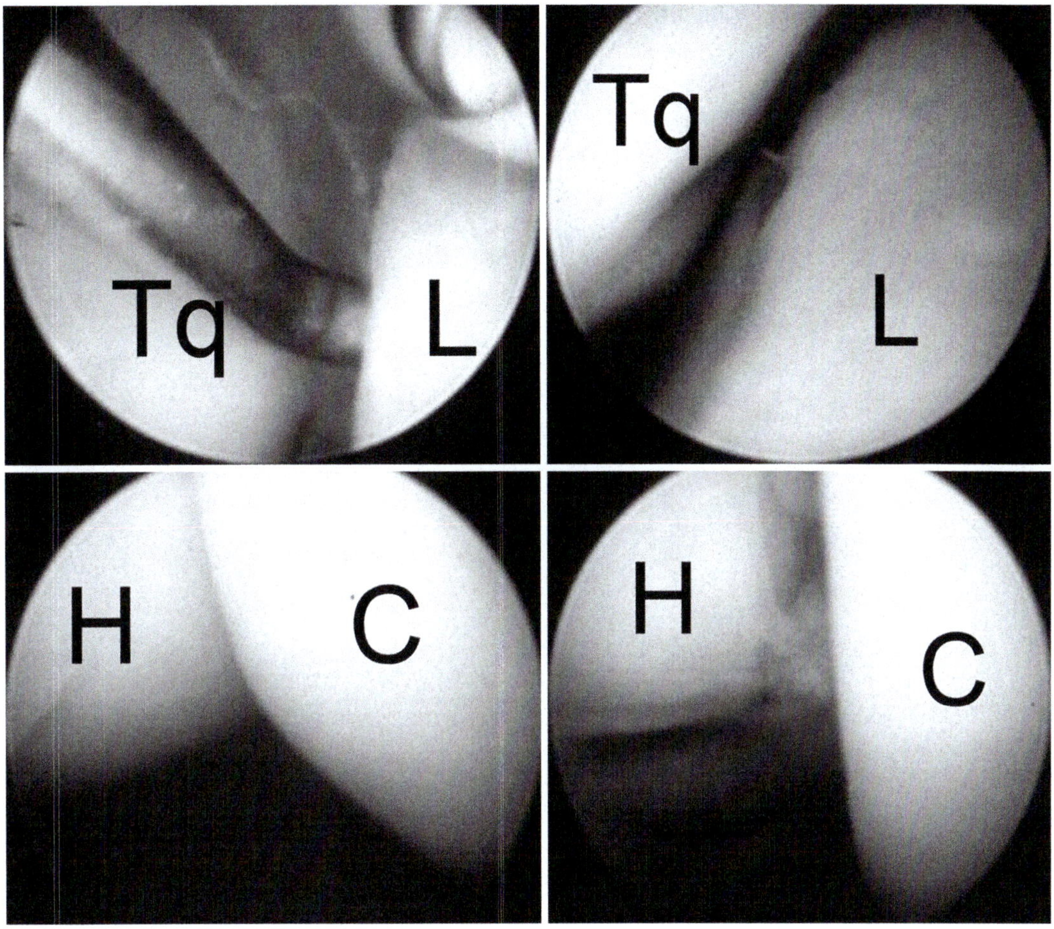

Fig. 21.7 Wrist arthroscopy demonstrating LT grade III instability (*upper left and right*) and capitohamate grade II instability (*lower left and right*). Note the easy admittance of the arthroscopic probe into the capitohamate articulation (*Tq* triquetrum, *L* lunate, *H* hamate, *C* capitate)

ligaments are healed or till the surgical reconstructions performed are stable.

Conclusion

Capitohamate dynamic axial carpal instability is a rare cause of chronic ulnar-sided wrist pain. Typical mechanisms of injury include fall on the ulnar side of the hand, punching injuries with loading on the ulnar side of the wrist, or mild to moderate crush injuries. Patients typically have chronic dorso-ulnar wrist pain with tenderness in and around the capitohamate region. Capitohamate ballottement may be positive for pain. Grip strength is often reduced. Radiographs often do not reveal any abnormalities. Bone scans may show increased uptake in the ulnar carpus but is often nonspecific. Magnetic resonance imaging and computed tomographic scans of the wrist are usually more helpful in finding associated abnormalities such as scapholunate or lunotriquetral ligament injuries. Diagnosis of capitohamate axial instability can only be confirmed at this point by direct visualization during midcarpal wrist arthroscopy. The severity of it can be graded using Geissler's classification. Treatment is with capitohamate fusion using autologous cancellous bone graft with implant fixation. Capitohamate axial instability is often associated with lunotriquetral or scapholunate instability producing a perihamate peritriquetral or perihamate perilunate type of axial carpal dynamic instability. These associated proximal carpal row instabilities need to be managed accordingly, depending on their severity.

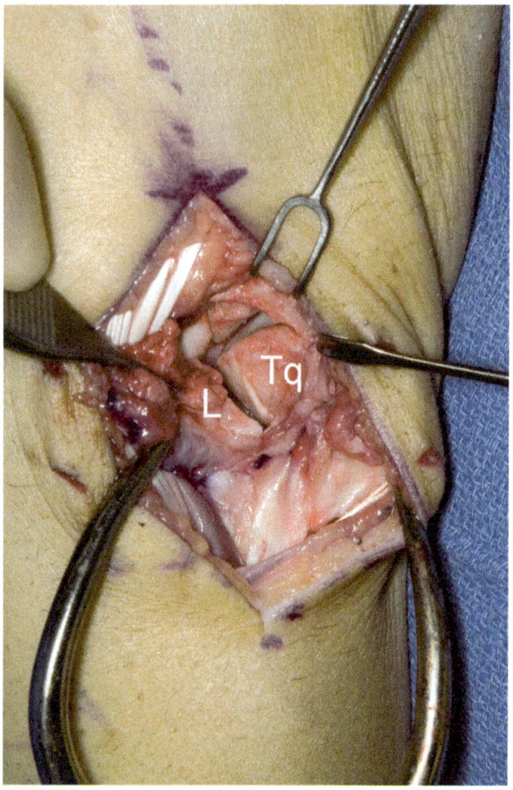

Fig. 21.8 Gross lunotriquetral joint instability (*L* lunate, *Tq* triquetrum)

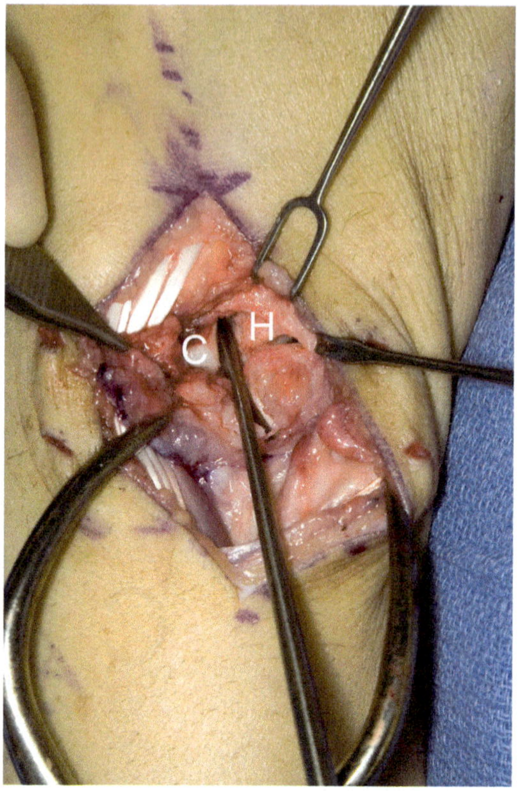

Fig. 21.9 Gross capitohamate joint instability. This is clearly a case of perihamate peritriquetral axial-ulnar carpal dynamic instability (*C* capitate, *H* hamate)

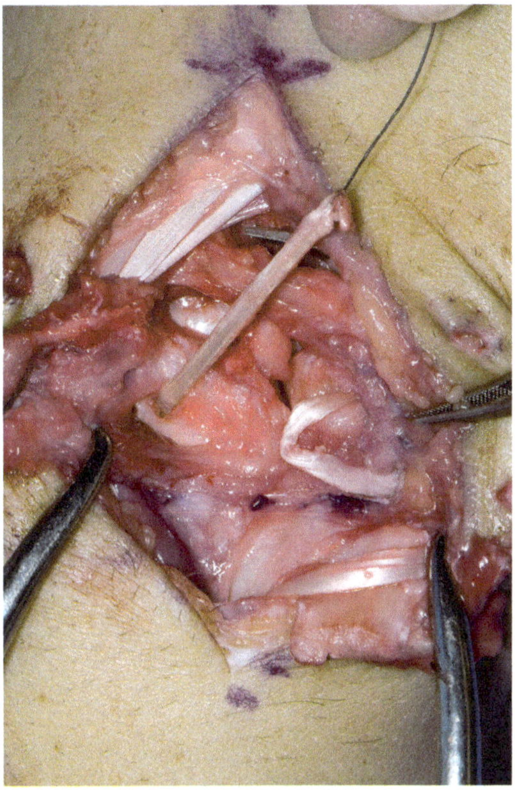

Fig. 21.10 Distally based extensor carpi ulnaris hemi-tendon used to reconstruct the incompetent lunotriquetral ligament

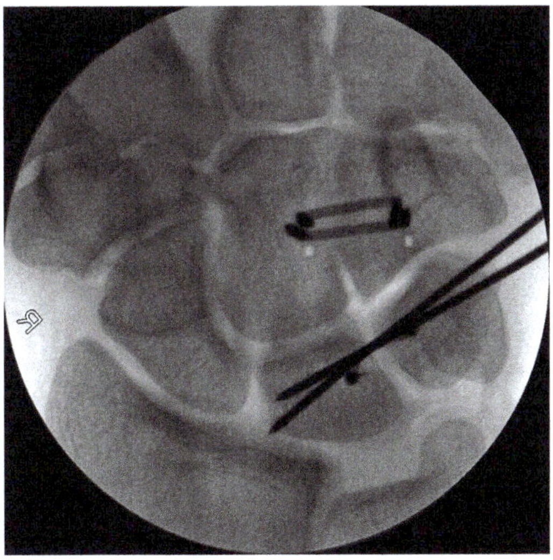

Fig. 21.11 Immediate postoperative radiograph demonstrating the capitohamate fixation with a staple as well as the LT reconstruction with temporary K-wire fixation

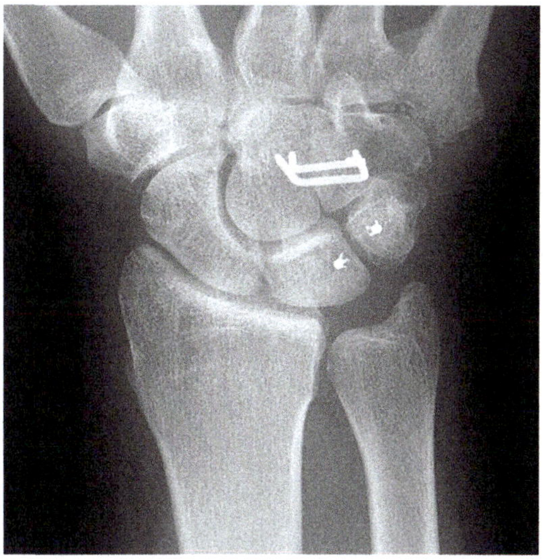

Fig. 21.12 Follow-up radiograph 6 months post surgery with K-wires removed

References

1. Berger RA (2007) A method of defining palpable landmarks for the ligament-splitting dorsal wrist capsulotomy. J Hand Surg Am 32(8):1291–1295. doi:10.1016/j.jhsa.2007.07.023
2. Cooney WP, Bussey R, Dobyns JH, Linscheid RL (1987). Difficult wrist fractures. Perilunate fracture-dislocations of the wrist. Clin Orthop Relat Res 214:136–147
3. de Lange A, Kauer JM, Huiskes R (1985) Kinematic behavior of the human wrist joint: a roentgen-stereophotogrammetric analysis. J Orthop Res 3(1):56–64
4. Garcia-Elias M, An KN, Cooney WP, Linscheid RL, Chao EY (1989) Stability of the transverse carpal arch: an experimental study. J Hand Surg Am 14(2 Pt 1):277–282
5. Garcia-Elias M, Dobyns JH, Cooney WP, Linscheid RL (1989) Traumatic axial dislocations of the carpus. J Hand Surg Am 14(3):446–457
6. Geissler WB, Freeland AE, Savoie FH, McIntyre LW, Whipple TL (1996) Intracarpal soft-tissue lesions associated with an intra-articular fracture of the distal end of the radius. J Bone Joint Surg Am 78-A(3):357–365
7. Gunther SF (1984) The carpometacarpal joints. Orthop Clin North Am 15(2):259–277
8. Ritt MJ, Berger RA, Bishop AT, An KN (1996) The capitohamate ligaments. A comparison of biomechanical properties. J Hand Surg Br 21(4):451–454
9. Ritt MJ, Berger RA, Kauer JM (1996) The gross and histologic anatomy of the ligaments of the capitohamate joint. J Hand Surg Am 21(6):1022–1028
10. Shin AY, Glowacki K, Bishop A (1999) Dynamic axial carpal instability: a case report. J Hand Surg Am 24(4):781–785
11. Tay SC, Shin AY (2006) Surgical approaches to the carpus. Hand Clin 22(4):421–434

22 Ulnar Injuries in Distal Radius Fractures

J. Henk Coert

Introduction

In the time of Hippocrates and Galen, distal radius fractures were thought to be dislocations of the wrist. In France, Pouteau was the first to differ from this view when he described in 1783 a variety of forearm fractures in the French literature, including distal radius fractures. Pouteau presented a muscular theory of fracture pattern etiology, but one that is useful in the understanding of the displacement of the bone fragments. His ideas were directed to the concept that in sprains and dislocations, ligamentous injuries should be considered in the differential diagnosis of forearm injury. As a result, distal radius fractures were initially termed Pouteau fractures in the French-speaking world [17].

These ideas stress that it is important to realize that other problems may be involved with the injury than just the fracture. An opposite view is that a distal radius fracture is a soft-tissue injury surrounding a broken bone and the radiographic diagnosis should not distract the surgeon from carefully assessing forearm soft-tissue issues [8].

New diagnostic tools, like arthrography and MRI, have improved imaging and understanding of these injuries. However, wrist arthroscopy has been the latest and most significant milestone, not only in diagnosing, but also in the minimally invasive treatment of ulnar injuries [36].

When the distal radius fracture has been treated in the (sub) acute phase, concomitant injuries can be detected by examination under anesthesia and preferably by wrist arthroscopy as plain films are usually not helpful [14, 15]. Destabilizing ligamentous injuries are thought to be an important cause of residual problems [16].

This chapter will discuss the acute and chronic ulnar injuries that can occur in distal radius fractures and can cause ulnar-sided wrist pain. Apart from the traditional work-up with physical examination and additional imaging (mostly MRI), the focus will be on the benefits of wrist arthroscopy. Arthroscopy has the unique possibility to diagnose and to treat pathology in the same procedure! On the other hand, ligaments can be visualized and tested for their mechanical integrity.

Work-Up

When evaluating the patient, the medical history should include the mechanism of injury. This may alert the hand surgeon towards ulnar injuries due to the excessive loading of the ulnar side. In the acute setting, physical examination is usually not helpful especially when the fracture will be treating conservatively. The wrist cannot be examined adequately because of pain and swelling. With closed or open reduction and fixation, the stability of the distal radioulnar joint and the lunate-triquetrum interval can only be evaluated

J.H. Coert, M.D., Ph.D.
Department of Plastic Surgery,
Erasmus Medical Center and Sint Franciscus Gasthuis,
Rotterdam, The Netherlands
e-mail: j.coert@erasmusmc.nl

F. del Piñal et al. (eds.), *Arthroscopic Management of Ulnar Pain*,
DOI 10.1007/978-3-642-30544-3_22, © Springer-Verlag Berlin Heidelberg 2012

properly under regional or general anesthesia. Comparison with the contralateral side is essential. Early diagnosis in the acute setting will therefore only be feasible, when fractures are not being treated conservatively.

In the chronic setting with persisting pain, the focus should be on ulnar structures.

The physical examination of a patient with ulnar-sided wrist pain begins with inspection. Symmetry of the wrist compared with that of the contralateral extremity and symmetry of the ulnar-sided digits compared with that of the radial-sided digits should be noted. In the acute setting, erythema, cyanosis, and edema may be present and should be noted. A focal area of swelling around the wrist may suggest a ganglion in the chronic case. Previous surgical or traumatic scars are important to note. Atrophy can be assessed by comparison with the contralateral extremity, and its presence is suggestive of nerve pathology. Atrophy of the hypothenar eminence may result from ulnar nerve compression in Guyon's canal or more proximally and can be expected to cause sensory disturbances in the ulnar nerve distribution [33, 34]. One should consider pathology of the extensor carpi ulnaris tendon (ECU) for chronic tendinitis, (sub)luxation or partial laceration (see also Chap. 25). Midcarpal instability should be considered when the patient complains of a so-called wrist clunk. This can be assessed by bringing the wrist under axial loading and moving the wrist from ulnar to radial (Lichtman test) [9]. A painful clunk may direct the diagnosis towards this problem. It is imperative to compare to the contralateral side.

Plain films of acute injuries can detect bony injuries or dislocations. Fractures like Galeazzi fractures, intra-articular fracture involving the DRUJ, or ulnar styloid fractures will reveal ulnar pathology. Unfortunately, almost all fractures of the distal radius may involve soft-tissue injuries that are not visible on plain films. Attention should be given to the ulna plus situation after distal radius fractures, and comparison between both wrists is very helpful. In the chronic setting, examination with a fluoroscan may show these dynamic instabilities as well as ulnar abutment if they are not visible on the conventional views.

In the chronic situation, stabilities of the lunate-triquetrum interval, the DRUJ, and the ECU tendon within the sheath are critical factors to locate pathology causing ulnar pain.

When ulnar wrist pain exists without clinical instability on the ulnar side, additional work-up should be considered. MRI with or without intra-articular contrast is the choice. Pathology of the TFCC, lunate-triquetrum interval, ECU and subsheath, quality of cartilage on the lunate fossa, lunate, DRUJ, and distal ulna, and synovitis can be seen. High-resolution MRI using a microscopy surface coil allowed assessment of each TFCC component and showed a higher accuracy for diagnosing injuries to the radial attachment and the disc of the TFCC compared with previous studies. High-resolution MRI was not able to diagnose distal radioulnar ligament (DRUL), palmar radioulnar ligament (PRUL), or ulno-lunate ligament injuries accurately [27]. The major limitations are asymptomatic tears in the central and/or peripheral TFCC and the lunate-triquetrum ligament due to normal wear. For pathology of Palmer 1B or 1C, MRI may give false-negative results.

Figure 22.1 contains a list of differential diagnoses for possible causes of ulnar-sided wrist pain associated with distal radius fractures [6].

Figures 22.2, 2.3, 22.4, and 22.5 show schematic drawings of, respectively, ulnar impaction, ulnar styloid fracture, distal radioulnar osteoarthritis, and lunate-triquetrum ligament injury.

Ulnar-sided pain can also be seen as two separate entities: with and without symptomatic clinical instability. It is critical to compare to the contralateral side and to ascertain that the instability is symptomatic as some patients may have (usually bilateral) asymptomatic instability. In the group of patients without instability, localizing the pathology may be more difficult. In these cases, three-phase bone scans may be helpful to locate the origin of pain and to exclude an osseous etiology (Fig. 22.6).

Figure 22.7 shows the possible causes of ulnar pain divided into stable or unstable. Extensor carpi ulnaris subluxation is not a true instability, but the click may be perceived as instability by the patient (Fig. 22.8).

Fig. 22.1 This table lists differential diagnoses for ulnar-sided wrist pain

Structure	Diagnosis
Bone	• Fracture: ulnar styloid, triquetrum, hamate, metacarpal base, pisoforme • Kienbock's disease
TFCC	• Classification Palmer 1 A-D or Class I-V
Joint	• Osteo-arthritis, DRUJ instability, ulno-carpal impingement, ganglion, pisiforme-triquetrum arthritis
Carpal ligament	• Lunate-triquetrum instability, midcarpal instability
Nerve	• Ulnar nerve compression, dorsal branch ulnar nerve neuralgia
Tendon	• Extensor carpi ulnaris tendinitis, subluxation or (partial) rupture, flexor carpi ulnaris tendinitis

Causes of pain may be an occult fracture, osteoarthritis, and ulnar impaction syndrome [22]. Especially, early osteoarthritic changes may be detected by bone scans [5] (Figs. 22.9 and 22.10 and 22.11).

Technique

The patient is in a supine position with the elbow on the arm table. I prefer to use a commercially available traction tower. This device allows pivoting the arm into a horizontal position while the wrist remains in traction. This may be helpful if a power drill is needed.

This will also facilitate the reduction and fixation of the distal radius fracture if the fracture and ligament injuries are being treated simultaneously in the acute setting.

Before applying the traction and draping, I prefer to redo the wrist examination on both wrists. The stability of the TFCC in full pronation, full supination, and neutral is being compared to the contralateral side. The lunate-triquetrum interval should be assessed again bilaterally. Especially maneuvers that would have provoked pain during normal physical examination can be tested now, e.g., midcarpal instability or ECU subluxation. Special attention is given to clunks and clicks that may be provoked by moving the wrist. Before mounting the arm in the traction device, the landmarks for arthroscopy and the dorsal veins are drawn with a marker. Under tourniquet and 6–7-kg traction, a standard diagnostic arthroscopy is performed. It is imperative to be systemic to avoid overlooking pathology. This has been called "satisfaction of search": one misses a second (typically subtle) abnormality after finding the first. These types of errors are due primarily to a lack of attention to an important region of the image during the search. Especially, in the radiology literature, this has given considerable attention [3, 24].

A standard radiocarpal and midcarpal arthroscopy should be performed as described in Chap. 4. In ulnar wrist pain, injuries to the lunate-triquetrum

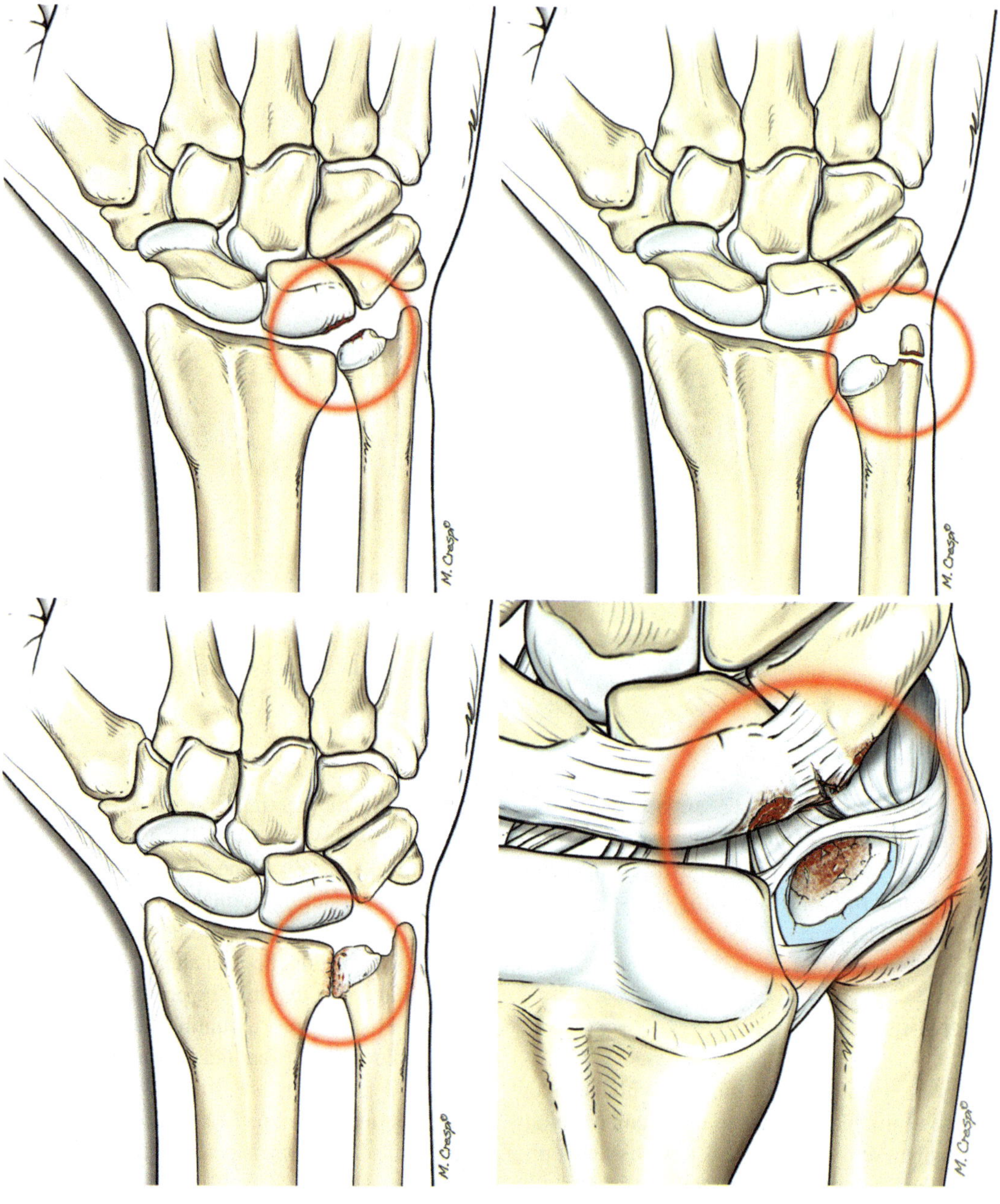

Figs. 22.2, 2.3, 22.4, and 22.5 These schematic drawing are showing, respectively, ulnar impaction, ulnar styloid fracture, distal radioulnar osteoarthritis, and lunate-triquetrum ligament injury with concomitant ulnar impaction

ligament should be assessed via the radiocarpal and midcarpal portals. A small wrist probe could be used to assess the stability of the space between the lunate and the triquetrum.

While the wrist is in traction, the Reagan test can be performed. Mechanical integrity can be judged at direct visualization. Synovitis in this area could also be indicative of injury to this ligament with symptomatic instability (see also Chap. 17). A small blue blade shaver is used to clear scar tissue and loose bodies. For the removal of synovitis, an arthroscopic cautery can be used. The triquetrum should be inspected to detect cartilage damage that may have occurred because of

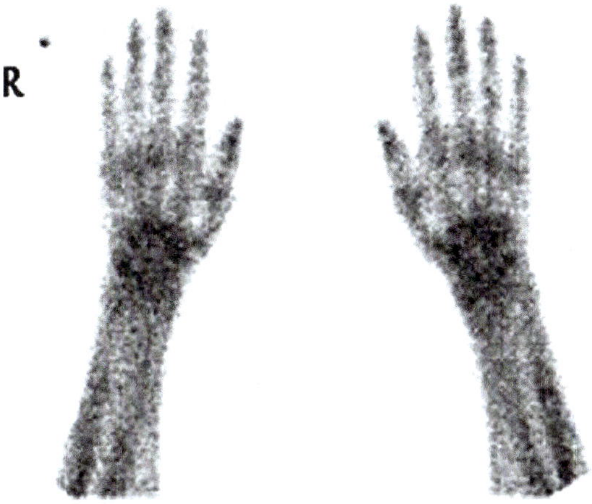

Fig. 22.6 This image shows a negative bone scan in the work-up for ulnar-sided pain

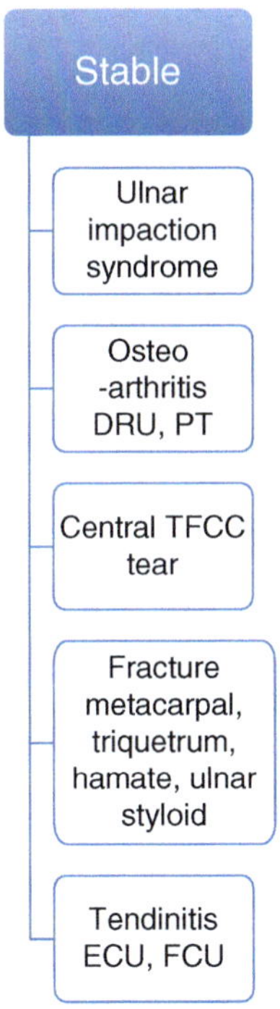

Fig. 22.7 This table lists causes for ulnar pain divided into stable and unstable

ulnar impaction (see also Chap. 15). Then we should focus on pathology related to the distal radioulnar joint. For this, additional portals could be useful: 6U and dorsal DRU portals. When a foveal detachment has been seen, a direct foveal (DF) incision is preferred.

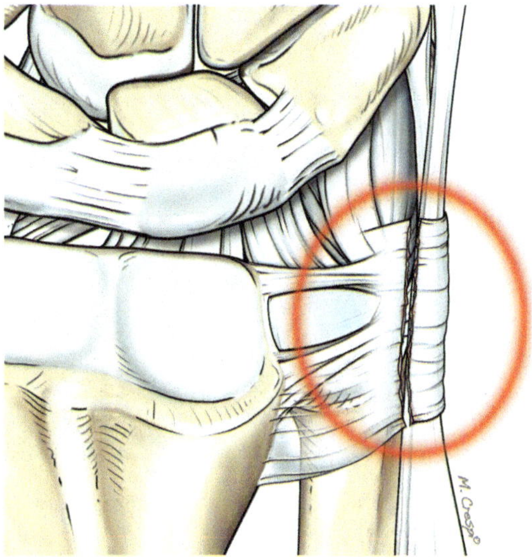

Fig. 22.8 This shows schematically a tear of the ECU subsheath

The TFC complex should be assessed for integrity of the central part and stability (Figs. 22.12, 22.13, and 22.14). In central lesions, synovitis may indicate that this lesion is the cause of the pain. Degenerative wear may also cause central lesions without symptoms.

This can be tested using a wrist probe by performing a "ballottement" (trampoline test) and the "hook test" to judge proximal injuries for the foveal attachment [2]. An ECU subsheath injury cannot be seen via wrist arthroscopy as it is located extra-articular. It is mostly a clinical diagnosis. In some cases, ECU subsheath injuries occur simultaneously. Their close anatomical relation can explain these concurrent injuries.

For suspected pathology of the distal radioulnar joint, the direct DRU portal, can be very useful to assess osteoarthritis or removal of loose bodies. Also, a volar portal has been described to assess the dorsal aspect of the DRU [26] (see also Chaps. 6, 7, 8, 9, 10, and 11).

Discussion

The etiology of ulnar-sided pain after distal radius fractures may very well be the underwater part of an iceberg that only presents itself when you "run

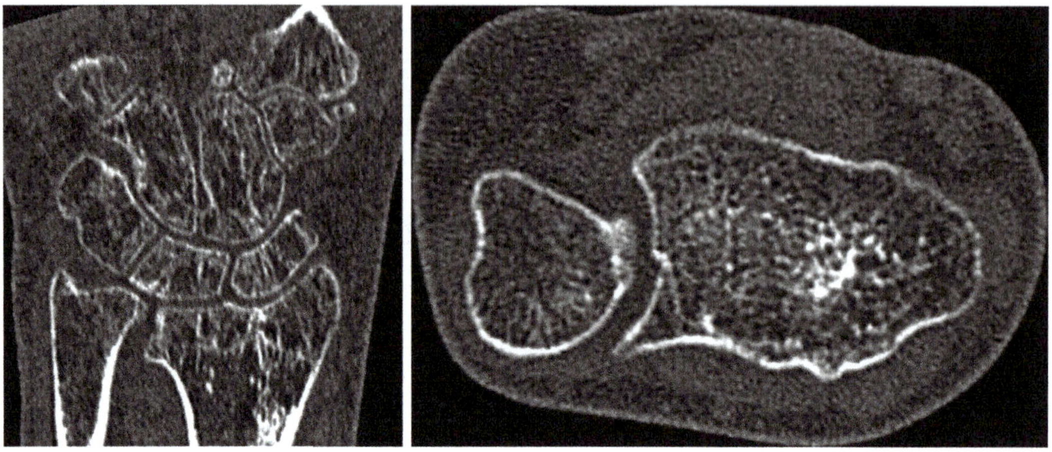

Fig. 22.9 and 22.10 This shows CT scan images of an osteoarthritis distal radioulnar joint and ulnar impaction without clinical instability

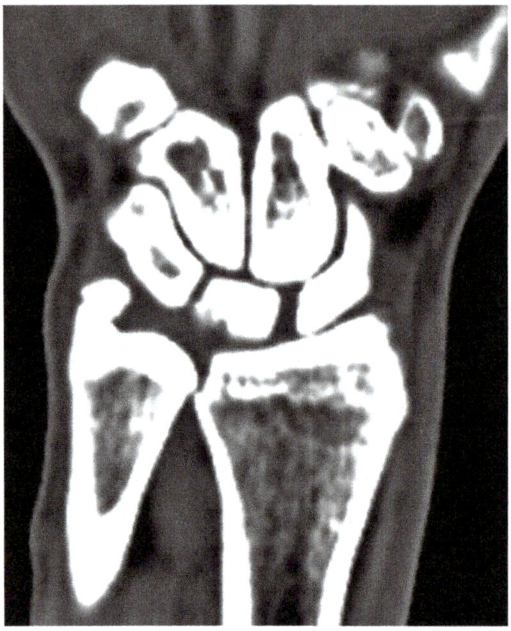

Fig. 22.11 This shows a CT scan image of osteoarthritis distal radioulnar joint with clinical instability

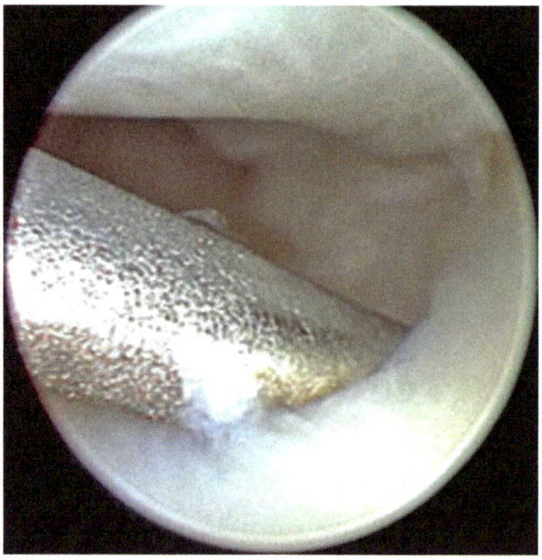

Fig. 22.12 Central TFCC tear

into it" with symptoms. The exact incidence of ulnar injuries after distal radius fracture is not known. Especially, when distal radius fractures have been treated conservatively, the assessment of concomitant injuries cannot perform in the acute setting.

In a group of 36 patients that we treated for Atzei's class 4 TFCC injuries (distal radioulnar instability without healing potential), 18 patients had had distal radius fracture and 14 patients had had an ulnar styloid fracture in their previous medical history. These patients were seen with a chronic instability demonstrating that the ulnar pathology had not been recognized previously. Interestingly, two patients had persisting ulnar pain after stability had been restored. In both cases, this was caused by osteoarthritis of the distal radioulnar joint.

MRI is frequently used to diagnose ulnar pain, in particular for injuries to the TFCC.

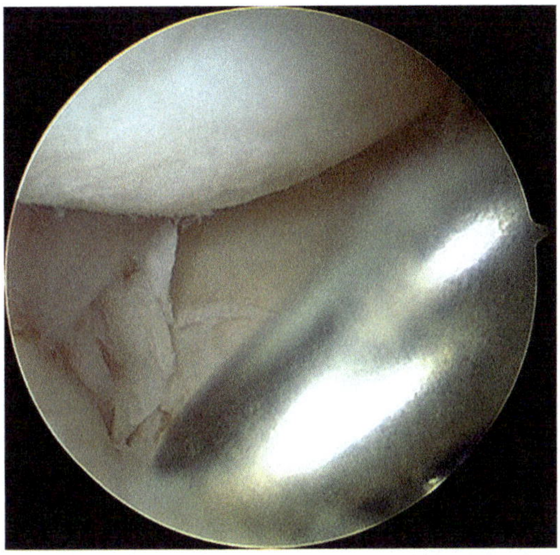

Fig. 22.13 Central tear with probe

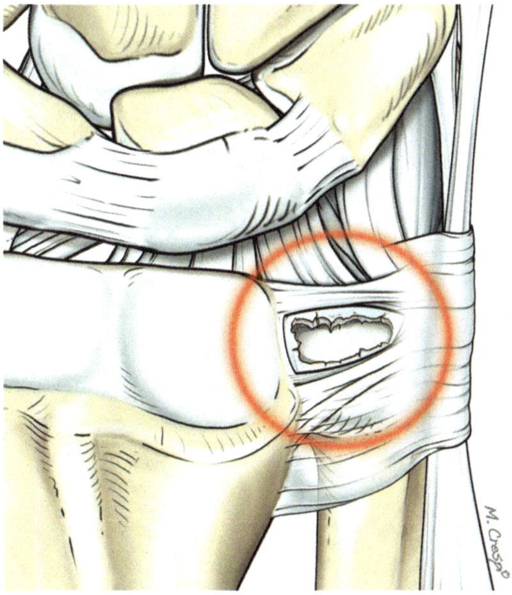

Fig. 22.14 Schematic drawing, central tear

When comparing to wrist arthroscopy, 3 Tesla MRI has shown to have sensitivity for detection of TFCC tears of 86 % and for lunate-triquetrum tears of 82 %. When arthrography was added, sensitivity for detection of ligament and TFCC tears was 100 %. MRI is sensitive and specific for detection of wrist ligament tears. However, MR arthrography can result in false-positive findings because of asymptomatic (micro)perforations [19]. On the other hand, MR imaging cannot adequately show the peripheral attachment of the triangular fibrocartilage complex. The sensitivity for evaluation of the peripheral triangular fibrocartilage complex tear was found to be 17 %, with a specificity of 79 % and an accuracy of 64 %. High signal intensity at the ulnar insertion of the triangular fibrocartilage complex as a marker for tear showed a sensitivity of 42 %, a specificity of 63 %, and an accuracy of 55 % [10]. Conflicting reports on the value MR arthrography has been reported in depicting of peripheral tears of the ulnar attachment of the triangular fibrocartilage. Rüegger reported that these tears often appear as noncommunicating tears extending from the distal radioulnar joint into the triangular fibrocartilage [23].

Also, the CT arthroscopy has been shown to be useful for detecting scaphoid-lunate ligament, lunate-triquetrum ligament, and central TFCC tears with high sensitivity and specificity. It is not as accurate at identifying peripheral tears [4].

For these injuries, arthroscopy still remains the gold standard.

This has been confirmed by others: when compared with arthroscopy of the wrist, the sensitivity, specificity, and accuracy of triple-injection cinearthrography in detecting tears of the scaphoid-lunate ligament, lunate-triquetrum ligament, and triangular fibrocartilage, as a group, were, respectively, 56, 83, and 60 % [35].

If an ulna plus situation is present after a distal radius fracture, this may cause ulnar pain. It has been shown that patients with ulna plus present with significantly higher numbers of apoptotic cells in degenerative lesions in comparison to patients with ulna neutral. The apoptotic cells were evenly distributed throughout the entire specimen. The results of this study revealed that increased length of the ulna is related to increased cell death. Techniques that decrease the ulna variance would appear to be appropriate and would improve the clinical situation by preventing further cell death [30]. High-resolution MRI with a microscopy coil is a useful tool for evaluating the relationship between ulnar variance and ulnar side structures.

Ulnar variance and TFCC angle were positively correlated, and ulnar variance and TFCC

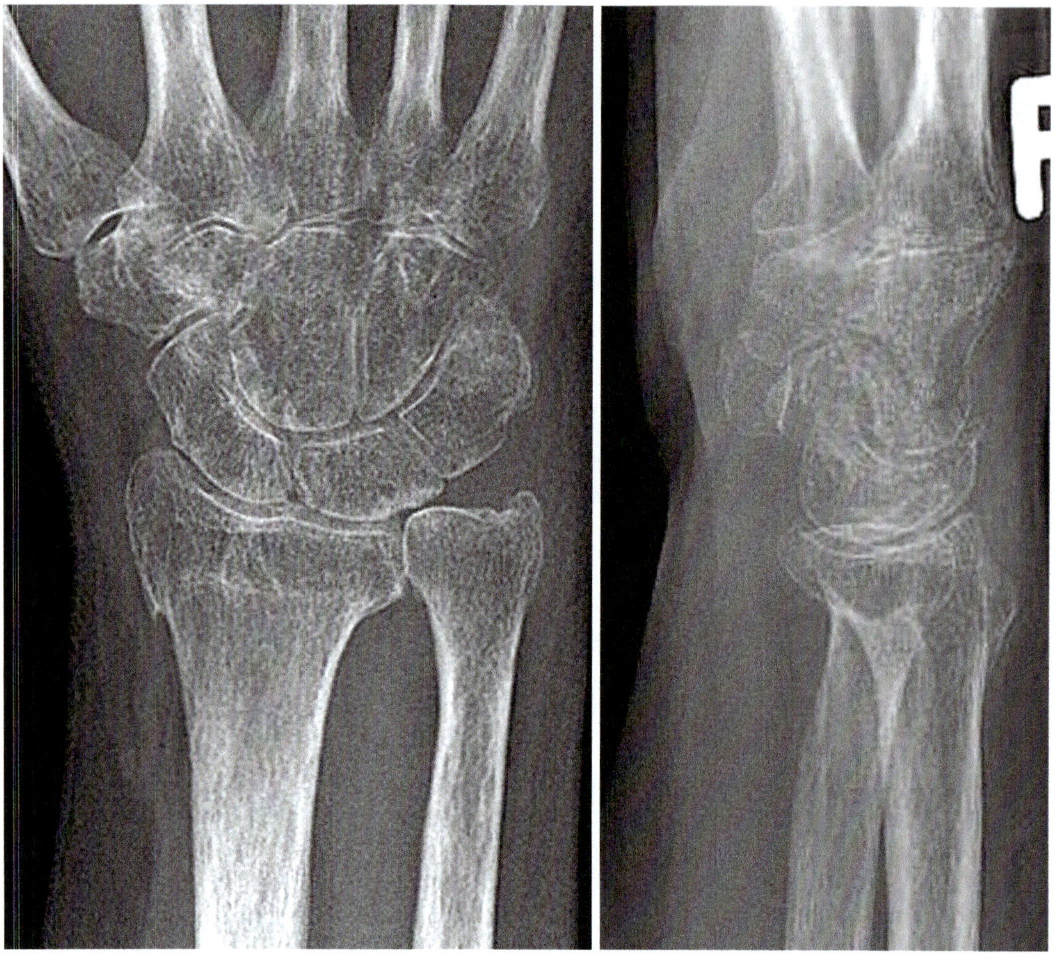

Fig. 22.15 and 22.16 Ulna positive variance with impaction after distal radius fracture

thickness were negatively correlated. However, ulnar variance and lunate or ulnar head cartilage thickness were not significantly correlated.

The relation of ulnar variance and the TFCC and ulnar cartilage has been a matter of debate. Central lesions have associated to positive ulnar variance after trauma. However, it has been reported that the length of the ulna does not play a role in the healing potential [31, 32] (Figs. 4 and 22.15 and 22.16).

Extensor carpi ulnaris pathology is one of the differential diagnoses of ulnar pain. This pathology has been described to occur with coexisting pathology of the TFCC or lunate-triquetrum ligament [1]. Ultrasound has been shown to be helpful in diagnosing dislocation or subluxation of the ECU tendon [18]. Also, a partial rupture of the ECU tendon has been described [7] (Fig. 22.17).

Ulnar variance and TFCC angle are positively correlated, but ulnar variance and TFCC thickness are negatively correlated. Ulnar variance and lunate or ulnar head cartilage thickness are not significantly correlated. MRI with a microscopy coil is a useful tool for evaluating the relationship between ulnar variance and ulnar side structures [37]. Unilateral symptomatic positive ulnar variance may be a cause of ulnar pain. Ulnar impaction may not always be obvious on the plain films, CT or MRI. Patient's pain can improve by an arthroscopic debridement and wafer resection [28]. An ulna-shortening

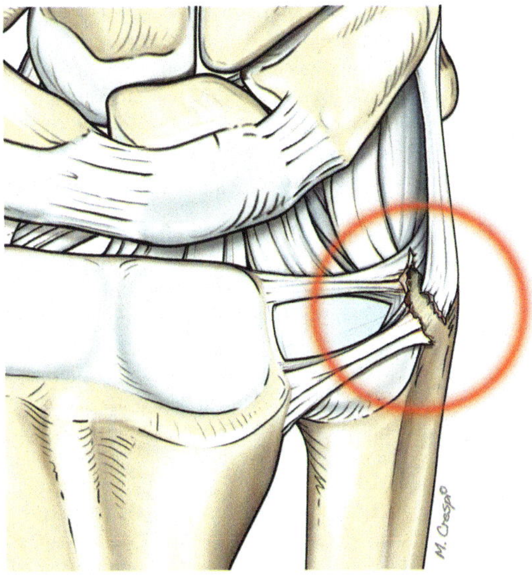

Fig. 22.17 Schematic drawing, Palmer 1B tear

osteotomy should be considered for patients whose previous arthroscopic debridement for central or nondetached peripheral TFCC was unsuccessful in eliminating ulnar-sided wrist pain [11].

Central lesions of the TFCC may be caused by trauma or by degenerative processes. The poor healing potential of the central part has been reported [31, 32]. An apoptotic cascade has been suggested of cells in the central part as result of a trauma [29]. Degeneration phenomena can be found in patients with trauma having occurred more than 18 months ago. The degree of degeneration correlated with the length of time passed since the occurrence of trauma [29]. This may explain persisting ulnar pain some years after a distal radius fracture. Arthroscopic debridement of the central portion of the TFCC for class 1A lesions and the wafer procedure for class 2C lesions has proved to be successful [12, 20, 21]. Laser may be helpful in these offering benefits as hemostasis and exact debridement [13].

Ulnar styloid fracture can be divided into type 1: distal to the base where superficial horizontal fibers of the TFCC insert, as well as the dorsal UT ligament; type 2: base fracture, goes through a line perpendicular to the ulnar shaft and into the proximal limitation of the fovea, but does not involve the articular surface of the ulnar head; and type 3: proximal to a type 2 fracture [25].

Conclusions

Ulnar injuries after distal radius may puzzle the hand surgeon. A variety of pathology can cause ulnar-sided wrist pain. The causes should be divided in injuries with and without clinical wrist instability. Instability is usually caused by damage to the TFCC or lunate-triquetrum ligament. When a thorough medical history, physical examination, and plain films do not lead to a diagnosis, until recently, MRI was the ultimate work-up. However, the sensitivity and specificity of MRIs is limited for the periphery of the TFCC. Wrist arthroscopy has shown superior qualities not only in diagnosing but also in the treatment of ulnar injuries.

Acknowledgment I would like to thank Tyson K. Cobb, M.D. for supplying some of the illustrations.

References

1. Allende C, Le Viet D (2005) Extensor carpi ulnaris problems at the wrist –classification, surgical treatment and results. J Hand Surg Br 30:265–272
2. Atzei A (2009) New trends in arthroscopic management of type 1-B TFCC injuries with DRUJ instability. J Hand Surg Eur 34:582–591
3. Berbaum KS, El-Khoury GY, Ohashi K, Schartz KM, Caldwell RT, Madsen M, Franken EA Jr (2007) Satisfaction of Search in Multi-trauma Patients: Severity of Detected Fractures. Acad Radiol 14:711–722
4. Bille B, Harley B, Cohen H (2007) A comparison of CT arthrography of the wrist to findings during wrist arthroscopy. J Hand Surg Am 32:834–841
5. Buckland-Wright JC, Macfarlane DG, Lynch JA (1995) Sensitivity of radiographic features and specificity of scintigraphic imaging in hand osteoarthritis. Rev Rheum Engl Ed 62(Suppl 1):14S–26S
6. Cerezal L, Abascal F, García-Valtuille R, Del Piñal F (2005) Wrist MR arthrography: how, why, when. Radiol Clin North Am 43:709–731
7. Chun S, Palmer AK (1987) Chronic ulnar wrist pain secondary to partial rupture of the extensor carpi ulnaris tendon. J Hand Surg Am 12:1032–1035
8. Davis DI, Baratz M (2010) Soft tissue complications of distal radius fractures. Hand Clin 26:229–235

9. Feinstein WK, Lichtman DM, Noble PC, Alexander JW, Hipp JA (1999) Quantitative assessment of the midcarpal shift test. J Hand Surg Am 24:977–983
10. Haims AH, Schweitzer ME, Morrison WB, Deely D, Lange R, Osterman AL, Bednar JM, Taras JS, Culp RW (2002) Limitations of MR imaging in the diagnosis of peripheral tears of the triangular fibrocartilage of the wrist. AJR Am J Roentgenol 178:419–422
11. Hulsizer D, Weiss AP, Akelman E (1999) Ulna-shortening osteotomy after failed arthroscopic debridement of the triangular fibrocartilage complex. J Hand Surg Am 22:694–698
12. Husby T, Haugstvedt JR (2001) Long-term results after arthroscopic resection of lesions of the triangular fibrocartilage complex. Scand J Plast Reconstr Surg Hand Surg 35:79–83
13. Infanger M, Grimm D (2009) Meniscus and discus lesions of triangular fibrocartilage complex (TFCC): treatment by laser-assisted wrist arthroscopy. J Plast Reconstr Aesthet Surg 62:466–471
14. Lindau T (2005) Treatment of injuries to the ulnar side of the wrist occurring with distal radial fractures. Hand Clin 21:417–425
15. Lindau T, Adlercreutz C, Aspenberg P (2000) Peripheral tears of the triangular fibrocartilage complex cause distal radioulnar joint instability after distal radial fractures. J Hand Surg Am 25:464–468
16. Lindau T, Hagberg L, Adlercreutz C, Jonsson K, Aspenberg P (2000) Distal radioulnar instability is an independent worsening factor in distal radial fractures. Clin Orthop Relat Res 376:229–235
17. Liverneaux P (2004) What wrist fracture did Pouteau actually describe? Chir Main 6:298–304
18. MacLennan AJ, Nemechek NM, Waitayawinyu T, Trumble TE (2008) Diagnosis and anatomic reconstruction of extensor carpi ulnaris subluxation. J Hand Surg Am 33:59–64
19. Magee T (2009) Comparison of 3-T MRI and arthroscopy of intrinsic wrist ligament and TFCC tears. AJR Am J Roentgenol 192:80–85
20. Osterman AL (1990) Arthroscopic debridement of triangular fibrocartilage complex tears. Arthroscopy 6:120–124
21. Palmer AK (1990) Triangular fibrocartilage disorders: injury patterns and treatment. Arthroscopy 6: 125–132
22. Querellou S, Moineau G, Le Duc-Pennec A, Guillo P, Turzo A, Cotonea Y, Le Nen D, Salaun PY (2009) Detection of occult wrist fractures by quantitative radioscintigraphy: a prospective study on selected patients. Nucl Med Commun 30:862–867
23. Rüegger C, Schmid MR, Pfirrmann CW, Nagy L, Gilula LA, Zanetti M (2007) Peripheral tear of the triangular fibrocartilage: depiction with MR arthrography of the distal radioulnar joint. AJR Am J Roentgenol 188:187–192
24. Samuel S, Kundel HL, Nodine CF, Toto LC (1995) Mechanism of satisfaction of search: eye position recordings in the reading of chest radiographs. Radiology 194:895–902
25. Scheer JH, Adolfsson LE (2011) Pathomechanisms of ulnar ligament lesions of the wrist in a cadaveric distal radius fracture model. Acta Orthop 82:360–364
26. Slutsky DJ (2007) Distal radioulnar joint arthroscopy and the volar ulnar portal. Tech Hand Up Extrem Surg 11:1–7
27. Tanaka T, Yoshioka H, Ueno T, Shindo M, Ochiai N (2006) Comparison between high-resolution MRI with a microscopy coil and arthroscopy in triangular fibrocartilage complex injury. J Hand Surg Am 31A: 1308–1314
28. Tomaino MM, Weiser RW (2001) Combined arthroscopic TFCC debridement and wafer resection of the distal ulna in wrists with triangular fibrocartilage complex tears and positive ulnar variance. J Hand Surg Am 26:1047–1052
29. Unglaub F, Fellenberg J, Germann G, Bickert B, Sauerbier M, Richter W (2007) Detection of apoptotic cartilage cells in symptomatic central tears of the triangular fibrocartilage. J Hand Surg Am 32: 618–622
30. Unglaub F, Wolf MB, Thome MA, Germann G, Sauerbier M, Reiter A (2008) Correlation of ulnar length and apoptotic cell death in degenerative lesions of the triangular fibrocartilage. Arthroscopy 24: 299–304
31. Unglaub F, Thomas SB, Kroeber MW, Dragu A, Fellenberg J, Mittlmeier T, Wolf MB, Horch RE (2010) Expression of TRAIL and death receptor DR4 in Palmer type 2 TFCC lesions. Arch Orthop Trauma Surg 130:1215–1220
32. Unglaub F, Thomas SB, Wolf MB, Dragu A, Kroeber MW, Mittlmeier T, Horch RE (2010) Cartilage cell proliferation in degenerative TFCC wrist lesions. Arch Orthop Trauma Surg 130:953–956
33. Vezeridis PS, Yoshioka H, Han R, Blazar P (2010) Ulnar-sided wrist pain. Part I: anatomy and physical examination. Skeletal Radiol 39:733–745
34. Watanabe A, Souza F, Vezeridis PS, Blazar P, Yoshioka H (2010) Ulnar-sided wrist pain. II. Clinical imaging and treatment. Skeletal Radiol 39:837–857
35. Weiss AP, Akelman E, Lambiase R (1996) Comparison of the findings of triple-injection cinearthrography of the wrist with those of arthroscopy. J Bone Joint Surg Am 78:348–356
36. Whipple TL, Marotta JJ, Powell JH 3rd (1986) Techniques of wrist arthroscopy. Arthroscopy 2: 244–252
37. Yoshioka H, Tanaka T, Ueno T, Carrino JA, Winalski CS, Aliabadi P, Lang P, Weissman BN (2007) Study of ulnar variance with high-resolution MRI: correlation with triangular fibrocartilage complex and cartilage of ulnar side of wrist. J Magn Reson Imaging 26:714–719

23 Arthroscopic Arthrodesis for Ulnar Wrist Instability and Arthritis

P.C. Ho

Introduction

The role of partial wrist fusion in the treatment of chronic ulnar wrist pain is relatively limited. It may be indicated in various forms of carpal instability or limited form of arthritis in the ulnar side of the wrist. The rationale of the partial wrist fusion is to eliminate the motion in the diseased segment of the wrist while to retain useful motion and function in the remaining unaffected part of the wrist. It helps to provide pain relief, to prevent progressive mechanical collapse of the carpal linkage as well as to control the progression of arthritis. The conventional open approach creates major surgical insult to the vital soft tissue envelope and connections of the wrist, potentially increases the degree of instability on one hand and on the other hand creates excessive stiffness of soft tissue that may compromise the final range of motion and the functional outcome of the wrist. Recent advance in arthroscopic and percutaneous fixation technique enables most fusion procedures to be conducted and accomplished through the small surgical accesses. This minimizes the surgical trauma and preserves maximal degree of motion pertained to the specific procedures.

P.C. Ho, MBBS, FHKCOS, FHKAM (Orthopaedics), FRCS(Edinburgh)
Department of Orthopaedics and Traumatolgy, Chinese University of Hong Kong, Prince of Wales Hospital, Shatin, Hong Kong SAR
e-mail: pcho@ort.cuhk.edu.hk

Carpal Instability

Carpal instability can be classified as dissociative and non-dissociative [7]. The former involves the disruption of interosseous ligament connecting carpal bones of the same row, with or without extrinsic ligament damage. Examples involving ulnar side of the wrist include lunotriquetral instability, capitohamate instability, chronic perilunate instability, and pisotriquetral instability. The latter implies a primary dysfunction of the extrinsic ligaments connecting the forearm skeleton and carpal bones, or between the two rows of carpal bones, in the absence of intrinsic ligament abnormality. Examples include palmar midcarpal instability and capitolunate instability. Symptomatic carpal instability can produce painful clunk, weakness of grip, sense of instability, reduced motion, and, in chronic situation, induce early arthritis of the wrist. Carpal instability in the absence of significant arthritis can be treated with ligament reconstruction or soft tissue plication. However, soft tissue reconstruction is often recognized to be difficult to achieve and is prone to recurrence and failure. Alternative solution includes fusion of the diseased segments so as to attain permanent control of the instability while to permit limited but useful functional motion to be preserved. For intrinsic ligament instability, this can be in the forms of lunotriquetral fusion, capitohamate fusion, and pisotriquetral fusion. For extrinsic instability, this can be treated by capito-lunate-hamate-triquetral fusion (four corner fusion) or triquetrohamate fusion.

F. del Piñal et al. (eds.), *Arthroscopic Management of Ulnar Pain*,
DOI 10.1007/978-3-642-30544-3_23, © Springer-Verlag Berlin Heidelberg 2012

Distal Radioulnar Joint Instability

Chronic distal radioulnar joint (DRUJ) instability is commonly caused by disruption of the TFCC with or without involvement of other secondary anatomical constraints. In the absence of significant arthritis involving the DRUJ, stability of the joint can be reliably restored by anatomical reconstruction of the TFCC using tendon graft weaving through bone tunnels in the distal radius and distal ulna as in the open procedure described by Adams [2] or in arthroscopic procedure described by Ho [15]. In severe symptomatic case that failed to respond to ligament reconstruction, Sauvé-Kapandji procedure has been suggested as an alternative solution to control the pain and instability [27, see also Chap. 24].

Wrist Arthritis

Isolated arthritic involvement of the midcarpal joint has been identified as a cause of chronic ulnar wrist pain [20]. This can be alleviated by four corner fusion with or without resection of the scaphoid, provided that there is no arthritis in the radiocarpal joint. Severe posttraumatic arthritis of the fifth carpometacarpal joint due to previous reverse Bennett's fracture can present as ulnar wrist pain. It can be treated with fusion of the fifth carpometacarpal joint. Pisotriquetral arthritis is conventionally treated by pisiform excision. There are, however, case reports on the use of pisotriquetral fusion as a solution for those patients with high demand on the wrist, such as in gymnast. Primary osteoarthritis or posttraumatic arthritis of the DRUJ can be salvaged by the Sauvé-Kapandji procedure, as an alternative solution to hemi-resection arthroplasty or ulnar head replacement.

Principle of Arthroscopic Partial Wrist Fusion

Partial wrist fusion is conventionally performed by open surgical approach which requires much soft tissue dissection including tendon, capsular, and ligament incisions around the wrist to expose the diseased intervals and to achieve fusion fixation. This may lead to capsular contracture and stiffness of the joint on top of the mechanical constraint rendered by selected carpal fusion. The expected loss of motion can be predicted theoretically from the biomechanical models, though in practice the final range of motion retained clinically will also rely on the degree of soft tissue contracture and the amount of compensatory hypermobility of the adjacent mobile segments. Thus, it is desirable to minimize surgical insult to soft tissue so as to maximize the motion preservation which is always the interest of both the patients and the surgeons.

Arthroscopic intervention in partial wrist fusion has the potential advantages of minimal surgical damage to the supporting ligaments and capsular structures of the wrist while allowing an unimpeded view to most articular surfaces of the joints and important soft tissue elements. This ensures a more accurate staging of the arthritis and facilitates clinical decision making on the most appropriate choice of fusion. The articular surfaces to be fused are denuded of cartilage down to subchondral level. Appropriate autogenous bone graft or artificial bone substitute is inserted into the bony interval through the arthroscopic portals. Definitive fixation is accomplished through percutaneous devices such as cannulated screws or K wires under the guidance of image intensifier. By limiting the extent of soft tissue dissection, the remaining carpal motion can be maximized and postoperative pain reduced which favors rehabilitation. There is also cosmetic benefit with the minimal surgical scar.

Contraindications

Contraindications for partial wrist fusion include active infection of the joint, panarthritis involving all or most compartments of the wrist and rapidly progressive inflammatory arthritis at proliferative stage. Patients who would like to have high level of certainty on pain control without major concern on motion preservation are better candidates for total wrist fusion. Arthroscopic partial wrist fusions are technically demanding procedures and should not be lightly taken by surgeons without much experience in therapeutic arthroscopy of the wrist. The choice of implant fixation is also more restricted using the existing percutaneous fixation systems. Patients with preexisting extensor tendon pathology over the wrist region may have higher incidence of tendon complications associated with complex arthroscopic wrist reconstruction procedures. Severe arthrofibrosis, joint contracture and long-standing carpal collapse, or wrist deformity may also pose additional difficulty and risk for surgeons in using the arthroscopic approach.

Technique

The general principles in all forms of arthroscopic partial wrist fusion should include the following steps:

1. Set up and instrumentation
2. Arthroscopic surveillance for final staging of the disease
3. Cartilage denudation
4. Provisional fixation of fusion intervals
5. Arthroscopic bone grafting
6. Definitive fixation

General Approach

Setup and Instrumentation

Operation is performed under general anesthesia for convenience and comfort in harvesting the bone graft if necessary. It can be done under regional anesthesia if bone substitute is employed or when no bone graft or substitute is being used. Either injectable or small granule form of bone substitute is suitable for the purpose. There is tendency not to use any bone graft or substitute augmentation if rigid fixation device such as cannulated compression screws can be applied to the fusion site. C-arm fluoroscopy should be available in all cases for intraoperative assessment. List of essential instrumentation includes motorized full-radius shaver and burr system of diameters ranging from 2 to 3-mm; small angled curette; 2.5-mm suction punch; radio-frequency thermal ablation system, and small cannulated screw system.

Patient is put in supine position while the operated arm is supported on a hand table. Either side of the iliac crest region is draped for bone graft harvesting depending on the patient's preference. Arm tourniquet is applied loosely but does not need to be inflated routinely. A tight application of the tourniquet without inflation leads to venous engorgement and can induce more troublesome bleeding. Most of the procedures can be done without the use of tourniquet. Piñal advocates the use of dry arthroscopy to avoid the problem of swelling and extravasation of fluid, but the use of tourniquet becomes mandatory throughout the procedure which may take extended time [6]. Vertical traction of 4–6-kg force is applied through plastic finger trap devices to the middle three fingers for joint distraction via wrist traction tower. We employ continuous saline irrigation and distension of the joint by using 3 l bag of normal saline solution suspended at 1–1.5 m above the operating table and instills with aid of gravity to maintain a clear arthroscopic view. Infusion pump is not necessary and is potentially harmful in causing extravasation of fluid. In wrist arthroscopy, it is mainly the distraction device that keeps the joint opened, not the fluid irrigation like in the shoulder joint.

Arthroscopic Surveillance

We perform routine inspection of both radiocarpal joint through 3–4 portal and midcarpal joint through MCR portal using a 2.7- or 1.9-mm video arthroscope. Adrenaline solution of 1 in 200,000 dilution is injected to the portal site skin and capsule to reduce bleeding associated with incision [14] (Fig. 23.1). Intra-articular injection is optional and may reduce bleeding associated with the arthroscopic procedures. Outflow portal is established at 6U portal just volar to the ECU tendon using 18-G needle. Particular attention is paid to note the status of interosseous ligament and the TFCC, degree of synovitis, and articular cartilage

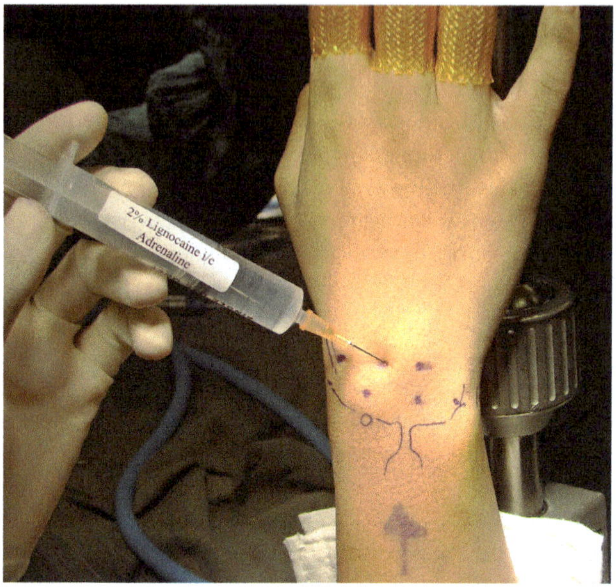

Fig. 23.1 Two percent Lignocaine with adrenaline solution in 1:200,000 dilution is injected to portal sites for hemostasis effect

condition of the joints intended to be fused and the other uninvolved joint compartments of the wrist. The latter is essential to determine whether the proposed fusion is appropriate or not. Frequently associated localized posttraumatic synovitis in the area may obscure the observation of cartilage condition. The synovial growth needs to be eliminated by using 2 mm shavers or small radio-frequency probe inserted from 4–5 portal. It may be necessary to swap the portal of the arthroscope and instrument in order to obtain a better attacking angle of the instrument for a more efficient synovectomy. The articular cartilage of the proximal surface of the triquetrum and ulnar aspect of lunate is best observed through 4–5 or 6R portal.

The midcarpal joint is approached through the MCR portal. Routinely, the STT joint, scaphocapitate joint, capitolunate joint, and triquetrohamate joint are inspected for cartilage lesion and synovitis. The scapholunate and lunotriquetral joints are assessed for stability with 2-mm probe introduced from the MCU portal. Any instability is graded according to the Geissler classification. Synovial overgrowth should be debrided by using a shaver or radio-frequency probe to adequately expose the underlying cartilage area for assessment of the true extent of chondral damage and subchondral bone exposure.

Cartilage Denudation

The articular surfaces of the joint compartments to be fused are then prepared. The extent and depth of cartilage denudation should be precisely controlled using 2.9-mm arthroscopic burr. In debriding carpal interval of the same carpal row, such as lunotriquetral or capitohamate interval, smaller burr such as 2 mm should be used to cater for the narrower joint space to avoid excessive cartilage and subchondral bone removal. Either forward or reverse blade rotation mode should be adopted at a speed of 2,000–3,000 rpm. Oscillating mode is not as effective as compared to unidirectional mode. One should be cautious about the jumping phenomenon when using a burr to attack a particularly sclerotic bone surface. The burr may get caught in the area of hard subchondral bone during high-speed revolution. The resultant force will bounce the burr off the bone and may lead to accident damage of the articular surface of the surrounding or opposing carpal bones. To have better control of the instrument, it is recommended to hold the arthroscopic burr near the far end with the surgeon's thumb and index finger, while using the middle finger to firmly anchor the burr over the skin around the portal site (Fig. 23.2). There should be maximal preservation of the subchondral bone so as to maintain carpal height. Burring is completed when subchondral cancellous

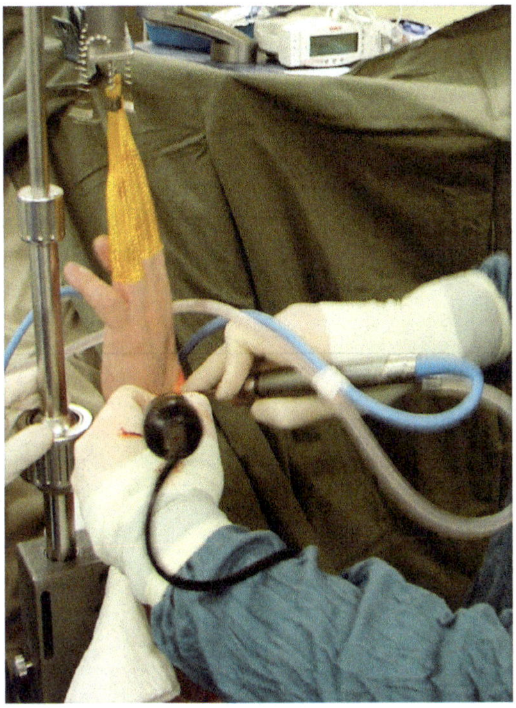

Fig. 23.2 To have better control of the instrument, the arthroscopic burr is being held near the far end with the surgeon's thumb and index finger, while the middle finger firmly anchors the burr over the skin around the portal site

bone with healthy punctate bleeding is reached. This phenomenon can be easily observed if tourniquet is not used during this process (Fig. 23.3). Usually, bleeding is limited and can be well controlled with hydrostatic pressure applied through the irrigation system. If bleeding is profuse, one may further elevate the suspension of the instilling saline bag to increase the hydrostatic pressure or use the coagulation mode of the radio-frequency apparatus. During the burring process, suction is switched on and off intermittently to remove any accumulated bone debris which may block the visual field. If suction is applied continuously during the burring process, excessive air bubbles drawn in will severely compromise the visibility of the operating site.

Provisional Fixation of the Carpal Fusion

The wrist is dislodged from the wrist traction tower and is placed horizontally over a hand table

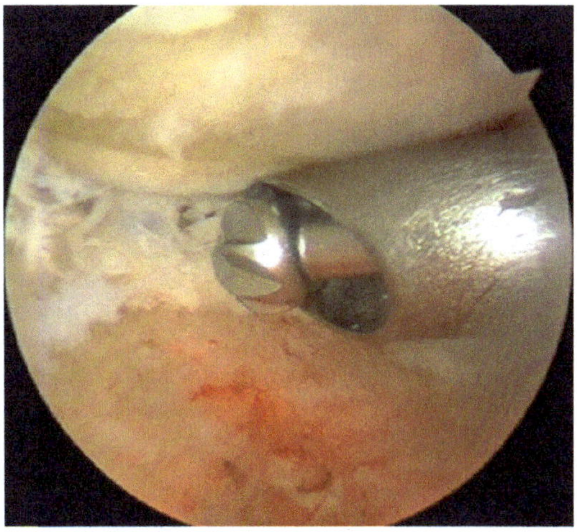

Fig. 23.3 Punctate bleeding can be readily seen from the subchondral bone during burring without the use of tourniquet

for provisional fixation. The carpal interval(s) to be fused is temporarily fixed with 1.1-mm K wire percutaneously using a powered driver in anatomical position as far as possible. Alignment is confirmed with intraoperative image intensifier. The K wires can be used as definitive fixation device or it can be used as the guide pin for subsequent conversion into percutaneous cannulated screw fixation. The pin is then withdrawn to be freed from the joint to be fused while it is maintained in position in the carpal bone. Externally, the pin should be protected with pin cap to avoid accidental injury to the surgeon's hand in the remaining process. The joint is then ready for grafting with autogenous cancellous bone or bone substitutes.

Arthroscopic Bone Grafting

Autogenous bone graft or bone substitute is frequently required to fill up voids between the articular surfaces to be fused. As vascularity and bone quality of the fusing bones are usually adequate, autogenous graft may not be essential and there is increasing role of using bone substitutes to reduce potential donor site morbidity with similar outcome. Both injectable form and small granule form are suitable for the purpose.

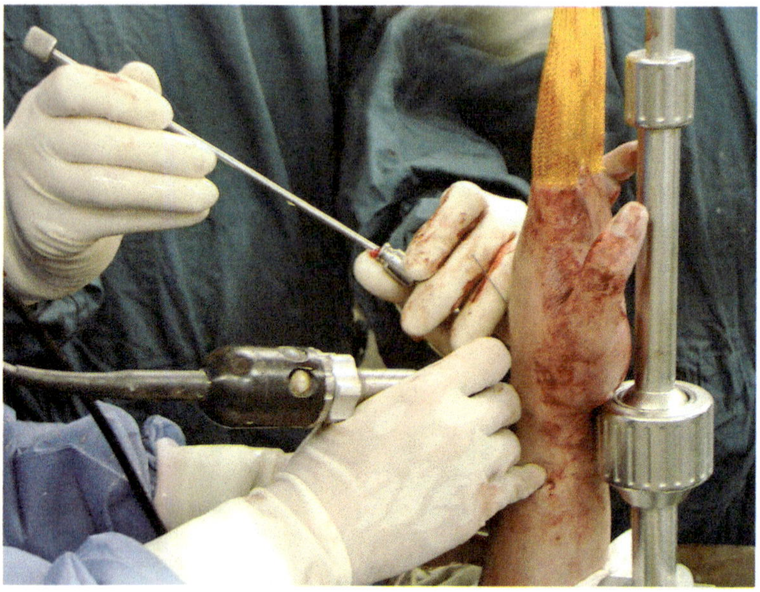

Fig. 23.4 Bone graft is delivered through a cannula with a slightly undersized trocar of flat end such as bone biopsy trocar into the joint cavity

An arthroscopic cannula is introduced through appropriate portal directly opposing the fusing surfaces. If autogenous graft is to be used, cancellous bone graft is harvested from the iliac crest either using trephine technique or open approach through small incision. The bone graft is then cut into small chips using a scissor and delivered through the cannula with a slightly undersized trocar with a flat end such as bone biopsy trocar into the joint cavity (Fig. 23.4). Trocar with roundish end is not effective enough. Too exact fitting of the trocar in the cannula will cause easy trapping of bone graft substance between the trocar and cannula wall and lead to delivery problem. So a slightly undersized trocar is more desirable. The bone graft is impacted with the trocar till satisfactory volume of graft is achieved (Fig. 23.5). This process requires two assistants to execute smoothly. One assistant helps to maintain the position of the arthroscope to provide optimal vision of the fusion site. The operating surgeon controls the arthroscopic cannula and trocar. A second assistant is responsible for delivering the bone graft or bone substitutes into the opening of the cannula in small volume every time. The operating surgeon then drives the bone graft or substitute into the fusion site under direct arthroscopic monitor (Fig. 23.6). The speed of the process can be enhanced by using a cannula of wider bore such as 4.5 or 5 mm so that each time more graft can be accommodated. If injectable bone substitute is to be used, joint irrigation should be ceased and all joint fluid evacuated with suction. A wide bore needle connecting the syringe containing the bone substitute is inserted through appropriate portal to reach the fusion site. Injection of the bone substitute can then be performed under direct vision till cavity is filled up completely. If necessary, intraoperative fluoroscopy can help to confirm the completeness of the filling process.

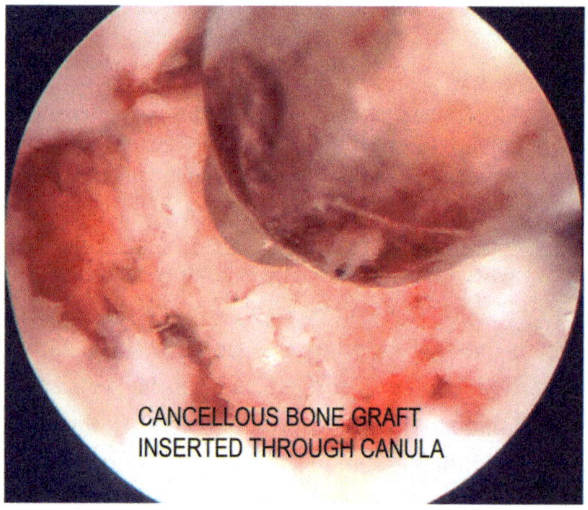

Fig. 23.5 Impaction of graft with blunt trocar at fusion site

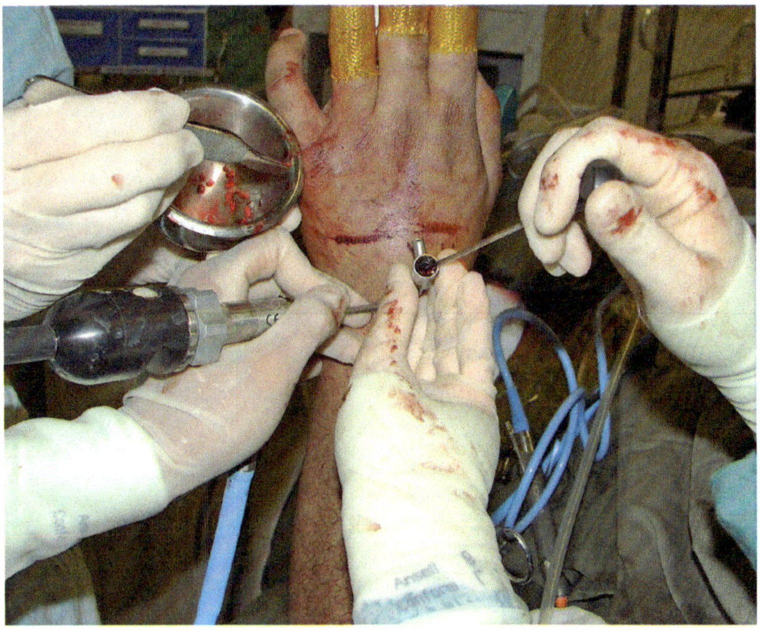

Fig. 23.6 With the help of two assistants, the operating surgeon controls the arthroscopic cannula and trocar and drives the bone graft or substitute into the fusion site under directly arthroscopic monitor

Definitive Fixation

The wrist is taken off from the traction tower again and placed in the hand table. Definitive fixation is performed by driving the K wire across the bony interval to be fused and in correct carpal alignment. If cannulated screw is preferred, the K wire will then serve as guide pin. After measuring the length of the screw required, the pin tract is drilled using a cannulated drill bit. Stable internal fixation can then be achieved with compression screw using appropriate percutaneous cannulated screw system, preferably headless system to avoid screw head impingement. The final carpal alignment, screw position, and length should be assessed by using image intensifier. In older patient with osteopenic bone, multiple K wire fixation is preferred over screw fixation to avoid hardware problem, such as protrusion of screw tip into the joint (Fig. 23.7). Percutaneous K wires should be cut short and buried underneath the skin. They are removed under local anesthesia when bone healing is complete. Exposing pins outside skin may predispose to pin tract infection. The wrist is then immobilized with plaster slab.

Specific Fusion Technique and Rehabilitation

Four-Corner Arthrodesis

Four corner arthrodesis is commonly indicated in chronic pathology related to scaphoid problem, such as advanced SNAC or SLAC wrist. Under these circumstances, the scaphoid is usually removed surgically as a concomitant procedure with the four corner arthrodesis. For pathology that does not involve radioscaphoid arthritis, the indications include midcarpal instability, isolated midcarpal arthritis, or lunotriquetral dissociation with fixed volar intercalated segmental instability alignment of the lunate. When performing four corner arthrodesis in cases without radioscaphoid arthritis, Taleisnik [28] favored scaphoid inclusion and Weiss et al. [31] preferred scaphoid retention. In a cadaveric study carried out by Kobza et al. [18], it was shown that simple four corner arthrodesis with scaphoid retention led to a significant decrease in extension, radial deviation, and ulnar deviation. Four corner arthrodesis with scaphoid excision allowed significantly greater radial deviation but also led to significant

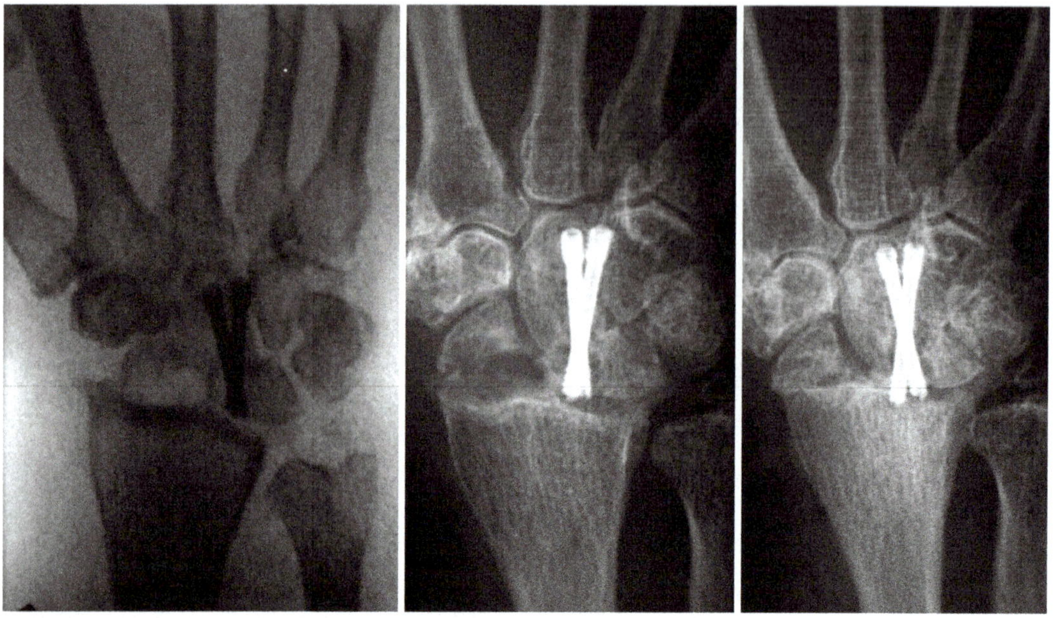

Fig. 23.7 Self-tapping headless screw may protrude into the joint gradually during healing process of the fusion site in old patient with osteopenic bone

increase in radiolunate contact area and mean contact pressure. However, the clinical impact was not known.

In 1988, Trumble et al. described six patients receiving partial wrist fusion to treat static and dynamic volar intercalated segmental instability, including 4 four corner fusions and two limited ulnar sided carpal arthrodesis [29]. Five of the six patients got relief of symptom, but only two returned to their previous occupations. In 1993, Lichtman et al. compared the results of their midcarpal fusions with soft tissue reconstruction in 13 patients who had 15 surgical procedures carried out between 1981 and 1989 [19]. Six patients received limited midcarpal arthrodesis, and nine patients had one of the four different soft tissue reconstruction procedures, addressing the ulnar arm of the arcuate ligament as a portion of the procedures. The limited carpal fusion included three triquetrohamate arthrodesis and 3 four corner arthrodesis. They were all rated as clinical successes and all patients could return to their former occupations. Six out of the nine soft tissue reconstruction procedures failed, with recurrence of the painful midcarpal clunk. Lichtman concluded that the limited midcarpal arthrodesis could provide definitive treatment. Goldfarb et al. reported results similar to those of Lichtman in 2004, with seven out of eight patients with palmar midcarpal instability satisfying with four corner arthrodesis they received and six of eight patients had no or mild residual pain [11]. The average wrist flexion/extension arc of motion decreased with surgery from 135° to 75°. The average grip strength increased significantly with surgery from 20 to 32 kg; however, grip strength remained significantly lower than the opposite side strength of 54 kg.

We reported four cases of arthroscopic four corner fusion with scaphoidectomy in 2008 [13]. All cases were indicated for either advanced SLAC wrist or SNAC wrist. We have no experience in using four corner fusion for treatment of midcarpal instability, as we believe that ligament reconstruction can produce predictably satisfactory outcome. Nevertheless, similar principle can be applied in cases for palmar midcarpal instability. Operation should begin with a surveillance of the radiocarpal joint to confirm an intact radiolunate articulation and preferably intact proximal articular surface of triquetrum. Arthroscopic scaphoidectomy is not necessary. However, it may be indicated if the patient wishes to have larger degree of radial and ulnar deviation motion. With arthroscope introduced from MCU portal, an arthroscopic burr of 2.9 mm is inserted into the MCR portal and directed towards the proximal and mid scaphoid region. The scaphoid is burred at high speed from articular surface down to the core cancellous bone. Bone debris is removed by intermittently applied suction. To avoid accidental damage of the adjacent articular surfaces to be preserved, a shell of cartilage can be left intact until majority of the cancellous bone is removed. This shell of cartilage can help to separate the burr from the adjacent carpal bone during the burring process (Fig. 23.8). This can be removed piecemeal at the end of the scaphoidectomy procedure by using a small pituitary rongeur or arthroscopic punch (Fig. 23.9). When taking out the larger piece of bone fragment, it is advisable not to use excessive violence in order to avoid damage to the attaching ligament and soft tissue structure. One trick is to firmly grip on the bone fragment with the small rongeur using both hands while to twist around its own axis and maintain a gentle pulling force. The fragment will gradually lose its connection to the soft tissue and can be delivered smoothly out of the joint. During the delivery process, the surgeon has to maintain a sustained and firm grip on the bony fragment or otherwise it may get lost in the juxta-articular or subcutaneous tissue plane. Under such situation, the surgeon may be forced to enlarge the surgical wound in order to remove the retained bony fragment, which is not desirable (Fig. 23.10). In order to speed up the process, arthroscopic burr of progressive increase in size such as 3.5 mm and even 4.5 mm can be used when there is more space open up

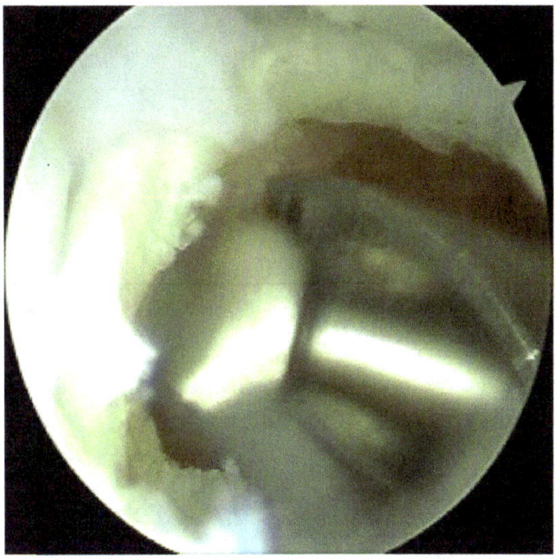

Fig. 23.8 Shell of cartilage left intact during burring of scaphoid to protect other uninvolved articular surface

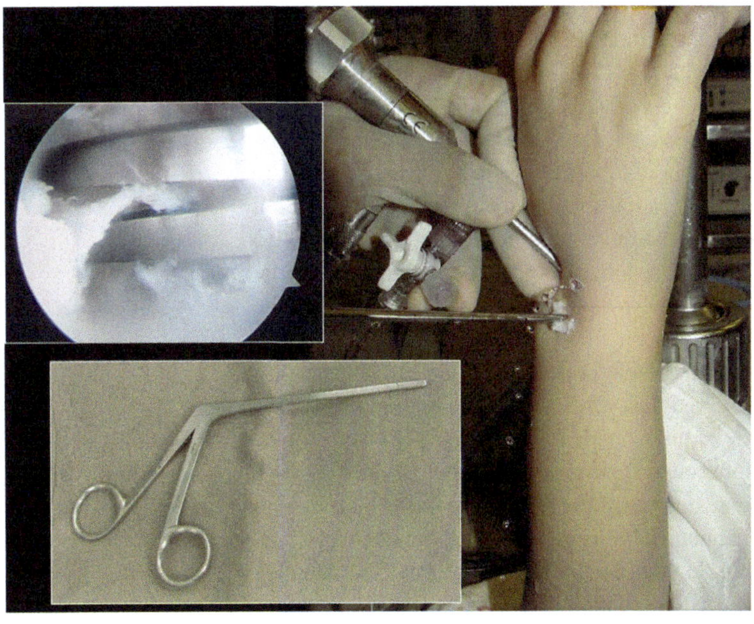

Fig. 23.9 Cartilage shell removed in piecemeal using small pituitary rongeur inserted through portals

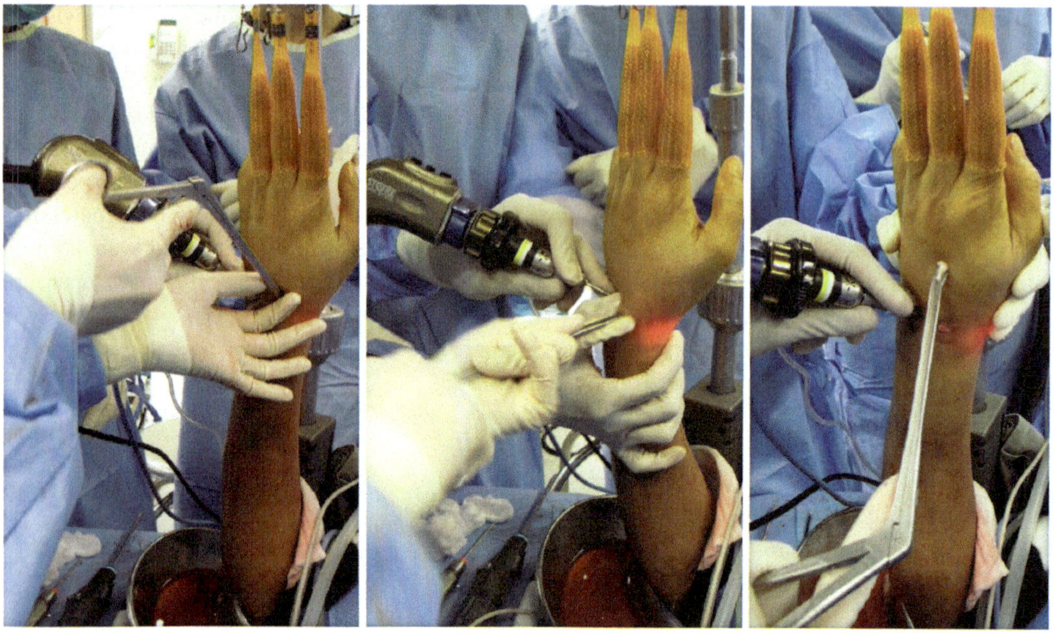

Fig. 23.10 The surgeon firmly grips on the bone fragment with the small rongeur using both hands while to twist around its own axis and maintain a gentle pulling force. The fragment will gradually lose its connection to the soft tissue and can be delivered smoothly out of the joint

after part of the scaphoid is removed (Fig. 23.11). The speed of scaphoid excision can often be double or even tripled. Alternatively, a small osteotome can also be used to break the bone into piecemeal for easier removal. Extreme care has to be exercised during insertion of the larger burr or osteotome to avoid iatrogenic injury to the extensor tendon and cutaneous nerve. The distal few millimeters of the scaphoid can be left in situ so as to preserve the scaphotrapezial ligament. The distal scaphoid tubercle does not normally articulate with the radial styloid, and hence its preservation will not cause impingement pain postoperatively.

Once scaphoid is cleared, attention can be paid to the fusion of the midcarpal joint at the four corners. The arthroscope is now inserted through MCR portal while the MCU portal is reserved for arthroscopic instruments. Usually, in palmar midcarpal instability, the space between triquetrum and hamate is abnormally wide due to excessive laxity of the volar arcuate ligament. The articular surface between the capitate, lunate, triquetrum, and hamate is denuded of cartilage with 2.9-mm burr. The joint surface

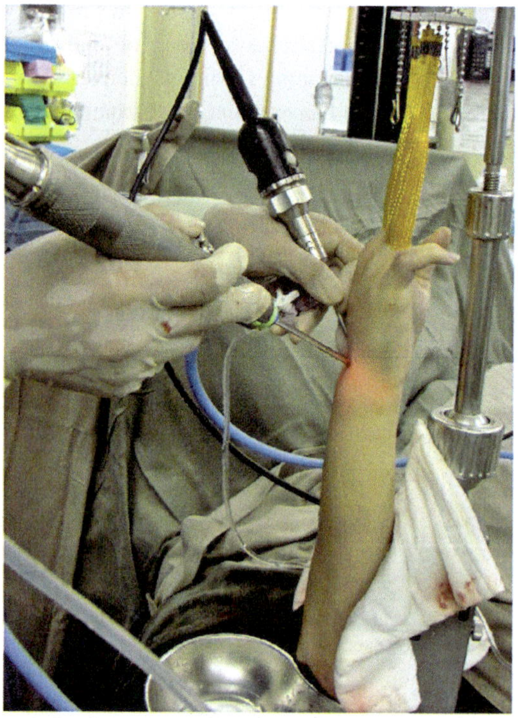

Fig. 23.11 Use of large 4.5-mm arthroscopic burr helps to speed up burring process

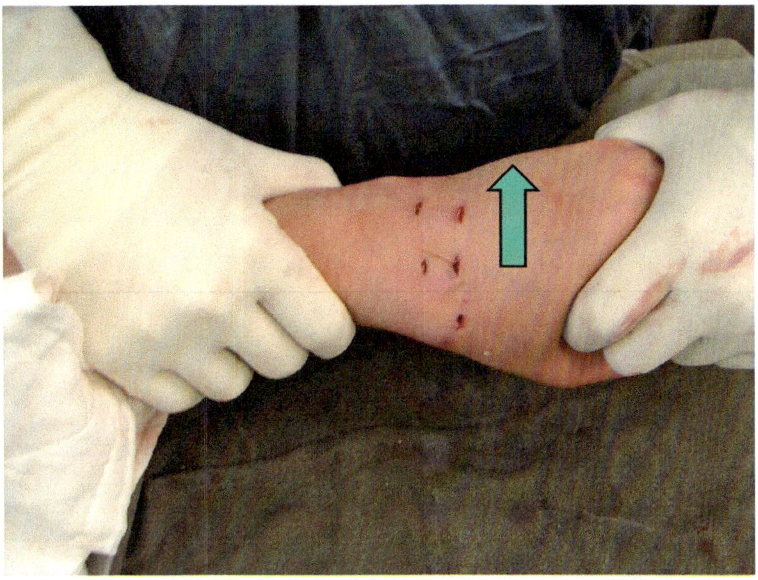

Fig. 23.12 The capitate is reduced by ulnar translation of the wrist so that it sits as much as possible on the distal lunate articular surface. The *arrow* depicts the direction of force to shift the distal carpal row ulnarward on the proximal row so as to maximize the contact between capitate and lunate

of the lunotriquetral joint is also burred. I do not routinely burr the articulation between hamate and capitate as the joint is very rigid normally.

Provisional fixation is performed under image intensifier's guide. If there is significant VISI deformity, the lunate is reduced by passive extension of the wrist so as to restore the normal radiolunate relationship. The lunate is then fixed to radius with percutaneous K wire of 1.1 mm inserted from distal radius.

After adequate cartilage destruction, capitate is reduced by ulnar translation of the wrist so that it sits as much as possible on the distal lunate articular surface (Fig. 23.12). A percutaneous K wire is inserted from dorsal surface of the capitate at the distal junction with the base of third metacarpal under image guide (Fig. 23.13). The mini stab wound should be bluntly dissected to avoid iatrogenic injury to the extensor tendon. With the help of lateral projection on image guide, the K wire is driven across the capitolunate joint to anchor into the lunate. The angle of attack has to be acute enough in order to catch the central part of the lunate to have better purchase of the bone. It is most crucial to obtain good surface contact of the capitolunate joint as the key point of the operation is to achieve solid fusion of the CL joint to avoid late collapse of the midcarpal joint and hence loss of the carpal height.

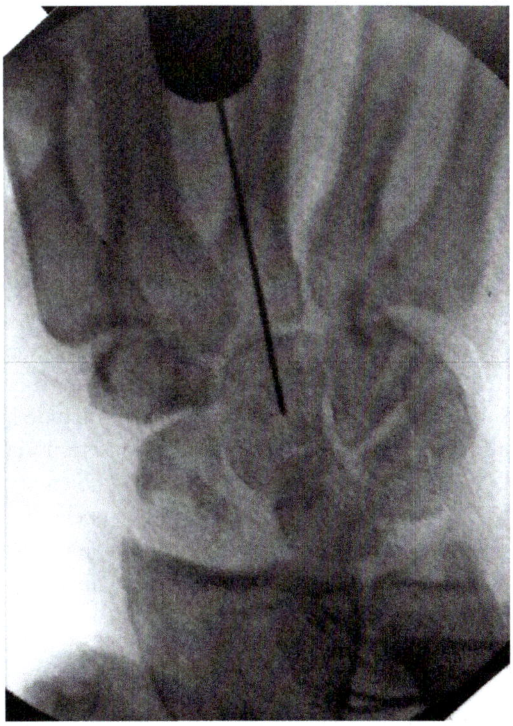

Fig. 23.13 Guide pin inserted through distal capitate to transfix capitolunate joint

If satisfactory alignment can be achieved, the K wire is withdrawn from lunate while still attaching to the capitate. This is then followed by

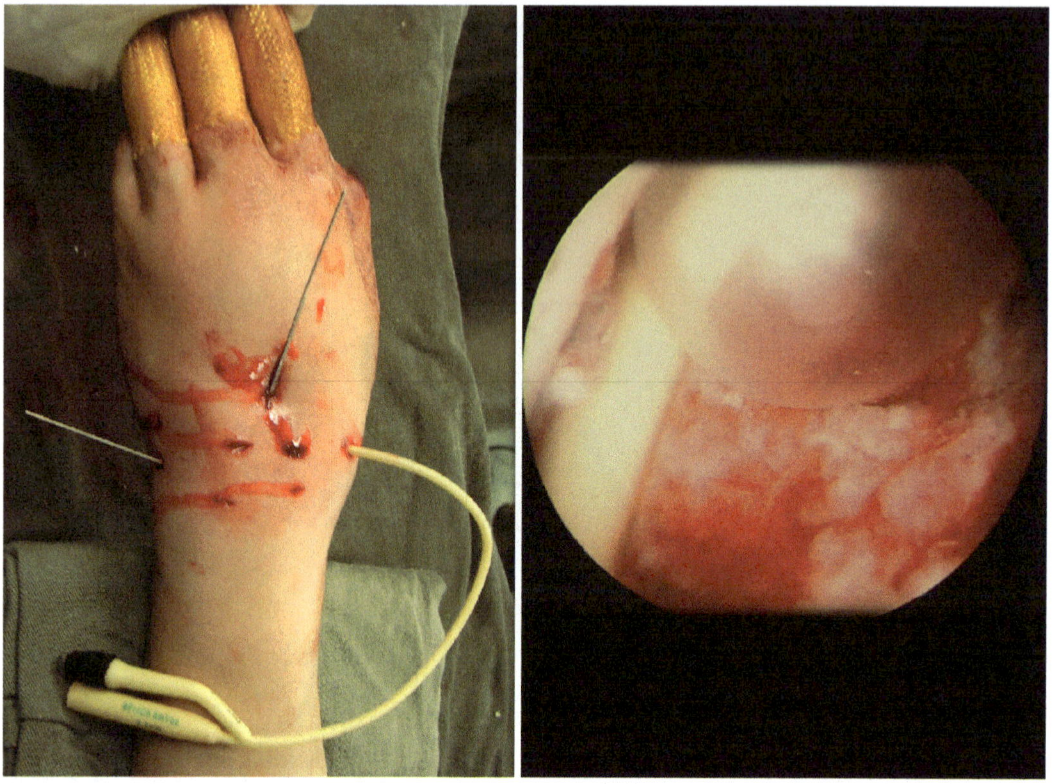

Fig. 23.14 A French-sized six Foley catheter is inserted via the 3–4 portal to completely obliterate the empty space left after the scaphoidectomy procedure

the bone grafting procedure at the midcarpal joint as described in session before. With the arthroscope held at MCR portal, the cannula can be inserted through the MCU portal for bone graft or substitute delivery. If scaphoidectomy is included, a French-sized six Foley catheter is inserted via the 3–4 portal to completely obliterate the empty space left after the scaphoidectomy procedure. The balloon is inflated while bone graft or substitute is being delivered to the ulnar midcarpal space (Fig. 23.14). The catheter can be removed after the bone grafting procedure or can be left in situ for a day or two to serve as a surgical drain.

After completion of bone grafting, the K wire over the capitate is driven back to lunate at the reduced position. Length of the K wire inserted is measured. This is followed by drilling of bone with cannulated drill bit and final insertion of headless self-tapped cannulated screw to fix the capitolunate joint. The screw tip should reach no less than two mm from the proximal surface of the lunate to avoid screw tip protrusion and iatrogenic damage to the radiolunate articulation. To avoid loss of reduction during the drilling action, an additional K wire can be inserted to the CL interval for temporary fixation. One has to be sure that the screw is completely buried in the capitate so that it will not cause impingement to the extensor tendons. Lateral and oblique X-ray views should demonstrate that the screw does not project beyond the proximal articular surface of the lunate so that no scratching of the articular surface of the distal radius will occur. This can also be checked with gentle passive movement of the wrist after the fixation procedure. The lunotriquetral joint and the capitohamate joint are then fixed with percutaneous K wires (Fig. 23.15). If the positions of the K wires are satisfactory, headless screws are inserted from ulnar aspect of the hand through small stab wounds to fix the carpal intervals (Fig. 23.16). Structures at risk include dorsal branch of ulnar nerve, EDM and ECU tendons.

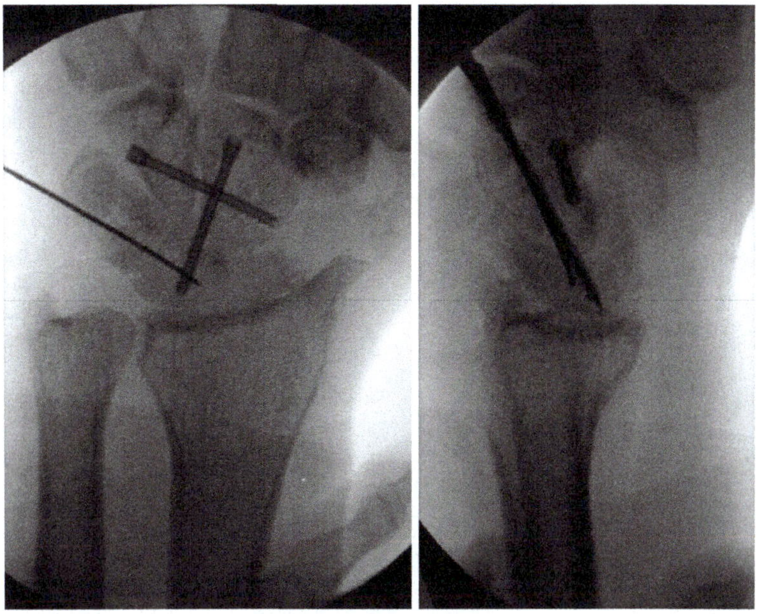

Fig. 23.15 The lunotriquetral joint and the capitohamate joint are fixed with percutaneous K wires

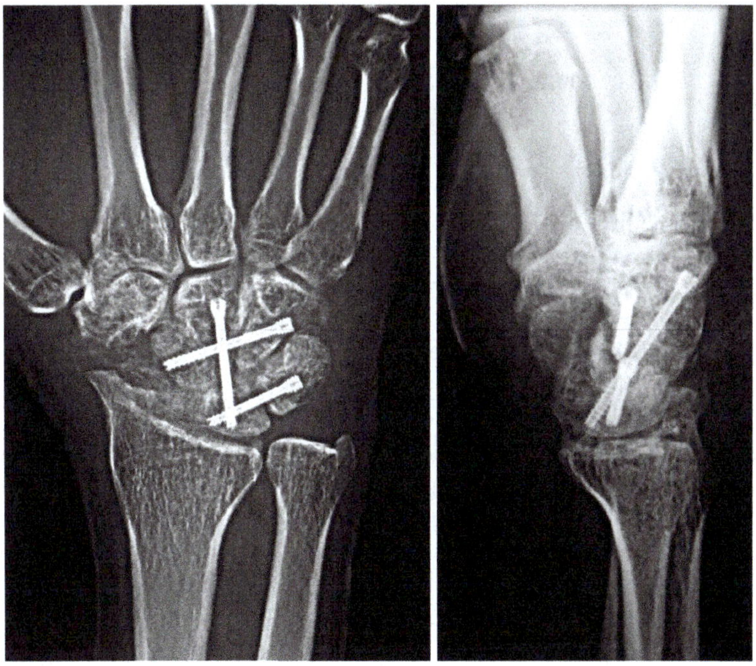

Fig. 23.16 Fusion of the four corner bones with percutaneous headless screws

Blunt dissection of the stab wound should be routine before insertion of guide wire to avoid iatrogenic injury to these important structures. In order to reduce the chance of hitting onto the screw fixing capitolunate joint, the guide wire for capitohamate fusion should aim at more volar aspect of the capitate, while that of the lunotriquetral fusion should aim at more dorsal aspect of lunate.

After solid fixation of the four corners bones, any K wire over the radiolunate joint can be left in situ for 2 weeks. The wire end is cut short and bent outside the skin. Wounds are closed with

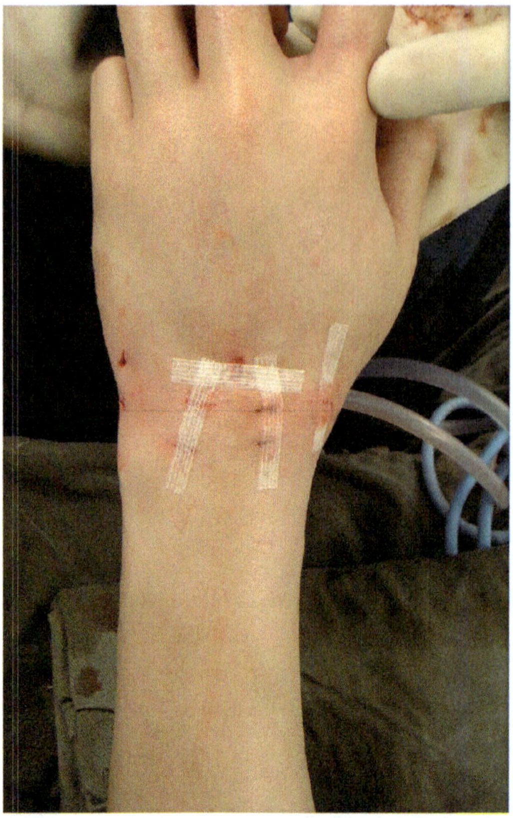

Fig. 23.17 Arthroscopic wounds are closed with steri-strips without stitch

steri-strip and a comfortable bulky dressing is applied supported with a short arm plaster slab (Fig. 23.17). The slab is changed to a removable wrist splint after the first week. After removal of the K wire over the radiolunate joint, active mobilization of the wrist can be initiated out of splint under supervision of hand therapist. Passive wrist mobilization and strengthening exercise can be offered when radiological and clinical union is evidenced, usually around 10–12 weeks post-op.

Lunotriquetral arthrodesis

Lunotriquetral (LT) arthrodesis is indicated for symptomatic chronic LT instability with or without ulnocarpal impaction syndrome [12, 30] In the latter condition, ulnar shortening osteotomy is often an accompanying procedure to decompress the ulnocarpal joint. In the absence of secondary chondral damage, an alternative option of LT ligament reconstruction can be considered, since failure to unite is common in surgical fusion of the LT joint, according to literature. In a meta-analysis of the outcome of intercarpal arthrodesis conducted by Siegel et al., the overall reported nonunion rate in 81 patients out of a total of 143 cases of LT fusion by open surgery in seven clinical series was 26 % [25]. Where reported, 46 % of patients have persistent postoperative symptom. Sennwald et al. also found disappointing high rate of pseudarthrosis of 57 % in 23 patients receiving LT fusion [23]. In their open procedure from a dorso-ulnar approach, they recommended routine use of corticocancellous bone graft to enhance union. They cautioned about prolonged rehabilitation with 6 months out of work at best and the significant loss of grip power particularly in male subjects, which might force them to change job nature.

Arthroscopic arthrodesis of the LT joint can be performed with midcarpal arthroscopic approach (Fig. 23.18). Routine radiocarpal joint arthroscopy is performed to evaluate the status of the TFCC, associated chondral lesions of the ulnar head, proximal lunate and triquetrum, and the LT ligament. If significant chondral lesion is present at the carpal bone surface, ulnar shortening or arthroscopic wafer procedure should be done in association with the LT fusion procedure.

The arthroscope is then directed to the midcarpal joint. With the arthroscope placed at the MCR portal, a small probe is inserted at the MCU portal to reach the LT joint to confirm instability. This is then replaced by a 2.0- or 2.9-mm arthroscopic burr, and debridement of the articular cartilage is performed from distal to proximal direction (Fig. 23.19). Attention should be paid at the dorsal aspect of the joint by rotating the 35-degree forward-slanting lens to a downward position. Difficulty may be encountered in burring this portion as the angle of attack of the burr is frequently restricted by the dorsal soft tissue of the wrist. A small angled curette may be found useful in removing cartilage at this area.

When burring is complete, provisional fixation of the LT interval is performed. A small wound is

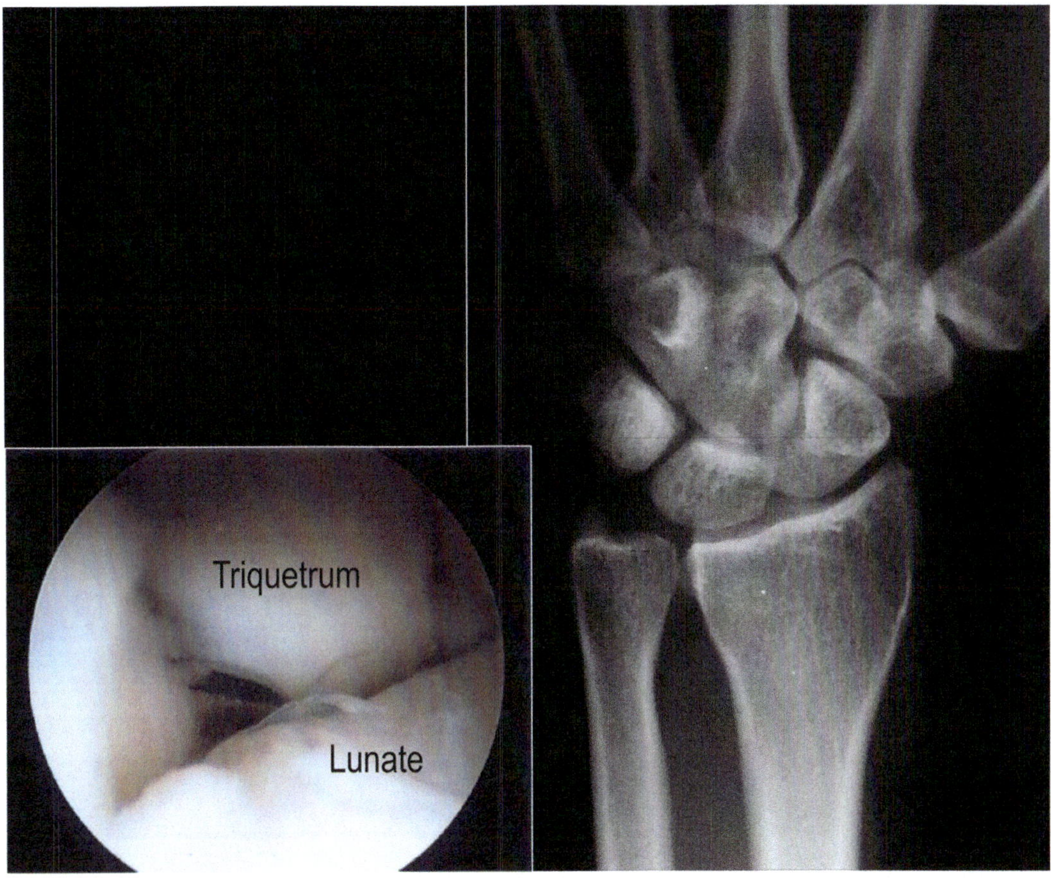

Fig. 23.18 Patient with painful ulnar wrist pain for 2 years. X-ray reviewed increased lunotriquetral interval. Arthroscopy confirmed Geissler grade 3 lunotriquetral instability

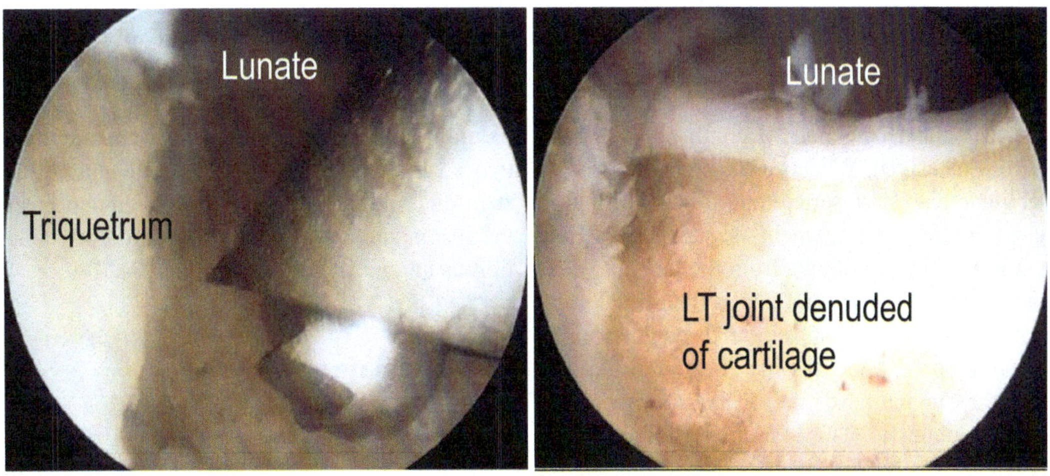

Fig. 23.19 Burring of the lunotriquetral joint before arthrodesis

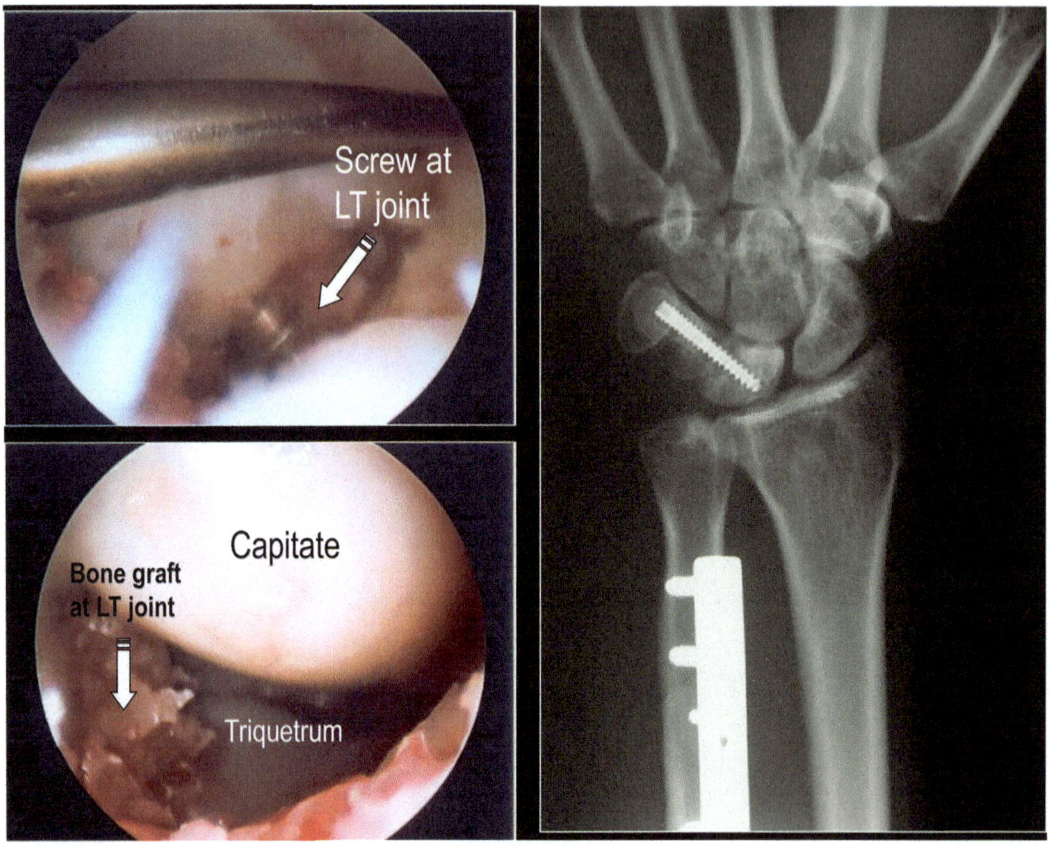

Fig. 23.20 Arthroscopic view of the screw in lunotriquetral joint, which was eventually covered with arthroscopic bone graft. X-ray showed good fusion position

made opposing the ulnar surface of triquetrum and bluntly dissected to free the overlying terminal branch of the dorsal sensory branch of ulnar nerve. Under image guide, a guide wire is inserted from the triquetrum across the LT joint to reach the lunate bone. Length of the guide wire is measured. Whenever feasible, two parallel guide pins are inserted to aim for two cannulated screws. If alignment is satisfactory, the guide pins are withdrawn from the lunate to free the joint space. The joint gap is then filled with bone graft or bone substitute through cannula inserted at the MCU portal. The former is preferred as nonunion of the fusion site is notoriously common. This is then followed by percutaneous fixation with compression cannulated screw inserted from the ulnar aspect of the hand. Cannulated drill bit is applied and a compression headless and self-tapping cannulated screw is inserted to compress the fusion site (Fig. 23.20). Preferably two screws should be inserted to obtain maximal stability of the fusion site (Fig. 23.21). Alternatively, a K wire can be used to augment the strength of a single screw fixation if the bone is too small to accommodate two screws. All wounds are closed with steri-strip, and a short arm plaster is applied to protect the fusion site until radiological union or stable fibrous union is achieved (Fig. 23.22).

Capitohamate arthrodesis

Capitohamate (CH) arthrodesis is considered as a surgical procedure for treating Kienböck disease combined with capitate shortening, with the aim to unload the lunate [3]. For ulnar wrist pain, CH instability is rarely reported as a clinical

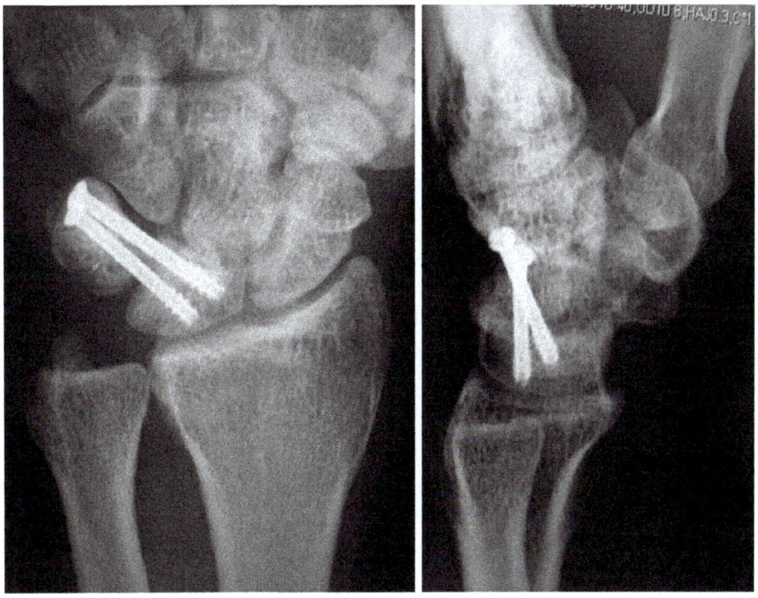

Fig. 23.21 Another patient with complete LT dissociation treated with arthroscopic LT arthrodesis using two compression screws

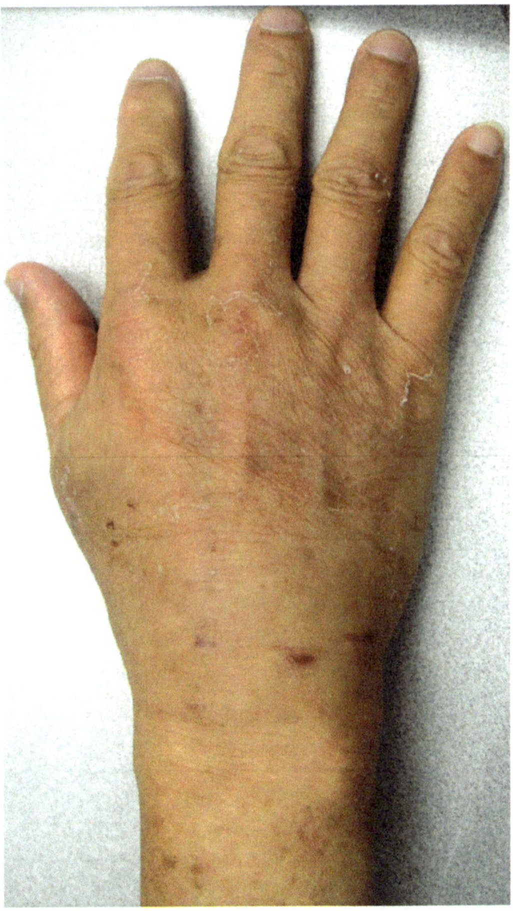

Fig. 23.22 Minimal scarring over surgical wounds

entity [24]. There are case reports of acute traumatic axial disruption of the carpus through the CH joint but chronic instability is rare [8, 9]. Detailed anatomical study by Garcia-Elias in 1989 and 1991 demonstrated three distinct and strong ligaments holding up the joint, namely, dorsal, deep, and palmar interosseous ligaments [8–10]. As a result, there is very limited motion at the CH joint of about 5° during extremes of ulnar deviation and finger flexion during grip power, as shown by Kaplan and Taleisnik [17]. Ritt et al. noted a larger degree of dorsopalmar rotation of the isolated CH joint of up to 17° but concluded that the motion will be more limited in vivo by other anatomical constraints [22]. CH instability could be the result of overzealous wedge osteotomy for carpal boss resection at the third and fourth carpometacarpal joint, damaging the dorsal CH ligament [16]. Packer presented a case of posttraumatic chronic symptomatic CH instability at a meeting (Greg Packer 2009, personal communication) in which there was clear arthroscopic evidence of instability of the CH joint upon probing. The logical treatment of this condition will be CH fusion. It is possible to accomplish this through the midcarpal arthroscopic portals and percutaneous fixation, with or without bone graft (see also Chap. 21).

Pisotriquetral Arthrodesis

Abrams first reported the use of pisotriquetral (PT) arthrodesis to treat a 14-year-old gymnast with chronic ulnar wrist pain caused by PT instability in 2006 [1]. Surgical approach was through the proximal ulnar aspect of the hand and wrist. Articular cartilage was curetted and joint surface was fixed with cannulated screw. Radiological fusion was achieved after 3 months. At 2 years of follow-up, she remained pain-free at arthrodesis site but developed painful popping sensation over volar-ulnar aspect of the wrist which was brought only by extreme wrist flexion coupled with forearm rotation. He suggested this was due to abutment of the fused pisiform and the distal ulna. Subsequently, Singer et al. reported the second case in 2011 in a professional mountain biker with complete pain relief and return to professional sport [26].

Arthroscopically, the PT joint can be approached in two ways. Cobb et al. described two portals placed ulnar to the PT joint, one proximal and one distal [5]. A small 30° arthroscope of 1.9 mm was inserted. Two-millimeter shaver and burr can be used to remove the synovitis and diseased articular surface. The other approach is through the 6R portal, in which the arthroscope is directed ulnarly, volarly, and distally through the pisotriquetral orifice just volar to the meniscus homologue of the TFCC, which is reported to be present in up to 88 % of the normal subject [4]. However, this approach can only reach the articular surface of the pisiform but not that of the triquetrum. In theory, PT fusion is possible with the direct arthroscopic approach. Extreme caution on the ulnar nerve which lies radial to the pisiform is essential. There is no report of arthroscopic fusion of the PT joint in the literature yet, and the author has no experience (see Chap. 17).

Triquetrohamate arthrodesis

Triquetrohamate (TH) arthrodesis has been used to treat palmar midcarpal instability to eliminate the abnormal catch-up clunk between triquetrum and hamate upon ulnar deviation of the wrist. Rao reported the result of treatment in 11 wrists of ten patients operated from 1981 to 1988 [21]. They all failed to either conservative treatment or soft tissue reconstruction procedures. The average duration of symptom was 16 months. Nonunion occurred in two cases. Based on a scoring system, excellent to good outcome was obtained in six wrists. Pain was completely eliminated in seven wrists, and painful wrist clunking was abolished in all patients. Four wrists continued to have varying degrees of pain. The range of motion compared to unaffected averaged 55 % flexion, 69 % extension, 61 % radial deviation, and 64 % ulnar deviation, and grip strength averaged 64 %. The author concluded that although TH arthrodesis could stabilize the midcarpal joint, a successful outcome might not be necessarily resulted in all cases as there was failure to control symptoms in almost 50 % of the cases. In theory, TH fusion can be performed through midcarpal arthroscopic portals, combined with percutaneous screw fixation. The author has no experience on this.

Conclusion

Partial wrist fusion is a valuable surgical option to treat a variety of instability and arthritis conditions around the ulnar side of the wrist. Arthroscopic surgery offers a very sound surgical principle and brings forth potential benefit in maximizing the resultant range of motion and functional outcome on the wrist by minimizing soft tissue damage and preserving vascularity. It is generally a more reliable procedure than soft tissue reconstruction and results in a more predictable outcome. At the present moment, experience on arthroscopic arthrodesis is still limited. Nevertheless, the surgical technique can be extended to a broader category of disorders and surgery, and the potential for development is enormous.

References

1. Abrams R, Tontz W (2006) Pisotriquetral arthrodesis as an alternative to excision for pisotriquetral instability in high-demand patients: a case report in a gymnast. J Hand Surg Am 31:611–614

2. Adams BD, Berger RA (2002) An anatomic reconstruction of the distal radioulnar ligaments for posttraumatic distal radioulnar joint instability. J Hand Surg Am 27:243–251
3. Almquist EE (1993) Capitate shortening in the treatment of Kienb ck's disease. Hand Clin 9:505–512
4. Aroya AP, Aulshreshtha R, Kakarala GK, Singh R, Compson JP (2007) Visualization of pisotriquetral joint through standard portals for arthroscopy of the wrist: a clinical and anatomical study. J Bone Joint Surg Br 89:202–205
5. Cobb T, Berber S, Badia A (2011) New frontiers in hand arthroscopy. Hand Clin 27:383–394
6. del Piñal F (2011) Dry arthroscopy and its applications. Hand Clin 27:335–345
7. Dobyns JH (1992) Carpal instability. In: Nakamura R, Linscheid RL, Miura T (eds) Wrist disorders: current concepts and challenges. Springer, Tokyo
8. Garcia-Elias M, An KN, Cooney WP, Linscheid RL, Chao EYS (1989) Stability of the transverse carpal arch: an experimental study. J Hand Surg Am 14:277–282
9. Garcia-Elias M, Dobyns JH, Cooney WP, Linscheid RL (1989) Traumatic axial dislocations of the carpus. J Hand Surg Am 14:446–457
10. Garcia-Elias M, Horii E, Berger RA (1991) Individual carpal bone motion. In: An KN, Berger RA, Cooney WP (eds) Biomechanics of the wrist joint. Springer, New York
11. Goldfarb C, Stern J, Kiefhaber T (2004) Palmar midcarpal instability: the results of treatment with 4-corner arthrodesis. J Hand Surg Am 29:258–263
12. Guidera PM, Watson HK, Dwyer TA et al (2001) Lunotriquetral arthrodesis using cancellous bone graft. J Hand Surg Am 26(3):422–427
13. Ho PC (2008) Arthroscopic partial wrist fusion. Tech Hand Up Extrem Surg 12:242–265
14. Ho PC, Lo WN (2003) Arthroscopic resection of volar ganglion of the wrist: a new technique. Arthroscopy 19(2):218–221
15. Ho PC, Hung LK (2004) Arthroscopic reconstruction of destabilizing TFCC lesions with tendon graft. In: Proceeding, 9th congress of the International Federation of Societies for surgery of the hand A-0362
16. Joseph RB, Linscheid RL, Dobyns JH, Bryan RS (1981) Chronic sprains of the carpometacarpal joints. J Hand Surg Am 6:172–180
17. Kaplan EB, Taleisnik J (1984) The wrist. In: Spinner M (ed) Kaplan's functional and surgical anatomy of the hand, 3rd edn. J.B. Lippincott, Philadelphia
18. Kobza P, Budoff J, Yeh ML, Luo ZP (2003) Management of the scaphoid during four-corner fusion – a cadaveric study. J Hand Surg Am 28:904–909
19. Lichtman DM, Bruckner JD, Culp RW, Alexander CE (1993) Palmar midcarpal instability: results of surgical reconstruction. J Hand Surg Am 18:307–315
20. Peterson B, Szabo R (2006) Carpal osteoarthritis. Hand Clin 22:517–528
21. Rao S, Culver J (1995) Triquetrohamate arthrodesis for midcarpal instability. J Hand Surg Am 20:583–589
22. Ritt MJPF, Berger RA, Bishop AT, An KN (1996) The capitohamate ligaments: a comparison of biomechanical properties. J Hand Surg Br 21(4):451–454
23. Sennwald GR, Fischer M, Mondi P (1995) Lunotriquetral arthrodesis: a controversial procedure. J Hand Surg Br 20(6):755–760
24. Shin AY, Glowacki KA, Bishop AT (1999) Dynamic axial carpal instability: a case report. J Hand Surg Am 24:781–785
25. Siegel J, Ruby L (1996) A critical look at intercarpal arthrodesis: review of the literature. J Hand Surg Am 21:717–723
26. Singer G, Ebrel R, Hoellwarth ME (2011) Pisotriquetral arthrodesis for pisotriquetral instability: case report. J Hand Surg Am 36:299–303
27. Slater R, Szabo R (1998) The Sauvé – Kapandji procedure. Tech Hand Up Extrem Surg 2:148–157
28. Taleisnik J (1984) Subtotal arthrodesis of the wrist joint. Clin Orthop 187:81–88
29. Trumble T, Bour CJ, Smith RJ, Edwards GS (1988) Intercarpal arthrodesis for static and dynamic volar intercalated segment instability. J Hand Surg Am 13:384–390
30. Vandesande W, De Smet L, Van Ransbeeck H (2001) Lunotriquetral arthrodesis, a procedure with a high failure rate. Acta Orthop Belg 67(4):361–367
31. Weiss LE, Taras JS, Sweet S, Osterman AL (2000) Lunotriquetral injuries in athletes. Hand Clin 16:433–438

Arthroscopic Ulnar Head Resection and Sauvé-Kapandji

24

Riccardo Luchetti

Introduction

Osteoarthritis of distal radioulnar joint (DRUJ) is a pathological condition that results in a painful wrist with limitation of the pronosupination and grip strength. Various surgical procedures have been described to treat this disabling condition, which include total resection of the ulnar head (Darrach procedure) [4], partial resection with interposition arthroplasty (Bowers and Watson technique) [2, 19], arthrodesis of the DRUJ with ulnar resection osteotomy proximal to the arthrodesis (Sauvé-Kapandji procedure) [15], and the ulnar head prosthesis [18]. The Darrach, Bowers, Watson, and Sauvé-Kapandji (S-K) procedures have become popular treatments for both primary and secondary arthritis of DRUJ and are currently well accepted in all the world with some criticism [17]. These techniques used for restoration of pronation and supination of the forearm are considered salvage procedures. The Darrach, Bowers, and Watson procedures are less demanding surgical techniques and more simple than the S-K procedure. The S-K procedure is considered advantageous over ulnar head resection as the essential ulnar supports of the wrist; i.e. the ulnar head, the distal radioulnar ligaments and the ulnocarpal ligaments are well preserved [17]. Another advantage of the S-K procedure is the shorter postoperative immobilization, which is an additional benefit for the patient.

However, the S-K procedure is not a simple technique, and the surgeon should take utmost care to maintain the correct anatomic alignment of the ulnar head with the radius, while the arthrodesis is performed. Furthermore, the position of ECU tendon in its osteofibrotic tunnel dorsally to the ulnar head should be well preserved. This concept is of great importance during the open surgery in which the operation is done with the wrist in pronation. It has the same value for the Darrach procedure, but it is considered less important for Bowers and Watson techniques in which the resection of the ulnar head is performed by limited surgical incision preserving the ECU tendon position dorsally to the ulnar stump. Many tips and tricks have been described by several authors [9] for all the techniques. Particularly for the S-K technique, it has been suggested to have a vertical position of wrist with 0° of pronosupination of the DRUJ [13] in order to perform an appropriate head resection or an arthrodesis of DRUJ and to prevent malpositioning of the ECU tendon and altered muscle tension of the pronator quadratus (PQ), two of the major stabilizers of this joint (Lluch and Garcia-Elias 2001).

Wrist arthroscopy used to treat such a degenerative condition of the DRUJ is rare, but we have seen that it satisfies the two requirements of the vertical position and selective working

R. Luchetti, M.D.
Rimini Hand Surgery and Rehabilitation Center,
Via Pietro da Rimini 4, 47900 Rimini, Italy
e-mail: rluc@adhoc.net

F. del Piñal et al. (eds.), *Arthroscopic Management of Ulnar Pain*,
DOI 10.1007/978-3-642-30544-3_24, © Springer-Verlag Berlin Heidelberg 2012

on the ulnar head both preserving the ECU position [10–12].

The aim of the present work is to describe the two novel arthroscopic techniques for (1) the resection of the ulnar head and (2) the arthrodesis of DRUJ followed by proximal resection pseudoarthrosis of ulna.

General Indications

The techniques can be successfully used for the treatment of any pathology involving the DRUJ, the most common indications being a primary or secondary degenerative arthritis of the DRUJ. Instability and incongruency after a distal metaphyseal radius fracture are also good indications; however, stability of the ulnar stump should always be given special attention.

These techniques are also indicated for the treatment of the DRUJ degeneration in rheumatoid patients [1, 14]. In these patients with the ulnar head completely dislocated, the resection procedures do not provide any ligamentous stability as the ligaments are damaged and already destroyed. The S-K will give a bony support for the carpus in comparison with the ulnar resection. A radiolunate arthrodesis performed simultaneously with this procedure may be beneficial in providing more bony contact between the lunate and distal radius and ulna, thereby enhancing the stability of wrist.

Another indication for the procedures is the ulnocarpal impaction syndrome due to a positive variance of ulna secondary to a fracture of the distal radius involving the DRUJ, too. However, both the Bowers, Watson, and S-K techniques allow for correction of the ulnar length while preserving the TFCC and ulnocarpal ligaments. The first two techniques allow the correction of the ulnar length only through the ulnar head resection; in the S-K procedure, the correction of the ulnar length can be reached through two possibilities depending on the amount of the ulna plus (1) wafer resection and (2) arthrodesis of DRUJ with proximal shifting of the ulnar head after the resection osteotomy of the ulna proximally to the arthrodesis.

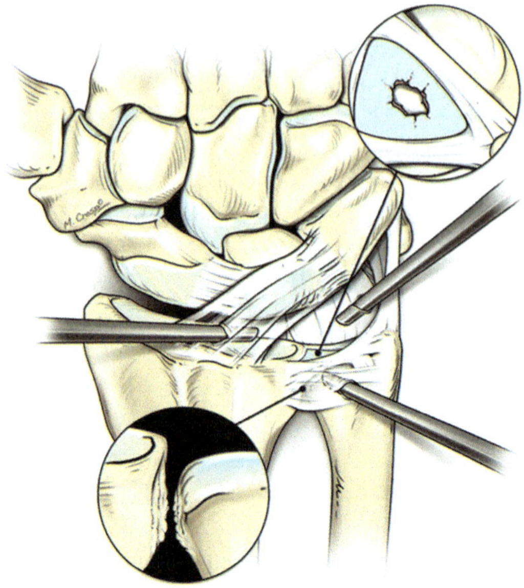

Fig. 24.1 The three main scope entrance portals for radiocarpal, ulnocarpal, and DRUJ arthroscopy. Note the central lesion of the TFCC frequently encountered and the chondral damage of both the sigmoid notch and ulna

Surgical Technique for S-K Procedure

The wrist is maintained in the usual vertical position during the wrist arthroscopy. The radiocarpal joint is explored first, followed by the DRUJ (Fig. 24.1). During the radiocarpal arthroscopy, attention is also focused to the ulnocarpal (UC) joint. For the scope, 3–4 portal is used and 6R for the probe. The UC joint should be explored completely to verify the condition of the triangular fibrocartilage complex (TFCC) and cartilage of both the lunate and the triquetrum. Many times an ulnocarpal impaction coexists (Fig. 24.2), and it should be treated during the same sitting to avoid persistent ulnar sided wrist pain after DRUJ surgery. Specific treatment for the UC conflict is described in Chap. 13.

If the TFCC is intact, its central part should be excised in order to expose the ulnar head reaching the DRUJ (Fig. 24.3a–d).

The surface of ulnar head is characteristically smooth under the intact TFCC. On the contrary, the part that articulates with the sigmoid notch shows severe chondral damage and exposed subchondral bone (Fig. 24.1), and this explains the wrist pain during DRUJ movements and the positivity of the specific test (pain at squeezing test during pronosupination maneuver).

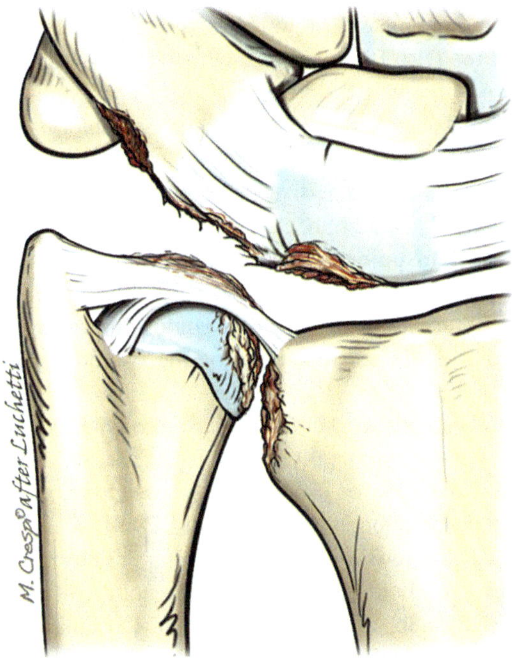

Fig. 24.2 Ulnocarpal impaction syndrome associated with DRUJ arthritis

The conventional wrist arthroscopy portals are not useful for managing the DRUJ arthritis but only to treat the distal part of the ulnar head. Wafer resection (Fig. 24.4a) along with the chondroplasty of the lunate and/or triquetrum is, in fact, a mandatory procedure for the UC conflict using the 3–4 and 6R portals (Fig. 24.4b).

The double approach (UC and DRUJ) is used to remove the remnant cartilage both on the ulnar head and the sigmoid notch (Fig. 24.5a, b). This is performed using a motorized "burr" and radiofrequency device. Frequent changes in the work portals should be done for a better visualization and effective instrumentation. As the distal part is finished, arthroscope is positioned at the 6R portal and instrumentation at the distal DRUJ portal (Fig. 24.5c, d).

Arthroscopic synovectomy is the first step before using the burr to remove the damaged cartilage. Cartilage should be removed only when the burr is perfectly seen to be in contact with the articular surface through the scope positioned in the 3–4 portal (Fig. 24.5b, d). Debrided cartilage is removed using suction through the burr. Suction through a small burr (2.9 mm) often gets blocked, and hence a 3.5 mm burr is recommended, keeping in mind the mechanical risk in this small area. The risk is on the volar side being the ulnar neurovascular bundle and on the dorsal side the tendons of ECU and EDM.

Dry arthroscopy can also be used [5]. Cartilage should be removed from the ulnar head almost completely, the most important part being in front of the sigmoid notch with the wrist in "0" posi-

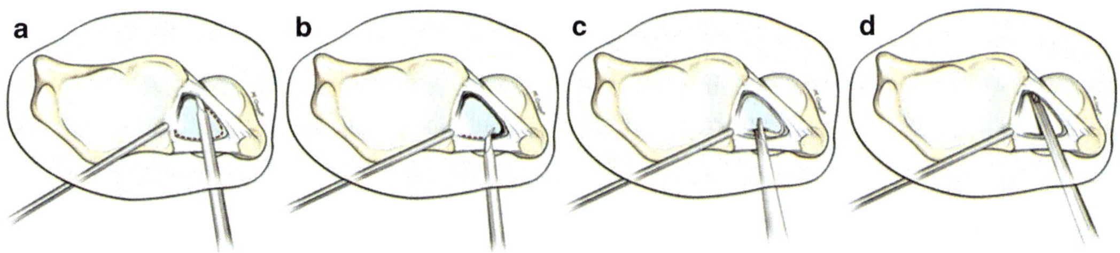

Fig. 24.3 (**a**–**d**) The excision of central part of TFCC to expose the ulnar cartilage (**a**–**c**) and reach DRUJ (**d**)

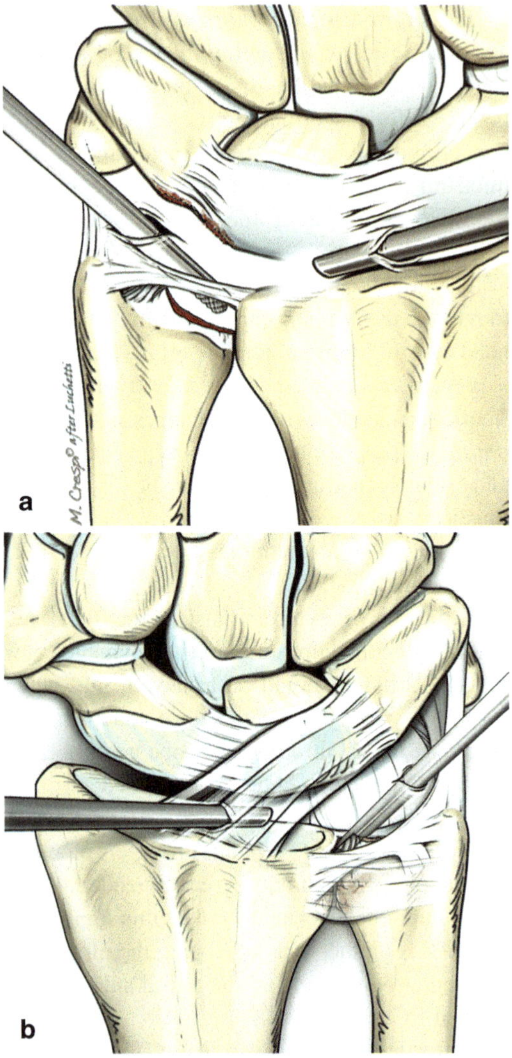

Fig. 24.4 (**a**) The arthroscopic wafer resection. (**b**) The technique to remove the cartilage from DRUJ and ulnar head. Scope in 3–4 portal and burr in the 6R portal

tion of pronosupination. This is an important site of articular contact while the arthrodesis is performed. This part of the cartilage can be easily removed while rotating the wrist in pronation pushing the ulnar head anteroposteriorly (Fig. 24.6a, b). In this position, the appropriate part of the ulnar head cartilage is exposed and easily removed by the burr. Sometime it is needed the resection of the TFCC dorsal branch to permit the exposition of the ulnar head (Fig. 24.6c).

The cartilage of the sigmoid notch is exposed with the DRUJ in supination and with a gentle maneuver of pushing the ulnar head posteroanteriorly (Fig. 24.6d).

Different sizes of burrs can be of immense help in this important procedure by reaching the most difficult part of the joint. When a sufficient area of cartilage on both the articular surfaces has been removed, fixation of DRUJ can be done.

A short vertical skin incision is made on the ulnar aspect of the wrist over the ulnar head and under fluoroscopy control; the DRUJ is temporarily fixed using a K-wire (Fig. 24.7a, b).

The joint is fixed and stabilized by a 2.5–3.0-mm cannulated screw (Fig. 24.8a). Arthrodesis of the DRUJ is performed while maintaining the wrist in a vertical position at 0° of pronosupination. The screw should be positioned anterior to the ECU tendon (Figs. 24.7 and 24.8a). At this time, the DRUJ is fixed and pronosupination is blocked (Fig. 24.8b, c).

Pronosupination can be permitted only by an ulnar osteotomy that should be done just proximal to the ulnar neck. Under fluoroscopic control, the correct level of the osteotomy is checked.

The vertical skin incision given on the ulna is continued proximally to the ulnar neck, and with an osteotome or oscillating saw, a 0.5–1 cm of ulnar resection is performed (Fig. 24.9).

The screw through the DRUJ is initially used just to hold the bones, but not tightened (Fig. 24.8b, c). After resection of the ulna, the screw is firmly tightened to achieve the compression at DRUJ (Fig. 24.10a, b).

A 2.0-mm K-wire is used in addition to the cannulated screw to provide additional reinforcement to the screw fixation (Fig. 24.11a, b). It can be placed proximal or rarely distal to the screw.

After removing the osteotomized bone, it is possible to test the pronosupination of the wrist (Fig. 24.12a, b) and evaluate the stability of the ulnar stump. At the end of the procedure, a final arthroscopic evaluation can be done, and with the probe, a good fixation and stability of the DRUJ can be appreciated (Fig. 24.13).

During all the arthroscopic surgery, the DRUJ is never surgically exposed. The pronator quadratus

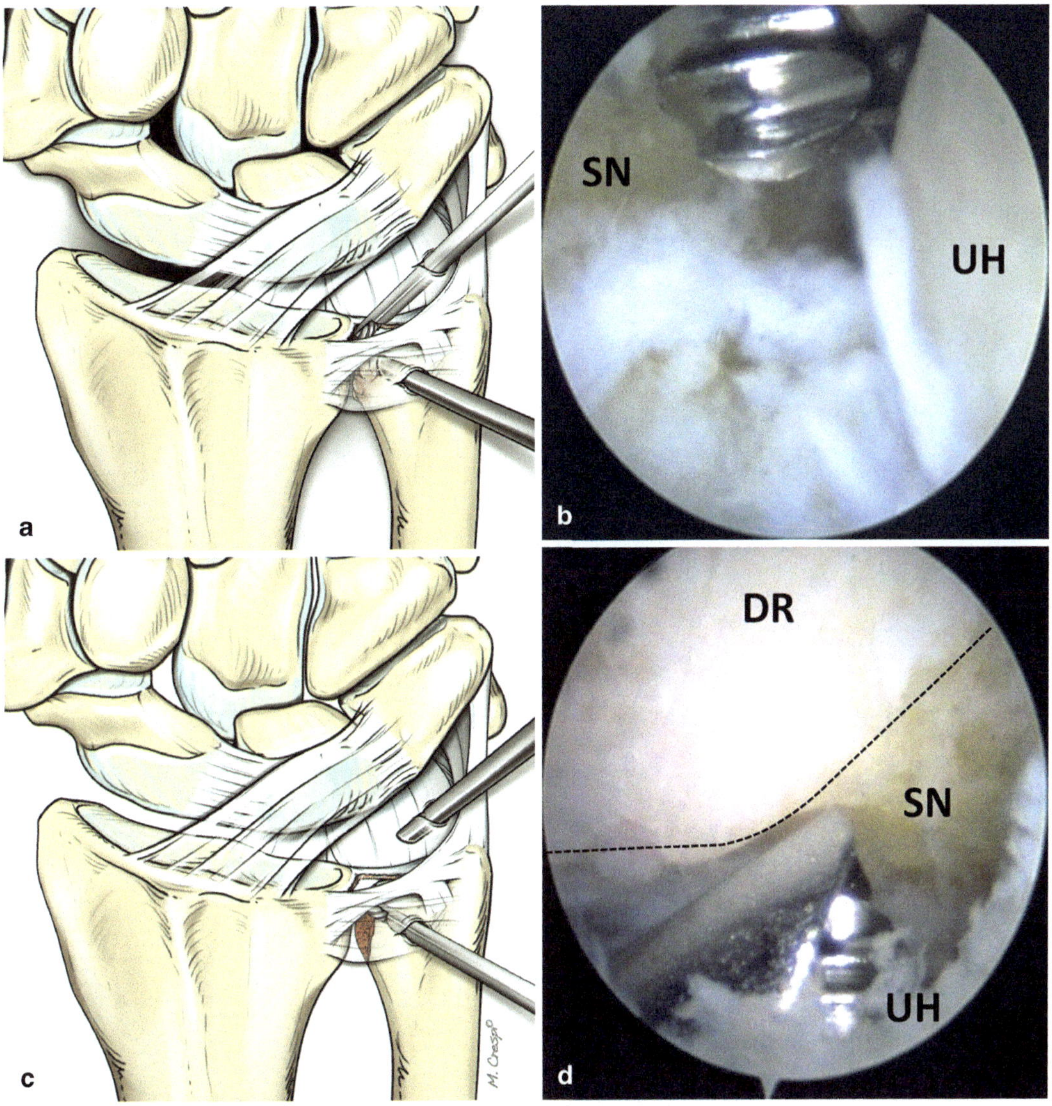

Fig. 24.5 (**a**) The arthroscope positioned at the DRUJ portal and instrumentation at 6R portal. (**b**) Arthroscopic view of resection of the ulnar head (*UH*). *SN* sigmoid notch. (**c**) The arthroscope positioned at the 6R portal and instrumentation at DRUJ portal. (**d**) Arthroscopic view taken from the scope in 6R portal: burr is removing the cartilage from the ulnar head (*UH*). The *dotted line* corresponds to the border between the distal radius (*DR*) and the sigmoid notch (*SN*)

muscle is not interposed at the site of osteotomy of the ulna as done during the conventional open surgery.

Postoperatively, an above elbow cast is given for 2 weeks with the wrist in 0° of pronosupination and the elbow flexed at 90°. Rehabilitation and physical therapy is continued for 1 month after the removal of the cast.

Complications

No complications were seen over four cases operated on; however, there are still some potential complication that can be encountered, such as incomplete resection of the articular surface of the DRUJ leading to failed arthrodesis, incorrect placement of the K-wire and/or screw, too

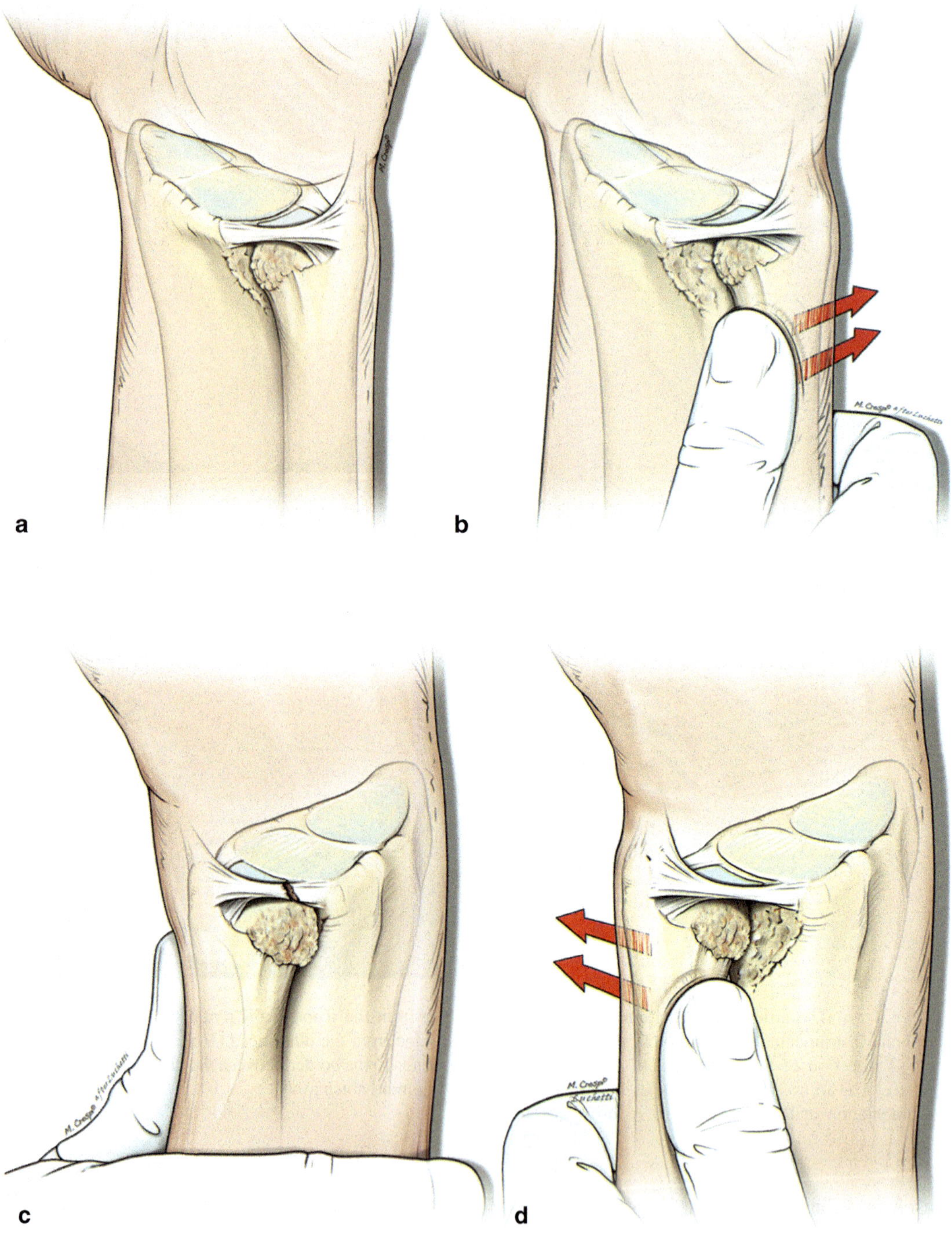

Fig. 24.6 (**a**) A clear DRUJ arthritis. (**b**) The pushing maneuver of the ulnar head from volar to dorsal. This maneuver allows to expose the ulnar head dorsally (*red arrows*). (**c**) As the section of the dorsal branch of the TFCC ligament can increase the dorsal translation of the ulnar head with the pushing maneuver. (**d**) The pushing maneuver of the ulnar head from dorsal to volar that increases the exposition of the sigmoid notch (*red arrows*)

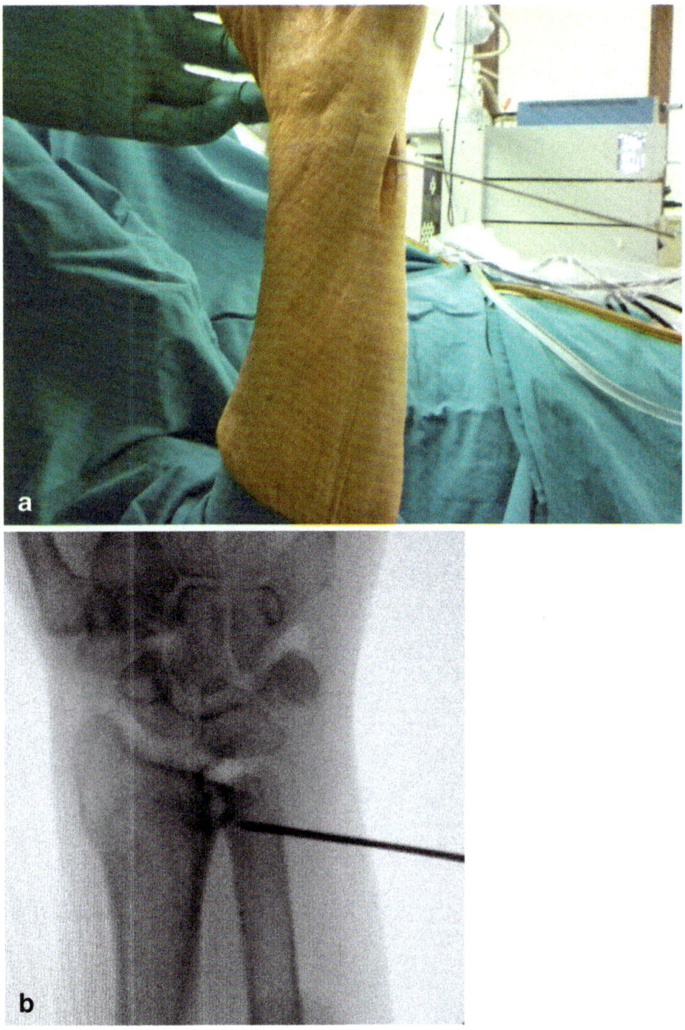

Fig. 24.7 (a) Intraoperative image showing the K-wire introduced from the ulnar head to the radius, blocking the DRUJ at 0° of pronosupination position maintained the wrist in vertical position. K-wire is placed volar to the ECU tendon. (b) X-ray image showing the introduction of the K-wire in the ulnar head with a proximal to distal direction through the DRUJ

proximal or too distal resection of the ulna, instability of the ulna stump with radioulnar impingement, and infection.

Clinical Cases

From 2003 to 2010, three patients (four cases) were operated on. Two females were operated at right and left side, respectively; male was operated bilaterally: mean age was 54 years (ranged from 32 to 78 years old).

The male patient had a primary arthritis of the DRUJ without sign of articular degeneration at the RC and MC joint. The youngest female had post-traumatic DRUJ and LT instability. She was operated for both instabilities, but the DRUJ instability failed twice (arthroscopic and open surgery, respectively). At the last wrist (DRUJ) arthroscopy, ulnar head chondropathy was seen without radiological signs of DRUJ degeneration. The last patient had a DRUJ rigidity due to post-traumatic arthritis with ulna dorsal subluxation and ulnocarpal abutment due to previous wrist fracture (Fig. 24.14a–j). In this case, an arthroscopic wafer resection was associated to the arthroscopic-assisted S-K procedure.

All the cases were preoperatively and postoperatively evaluated using the Mayo Wrist Score modified by Cooney (pain, wrist ROM, grip strength, and work status) [3].

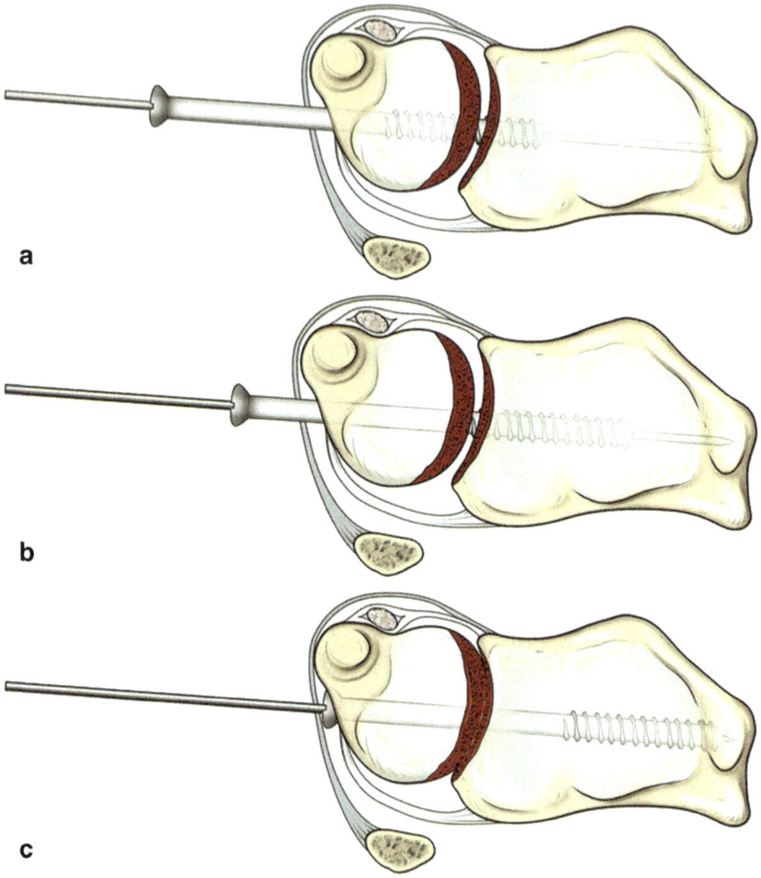

Fig. 24.8 (a–c) The progression time of introduction of the cannulated screw through the DRUJ. Note the position of the head of the screw (c) when the DRUJ is fixed. It must be (1) volar to ECU tendon, (2) under the extensor retinaculum not to interfere with its normal sliding and (3) against the ulna to determine a good compression of the DRUJ

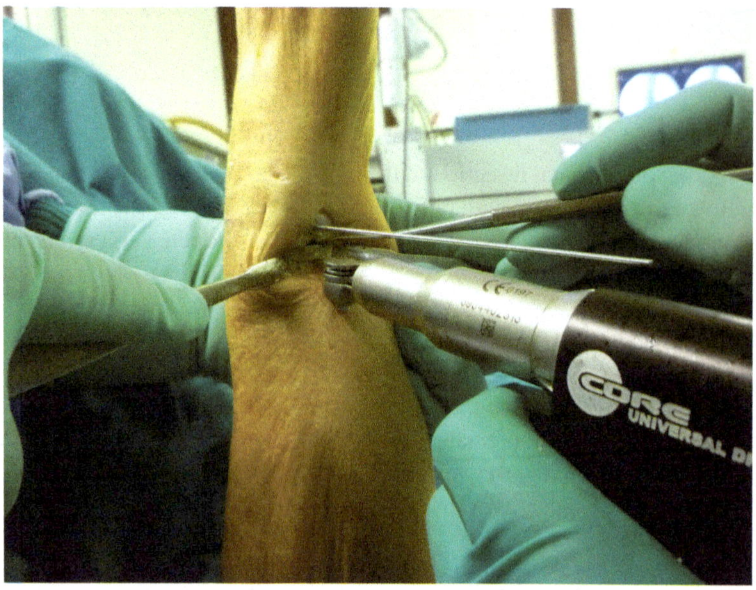

Fig. 24.9 Intraoperative image showing the ulnar osteotomy. It is performed through the small longitudinal skin incision and proximal to the K-wire position

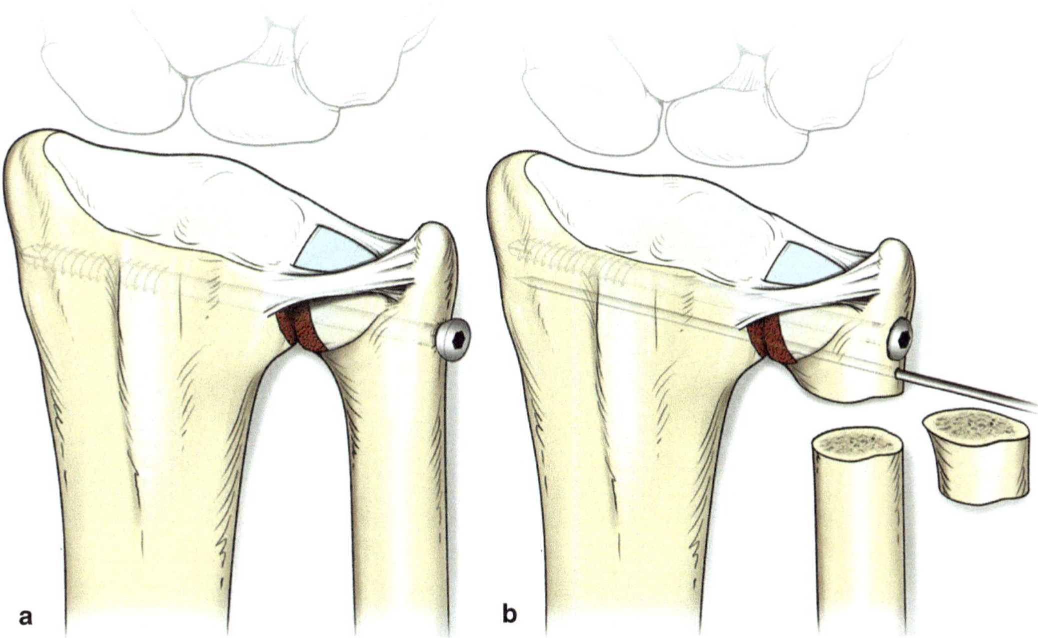

Fig. 24.10 (**a**) The position of the screw through the DRUJ in a posterior anterior view. (**b**) Strong fixation of the DRUJ through tightening of the screw is performed after the proximal ulnar resection/osteotomy. A K-wire is added to increase the stability of the DRUJ fixation

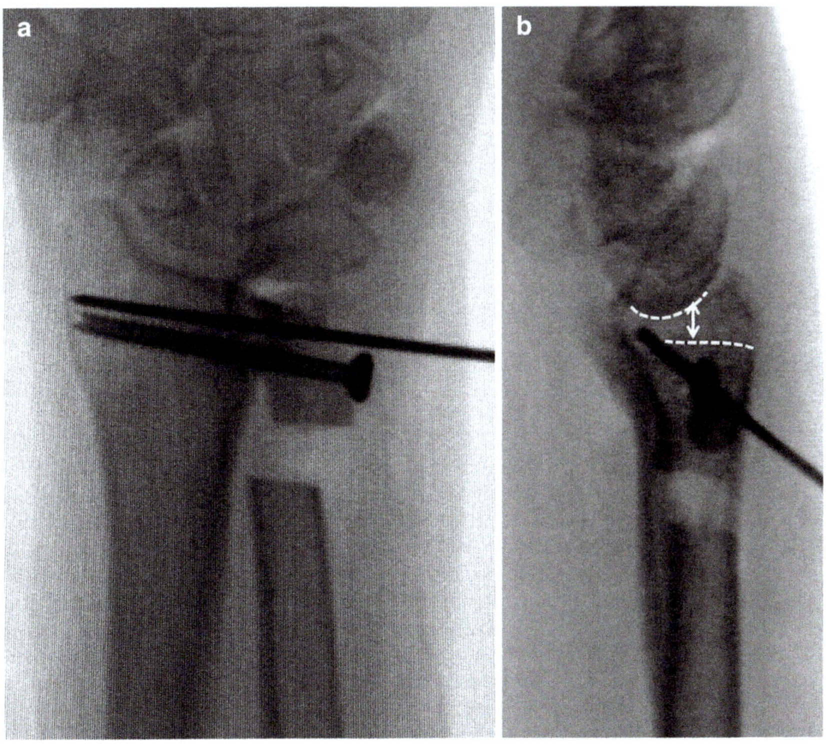

Fig. 24.11 (**a**) Radiograph showing the right position of the screw through the DRUJ in an AP view and the additional reinforcement with a K-wire. *Note*: K-wire has been introduced distally to the screw. (**b**) Radiograph showing the right position of the ulnar stump collinear with the radius. The *double side arrows* shows the correct distance between the ulna head and the carpal bones due to proximal translation of the ulna head in doing the DRUJ arthrodesis

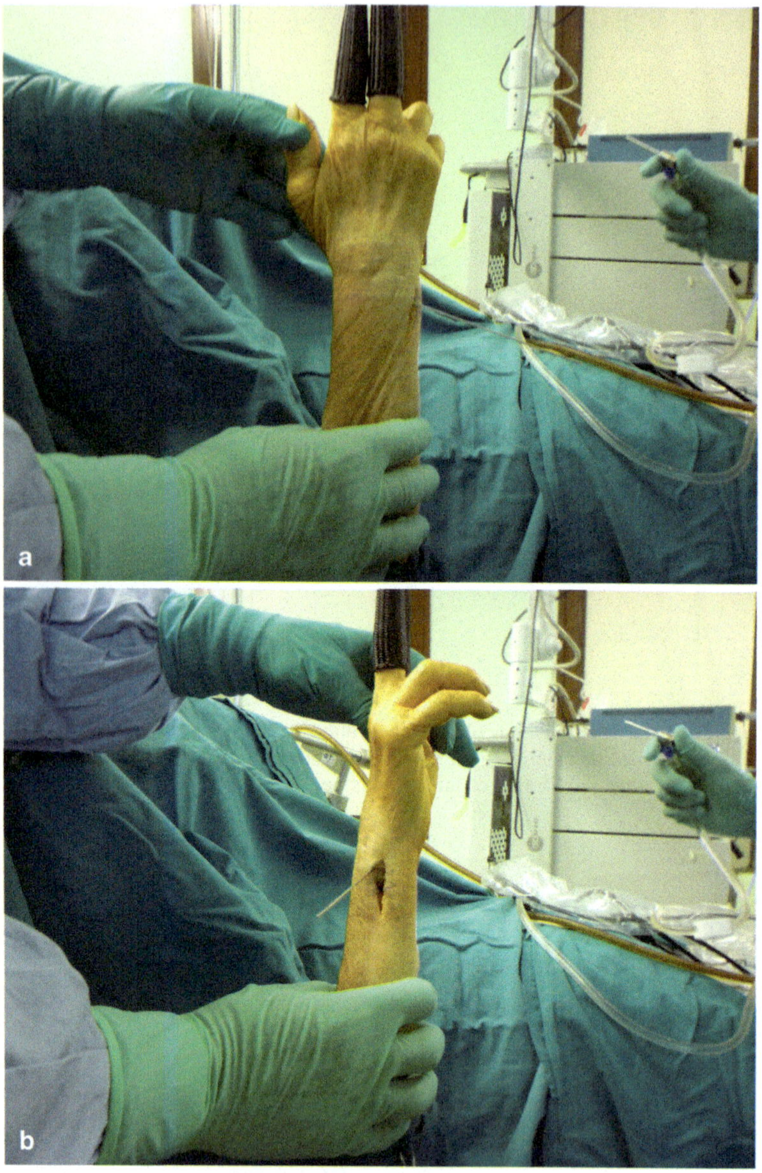

Fig. 24.12 (**a**, **b**) Photographs showing the testing of pronosupination wrist motion at the end of the procedure. (**a**) Supination and (**b**) pronation

Fig. 24.14 (**a**) Preoperative wrist range of motion of 75-year-old female patient affected by post-traumatic DRUJ arthritis. Minimal decrease of ROM of the right wrist is evident. (**b**) Pain location at the DRUJ showed by the same patient. (**c**) X-rays of the right wrist. In the AP view, it was quite evident both the arthritis of the DRUJ (*red arrows*) and the ulnocarpal conflict (*yellow arrows*). (**d**) Intraoperative view of the arthroscopic resection of the DRUJ cartilage. Scope is in 3–4 portal, and burr in the DRUJ portal. To obtain a better arthroscopic vision, the scope was turned to 180° (*red arrow*). (**e**) Intraoperative view of the arthroscopic resection of the DRUJ cartilage. Scope in DRUJ portal and burr in 6R portal. Note the almost vertical position of the burr. (**f**) Fixation of the DRUJ with K-wire under fluoroscopic control. (**g**) Drilling with a cannulated drill of the DRUJ along the K-wire previously introduced. (**h**) View of the right wrist 2 days after operation. Note the K-wire (*red arrow*). (**i**) Post-op X-rays of the wrist with complete fusion of the DRUJ and absence of signs of radioulnar conflict (3 months of follow-up). (**j**) Functional result at 3 months of follow-up

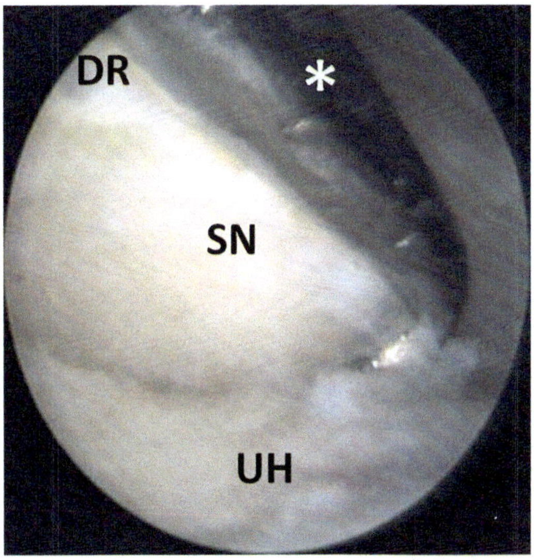

Fig. 24.13 Arthroscopic view of the DRUJ fixation (arthrodesis). Note that the probe (*asterisk*) cannot enter into the DRUJ. *UH* ulnar head, *SN* sigmoid notch, *DR* distal radius

At a mean follow-up of 52 months (ranged from 10 to 96 months), all the patients healed. No complication was shown. Mean pain passed from 7 to 0 at rest and from 9 to 2 after heavy work. Mean range of motion (pronosupination) and grip strength increased consistently.

All patients returned to their previous manual work. X-ray images demonstrated complete fusion of the DRUJ.

Ulnar Head Resection

The arthroscopic ulnar head resection preserves the ulnar styloid in continuity with the ulnar shaft; thus it creates a form of Bowers procedure. The idea of such of arthroscopic surgery comes from the technique of wafer resection and represents an extension of this procedure proximally on the ulnar head. The procedure starts with the

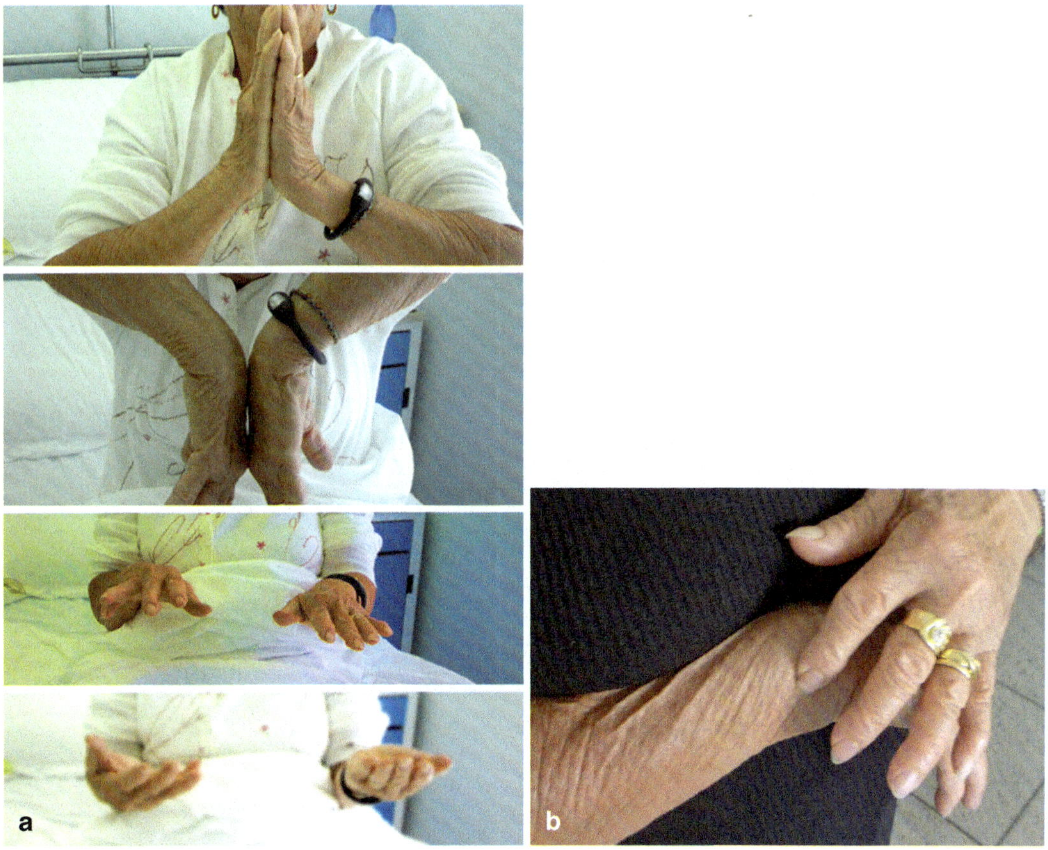

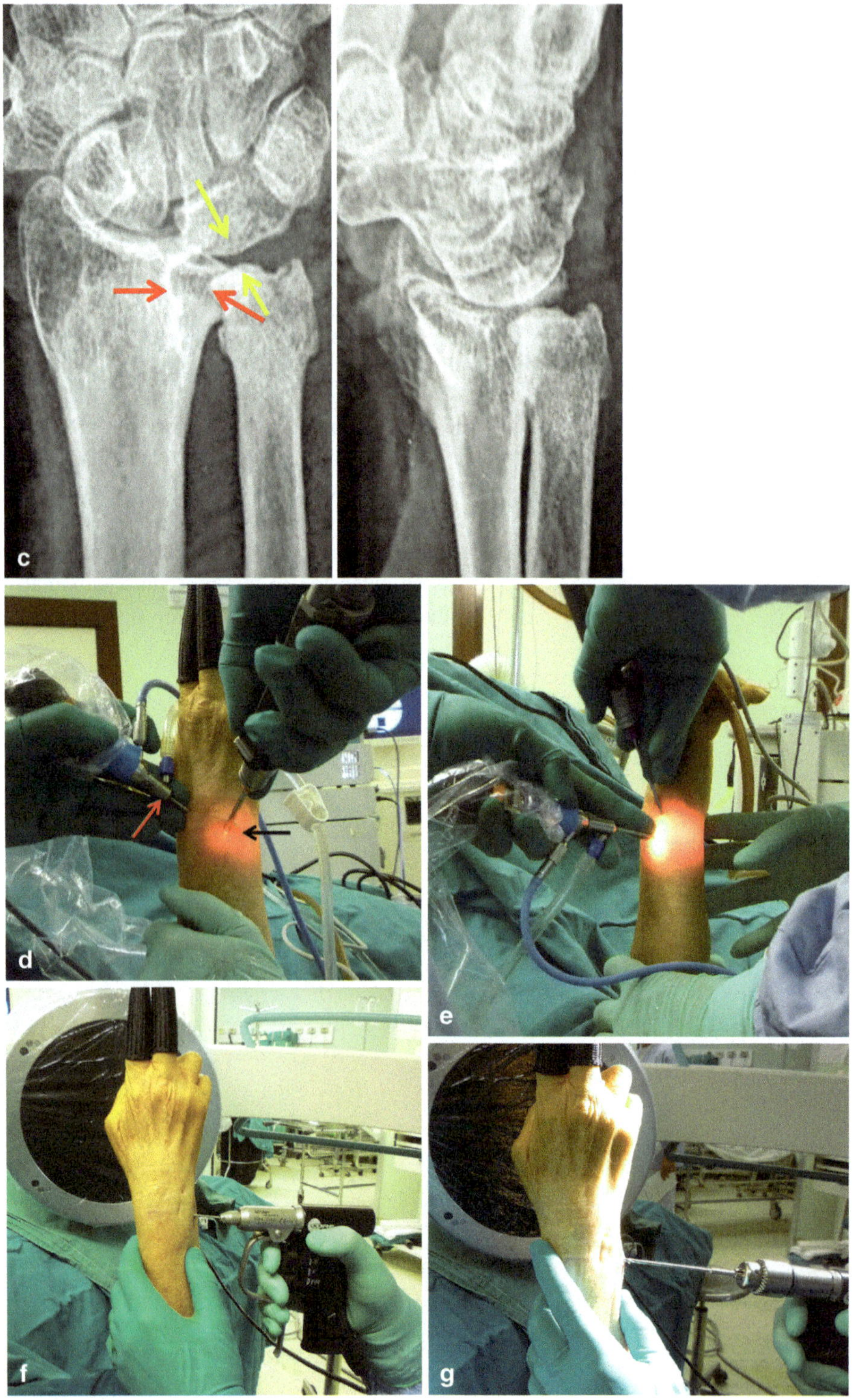

Fig. 24.14 (continued)

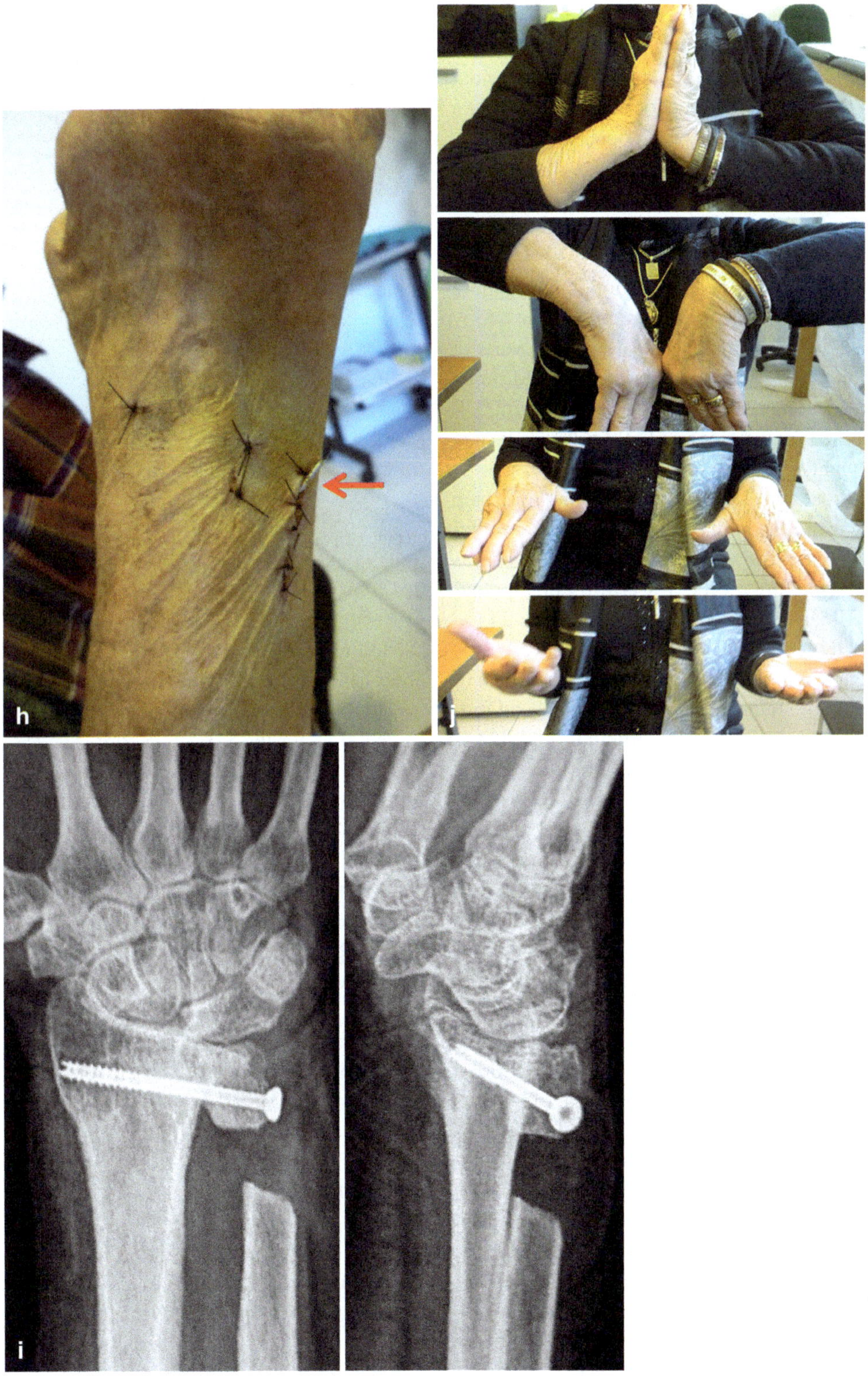

Fig. 24.14 (continued)

resection of the distal ulna head and continues proximally along the DRUJ resecting the portion of the ulnar head that articulates with the sigmoid notch. However, such a procedure is not aware from complications as for the open surgery [17].

Surgical Technique

Arthroscopic ulnar head resection is much more simple than the S-K procedure. Dry arthroscopy can also be used [5]. The wrist is in the vertical position for the arthroscopy. Traditional arthroscopic investigation is performed with 3–4 portal used for the scope and 6R for the probe and instruments.

Arthroscopic synovectomy is the first step before using the burr: 2.9–3.5 mm burrs are recommended. The UC joint is managed as described before for the S-K arthroscopic procedure. Ulnar head is exposed through the TFCC even if it is intact (Fig. 24.2a–d). Wafer resection is the first step of the procedure with the intent of resecting the remnant part of the ulnar head preserving the ulnar styloid. Particular attention is placed to preserve the volar and the dorsal branches of the TFCC and its foveal insertion in order not to provoke a secondary DRUJ instability. Instrumentations (full-radius, motorized "burr" and radio-frequency device) at the 6R portal progressively passed from an oblique to a vertical position (Fig. 24.15) to resect completely the ulnar head going from the UC joint to the DRUJ as the joint space increases. The ulnar head is resected in a rounded fashion using the same strategy of wrist pronosupination motion used for the wafer resection (Fig. 24.16a–c). As the resection of the ulnar head proceeds (Fig. 24.17), the pronosupination of the wrist increases. Sometime a larger burr, as for example, the burr for shoulder arthroscopy, is needed to quickly remove the ulnar head. If it is used, particular attention must be placed to the neurovascular structures around the DRUJ, particularly for the ulnar nerve and its dorsal branch.

From a theoretical point of view, the volar and/or dorsal portals of the DRUJ can also be

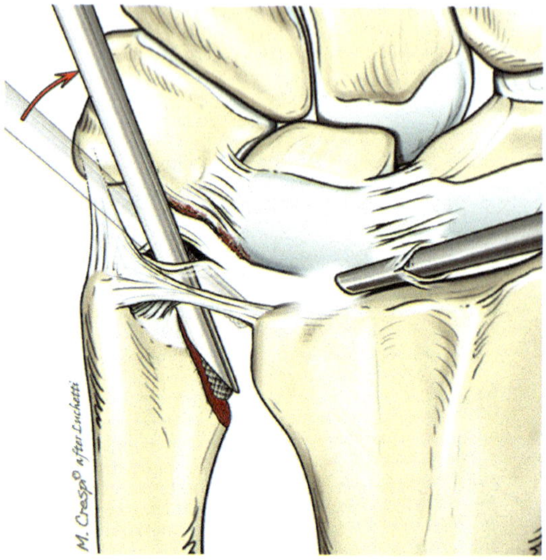

Fig. 24.15 The resection of the ulnar head. Note the change of position of the burr from an almost horizontal (valid for the wafer resection) to an almost vertical one (*red arrow*)

used to resect or to complete the resection of the ulnar head, above all of the proximal part.

The maneuvers of ulnar head pushing are not so useful as for the S-K procedure. The sigmoid notch remains untouched. Fluoroscopy could be useful to check the correct ulnar head resection (Fig. 24.18).

When a sufficient part of ulnar head is removed and a sufficient pronosupination of the DRUJ is obtained, the surgery is ended.

Postoperatively, an above elbow cast is given for 2 weeks with the wrist in 0° of pronosupination and the elbow flexed at 90°. Rehabilitation and physical therapy started after 2 weeks, and it is continued for 1 month after the removal of the cast.

Complication

Due to insufficient experience, only potential complications can be postulated. As for the ulnar head resection performed by open surgery, limited instability of remnant distal ulna should be expected even the TFCC insertion is preserved. Anteroposterior instability is minimal, but lateral

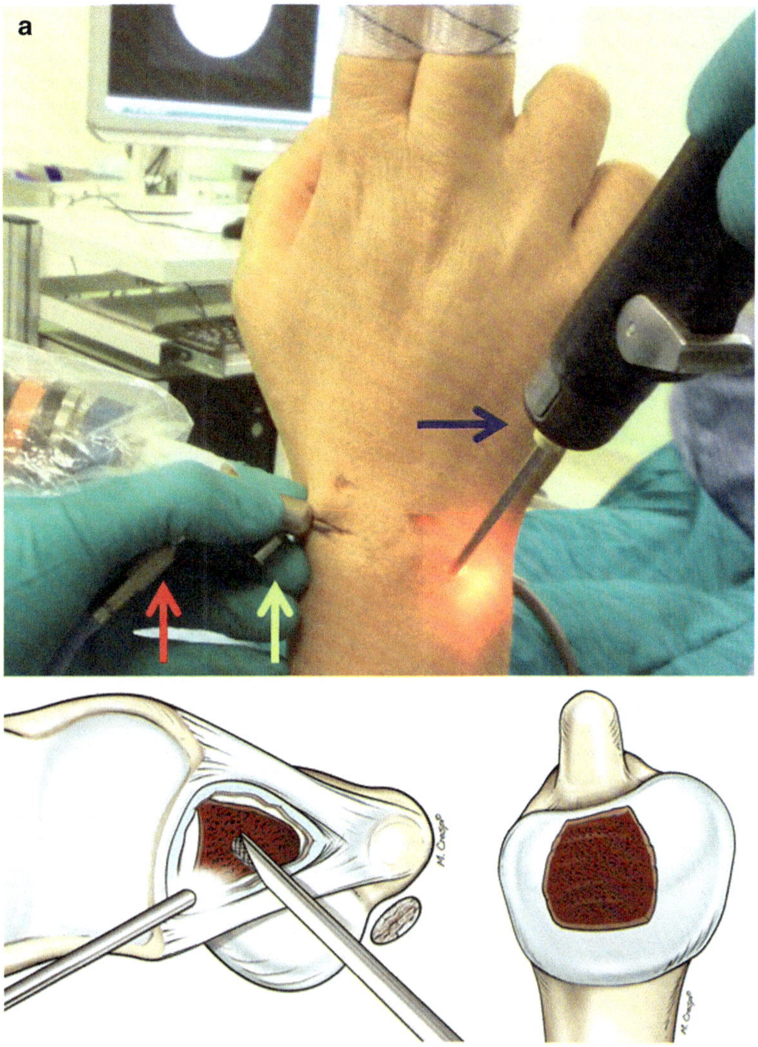

Fig. 24.16 (**a**) Assembled image showing the intraoperative view of ulnar head resection (*top*) and illustration of starting technique (*bottom*). Dry arthroscopy is being used (*red and yellow arrows*); burr is positioned in the 6R portal (*blue arrow*). (**b**) Turning the wrist in pronation (*yellow arrow*) and maintaining the scope in the same position (*red arrow*), the volar side of the ulnar head is exposed permitting its resection (*bottom*). (**c**) Turning the wrist in supination (*yellow arrow*), it is possible to resect the dorsal side of the ulnar head

Fig. 24.16 (continued)

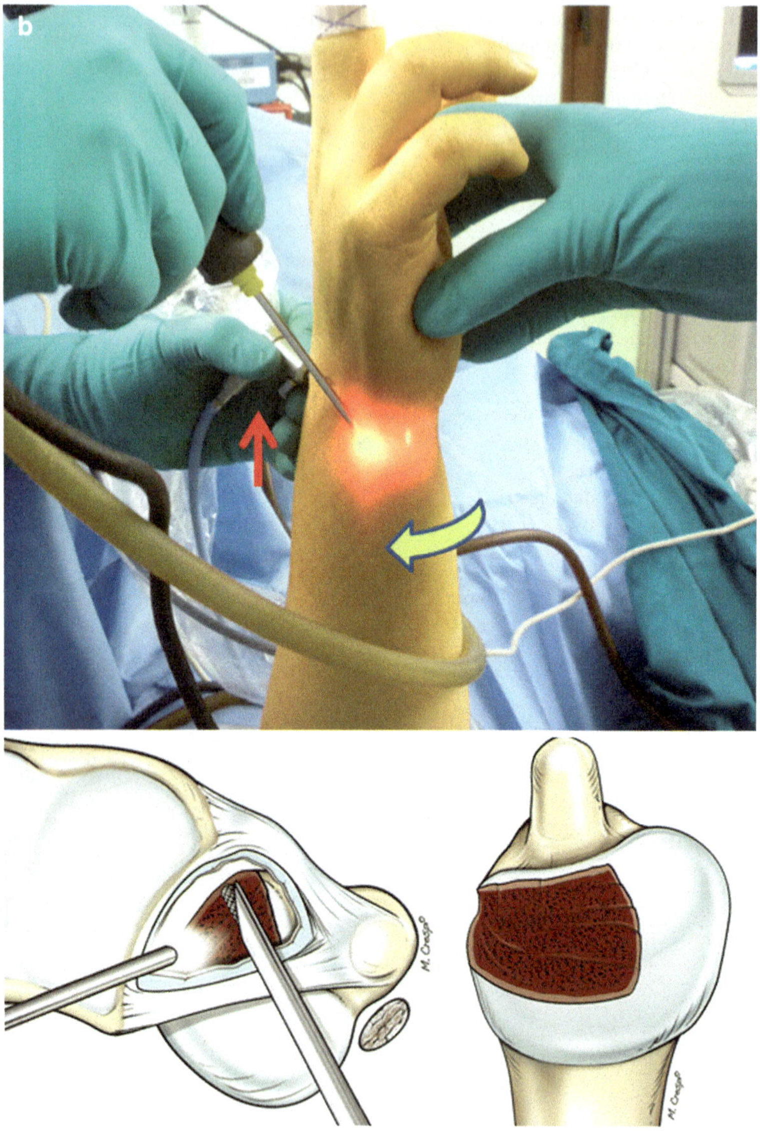

Fig. 24.17 Arthroscopic images showing the resection of the ulnar head (*UH*) in two different steps. Initial resection (**a**) of it in which the contact between the UH and the sigmoid notch (*SN*) is still evident and; (**b**) a more advanced stage of UH resection in which the SN is exposed; space is created between the UH and SN (*black double arrow*). Margins of the UH have to be still resected. *DR* distal radius. *Blue arrow* shows the direction to which the ulnar head (UH) must be turned (pronation) to permit the resection of the volar part of the UH

Fig. 24.16 (continued)

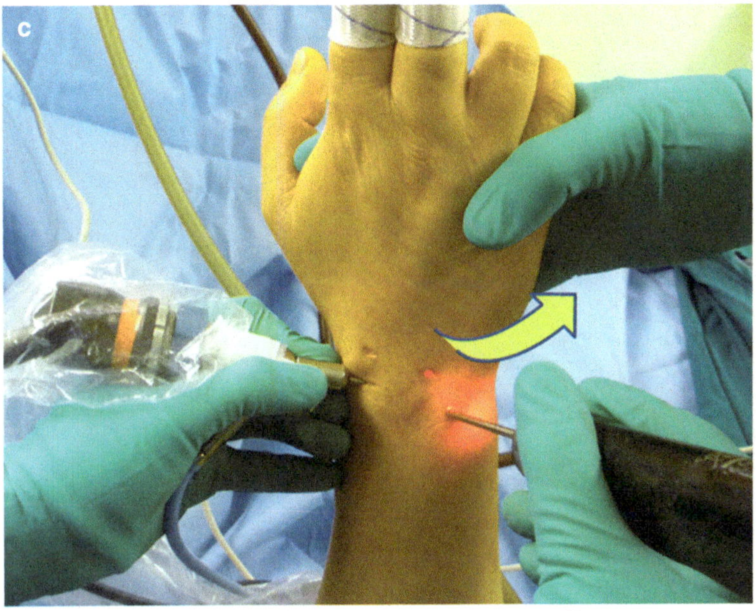

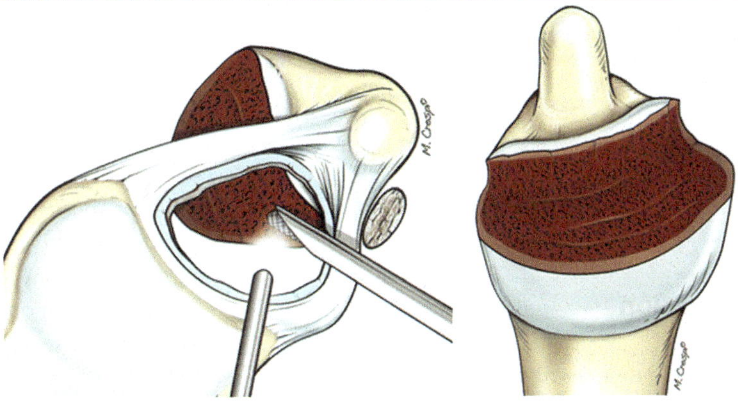

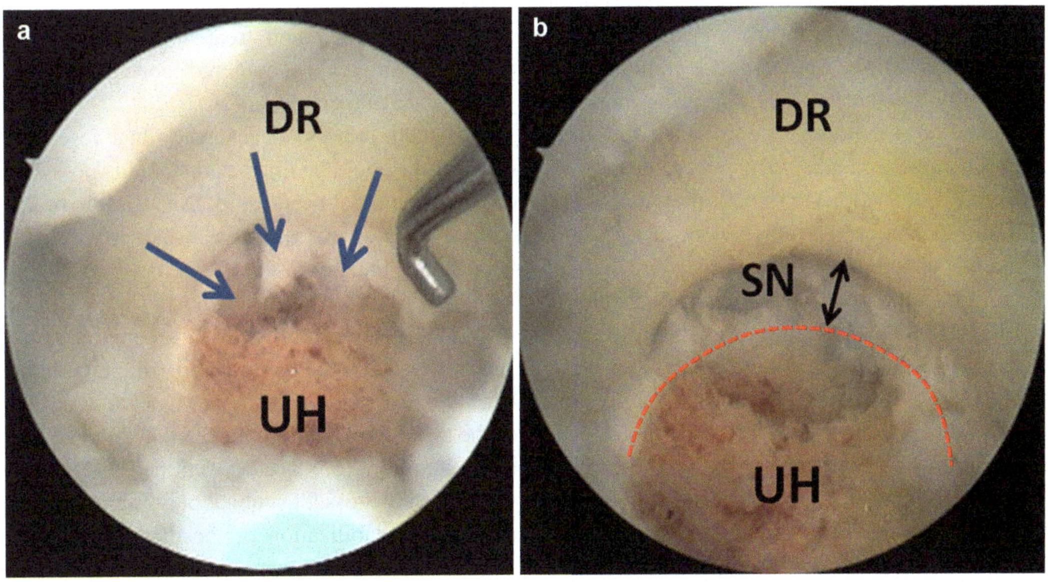

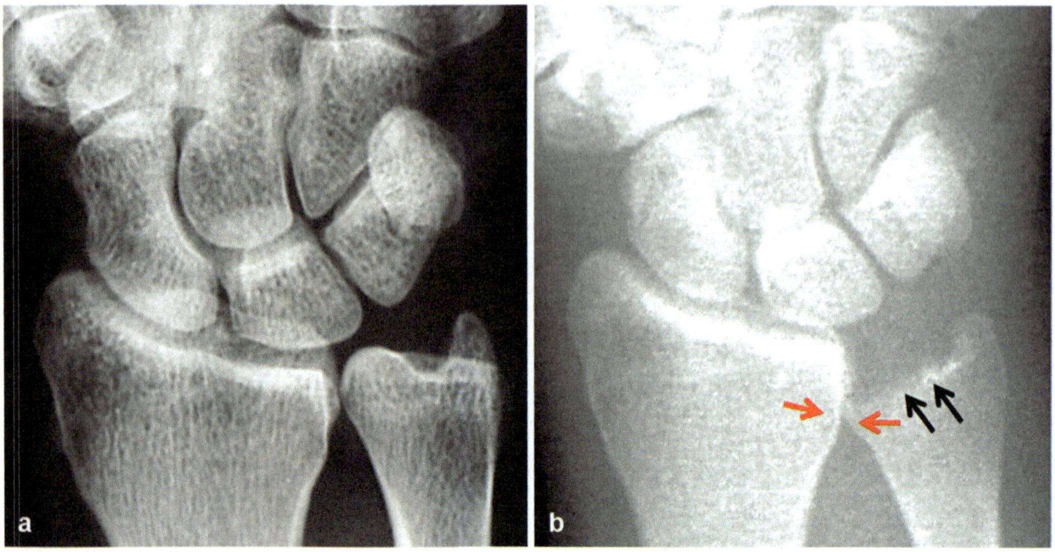

Fig. 24.18 Preop (**a**) and postop (**b**) X-ray images of the wrist. Note the type of the UH resection: it has been done preserving the proximal part in order to maintain a sort of articular contact between the two bones (radius and ulna). *Red arrows* show the maintenance of the proximal part of the ulnar head, *black arrows* show the resection of the ulnar head in an oblique shape

instability implies possible radial conflict or stylocarpal impingement.

Discussion

Arthroscopic-assisted S-K procedure and resection of the ulna head are a safe and promising technique, and they can be successfully used for primary or secondary arthritis of DRUJ. The S-K procedure is a more demanding technique. The noteworthy advantages of the arthroscopic S-K procedure are the preservation of fifth and sixth extensor compartments, more anatomical position of DRUJ, and a faster rehabilitation.

These techniques permit to work in a vertical position of wrist throughout the procedure without opening the joint, which has two major advantages. For the arthroscopic S-K procedure, firstly, there is no rotation of the DRUJ, and arthrodesis is done in a neutral pronosupination position maintaining the ECU tendon, PQ muscle, FCU tendon, and ligaments in the respective anatomical positions and tension. Furthermore, the vertical position of the forearm and wrist permits the introduction of the screw volarly to the ECU tendon which is the ideal position as suggested by many authors [8, 9].

The second advantage is that there is no devascularization of any part of the DRUJ, as could happen during an open surgery. Thus the healing potential of the regenerating bone tissue, which is mandatory for the arthrodesis, is not compromised. Arthroscopy also permits a contemporary wafer resection when needed in order to treat the ulnocarpal conflict and treat at the same time other pathologies encountered during the first step of the arthroscopy.

As some authors suggest, the ulnar resection osteotomy should be done as distally as possible, closer to the ulnar head [8, 9]. Localization of the correct position for the ulna osteotomy can be done using the fluoroscopy. It must be remembered that the deep head of the PQ muscle provides stabilization of the DRUJ originating more anteriorly on the ulna as compared to the superficial head and inserts into the whole of the ulnar border of the distal radius, filling the "axilla" of the distal radioulnar joint [6, 8]. Moreover, the ECU tendon within its fibro-osseous tunnel plays an important role in the stabilization of the distal radioulnar joint [16]. If the ulnar head has been arthrodesed to the distal radius, it does not need the ECU for stabilization; however, it will still provide some stability to the proximal ulnar stump. This will be more effective when the osteotomy is done very close to the ulnar head, the ECU sheath is not disrupted from the ulna, and the ECU is placed dorsal to the osteotomy [8].

The advantage of the arthroscopic ulnar head resection is the improvement of the wrist pronosupination. An intact TFCC is the prerequisite for this procedure. However, the ulnar head resection [17] procedure, as the open technique, can lead to radioulnar or stylocarpal impingement [17]. Even if the TFCC foveal and radial insertions are preserved, the DRUJ stability cannot be completely maintained because of the ulnar head resection. The absence of the ulnar head determines the lack of the anatomical contact between the two bones producing decrease of the capsule-ligament tension around the ulnar head with secondary limited DRUJ instability. To obviate to that type of consequence (ulnar radial or stylocarpal impingement), the proximal part of the ulnar head can be preserved maintaining a contact with the sigmoid notch. However, two main anatomical conditions must be considered: (1) absence of chondropathy in the preserved (unresected) ulnar head and (2) absence of ulnar head subluxation. If one or both of the conditions are present, pain and/or rigidity are maintained. In these circumstances, it is better to remove the ulnar head entirely as the traditional method proposes.

Summarizing, the S-K procedure will work very well if the arthrodesis is done with the ideal positioning of the ulnar head, maintaining the ulnocarpal ligaments and muscles in appropriate tension, and the proximal stump of the ulna will be stable if the ulnar resection osteotomy is very close to the head of the ulna and if the ECU and FCU tendons and PQ muscle remain untouched. All these surgical tips permit a rapid patient recovery, within about 2 weeks.

However, occasionally the instability of the ulna stump appears after the ulnar resection osteotomy and persists after the arthrodesis. This could be due to a concomitant lesion of the interosseous membrane, and the proximal stump should be treated by a tenodesis using the slip of ECU or FCU tendons [7], depending on direction of the instability of proximal ulnar stump.

The arthroscopic procedure of ulnar head resection has the same advantages of the S-K concerning the vascularization of the DRUJ and ECU tendon preserving position. The technique is less demanding and easier to do, but more problems should be taken into consideration as consequence of the complete or partial resection.

References

1. Baldwin WI (1921) Orthopaedic surgery of the hand and wrist. In: Jones R (ed) Orthopaedic surgery of injuries. Henry Frowde and Hodder & Stoughton, London, pp 241–282
2. Bowers WH (1985) Distal radioulnar joint arthroplasty: the hemiresection- interposition technique. J Hand Surg 10A:169–178
3. Cooney WP, Bussey R, Dobyns JH, Linscheid RL (1987) Difficult wrist fractures. Perilunate fracture-dislocation of the wrist. Clin Orthop 214:136–147
4. Darrach W (1913) Partial excision of the lower shaft of the ulna for deformity following Colles's fracture. Ann Surg 57:764–765
5. del Piñal F, Garcia-Bernal FJ, Pisani D, Regalado J, Ayala H, Studer A (2007) Dry arthroscopy of the wrist: surgical technique. J Hand Surg 32A:119–123
6. Johnson RK, Shrewsbury MM (1976) The pronator quadratus in motions and in stabilization of the radius and ulna at the distal radioulnar joint. J Hand Surg 1:205–209
7. Jupiter JB (2008) Tendon stabilization of the distal ulna. J Hand Surg 33A:1196–1200
8. Lluch AL, Garcia-Elias M (1995) The Sauvé-Kapandji procedure: technical considerations. Orthop Surg Tech 9:67–70
9. Lluch AL, Garcia-Elias M (2004) Arthrodesis of the distal radioulnar joint with pseudoarthrosis of the distal ulna: the Sauvé-Kapandji procedure. In: EFFORT (ed) Surgical techniques in orthopaedics and traumatology. Elsevier SAS, Paris: 55Y 290-A-20
10. Luchetti R, Atzei A (2001) Artroscopia di polso. Mattioli 1885 Editore, Parma
11. Luchetti R, Atzei A, Da Rin F, Borelli PP, Mathoulin C (2006) Trattamento dell'artrosi dell'articolazione radio ulnare distale mediante assistenza artroscopia. Riv Chir Mano 43:389–392
12. Luchetti R, Khanchandani P, Da Rin F, Borelli PP, Mathoulin C, Atzei A (2008) Arthroscopically assisted Sauvé-Kapandji procedure: an advanced technique for distal radioulnar joint arthritis. Tech Hand Up Extrem Surg 4:216–220

13. Luchetti R, Cozzolino R, Da Rin F, Atzei A, Khanchandani R (2009) Arthroscopic assisted Sauvé-Kapandji procedure. In: Herzberg G (ed) Avant-bras post-traumatique, arthroscopie – arthroplasties. Sauramps Medical, Montpellier-Paris, pp 297–306
14. Rothwell Ag, O'Neill L, Cragg K (1996) Sauvé-Kapandji procedure for disorders of the distal radioulnar joint: a simplified technique. J Hand Surg 21A: 771–777
15. Sauvé L, Kapandji M (1936) Nouvelle technique de traitement chirurgical des luxations recidivantes isolees de l'extremite inferieure du cubitus. J Chir 47: 589–594
16. Spinner M, Kaplan EB (1970) Extensor Carpi ulnaris. Its relationship to the stability of the distal radio-ulnar joint. Clin Orthop 68:124–129
17. Taleisnik J, Ruby LIL (1998) Arthritis deformity: resection, arthroplasty and fusion. In: Cooney WP, Linscheid RL, Dobyns JH (eds) The wrist. Mosby, St Louis, pp 788–818
18. Van Schoonhoven J, Fernandez D, Bowers WH, Herbert TJ (2000) Salvage of failed resection arthroplasties of the distal radioulnar joint using new ulnar head prosthesis. J Hand Surg 25A:438–446
19. Watson HK, Ryu JY, Burgess RC (1986) Matched distal ulnar resection. J Hand Surg Am 11:812–817

25 Extra-articular Ulnar-Sided Wrist Pain

Carlos Heras-Palou

Introduction

One fourth of patients referred to a dedicated wrist clinic do not present with a wrist or distal radio-ulnar joint problem. In these cases, the origin of the problem is outside the joint, and the cause of pain can be neurological, vascular, tendinous or muscular.

These patients often present a diagnostic challenge, and standard investigations focused on the wrist joint may not provide the answer; in fact, incidental findings may misguide the surgeon. Clinical history and examination remain the key to the diagnosis.

Extensor Carpi Ulnaris Tendinopathy

The term tendinopathy includes a group of conditions affecting the tendons that can be caused by a discrete injury or by overuse. In many cases, it is more appropriate to use the term tendinosis, which indicates degeneration, rather than tendinitis which indicates inflammation of the tendon. Tenosynovitis, which is inflammation of the synovial sheath of the tendon, is often used to describe the findings in patients with rheumatoid or other inflammatory arthritis. Stenosing tenovaginitis or tendon entrapment may be a better term for cases where the problem is caused by narrowing or stenosis of the tendon sheath.

Tendinopathies often follow a pattern with three phases [4]. The first one is inflammation, starting after the injury and lasts up to two weeks, presenting with pain, swelling, redness and tenderness. The second phase is the proliferative stage, where new collagen is deposited, lasting about 2 weeks. The third phase is maturation, where healing is complete, and this lasts 6–12 weeks. Therefore, after an episode of injury, it may take several months for the symptoms to settle completely.

Extensor carpi ulnaris tendinosis is the second most common tendinopathy of the wrist, after de Quervain's. It is often precipitated by an injury, followed by increasing pain and swelling over the following 24 or 48 h. The pain may not be very localised, sometimes felt along the course of the tendon or deep in the joint, and can be severe at night and at rest.

This condition may coexist with TFCC tears (Fig. 25.1), non-union of the ulnar styloid, distal radio-ulnar joint degeneration, lunotriquetral instability, anomalous slips of the ECU or septation of the sixth extensor compartment (Fig. 25.2). It may also take place with ECU instability.

Patients with ECU tendinopathy present with dorso-ulnar wrist pain and a firm fusiform swelling of the sixth compartment, which is tender. The pain over this compartment can be provoked by resisted ulnar deviation of the wrist in pronation and resisted extension of the wrist in supination.

C. Heras-Palou, M.D.
Pulvertaft Hand Centre, Royal Derby Hospital, Derby, UK
e-mail: carlos.heras-palou@virgin.net

F. del Piñal et al. (eds.), *Arthroscopic Management of Ulnar Pain*,
DOI 10.1007/978-3-642-30544-3_25, © Springer-Verlag Berlin Heidelberg 2012

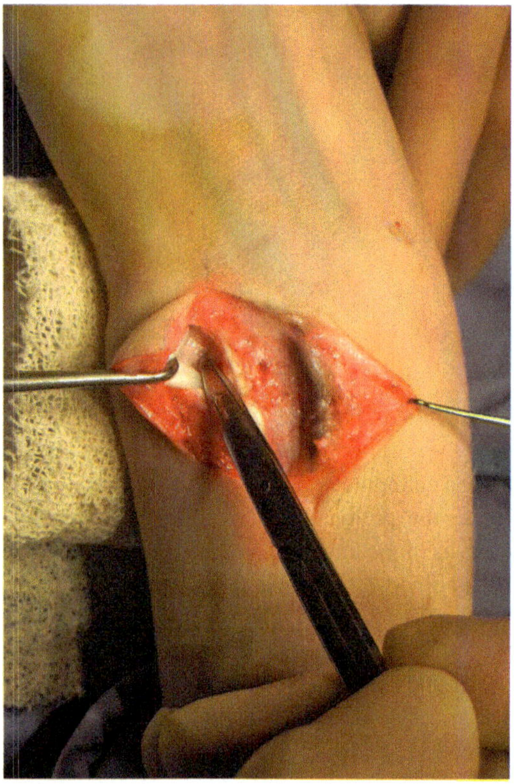

Fig. 25.1 This patient presented with pain and clicking in pronation and supination, 6 months after a twisting injury to the wrist. She had swelling and pain localised to the ECU sheath. A diagnosis of TFCC tear was made. During surgical exploration through a dorso-ulnar approach, the ECU sheath was opened and the ECU retracted to reveal a tear in the floor of the ECU tunnel, in continuity with the TFCC tear. The TFCC was reattached and the tear in the ECU sheath repaired

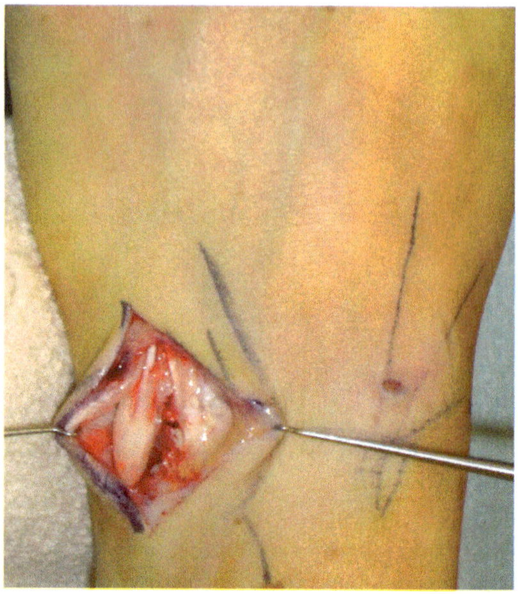

Fig. 25.2 This 22-year-old heating engineer presented with recurrent episodes of pain and swelling in the ulnar side of his left wrist. The symptoms settled with rest, steroid injection into the ECU sheath and splint, but recurred after a few weeks. Wrist arthroscopy did not detect any abnormalities. Exploration of the ECU revealed multiple slips of the tendon and septation of the distal part of the compartment

It is useful to confirm the clinical diagnosis with an injection of 1 ml of local anaesthetic into the sheath of the ECU tendon. Transient complete resolution of the symptoms indicates that the origin of the pain is in the tendon sheath and not in the wrist joint. Conservative treatment with splinting or casting, oral anti-inflammatories and ice usually provides good relief on symptoms in the acute phase. If the symptoms persist, injection of corticosteroid can be very helpful.

Occasionally, surgical treatment can be required in recalcitrant cases. Through a 3-cm incision over the ECU sheath, and parallel to the course of the dorsal sensory branch of the ulnar nerve, the sixth compartment is released. The tendon is trimmed if frayed. Any osteophyte or roughness in the groove is removed, and the retinaculum is repaired.

The extensor retinaculum is a different tissue layer to the ECU sheath, and it is therefore feasible to release the ECU sheath but repair the retinaculum over it, in order to prevent instability of the tendon, and this is what we recommend, although there are reports in the literature of complete release without reconstruction or repair and no instability of the tendon was noted postoperatively.

Extensor Carpi Ulnaris Instability

The extensor carpi ulnaris tendon has a unique fibro-osseous sheath that maintains the tendon in its position, deep to the extensor retinaculum. The extensor retinaculum does not insert in the ulna; it goes round to insert in the pisiform, triquetrum, fifth metacarpal and volar tissues.

During pronosupination, all the wrist and digital extensor tendons move with the radius, except the ECU that keeps its relationship to the ulna. With the wrist supinated, the ECU is dorsal and is therefore a pure extensor. While in pronation, the ECU is on the ulnar side of the wrist and its action is ulnar deviation. The main role of the ECU is to stabilise the wrist and allow powerful use of fingers and thumb. There is good evidence that the ECU is a very important dynamic stabiliser of the wrist and the DRUJ [8].

The ECU takes an angular path across the head of the ulna to its insertion on the fifth metacarpal base. This angle is more marked in supination and with the wrist in ulnar deviation.

Differentiating intra-articular from extra-articular pathology can be difficult. Two tests are specific for ECU pathology. The 'synergy test' is carried out by placing the forearm of the patient vertical, resting the elbow on a table top, with the forearm supinated, and during resisted abduction of the thumb, the ECU can be seen bowstringing [7]. Another provocation test is the 'sand scoop test', where the patient is asked to use his hand as if scooping sand. This combines wrist extension and ulnar deviation with supination of the forearm. When this movement is resisted by the examiner, the ECU is tested (Fig. 25.3).

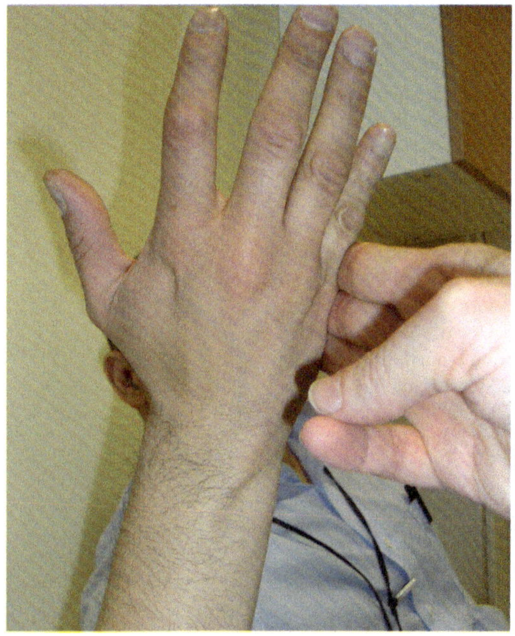

Fig. 25.3 During the 'sand scoop test', the patient is asked to move his hand as if he was trying to scoop sand against resistance. The forearm is supinated, the wrist slightly extended, and pushing against the ulnar side. Pathology around the ECU will be painful, and if the ECU is unstable, it can be seen subluxating out of the groove

ECU instability is often the result of an injury with the forearm in supination and the wrist in ulnar deviation and flexion. In this position, active contraction of the ECU muscle generates a moment that tends to pull the ECU tendon away from the ulna, placing considerable tension on the ECU sheath that is trying to contain the tendon. In a review of 12 cases with chronic ECU instability, three patterns of injury were identified (Inoue and Tamura 2001) (Fig. 25.4).

Acute cases can be treated conservatively by immobilisation in a splint, with the forearm in pronation and the wrist in neutral position for 6 weeks, and oral anti-inflammatories. Surgical repair is usually reserved for patients with persistent symptoms. Through a longitudinal dorsal incision, between the fifth and sixth extensor compartments, the ECU sheath is inspected, taking care to protect the dorsal branch of the ulnar nerve. The tendon and the groove are inspected. Any osteophytes or roughness in the groove is excised, and the sheath is assessed. On occasions, the sheath can be repaired, taking care not to over-tighten the compartment. To this effect, it is useful to place a paediatric feeding tube next to the tendon during the repair to reduce the risk of entrapment of the tendon after the surgery.

If the groove is too shallow, it can be deepened with a burr. There are several techniques to reconstruct the ECU sheath using a flap of retinaculum [9]. Suture anchors can be used along the ulnar edge to reconstruct the sheath [5].

A different approach has been proposed by Garcia-Elias, raising a capsular flap from the DRUJ and placing the ECU tendon in the groove, replacing the capsule over the tendon (Fig. 25.5). This has the advantage that the ECU remains in its anatomical position in relation to the ulna. The author has used this technique in a small series of cases with good results (Fig. 25.6).

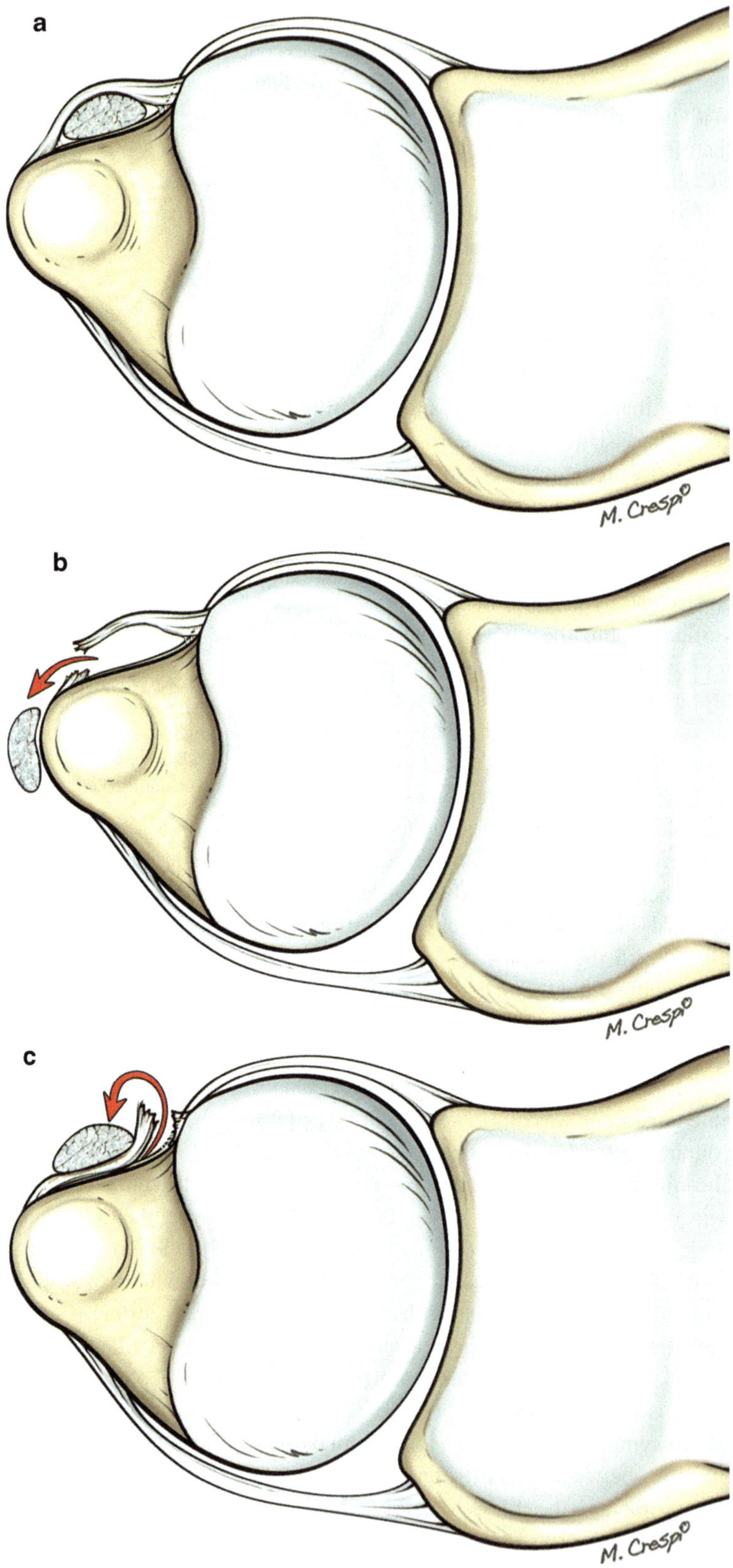

Fig. 25.4 (**a**) The ECU is contained in its fibro-osseous tunnel. Innoue described three types of disruption of the tendon sheath. (**b**) The first one is a rupture of sheath from the ulnar wall and dislocation of the tendon. (**c**) The second type is a disruption of the radial wall of the tunnel with dislocation of the tendon that returns to its position but lies on top of the sheath. (**d**) In the third type, the tendon dislocates into false pouch formed by stripping of the periosteum from the ulna

Fig. 25.4 (continued)

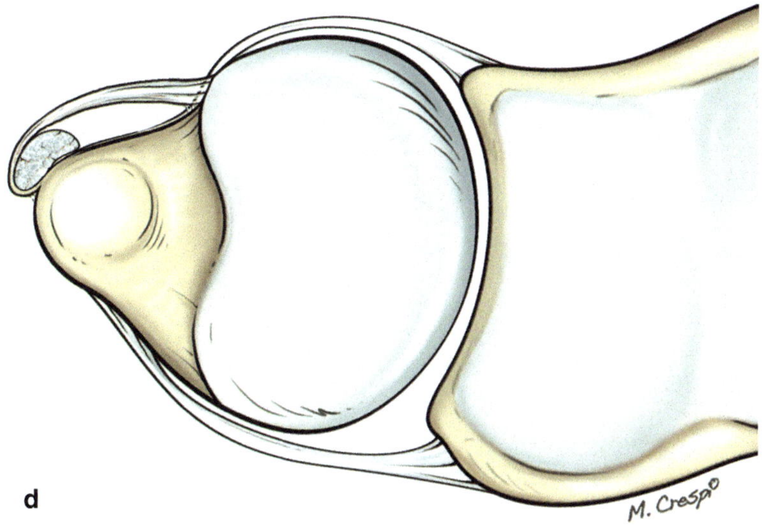

d

a

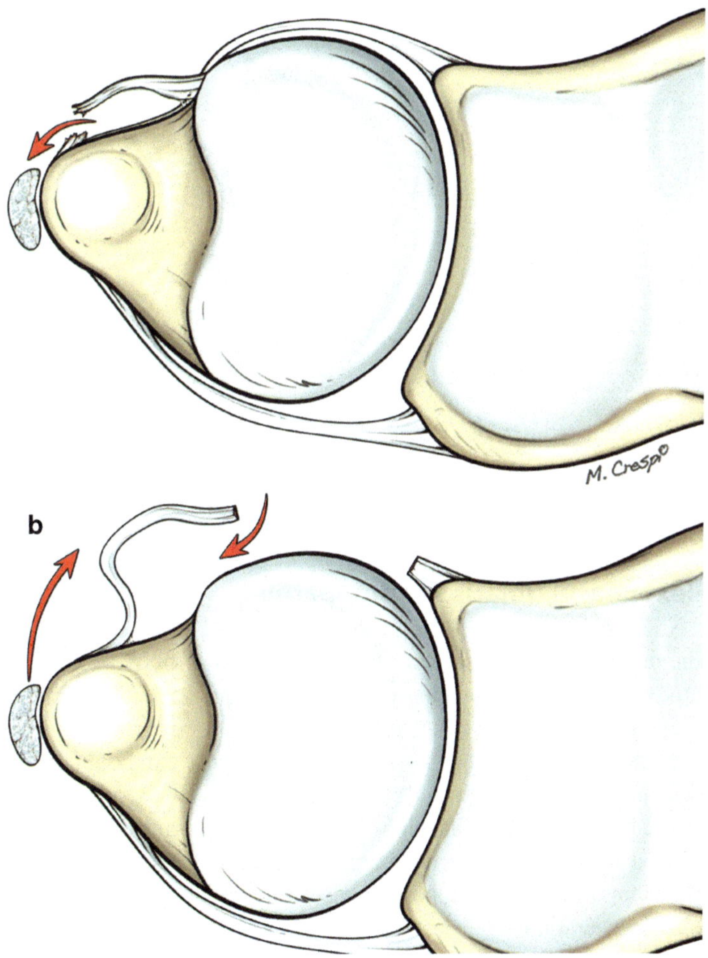

b

Fig. 25.5 (**a**–**d**) Through a dorsal approach to the DRUJ, a capsular flap is raised and the ECU tendon is placed in its groove under the capsule

Fig. 25.5 (continued)

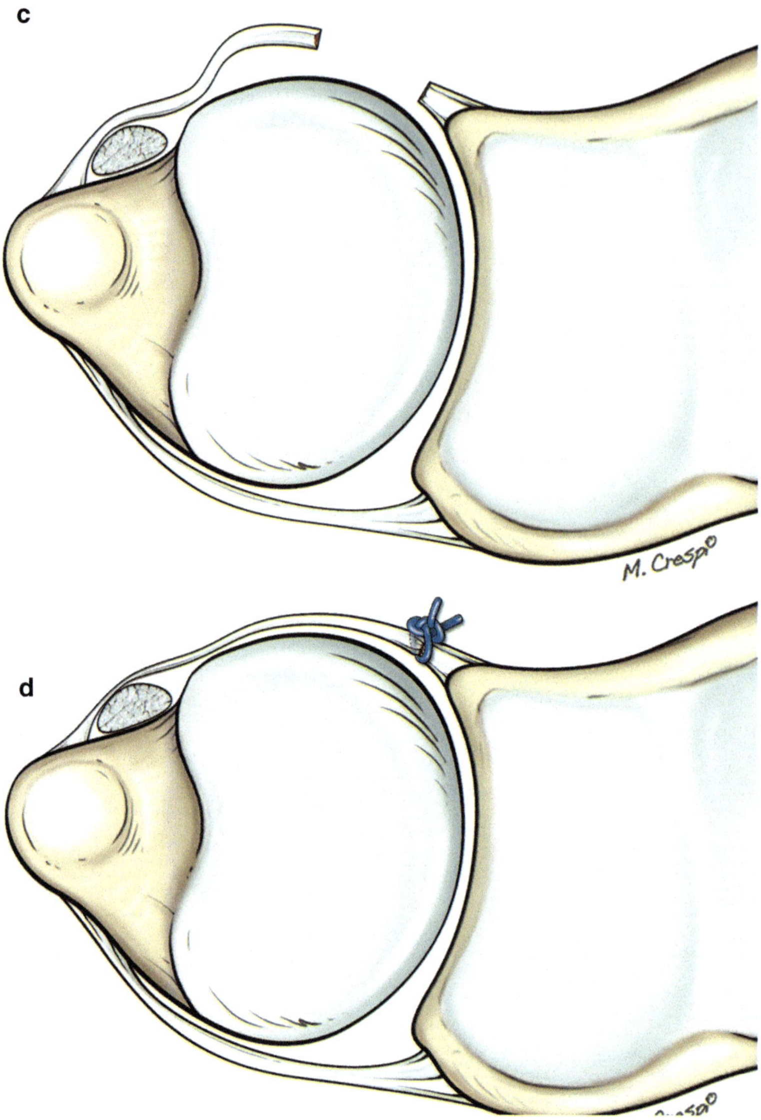

Flexor Carpi Ulnaris Tendinopathy

The most common wrist flexor to develop tendinitis is the flexor carpi ulnaris. It may present after repetitive activities that require wrist flexion in ulnar deviation of the wrist, although often may present without a history of trauma or unusual activity. The pain can be exacerbated by resisted flexion and ulnar deviation of the wrist. The main differential diagnosis is piso-triquetral joint degeneration.

Radiographs may show calcific deposition in the tendon (Fig. 25.7). This is due to deposition of hydroxyapatite, causing an acute inflammatory reaction. The aetiology is unknown. The florid reaction with severe pain, swelling and redness can be mistaken for an infection.

Conservative treatment with splint and oral anti-inflammatory is usually successful. Very rarely, resistant or chronic cases require surgical exploration. This reveals some degeneration of the tendon, and the deposited material can be extruded, resembling toothpaste in its consistency.

Digital Extensor Tendons Rupture

It is well known that rupture of the extensor tendons to the fingers, in particular of the extensor digiti quinti and extensor digitorum communis, can occur over the dorsum of the wrist in patients with inflammatory arthritis, typically rheumatoid arthritis. These patients present with a sudden inability to extend one or several fingers. Most frequently, the problem affects first the little finger, and if not treated then the ring and the middle fingers, but rarely all four fingers. It is sometimes thought that the rupture of these tendons is due to synovitis. However, the location and pattern of the ruptures is constant and predictable, always occurring over the dorsally subluxated ulnar head. The ulnar head is degenerated and has an osteophyte, often with a sharp edge, that causes attrition of the tendons during pronation and supination (Fig. 25.8). It is an interesting finding during surgical exploration that there is always a perforation of the dorsal capsule of the DRUJ caused by the same osteophyte, which indicates that the cause of tendon rupture is

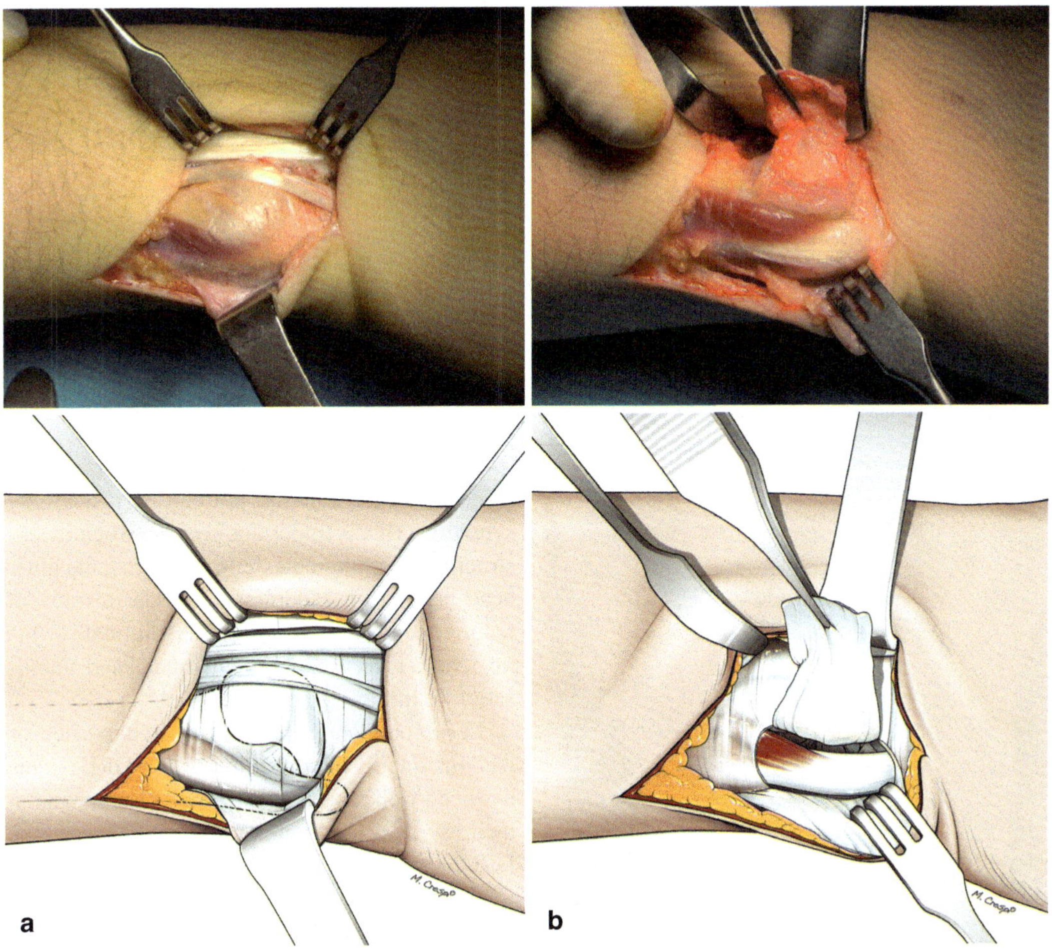

Fig. 25.6 (**a**, **b**) Dorso-ulnar approach through the fifth extensor compartment. Unstable ECU can be seen under the extensor retinaculum. (**c**, **d**) The ECU is retracted and an ulnarly based capsular flap is raised. (**e**, **f**) The ECU tendon is placed under the capsular flap. (**g**, **h**) Once the ECU tendon is relocated into its groove, the capsular flap is secured and the extensor retinaculum repaired

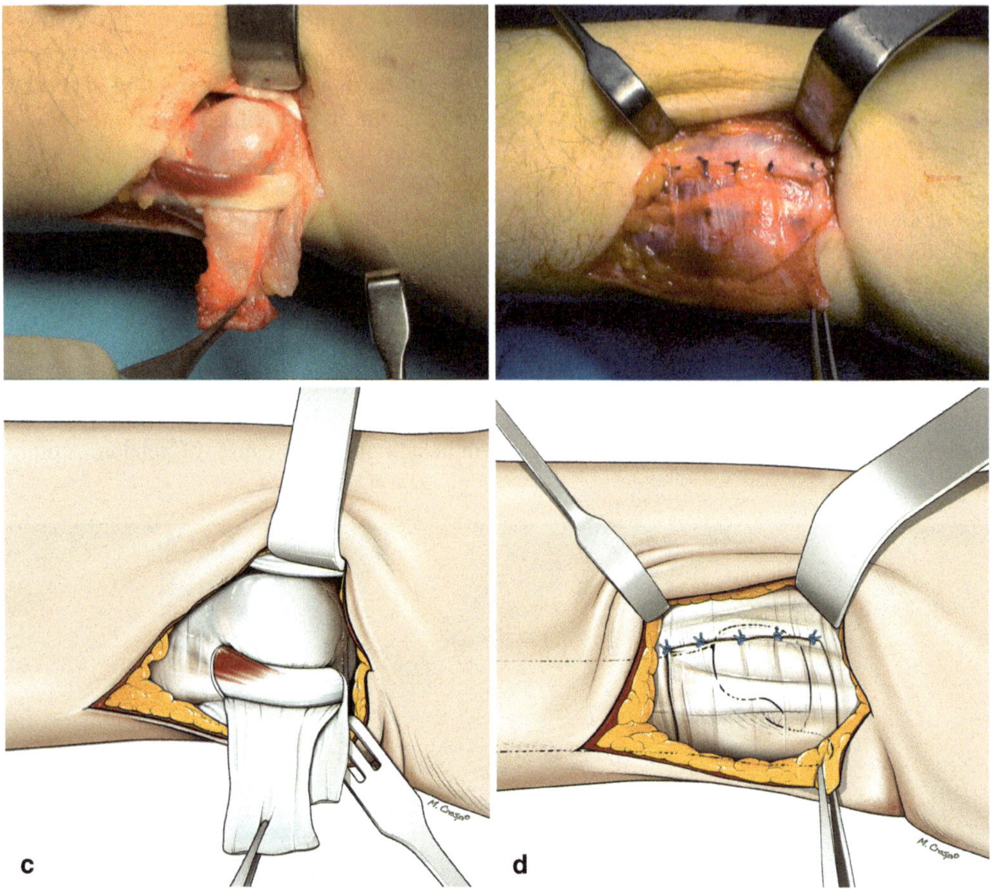

Fig. 25.6 (continued)

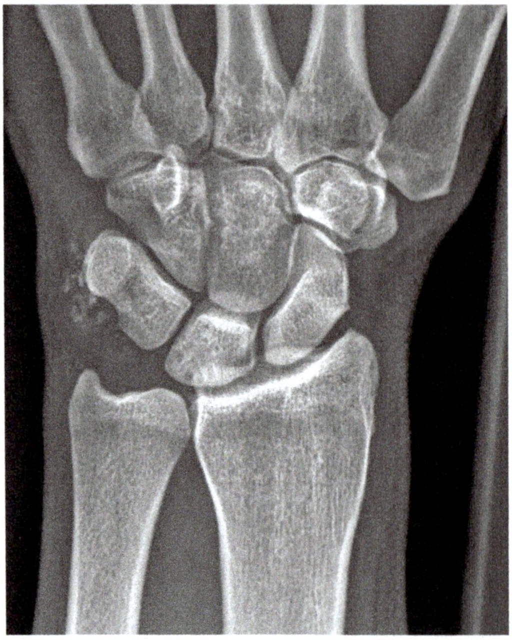

mechanical attrition and not caused just by the synovitis. This is important because when reconstructing the ruptured extensor tendons, the ulnar head needs to be addressed in order to prevent recurrence of the problem. Traditionally, this involves a resection of the ulnar head and stabilisation of the stump.

Less common is rupture of digital extensor tendons due to osteoarthritis of the DRUJ. This has been well reported by Carr and Burge, and in their study, the communication between the DRUJ and the extensor compartments was

Fig. 25.7 Calcific tendinitis can present as an acute episode of severe pain with redness and swelling. Plain radiographs may show areas of calcification in the FCU tendon

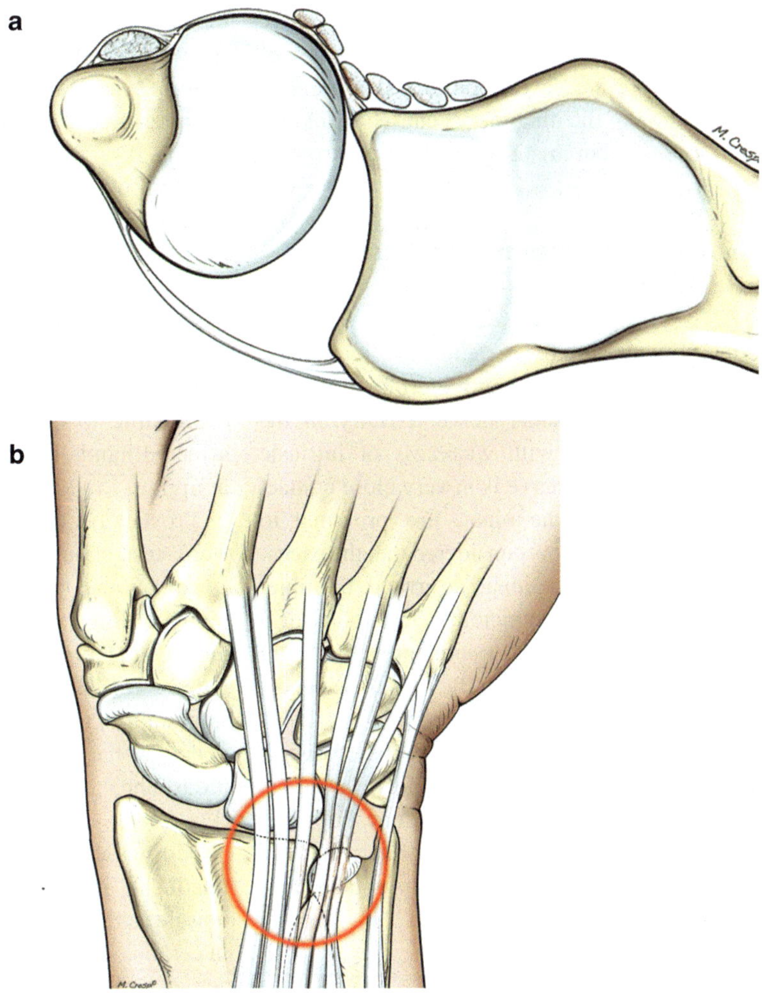

Fig. 25.8 Rheumatoid arthritis damages the stabilising structures of the DRUJ, resulting in dorsal subluxation of the ulna and supination of the hand on the forearm (**a**). This brings the digital extensor tendons towards the head of the ulna, causing attrition and rupture, starting with the most ulnar tendons. Later, the radial ones can be involved (**b**)

demonstrated by arthrography [2]. The principles of treatment are the same, reconstructing the tendons and dealing with the head of the ulna, although in these cases, an ulnar head replacement seems to provide better results.

Neurogenic Ulnar-Sided Wrist Pain

Patients often present with a main symptom of wrist pain; however, when taking a clinical history, it becomes apparent that the pain is not localised to the wrist, it radiates up or down the forearm or the whole arm, it is accompanied by paraesthesia and altered sensation, symptoms are severe at night and the pain does not necessarily get better with rest. This raises the suspicion that the pain can be neurogenic and not from the wrist joint.

Compression of the ulnar nerve at the wrist or at the elbow, problems with its dorsal sensory branch, thoracic outlet syndrome and even cervical root problems can present with a predominant symptom of ulnar-sided wrist pain.

Ulnar Nerve at Guyon's Canal

Guyon's canal or tunnel is approximately 4 cm in length, from the proximal edge of the transverse palmar ligament to the fibrous arch of the hypothenar muscles. Compression of the ulnar nerve at Guyon's canal is an uncommon condition, and it usually has an extrinsic cause, often a space-occupying mass. A ganglion is responsible for 85 % of these cases without a history of trauma. There are several published reports of compression of the ulnar nerve caused by anomalous muscles, but this is a very rare occurrence.

Ulnar Nerve Irritation Associated to Instability

Often, patients with distal radio-ulnar joint instability report paraesthesia and intermittent numbness affecting the ulnar nerve territory in the hand, occasionally with weakness of intrinsic muscles. The ulnar nerve is in very close contact with the head of the ulnar, just proximal to Guyon's canal, and it is considered that the excessive movement of the ulna can irritate the ulnar nerve and cause the symptoms. The solution in these cases seems to be treatment of the joint instability, and by removing the cause, the neurological symptoms will settle.

It can be difficult to differentiate these patients from those that have a primary nerve problem. Electrophysiological tests to examine the ulnar nerve and ultrasound scan of the area to exclude space-occupying lesions can help in establishing the diagnosis.

Dorsal Sensory Branch of the Ulnar Nerve

The dorsal sensory branch of the ulnar nerve wraps round the ulnar side of the wrist from volar to dorsal. It can be irritated by swelling of the wrist or by pressure from a ganglion. Its position leaves this nerve at risk during surgical approaches to the ulnar side of the wrist and arthroscopy [6]. Neuromas at this location can be very painful and troublesome. It is therefore very important to identify and protect this branch during open surgery to the ulnar side of the wrist.

Thoracic Outlet Syndrome

Thoracic outlet syndrome (TOS) results from the compression of the nerves at some point between the interscalene interval and the coracoid process. As well as affecting the brachial plexus, it can have a vascular component if the artery is compressed.

It is often related to position and it can present with wrist pain. Pain of the wrist and hand and numbness, often affecting the dorsum of the wrist and hand and the middle ring and little fingers, are common in these patients. The pain can be made worse by tasks that require elevation of the arm, for example, stacking a shelf, or by traction on the arm. Most patients are unable to carry a shopping bag with the affected hand. The symptoms are often severe at night.

Provocative tests like Adson's manoeuvre or Roos test should be interpreted with caution, since they can be positive in the normal population. The Roos elevation test can be enhanced by placing the probe of a pulse oximeter on the thumb. This will demonstrate a drop in oxygen saturation in the hand if there is a vascular component to the TOS. A duplex scan (Doppler and ultrasound) can confirm vascular compromise (Fig. 25.9).

Most cases of TOS improve with conservative treatment, including postural re-education and muscle retraining. Botulinum toxin can be useful in certain cases, for example, those with an overactive pectoralis minor muscle. A minority of patients may continue to have significant symptoms, and surgery may then be indicated, including scalenectomy, excision of cervical rib or excision of the first rib.

Other Neurological Conditions

Cervical root compression, cervical cord compression and previous injury to the ulnar nerve are rare causes of wrist pain (Fig. 25.10). However, they must be born in mind, and if there are neurological symptoms, examination of the neck and of the upper arm is warranted. Neck pain is very common in the general population, and MRI scan will often show degenerative changes in asymptomatic subjects. Therefore, investigations must be interpreted with caution.

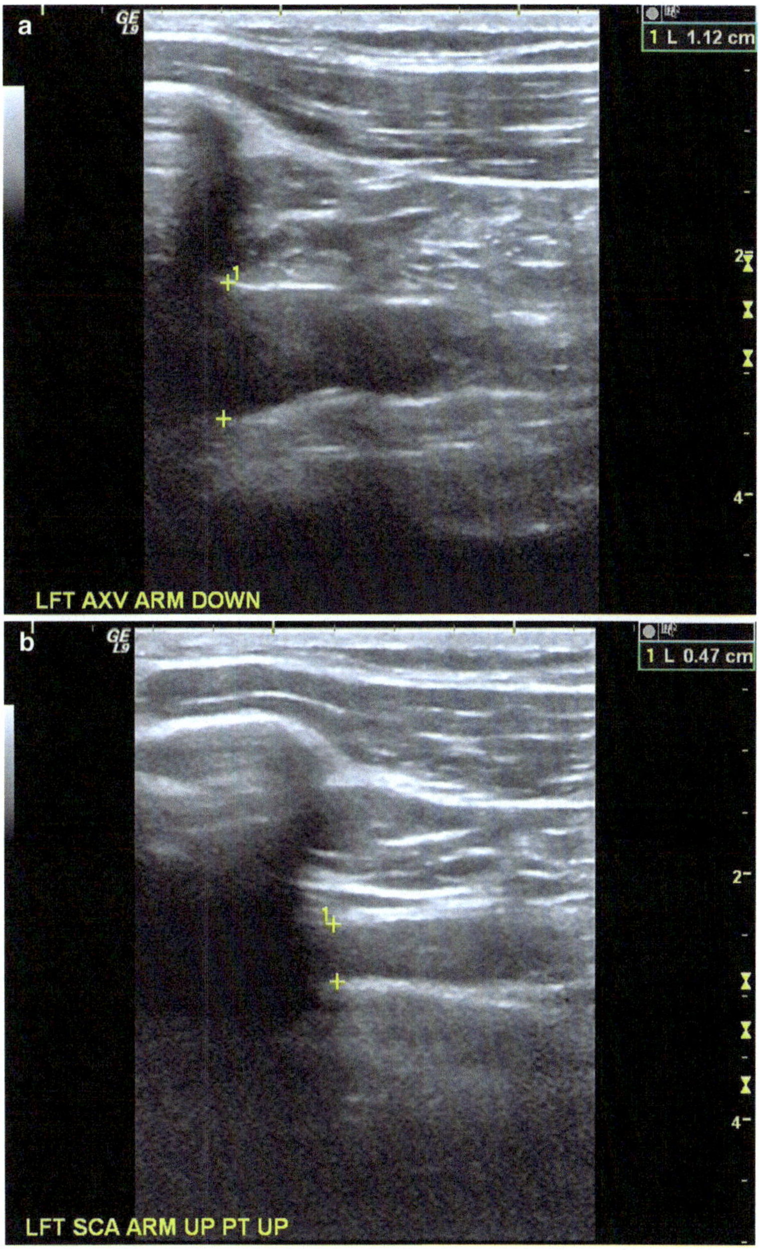

Fig. 25.9 This patient was referred with ulnar-sided wrist and forearm pain. She has significant pain at night, paraesthesia and numbness. Doing a Roos provocation test reproduced her symptoms. The pulse oximeter probe during this test showed a drop in saturation from 99 to 82 %. Ultrasound scan shows the diameter of the subclavian artery to be 1.12 cm with the arm of the patient by her side (**a**) and 0.47 cm with the shoulder abducted (**b**), confirming a significant compression of the artery and indicating a significant neurological compression

Hypothenar Hammer Syndrome

Hypothenar hammer syndrome refers to a group of symptoms caused by thrombosis and/or aneurismal dilatation of the ulnar artery within Guyon's canal, as a consequence of repeated blunt trauma to the artery. It is seen in men of employment age, and they usually have a clear occupational or recreational exposure to repeated trauma of the area, often using the hypothenar area of the hand as a hammer.

Compression of the adjacent ulnar nerve may cause pain in the ulnar side of the wrist and hand and paraesthesia and numbness in the little and ring fingers. Ischemia of the ulnar digits may develop from emboli, vasospasm or an incomplete arch, causing coldness, pallor and blanching.

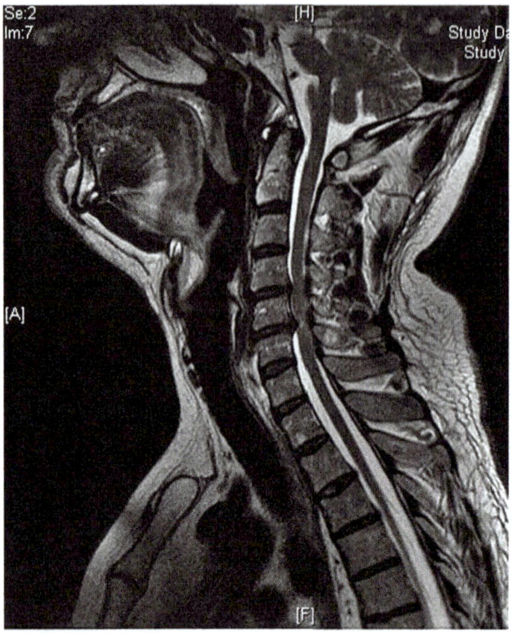

Fig. 25.10 This 42-year-old manual worker presented with severe wrist pain and weakness of his left hand. On questioning, it became clear that he had left arm pain, paraesthesia and weakness of intrinsic muscles, mild symptoms on the right arm but no symptoms in his legs. MRI scan of the cervical spine confirmed significant compression of the cervical spinal cord

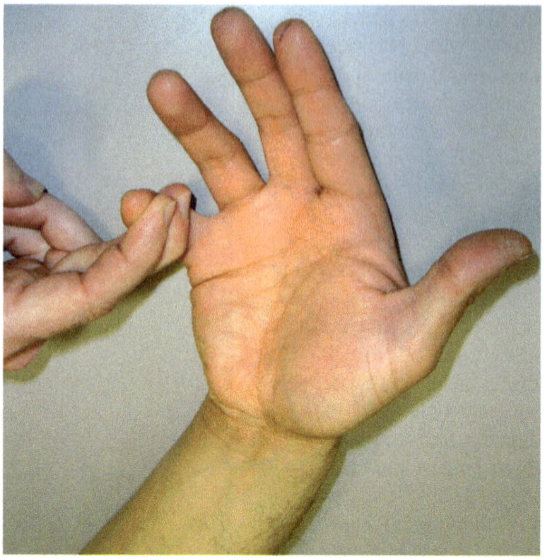

Fig. 25.11 With the wrist in ulnar deviation, the patient is asked to flex his little finger against resistance. The hook of the hamate works as a pulley for the digital flexors, and this movement puts pressure onto it, reproducing the patient's symptoms if there is a fracture or non-union of the hook of the hamate

Allen's test reveals no flow from the ulnar artery, and the diagnosis is confirmed with angiography, showing the aneurism or the occlusion of the distal ulnar artery. Resection of the affected segment of the artery removes the painful lump, relieves compression of the ulnar nerve, prevents further embolic episodes and produces a local periarterial sympathectomy. Reconstruction of the artery with a graft is done to restore vascularity.

Hook of the Hamate Fracture and Non-union

Fractures of the hook of the hamate represent between 2 and 4 % of carpal bone fractures. They are usually associated to a sport injury that involves handling a club, a bat or a racket: golf, baseball, tennis and squash. This can be caused by an incident where the swinging club comes into contact with the ground, transferring the energy to the hand in a strong grip, or, for example, when the racket of a squash player hits the wall. It is also considered in some cases that a stress fracture can be caused by the repetitive forces on the hook. The injury tends to be in the non-dominant hand of a baseball batter or a golfer, but in the dominant hand of a racket sport player [10]. The diagnosis is often missed since the deep location of the hook makes physical examination difficult and routine radiographic views do not show reliably the fracture. A history of injury as mentioned, with pain of resisted flexion of the little finger (Fig. 25.11), is suggestive of this lesion and requires further investigation. The carpal tunnel radiological view may show better the hook, but it is often painful and difficult to achieve, particularly in the acute situation. CT scan seems to be the best investigation (Fig. 25.12).

Acute fractures can be treated conservatively in a cast, and most undisplaced fractures seem to heal, while displaced fractures and those diagnosed late have a high rate of non-union. Acute internal fixation of this fractures and fixation with bone grafting for non-union have been described, but they offer little advantage over excision of the

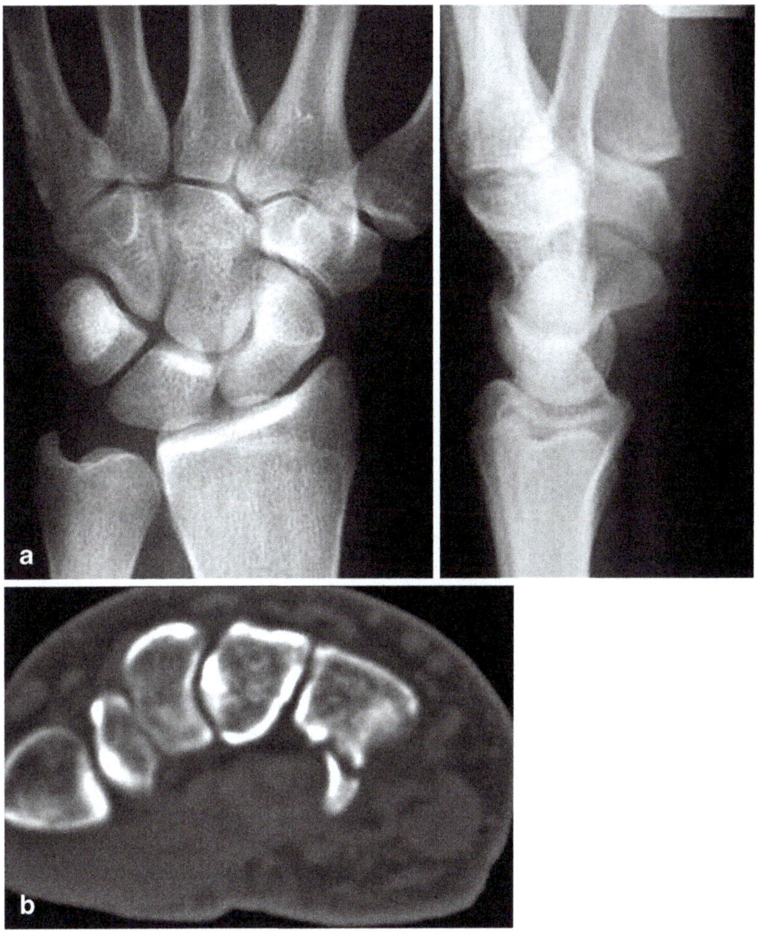

Fig. 25.12 (**a**, **b**) This keen golfer had pain in the hypothenar eminence for several months. Plain radiographs did not show the cause of his symptoms. Resisted flexion of the little finger reproduced his symptoms. A CT scan confirms the clinical impression of a non-union of the hook of the hamate

hook in the case of a symptomatic non-union [1]. In the author's experience, even professional golfers can return to the previous level of competition after excision of the hook of the hamate, and therefore internal fixation is not recommended.

References

1. Bishop AT, Beckenbaugh RD (1988) Fracture of the hamate hook. J Hand Surg (Am) 13:135–139
2. Carr AJ, Burge PD (1992) Rupture of extensor tendons due to osteoarthritis of the distal radio-ulnar joint. J Hand Surg Br 17B:694–696
3. Inoue G, Tamura Y (2001) Surgical treatment for recurrent dislocation of the extensor carpi ulnaris tendon. J Hand Surg Br 26B:556–559
4. Kiefhaber TR, Stern PJ (1992) Upper extremity tendinitis and overuse syndromes in the athlete. Clin Sports Med 11:39–55
5. MacLennan AJ, Nemechek NM, Waitayawinyu T, Trumble TE (2008) Diagnosis and anatomic reconstruction of extensor carpi ulnaris subluxation. J Hand Surg Am 33A:59–64
6. McAdams TR, Hentz VR (2002) Injury to the dorsal sensory branch of the ulnar nerve in the arthroscopic repair of ulnar-sided triangular fibrocartilage tears using an inside-out technique: a cadaver study. J Hand Surg Am 27A:840–844
7. Ruland RT, Hogan CJ (2008) The ECU synergy test: an aid to diagnose ECU tendonitis. J Hand Surg Am 33A:1777–1782
8. Salva-Coll G, Garcia-Elias M, Leon-Lopez MM, Llusa-Perez M, Rodríguez-Baeza A (2012) Role of the extensor carpi ulnaris and its sheath on dynamic carpal stability. J Hand Surg Eur 37:544–548.
9. Spinner M, Kaplan EB (1970) Extensor carpi ulnaris. Its relationship to the stability of the distal radio-ulnar joint. Clin Orthop Relat Res 68:124–129
10. Walsh JJ, Bishop AT (2000) Diagnosis and management of hamate hook fractures. Hand Clin 16:397–403

Appendices

Appendix A: Suturing Techniques: All-Inside Repair Techniques

Introduction

Wrist arthroscopy has developed rapidly in the last decade. From a purely diagnostic tool, it has become more and more a treatment tool. Distal radius fracture, osteotomies, or arthrodesis are now commonly performed under arthroscopy by the most active teams. The need to place sutures inside the joint is an everyday scenario in any busy arthroscopy practice. Suturing dorsal tears is undoubtedly one of the most common among them (Chap. 8).

Dorsal capsular tears have been treated by suturing the TFC proper to the dorsal capsule, placing the knot outside the joint over an external bolster or a button [3]. If the suture had been placed blindly, there was a risk of entrapping the dorsal branch of the ulnar nerve [7, 10], this occurring in up to 50 % of the cases in a cadaveric study [8]. Additionally, the button or bolster could cause skin irritation, skin necrosis, and even septic arthritis [11]. A mini-open approach minimized this risk, the nerve could be protected, and the suture placed on top of the capsule or the floor of the ECU sheath (see Chap. 8 and Appendix B). The knot, which needed several throws, created a new set of complications, namely, irritation of the ECU tendon or the nerve itself. A second operation may be needed to remove the knot, even if resorbable material was used [2, 9]. To circumvent these problems, several devices have been presented in the literature. In this appendix, I would like to describe in detail two methods for an all-in suturing in the wrist joint that leaves the knot inside and that requires no special equipment.

F. del Piñal, M.D., Dr. Med.
Hand-Wrist and Plastic Surgery,
Private Practice and Mutua Montañesa,
Paseo de Pereda 20-1°,
E-39004 Santander, Spain
email: drpinal@drpinal.com, pacopinal@gmail.com

All-Inside Variant 1 Mattress Suture with a Tuohy Needle (Fig. A.1)

The technique has been applied for capsular suturing, TFC frontal tears, reattachments to the fovea of the TFC in combination with anchors [5], and repair of volar structures such as the volar scapho-lunate ligament [6].

Step 1: A Tuohy needle loaded with a thread is inserted proximal to the tear perforating both the capsule and the TFC proper.

Step 2: The thread is pushed into the joint and the end (henceforth named end A) grabbed with grasper introduced from 6R. End A is now retrieved out of the joint and secured with a mosquito to avoid slippage.

At this moment, end A is outside the joint, the needle is loaded with the thread, and the other end of the suture (henceforth named B) is also outside of the joint.

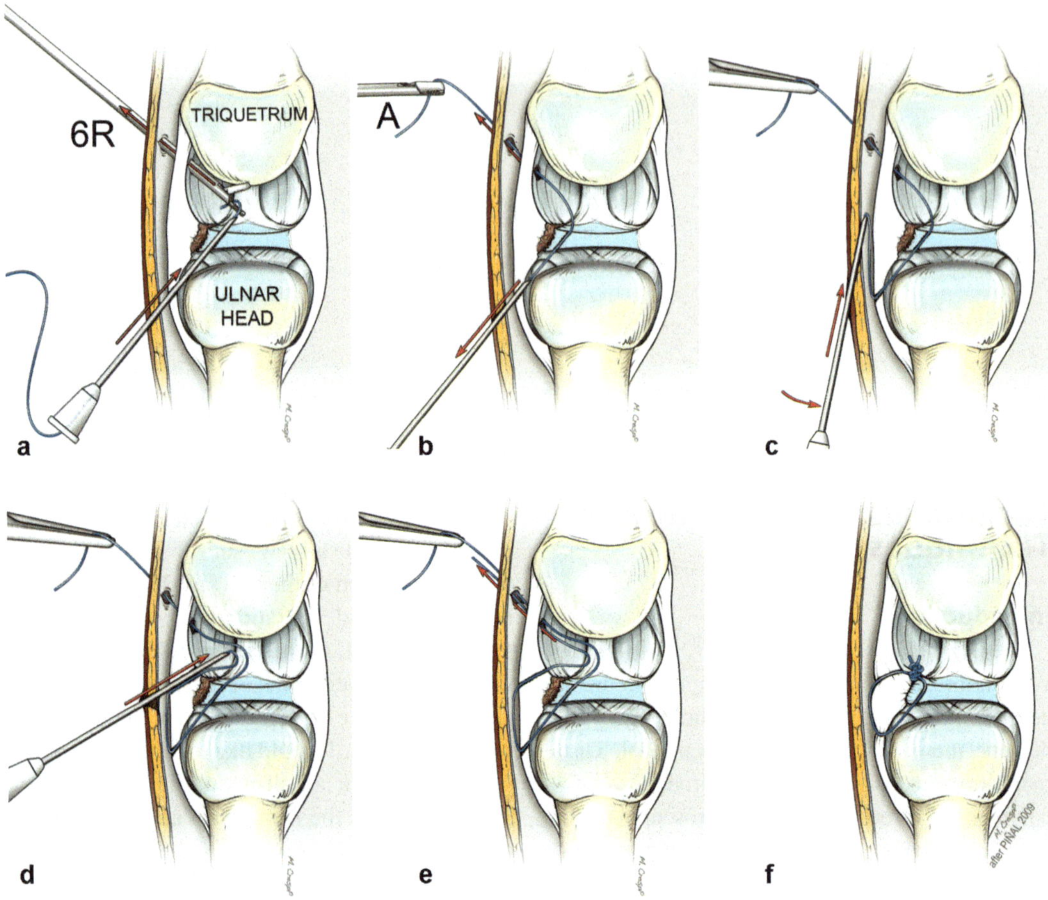

Fig. A.1 (**a–f**) All-inside repair technique applied for a dorsal TFC tear. See text for details (From del Piñal et al. [5]. © by the British Society for Surgery of the Hand with permission. 2010)

Step 3: The needle is now slowly withdrawn out of the joint under arthroscopic visualization, until it reaches the edge of the capsule. Once the tip of the needle is out of the joint, it is slid distally on top of the capsule perforating the dorsal capsule-ECU sheath distal to the first pass.

The outside of the capsule is easily recognized first by the scope visualization and, secondly, because the surgeon will be able to move the needle without resistance.

Step 4: The surgeon now pushes in the thread through the needle until a loop is inside the joint. The loop is now grabbed with a grasper introduced from 6R and pulled outside the joint, until "end B" of the thread is also out.

Both suture ends (A and B) will now be outside the joint through 6R portal, and the "loop" of the stitch is now penetrating the TFC anterior to the tear, around the capsule, and outside the joint and again penetrates into the joint.

Step 5: The surgeon makes one of the available sliding knots and pushes it in with a knot pusher. Two or three additional throws can be added as required. The ends are cut flush to the knot with a basket forceps or one of the available scissors.

Hints: One of the problems one may encounter is that each end of the thread comes out of the joint through the same portal, but leaving some tissue interposed (Fig. A.2). In this circumstance, tying the knot is not recommended because it will not sit properly in the joint. Furthermore, there lies the risk of entrapping a nerve branch, or a tendon, which may have become entangled. This

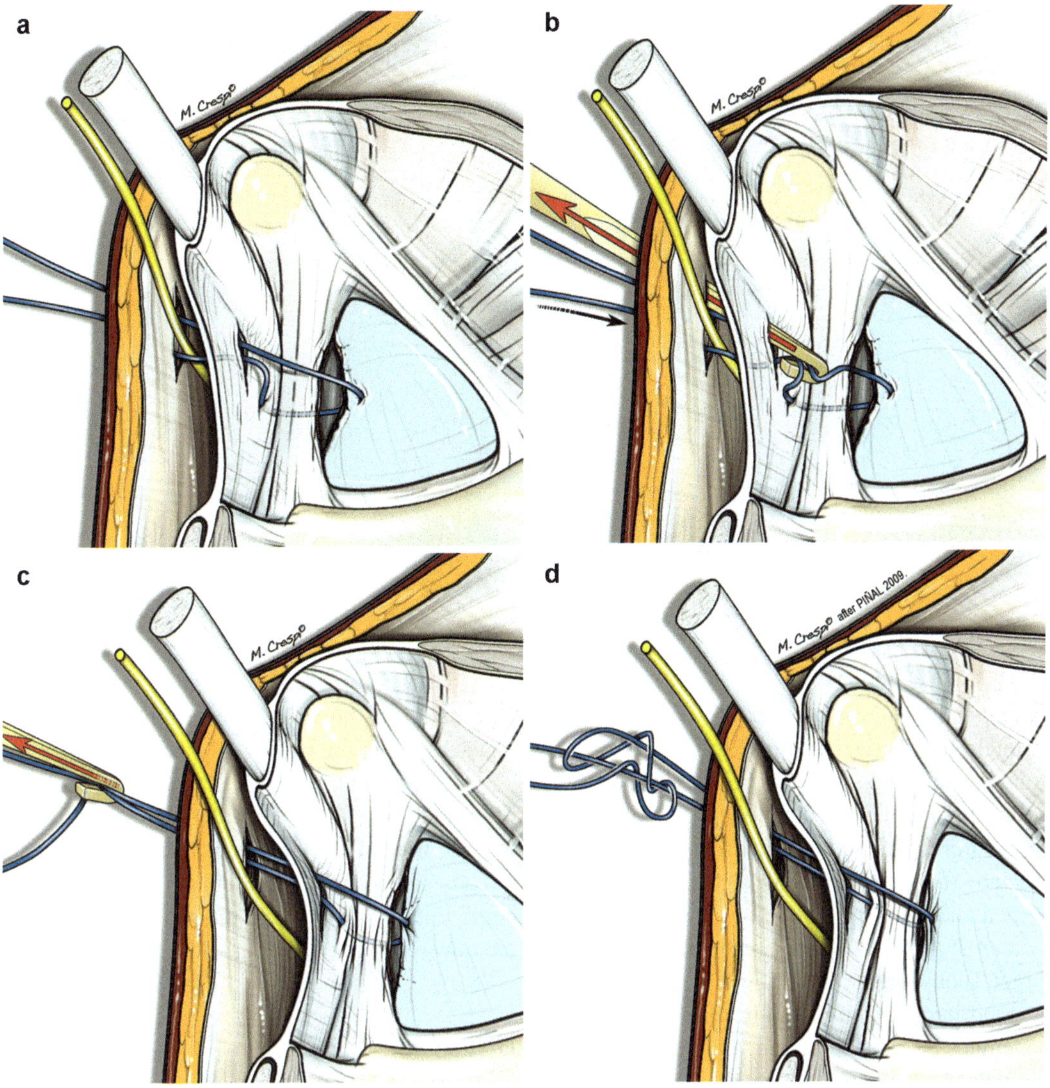

Fig. A.2 In this clinical case, a slip of the EDM tendon can be seen interposed between the two threads

trap can be solved by introducing a shoulder suture hook from 6R (or any portal), hooking both threads close to the TFC and pulling them out of the joint, now through the same path (Fig. A.3). If available, a Transporter® (Ref 014617, ACUFEX, Smith and Nephew Inc, Andover, MA, USA), or a similar device, can instead be used. The instrument is inserted into the joint, and after snaring both threads they will come out of the joint along the same path. In any instance, a sliding knot is placed and will now pass without any difficulty to the joint.

All-Inside Variant 2 (Figs. A.4 and A.5)

This procedure is a bit more awkward, but one has to resort to it when the surgeon does not have an appropriate angle to insert the Tuohy needle. It is a combination of several well-known suturing techniques, namely, the loop and the trick just described. It permits stitching in "impossible" places while keeping the knot inside the joint. It will be illustrated in a coronal tear (Chap. 16), but the limit is the surgeon's imagination.

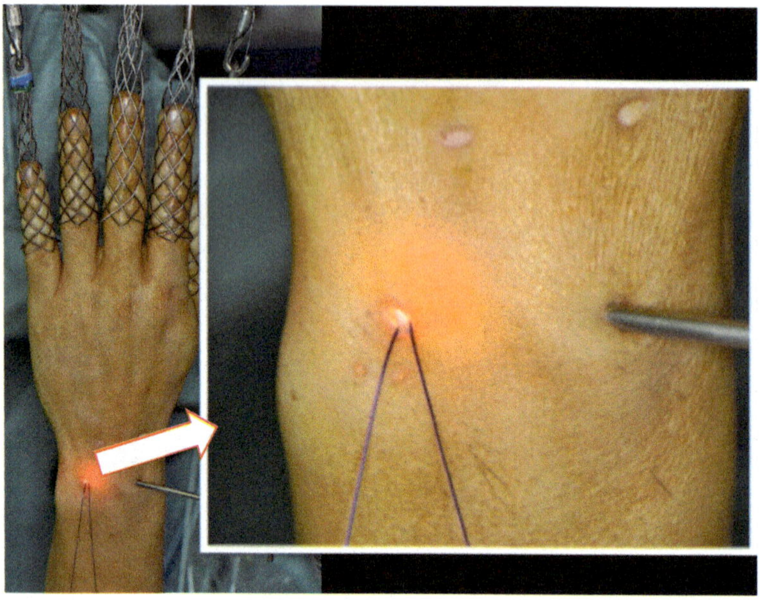

Fig. A.3 Method to retrieve the suture through the same path. See text for details (From del Piñal et al. [5]. © by the British Society for Surgery of the Hand with permission. 2010)

Step 1: An intramuscular needle is inserted through 6U portal and penetrates firstly the volar capsule and secondly the volar distal radioulnar ligament from distal to proximal. A 2/0 PDS colored thread is pushed through the needle into the joint (this end will be henceforth named end A)

Step 2: Another needle (in general I prefer the larger Tuohy needle) loaded with a nylon loop is inserted into the joint slightly ulnar to 6R. This penetrates the dorsal capsule, and then the dorsal radioulnar ligament, from distal to proximal. The nylon loop suture is pushed into the joint.

Step 3: A grasper is introduced from 6R portal, passes through the nylon loop, and grabs the end of the PDS suture (end A). End A is now pulled out of the joint through 6R. This is done so as to have sufficient length of thread to proceed to the next step.

Step 4: The surgeon now pulls the needle with the loop out of the joint. By doing so, the end A of the thread will automatically come out of the joint too.

At this stage, end A is outside the joint slightly ulnar to 6R portal while the other end (end B) is also outside but in 6U portal. The hitch of the PDS suture is, however, volar to the DRUL and on each side of the tear!

Step 5: A suture hook is now introduced from 6R portal and hooks both threads distal to the DRUL. By pulling the suture hook out with the threads snared on it, both ends of the PDS will come out of the joint via the same channel and are now ready for a gliding knot.

Discussion

The procedure we have presented above can be applied, or modified according to the scenario, to any situation where the knot is to be placed inside the joint. Although beyond the scope of this book, the technique can be applied for suturing volar tears in the vicinity of "dangerous" structures [6]. In all our cases, we carried out arthroscopy with the dry technique [4]. We have not found any reason to use water during our arthroscopies. Contrarily, water infiltrates the tissues, causing the surgeon to lose bony references and hindering smooth passage of the grasper in and out of the joint along the same path. With the dry technique, however, the inside of the joint can many times be seen from the skin, allowing accurate introduction of the grasper in and out.

We have used different suture materials in our surgery depending on the structure to be sutured. Unbraided material such as 2-0 polydioxanone or nylon will pass easily through the Tuohy needle. For threads of larger caliber or braided ones (such as FiberWire®) that are more difficult to pass through the Tuohy needle, which is 1.3 mm diameter, we use a Rodiera® needle. Both Tuohy and Rodiera's needles are readily available from anesthesiologists' supplies. The latter is also an epidural needle but of a slightly larger caliber (1.5 mm). It is important to insert the needle always with the bevel parallel to the course of the extensor tendons (i.e., vertical). As the tendon is under tension (because of the traction), the bevel of the needle will act as a sharp knife if inserted perpendicularly. However, if inserted parallel, it will only pierce the tendon. By the same token, the smaller Tuohy needle is preferred, if at all possible.

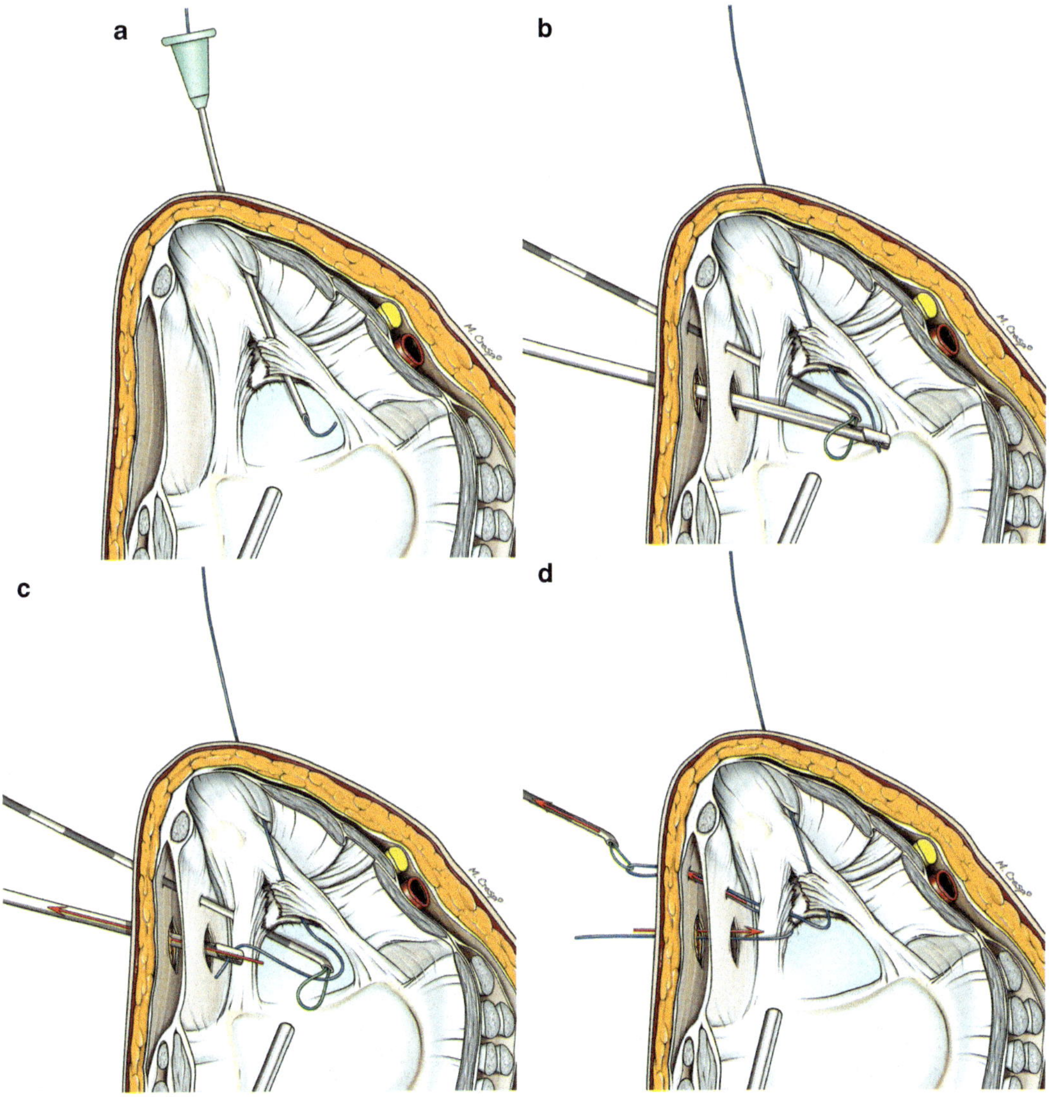

Fig. A.4 All-inside variant 2 (see text for details)

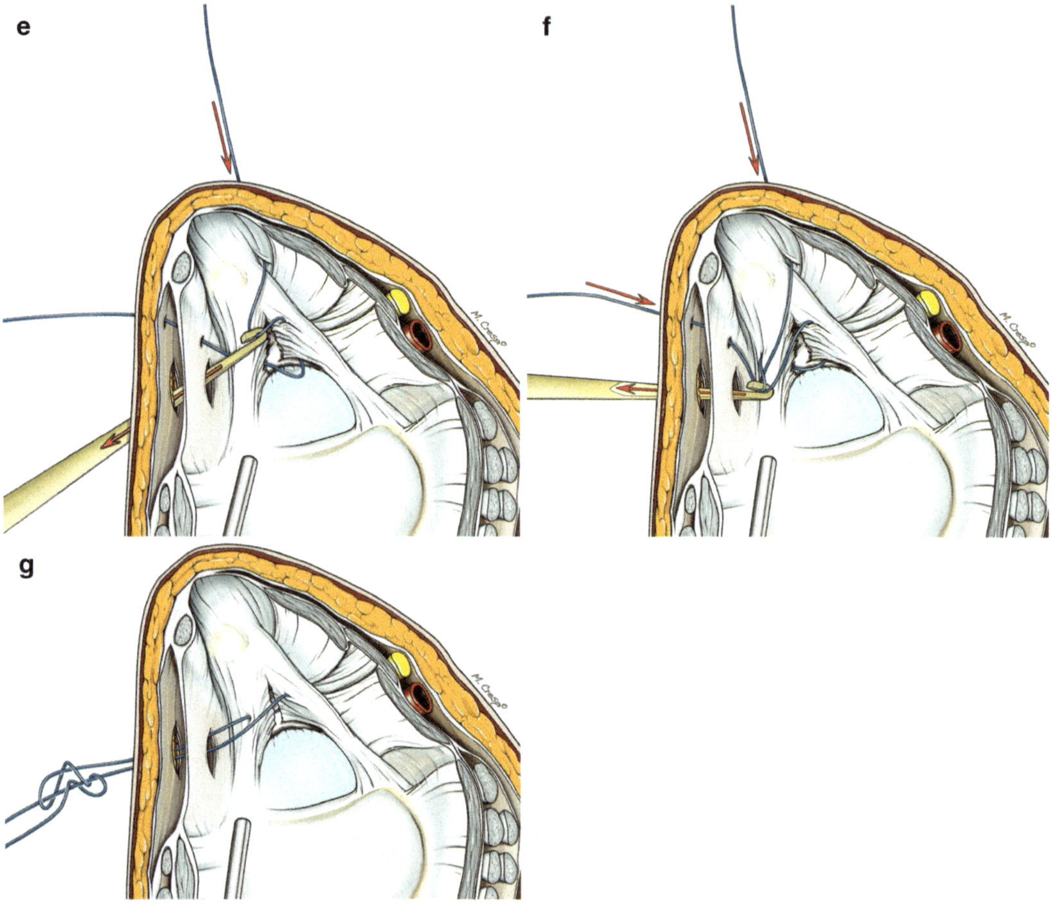

Fig. A.4 (continued)

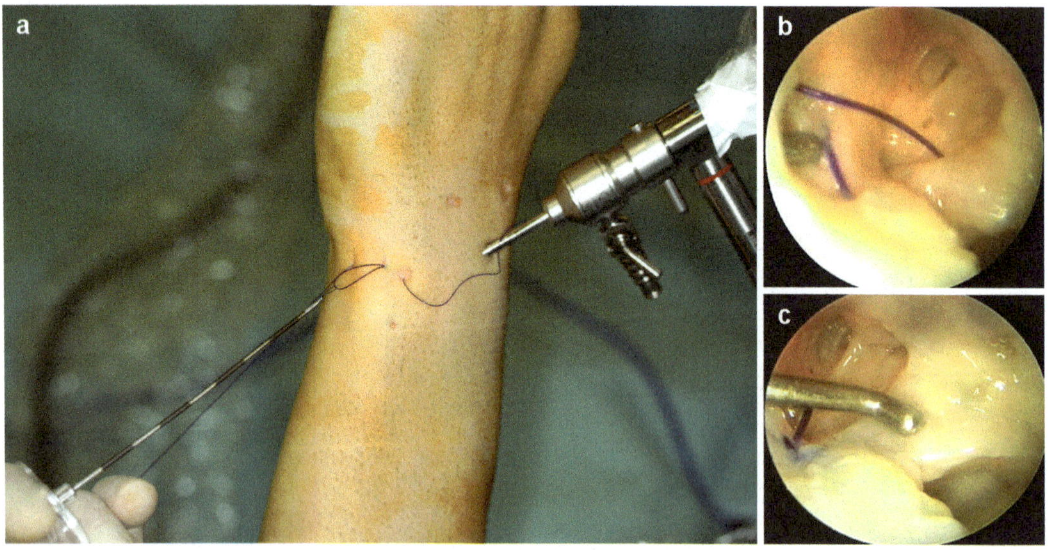

Fig. A.5 (**a**) Clinical case during suturing of a coronal tear corresponding to Fig. A.4d. (**b**) Arthroscopic view corresponding to Fig. A.4e. (**c**) Final result with the know inside

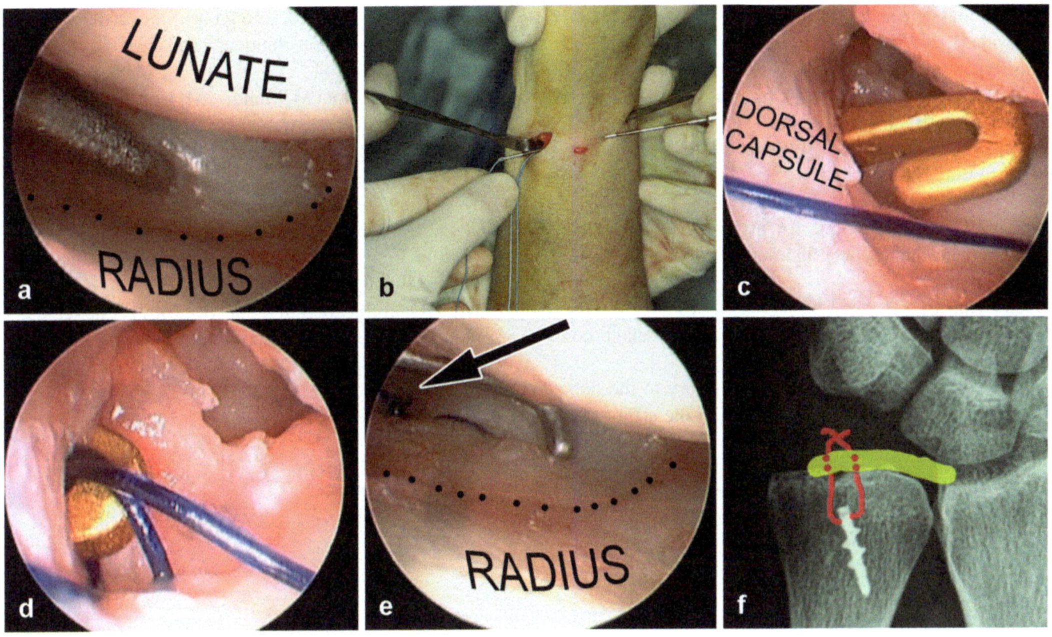

Fig. A.6 Technique for reattachment of the TFC at the fovea. The surgeon introduces a Tuohy needle at about 4–5 portal, pierces the TFC, and exits ulnarly near the fovea (**a**). The needle is then fed with one of the thread's ends of the bone anchor (**b**). The needle is retrieved, all the way out, having now the suture end out of the joint dorsally. The maneuver with the Tuohy needle is repeated, so as to have both suture ends out of the joint dorsally, although rarely through exactly the same channel. In order to have both suture ends through the same path, permitting a gliding knot, the shoulder suture hook is introduced through 6R (or any other portal) (**c**), retrieving both suture ends out of the joint (**d**). Finally, a sliding knot is carried out of the joint and slid in with the (shoulder) knot pusher. Traction is relieved during the knotting process in order to allow the TFC to sit in the fovea (*arrow* points the knot) (**e**, **f**) (From del Piñal et al. [5]. © by the British Society for Surgery of the Hand with permission. 2010)

Intravenous needles or intramuscular needles are not recommended for the all-inside technique we propose here. First of all, the inner core of the point is sharp, and in step 4 (of procedure 1), the thread can be cut, as there is some pulling required before end B is outside the joint. More importantly, however, is that they are too sharp, and besides cutting too much, they provide no "feel" when the surgeon has to creep with the tip of the needle on the dorsal capsule in step 3 (of procedure 1). The epidural needle is comparatively much blunter, and the surgeon will notice when the capsule has been passed and "feels" the tip of the needle when sliding on top of the hard surface of the capsule. It is critical that the surgeon stays immediately on top of the outer surface of the capsule when moving the needle distally. If the needle has been withdrawn too much, there will be a risk of entangling a tendon or a nerve branch when reintroducing the needle into the joint. If this were to accidentally happen, the suture should be removed and the process repeated.

The technique we present here bears no difficulty for an arthroscopist. We have used this procedure for TFC reattachment to the dorsal capsule, in combination with bone anchors for foveal reinsertion of the TFC ([1], Chapter 10, Fig. A.6).

References

1. Atzei A (2009) New trends in arthroscopic management of type 1-B TFCC injuries with DRUJ instability. J Hand Surg Eur 34:582–591
2. Bednar JM, Osterman AL (1994) The role of arthroscopy in the treatment of traumatic triangular fibrocartilage injuries. Hand Clin 10:605–614
3. de Araujo W, Poehling GG, Kuzma GR (1996) New Tuohy needle technique for triangular fibrocartilage complex repair: preliminary studies. Arthroscopy 12: 699–703

4. del Piñal F, García-Bernal FJ, Pisani D, Regalado J, Ayala H, Studer A (2007) Dry arthroscopy of the wrist: surgical technique. J Hand Surg Am 32:119–123
5. del Piñal F, García-Bernal FJ, Cagigal L, Studer A, Regalado J, Thams C (2010) A technique for arthroscopic all-inside suturing in the wrist. J Hand Surg Eur 35:475–479
6. del Piñal F, Studer A, Thams C, Glasberg A (2011) An all-inside technique for arthroscopic suturing of the volar scapholunate ligament. J Hand Surg Am 36: 2044–2046
7. Estrella EP, Hung LK, Ho PC, Tse WL (2007) Arthroscopic repair of triangular fibrocartilage complex tears. Arthroscopy 23:729–737
8. McAdams TR, Hentz VR (2002) Injury to the dorsal sensory branch of the ulnar nerve in the arthroscopic repair of ulnar-sided triangular fibrocartilage tears using an inside-out technique: a cadaver study. J Hand Surg 27A:840–844
9. Pederzini LA, Tosi M, Prandini M, Botticella C (2007) All-inside suture technique for Palmer class 1B triangular fibrocartilage repair. Arthroscopy 23:1130.e1–1130.e4
10. Tsu-Hsin Chen E, Wei JD, Huang VW (2006) Injury of the dorsal sensory branch of the ulnar nerve as a complication of arthroscopic repair of the triangular fibrocartilage. J Hand Surg 31-B:530–532
11. Yao J, Dantuluri P, Osterman AL (2007) A novel technique of all-inside arthroscopic triangular fibrocartilage complex repair. Arthroscopy 23:1357.e1–1357.e4

Appendix B: Suturing Techniques: Double Loop Technique for Large Dorsal TFCC Rupture

Introduction

According to the classification of Palmer and Werner [5], type I traumatic TFCC lesions are further classified into four types where 1B is a peripheral lesion at the ulnar insertion of the TFCC. These are the most frequent and well-known lesions.

On occasions, we have come across certain lesions which are not in standard classifications. The TFCC tear is much broader than in the classical type 1B lesions. The lesion begins in the prestyloid recess and ends almost at the radial insertion of the ligament. This leads to minor degrees of DRUJ instability, and the classic single stitch may be insufficient. Hence, we modified the classic suture to a double loop suture.

Arthroscopic Analysis

Classic TFCC arthroscopy is performed through a 3–4 radiocarpal portal and a probe through the 6R portal. The tension of the TFCC is evaluated using the so-called trampoline test – positive when the TFCC is lax, indicating a peripheral lesion.

The "hook test" involves traction on the ulnar part of the TFCC at the styloid recess with a probe. The test is positive if the TFCC can be brought toward the radial border of the radioulnar joint. This test detects foveal detachment, particularly if the distal component is intact. In this case, arthroscopic exploration of the radioulnar joint becomes necessary. Lesions of the distal and proximal components of the TFCC can be isolated or in association, and only DRUJ arthroscopy can show an isolated lesion of the proximal component (foveal attachment) of the TFCC.

Christophe Mathoulin
Institut de la main, Clinique Jouvenet,
6 square Jouvenet 75016 Paris, France
email: cmathoulin@orange.fr

When faced with a complete dorsal detachment without foveal detachment, traditional simple suture of the distal component can no longer suffice. We describe an original suture technique with a double loop, allowing easy repair of these extensive lesions.

Technique

This technique is usually performed as day surgery under axillary block anesthesia with an arm tourniquet. The arm is placed on a table, and traction is applied to the hand and forearm in the axis of the forearm. The joint is distended by saline injection, and a wrist arthroscope (2.4 mm) is introduced through the usual 3–4 radiocarpal portal. A probe is introduced through the 6R radiocarpal portal, and the trampoline and "hook" tests are performed.

The DRUJ may be explored through a radioulnar portal (RUP). This is a tight joint and arthroscopy is often difficult, especially if the proximal portion of the TFCC is intact. When detached, it is easy to explore the foveal insertion of the TFCC.

In case of an extensive peripheral lesion, reinsertion is carried out using the double loop technique (Fig. B.1a, b).

The scar tissue at the zone of the tear is first debrided and freshened using a synovial resector, and synovectomy is performed (Fig. B.2a, b). An intramuscular needle is inserted into the RUP via the capsule directed obliquely distally and laterally. Its exit is verified via the TFCC detachment zone exactly at the center. A loop of absorbable suture is passed through the needle from outside (Fig. B.3a, b), retrieved with a forceps and pulled out through the 6R radiocarpal portal (Fig. B.4a, b). We usually use a PDS 3.0 or 4.0 absorbable suture according to the size of the wrist. A second intramuscular needle is placed radially adjacent to the radial insertion of the TFCC through the same portal in the same direction through the capsule and the TFCC (Fig. B.5a, b). A second suture is passed through this needle and pulled out through 6R.

A third intramuscular needle is placed ulnarly adjacent to the styloid recess of the TFCC through the same approach in the same direction through

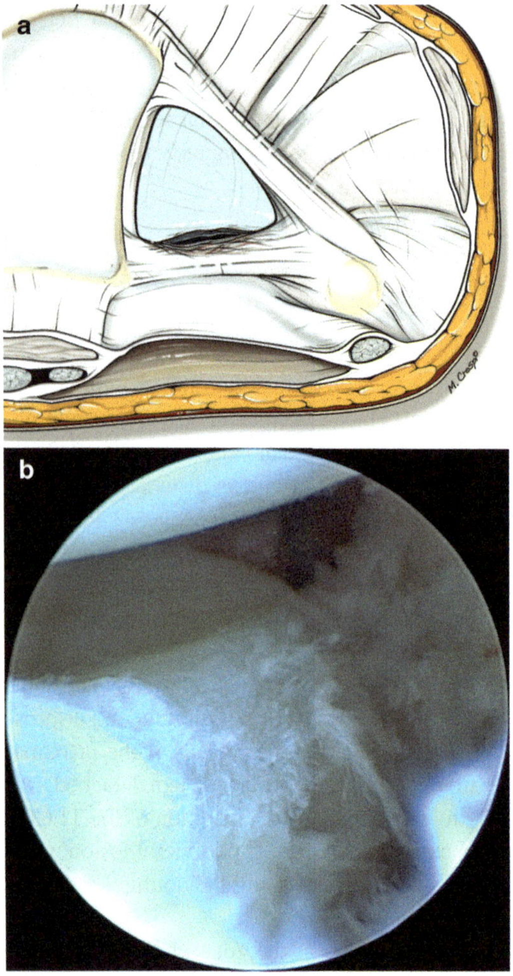

Fig. B.1 (**a**, **b**) Drawing and intra-articular operating view showing a large dorsal tear of TFCC

the capsule and the TFCC (Fig. B.6a, b, c), and a third absorbable suture through the needle is likewise pulled out through 6R.

Thus, at this stage, we have three sutures, two simple and one loop, passed via the DRU portal through the capsule and the TFCC (the loop in the center and the two simple sutures radial and ulnar) and retrieved through 6R to the exterior (Fig. B.7).

The two simple sutures are passed through the loop outside the joint. The loop is pulled out through the DRUJ portal pulling the two simple sutures through behind it at the center of the TFCC lesion where their ends can be retrieved at the DRUJ portal (Figs. B.8a, b, c and B.9).

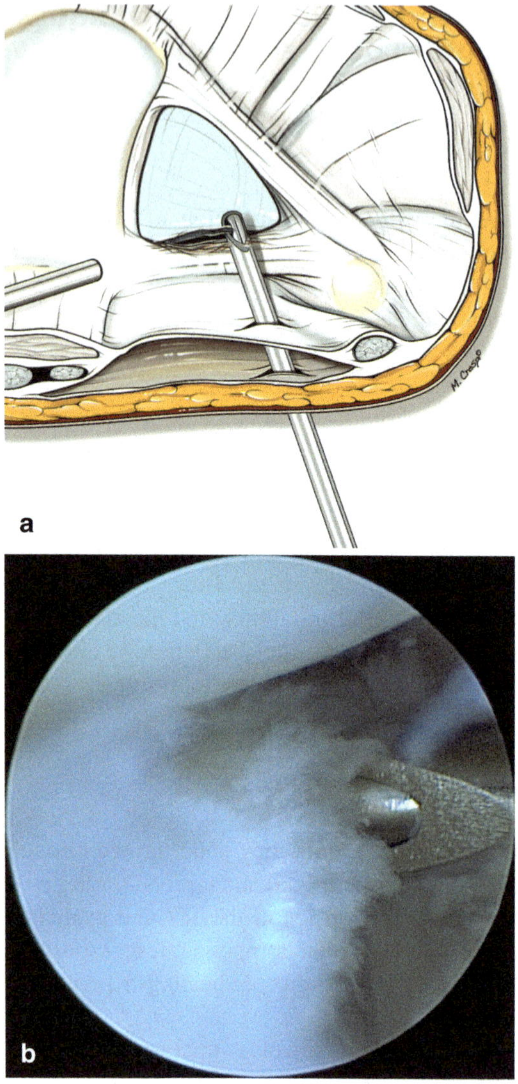

Fig. B.2 (**a**, **b**) Drawing and intra-articular operating view showing the position of the scope through the 3–4 radiocarpal portal to visualize TFCC detachment. A synovial resector is introduced through 6R to debride the ligament tear

AT this stage, we have two intra-articular loops, allowing a complete suture of the entire zone of the TFCC tear (Fig. B.10a, b, c).

The wrist traction is relieved, the wrist is positioned in slight extension and ulnar inclination, and the sutures at the DRU level are then tied. An anterior palmar splint is used to maintain this position for 6 weeks. Physiotherapy is started at 6 weeks in all cases.

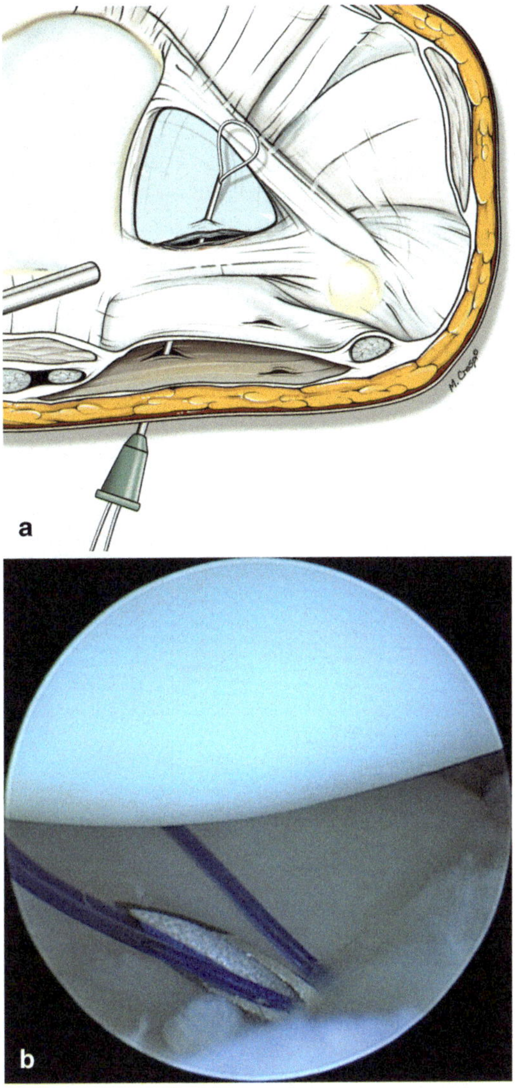

Fig. B.3 (**a**, **b**) Drawing and intra-articular operating view showing passage of the intramuscular needle through the dorsal capsule then the TFCC tear with a PDS loop

Discussion

The TFCC is more complex than it appears. Wrist arthroscopy allows a better understanding of the different insertions of this complex proximally and distally and detection of its lesions. Appropriate treatment of these lesions avoids the failures of classic arthroscopic reattachment and their associated persistent radioulnar instability since the problem had been only partially addressed. Numerous arthroscopic techniques of suturing the TFCC dorsal capsule have been proposed with the advantage of a direct suture of the distal medial portion of the TFCC lesions and often produce good results. In proximal TFCC lesions with clinical distal radioulnar instability, traditional arthroscopic suture techniques cannot restore stability, as reinsertion of the foveal attachment of this ligament is not possible. Open surgical technique has been recommended so far to achieve transosseous reinsertion of the TFCC. Despite the good results often reported, this operation often resulted in stiffness and limitation of pronosupination. With the advances in arthroscopy, this operation can be done with better results [4, 6].

The healing potential of the TFCC depends mainly on its blood supply – mainly, branches of the ulnar artery and palmar and dorsal branches of the anterior interosseous artery. Poor vascularization limits the possibility of a good quality repair as often seen in old TFCC lesions with retraction (stage 4). Blood supply is sometimes altered in some congenital malformations as, for example, styloid hypoplasia. Good quality cartilage is a condition (sine qua non) for TFCC repair. The classification proposed by Atzei under EWAS has shown the possibility of existence of isolated proximal lesions, formerly undetected [2]. Recent studies analyzing arthroscopic repair by the Hong Kong team [3] have shown that 51 % of their 35 patients could not be appropriated by the Palmer classification. With an average follow-up of 39 months, they had 26 % bad results. In 45 % cases, these bad results were due to DRUJ instability. More recently, the Mayo Clinic team has published a comparative study of results of the classic arthroscopic repair techniques and open surgery. In the arthroscopic series, there were 17 % reoperations for persistent DRUJ instability [1].

Extensive distal peripheral tears involving the entire dorsal insertion of the TFCC do exist in reality, even if rare. Simple peripheral suture techniques do not achieve good repair in this case. Double loop sutures using the “in-and-out” principle allow excellent healing.

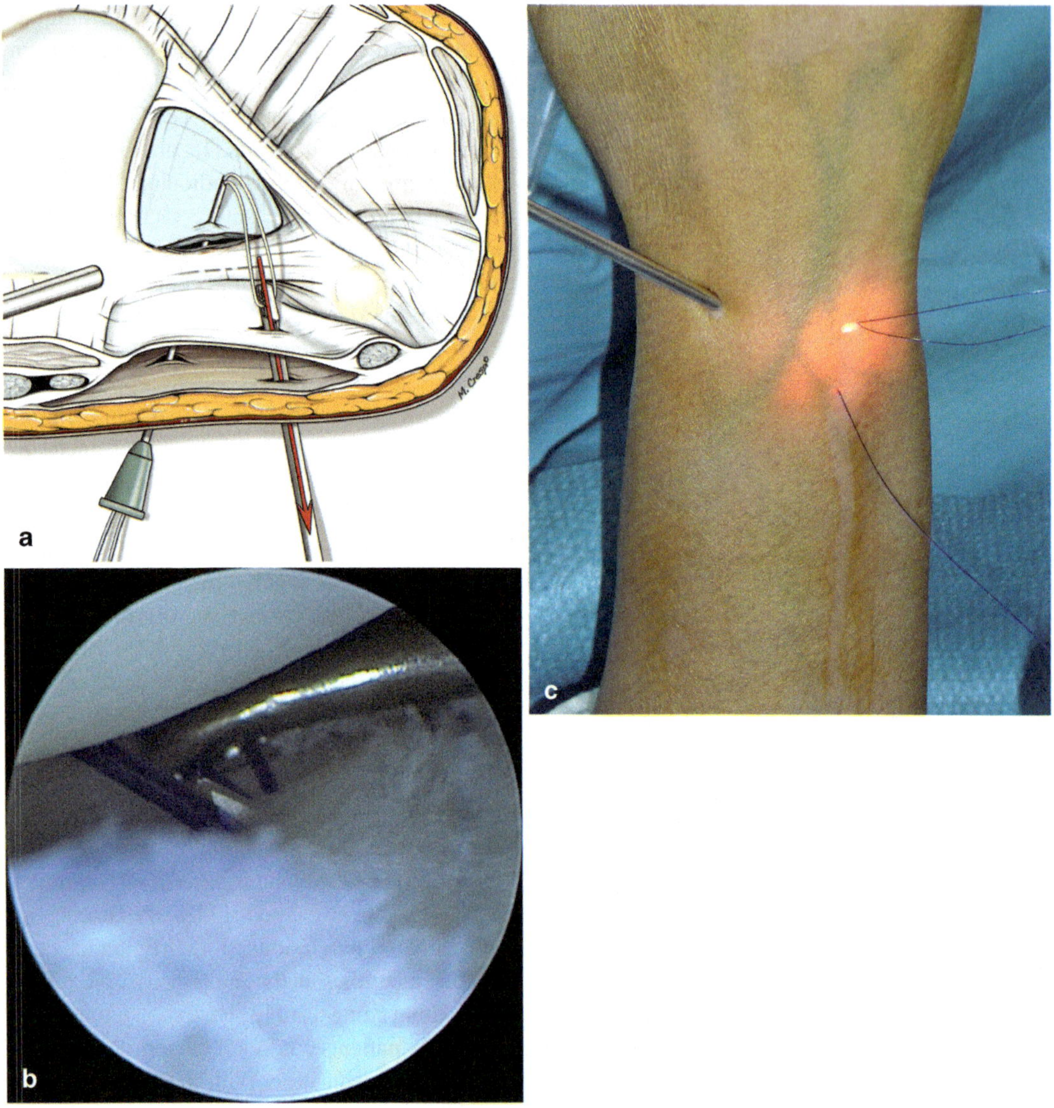

Fig. B.4 (**a**, **b**, **c**) Drawing, intra-articular operating view, and external operative view of the PDS loop retrieved using a forceps through 6R portal

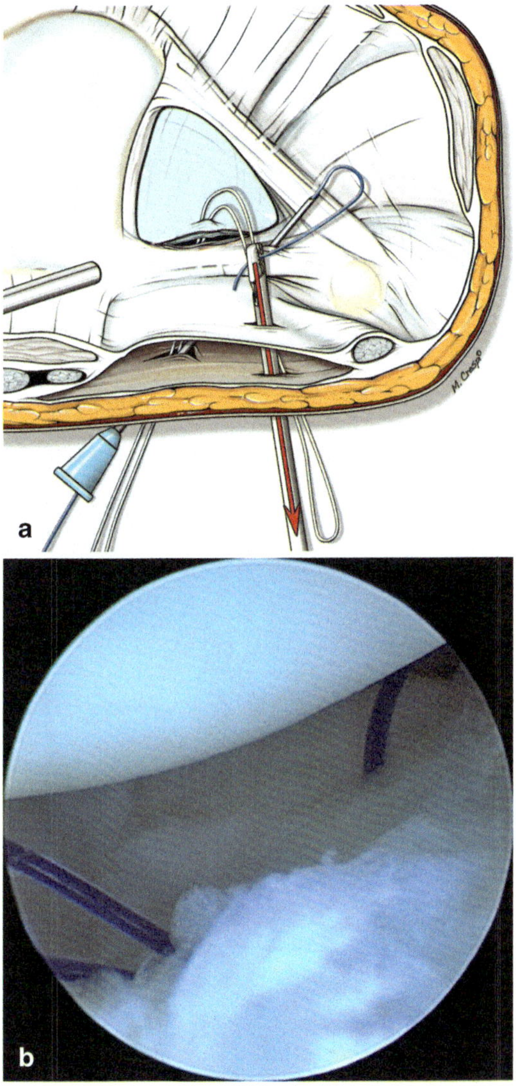

Fig. B.5 (**a**, **b**) Drawing and intra-articular operating view showing the passage of the second suture beside the first and similarly retrieved through 6R

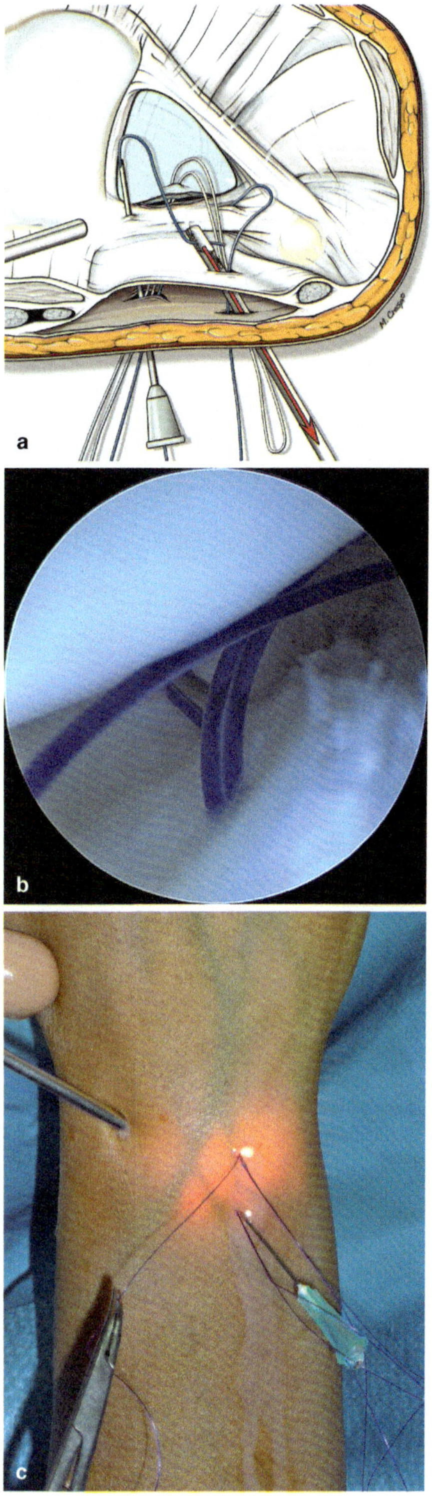

Fig. B.6 (**a**, **b**, **c**) Drawing, intra-articular operating view, and external operative view showing the passage of the third suture beside the others and similarly retrieved through 6R

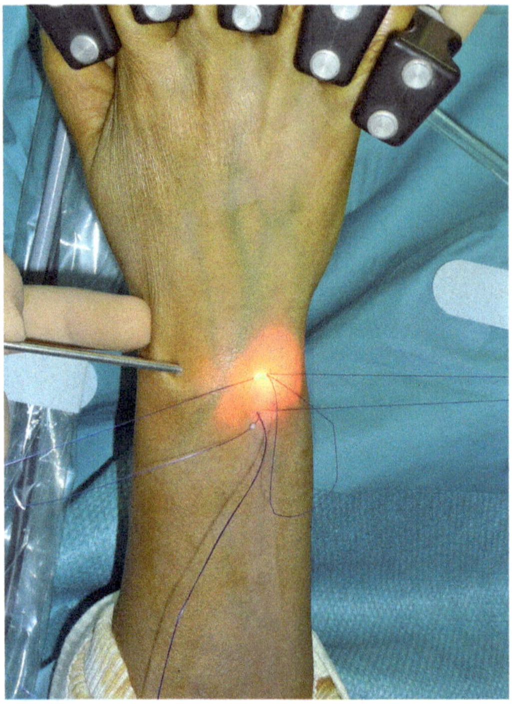

Fig. B.7 Operative view showing the three sutures, two simple and one loop, passed via the RUP through the capsule and the TFCC (the loop in the center and the two simple sutures radial and ulnar) and retrieved through 6R to the exterior

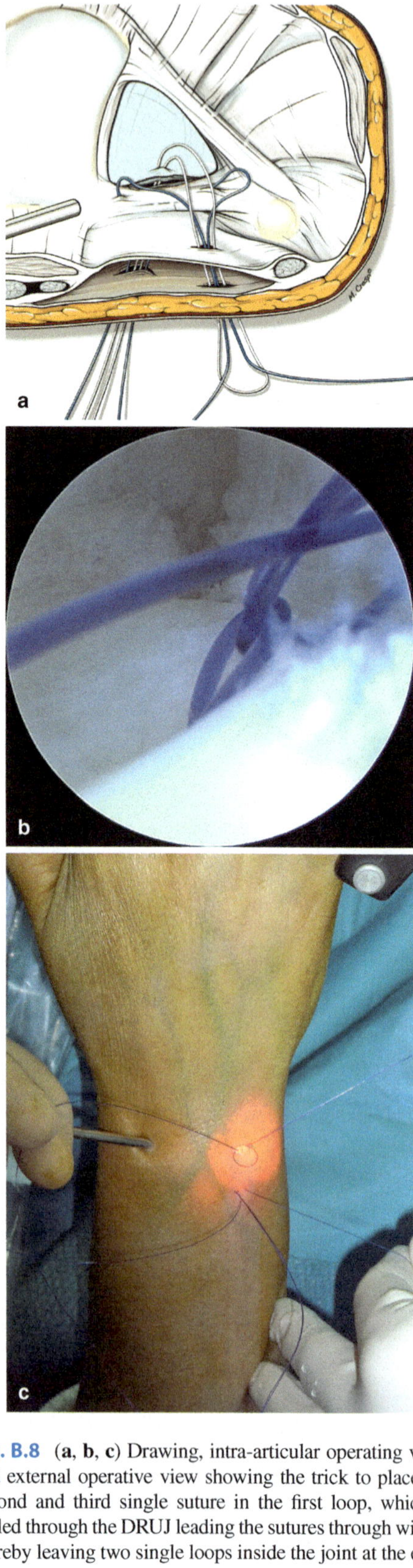

Fig. B.8 (**a**, **b**, **c**) Drawing, intra-articular operating view, and external operative view showing the trick to place the second and third single suture in the first loop, which is pulled through the DRUJ leading the sutures through with it, thereby leaving two single loops inside the joint at the end

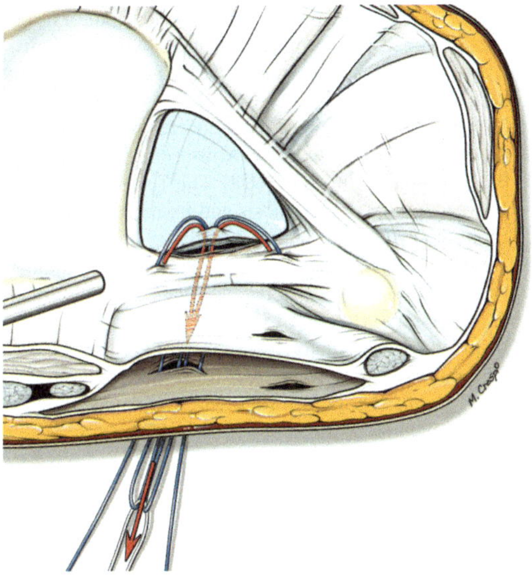

Fig. B.9 Drawing showing the two intra-articular loops before suture of the entire zone of the TFCC tear

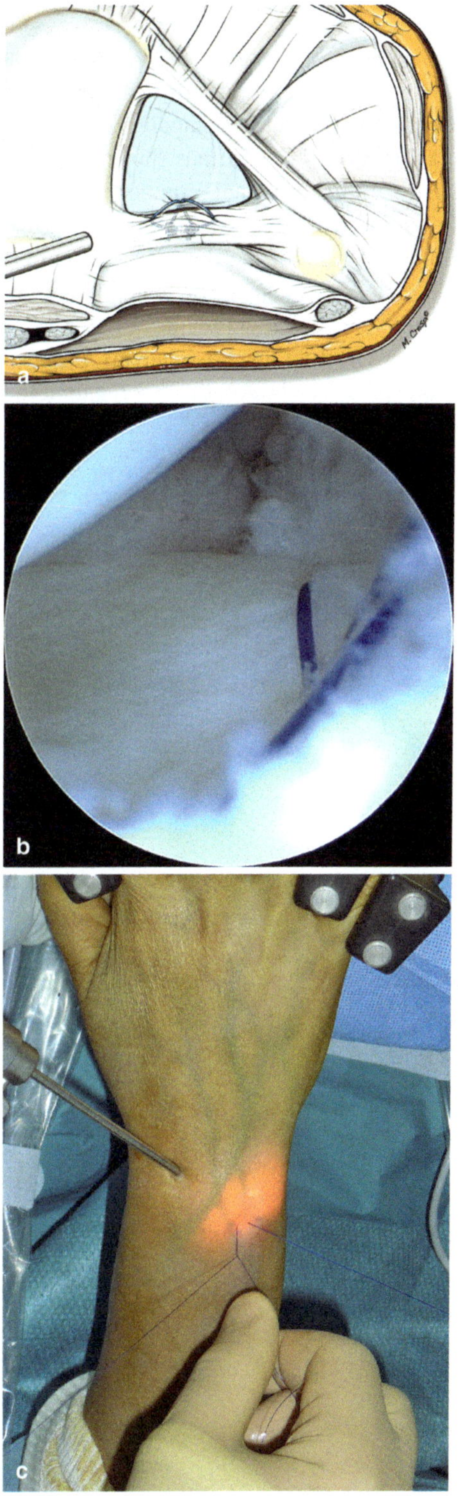

Fig. B.10 (**a**, **b**, **c**) Drawing, intra-articular view, and external operative view showing the two intra-articular loops after suture, allowing complete repair of the entire zone of the TFCC tear

Conclusion

Arthroscopic analysis of the radiocarpal and distal radioulnar joints has allowed better appreciation and understanding of the complexity of the TFCC. It has shown the importance of the proximal component and the foveal insertion for the stability of the DRUJ. Complete tears of the dorsal insertion of the TFCC are an example. The double loop suture allows simple efficient repair of these lesions. It allows healing for most patients, especially sports persons who can thereby regain a functional painless wrist.

References

1. Anderson LM et al (2008) Clinical comparison of arthroscopic versus open repair of triangular fibrocartilage complex tears. J Hand Surg 33A: 675–682
2. Atzei A et al (2008) Arthroscopic foveal repair of triangular fibrocartilage complex peripheral lesion with distal radioulnar joint instability. Tech Hand Up Extrem Surg 12(4):226–235
3. Estrella PE et al (2007) Arthroscopic repair of triangular fibrocartilage complex tears. Arthroscopy 23:729–737
4. Fulcher S, Poehling G (1998) The role of operative arthroscopy for the diagnosis and treatment of lesions about the distal ulna. Hand Clin 14:285–296
5. Palmer AK, Werner FW (1981) The triangular fibrocartilage complex of the wristVanatomy and function. J Hand Surg Am 6:153–162
6. Pederzini L, Luchetti R, Soragni O et al (1992) Evaluation of the triangular fibrocartilage complex tears by arthroscopy, arthrography, and magnetic resonance imaging. Arthroscopy 8:191–197

Index

DOI 10.1007/978-3-642-30544-3, © Springer-Verlag Berlin Heidelberg 2012

The manufacturer's authorised representative in the EU is Springer Nature Customer Service Centre GmbH, Europaplatz 3, 69115 Heidelberg, Germany. If you have any concerns regarding our products, please contact ProductSafety@springernature.com

Printed and bound by CPI Group (UK) Ltd, Croydon, CR0 4YY
07/01/2026
02030949-0017